Aquatic Rehabilitation

Aquatic Rehabilitation

Richard G. Ruoti, PhD, PT
Director
Bux-Mont Physical Therapy and Work Hardening Center
Warminster, Pennsylvania

David M. Morris, MS, PT
Assistant Professor
Division of Physical Therapy
University of Alabama at Birmingham
Birmingham, Alabama

Andrew J. Cole, MD, FACSM
Director, Research and Education
Puget Sound Sports and Spine Physicians
Bellevue, Washington
Assistant Clinical Professor
Department of Physical Medicine and Rehabilitation
Department of Physical Therapy
University of Texas Southwestern Medical Center
Dallas, Texas

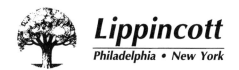

Lippincott
Philadelphia • New York

Acquisitions Editor: *Andrew Allen*
Editorial Assistant: *Patricia Moore*
Project Editor: *Sandra Cherrey Scheinin*
Production Manager: *Helen Ewan*
Production Coordinator: *Patricia McCloskey*
Design Coordinator: *Melissa Olson*
Indexer: *Victoria Boyle*

9 8 7 6 5 4 3 2 1

Library of Congress Cataloging in Publications Data

Aquatic rehabilitation / [edited by] Richard G. Ruoti, David M.
   Morris, Andrew J. Cole.
      p.   cm.
   Includes bibliographical references and index.
   ISBN 0-397-55152-5 (alk. paper)
   1. Hydrotherapy,   I. Ruoti, Richard G. (Richard Gene)
II. Morris, David M. (David Michael), 1960–   .   III. Cole, Andrew
J.
   [DNLM: 1. Hydrotherapy—methods.   2. Exercise Therapy—methods.
3. Rehabilitation—methods.   WB 520 A6558 1997]
RM811.A65   1997
615.8′53—dc20
DNLM/DLC
for Library of Congress   96-2682
                                                   CIP

Care has been taken to confirm the accuracy of the information presented and to describe generally accepted practices. However, the authors, editors, and publisher are not responsible for errors or omissions or for any consequences from application of the information in this book and make no warranty, express or implied, with respect to the contents of the publication.

The authors, editors and publisher have exerted every effort to ensure that drug selection and dosage set forth in this text are in accordance with current recommendations and practice at the time of publication. However, in view of ongoing research, changes in government regulations, and the constant flow of information relating to drug therapy and drug reactions, the reader is urged to check the package insert for each drug for any change in indications and dosage and for added warnings and precautions. This is particularly important when the recommended agent is a new or infrequently employed drug.

Some drugs and medical devices presented in this publication have Food and Drug Administration (FDA) clearance for limited use in restricted research settings. It is the responsibility of the health care provider to ascertain the FDA status of each drug or device planned for use in their clinical practice.

⊗ This Paper Meets the Requirements of ANSI/NISO Z39.48-1992 (Permanence of Paper).

Dedicated to my father,
the late Genero V. Ruoti,
and my mother,
Mary Rita

Richard Gene Ruoti

In memory of Shirley A. Shaddeau, MMSc, PT,
a valued clinician, researcher, teacher, and friend.
Shirley personified the heart of physical therapy.

Dave Morris

To my wife for her love and patience,
to my parents and sister for their support,
and to Marilou Moschetti and Richard Eagleston
for keeping my head above water

Andrew Cole

Contributors

Bruce E. Becker, MD
Vice President of Medical Affairs
Rehabilitation Institute of Michigan
Detroit, Michigan

Jolie Bookspan, PhD, MEd
Adjunct Researcher
University of Pennsylvania
Philadelphia, Pennsylvania

Judy Cirullo, BS, PT
Owner, Integrative Aquatic Therapy
Eugene, Oregon
Physical Therapist, BackCARE
Sacred Heart Medical Center
Eugene, Oregon

Annie Clement, PhD, JD
Professor, Sports Management
Cleveland State University
Cleveland, Ohio

Karen S. Congdon, MS, RN
Clinical Coordinator
EXERLIFE Cardiac Rehabilitation Program
University of Rhode Island
Kingston, Rhode Island

Jennifer Cunningham, BS, PT
Executive Director
Adapted Aquatic Center, Inc.
Lubbock, Texas

Kirk J. Cureton, PhD
Professor
Head, Department of Exercise Science
University of Georgia
Athens, Georgia

Harold Dull, MA
Director
School of Shiatsu and Massage at Harbin Hot
    Springs
Middletown, California

Emily Dunlap, PT
Director of Physical Therapy
Timpany Center
San Jose, California

Cheryl S. Fuller, MS, AT, C
Aquatics Director
University of Alabama Hospital
Spain Rehabilitation Center
Birmingham, Alabama

Gwendolyn Garrett, MAOTR/L
President
Aquatic Rehabilitation Consultants
Smithfield, Virginia
Director
Industrial Rehabilitation and Aquatics
Rehabilitation Management, Inc.
Richmond, Virginia

Christine L. Giesecke, PT
Physical Therapist, Bryn Mawr Rehab
Malvern, Pennsylvania
Physical Therapist, Bryn Mawr Rehab Services
Wayne, Pennsylvania
Adjunct Faculty, Beaver College
Glenside, Pennsylvania

Jean M. Irion, MEd, PT, SCS, ATC
Assistant Professor
University of Central Arkansas
Conway, Arkansas

Christine McNamara, PT
Director, Aquatic Therapy
Coordinator of Clinical Education
Cornell Physical Therapy
Cornell University
Ithaca, New York

Roxane McNeal, PT, BA, BS
President, Aquatic Therapy Services, Inc.
Abingdon, Maryland
Coordinator of Aquatic Physical Therapy
Co-owner, Vice President/Secretary
Harford Physical Therapy and Sports
    Rehabilitation
Forest Hill, Maryland

David M. Morris, MS, PT
Assistant Professor
Division of Physical Therapy
University of Alabama at Birmingham
Birmingham, Alabama

Marilou Moschetti, BSc, PTA

Executive Director
AquaTechnics Consulting Group
Aptos, California

Jane L. Styer-Acevedo, PT

Clinical Instructor, Department of Physical
    Therapy
Thomas Jefferson University
Philadelphia, Pennsylvania
Pediatric Coordinator, Prime Professionals
Bala Cynwyd, Pennsylvania

Lori A. Thein, MS, PT, SCS, ATC

Senior Clinical Specialist
Sports Medicine Center
University of Wisconsin Clinics
Research Park
Madison, Wisconsin

Thomas J. Tierney, BSEd

Owner
Aquatic Physical Therapy Resources
Woodridge, Illinois

Preface

Aquatic Rehabilitation has been developed to address the needs of professionals of diverse backgrounds. The editors have envisioned this text to be useful not only to students, but also to physical therapists, physicians, occupational therapists, nurses, athletic trainers, exercise physiologists, recreational therapists, and others who use aquatics as part of the rehabilitation process.

Within the past decade, aquatic rehabilitation has experienced a resurgence. This text, therefore, is timely, given the scarcity of material regarding this subject. A review of the literature has suggested that there are few texts available that encompass as wide a scope of rehabilitation aspects and client populations as *Aquatic Rehabilitation*.

The text is divided into four major divisions. It begins by addressing the basic foundations of aquatic rehabilitation: history, aquatic physics, and the physiologic basis of response to immersion and exercise in water.

The second section details aquatic rehabilitation techniques that can be applied by professionals who treat a variety of client populations. Topics covered include: orthopedics, neurology, athletics, degenerative diseases, obstetrics, pediatrics, spinal cord injuries, and cardiac care. While specific techniques are annotated, every effort has been made to present a rationale for treatment and to avoid a "cookbook" protocol.

Part three presents a unique opportunity for the reader to be exposed to various aquatic philosophies. We are especially pleased that one chapter, WATSU, was penned by the originator of the technique of Water Shiatsu.

The concluding section deals with important information required to supplement the design of an aquatic program. Risk management, facility design, and aquatic equipment are discussed in detail.

Conspicuous by its absence is a chapter covering aquatic rehabilitation research. It is difficult to imagine, yet true, that our review of the literature revealed a scarcity of studies dealing with specific pathologies and functional outcomes. The contributors to *Aquatic Rehabilitation* are keenly aware of this fact and have attempted to carefully document their material, while at the same time allowing us to benefit from their aquatic clinical expertise. Should a second edition come to fruition, we hope that enough direct client research will have accumulated by then so that an independent chapter on aquatic research can be included.

In our opinion, this book presents the work of twenty of the top aquatic rehabilitation experts in the United States and perhaps the world. We hope that this offering will be enlightening to students and clinicians, and that the readers will find some new idea or variation of technique to enable them to provide the excellence of care expected of the aquatic rehabilitation specialist.

Richard G. Ruoti, PhD, PT

Acknowledgments

There are numerous people to whom I always will be grateful for their contributions, time, guidance, and editorial review. My grateful appreciation is extended to Christine Fissel, MS, PT, Rosemarie T. Whelan, BA, James J. Whelan, BS, Christine Giesecke, PT, George Logue, MS, PT, Carol Lieber, PhD, PT, Jolie Bookspan, PhD, Kirk Cureton, PhD, Lori Thein, MS, PT, Robert Wilder, MD, Jamie Tomlinson, MS, PT, and Emily Dunlap, PT.

A special thank you is extended to my administrative assistant, Kelly A. Cern, for the time, diligence, support, and management skills she contributed while this work was in progress.

RGR

Contents

PART II

APPLICATIONS OF AQUATIC REHABILITATION,   57

INTRODUCTION

CHAPTER 1

Historical Overview of Aquatic Rehabilitation

Jean M. Irion

The use of water as a healing medium dates back many centuries, although its original use does not coincide exactly with our present perception of its use for rehabilitation purposes. It was not until the latter part of the 1890s that aquatic rehabilitation moved from a passive modality to one that involved active patient participation.

Throughout history, the name used to denote the concept of the use of water for healing and rehabilitation purposes changed often. Some of these "titles" were used synonymously: hydrotherapy, hydrology, hydratics, hydrogymnastics, water therapy, water therapeutics, and water exercise. The most commonly used terms today are "aquatic rehabilitation" or "aquatic therapy."

This chapter provides an overview of the history of the use of water in healing and as a form of therapeutic exercise in both Europe and the United States. The influences of England and Europe on aquatic rehabilitation in the United States are also discussed.

Origin of the Use of Water

In many cultures, the use of water was closely connected to the mystical and religious worship of water and its perceived power of healing. The use of hydrotherapy as a therapeutic modality is unknown, but records dating back to 2400 BC indicate that the Proto-Indian culture made hygienic installations.[1,2] It has been noted that early Egyptians, Assyrians, and Moslems used curative waters for therapeutic purposes.[1–3]

There is also documentation that the Hindus, in 1500 BC, used water to combat fever.[1,3] Throughout the historical records of the early Japanese and Chinese civilizations, there is significant mention of respect for and worship of running water and the submersion in baths for prolonged periods of time.[1,3] Homer mentions the use of water to treat fatigue, heal injuries, and combat melancholy.[1,3,4] The waters of Bath, England were used as early as 800 BC for healing purposes.[3]

Era of Water Healing, 500 to 300 BC

By 500 BC, the Greek civilization no longer viewed water from the standpoint of mysticism and began to use water more logically for specific physical treatments.[1,2] Schools of medicine came into existence near many of the baths and springs developed by the Greek civilization.[2] Hippocrates (460–375 BC) used hot and cold water immersion to treat many diseases, including muscle spasms and joint diseases.[3–5] Hippocrates recommended hydrotherapy for the treatment of a variety of disorders, including rheumatism, jaundice, and paralysis.[2]

The Lacedaemonians have been credited with establishing the first public bath system in 334 BC.[3] The Greeks and Romans engaged in the taking of long baths many years before the birth of Christ.[1,4] Greek civilization was the first to recognize and appreciate the relation between state of mind and physical well-being. The

Greeks developed bathing centers near natural springs and rivers; the primary purpose of these centers was for bathing and recreation.[1]

Use of Water During the Roman Empire

The Roman Empire further expanded the bath system developed by the Greeks.[1] The Romans were noted for their architectural and construction skills. As in the Greek system, the Roman baths were originally used by athletes for bathing and served the purposes of hygiene and prevention more than treatment.[2] The Roman system evolved into a series of baths at varying temperatures ranging from very hot (*caldarium*), to lukewarm (*tepidarium*), to the coldest (*frigidarium*).[5] Some of these baths were quite elaborate and covered large areas. For instance, the baths of Emperor Caracalla covered 1 square mile, with a swimming pool that measured 1050 × 1390 feet.[3] The baths began to be used by more people than just athletes. In addition to bathing, the baths became centers for health, hygiene, rest, and intellectual, recreational, and exercise activities.[1]

By AD 330, the primary purpose for the Roman baths was for healing and treating rheumatic disease, paralysis, and injuries.[1] However, the primary mode of use continued to be "taking of the waters,"[6] a passive means of using water that consisted of drinking and sitting in it.

Use of Water During the Decline of the Roman Empire and the Middle Ages

With the decline of the Roman Empire, the hygienic nature of the Roman baths began to deteriorate. This, coupled with the banning of the use of public baths by the early Christians, led to a decline in the use of the illustrious Roman bath system.[1] These elaborate bath systems fell into ruin over the course of decades, and by AD 500 they were no longer in existence.[3] Religious influence during the Middle Ages led to further decline in the use of public baths and water as a healing power. Christians during this time viewed the use of physical forces, such as water, as a pagan act.[1,3] This public attitude persisted until the 15th century, when there appeared to be a resurgence in the interest of the use of water as a healing medium.[1]

Use of Water During the Late 1600s and 1700s

In the 17th and 18th centuries, bathing for hygienic purposes was not an accepted practice. The therapeutic use of water, however, began gradually to increase. In the early 1700s, a German physician, Sigmund Hahn, and his sons advocated the idea of using water for "leg sores and itch" and many other medical problems.[2] This medical discipline began to be referred to as "hydrotherapy" and, as defined by Wyman and Glazer, consists of external application of water in any form for the treatment of disease.[7]

Some physicians in England, France, Germany, and Italy promoted the internal and external application of water for treatment of many conditions.[4] Most physicians at this time were devoting the greatest amount of their time and energy to diagnosing diseases. Less emphasis was placed on treatment protocols for diseases, particularly those that included the use of what were considered to be natural therapies.[1] Therefore, by the middle of the 17th century, few physicians used water for the treatment of diseases.

Baruch[8] credits Great Britain as the birthplace of scientific hydrotherapy, with the publication in 1697 of Sir John Floyer's treatise, "An Inquiry into the Right Use and Abuse of Hot, Cold, and Temperate Baths."[1,3] Floyer devoted much of his life to the study of hydrotherapy. Baruch[8] believes that Floyer's treatise influenced Professor Friedrich Hoffmann of Heidelberg University to include Floyer's doctrines in his teachings. From Heidelberg, these teachings were taken to France.[8] From there, Dr. Currie, of Liverpool, England, wrote works regarding hydrotherapy. Currie then attempted to give hydrotherapy a more scientific basis through experimentation.[2] These works were translated into several languages.[8,9] Although Currie's work was not well accepted in England, it was in Germany.[9]

John Wesley, the founder of Methodism, published a book in 1747 entitled *An Easy and Natural Way of Curing Most Diseases*. This book focused on the use of water as a healing medium.[1,3] The Scandinavian and Russian cultures popularized the use of cold baths after hot vapor baths. Hot vapor baths, followed by cold baths, remained a tradition and were popular for many generations.[3]

Resurgence of Water for Healing in the 1800s

The use of hydrotherapy at this point in history continued to be primarily passive in nature. The treatment techniques included sheet baths, wet packs, wet compresses, cold friction baths, sedative baths, hammock baths, and carbon dioxide baths.[8]

In 1830, a Silesian peasant, Vincent Priessnitz, developed treatment programs that primarily used outdoor baths.[1,5] His treatments consisted of cold water baths, showers, and packs.[3,10] Because Priessnitz possessed no credible medical credentials, he was not viewed favorably by all physicians during this time. The medical community attempted to discredit him and his treatment programs and viewed him and others of his kind as empirics.[1] These empirics called themselves *Naturaerzte* ("naturopaths").[3] Some "hydrotherapist–physicians" of this time traveled to Silesia to learn and research the techniques developed by Priessnitz.[2]

During this time, Sebastian Kniepp (1821–1897), a Bavarian priest, modified the treatment techniques of Priessnitz by alternating cold applications with warmer and even hot partial baths.[1,3,10] Kniepp's water treatments also consisted of drenching the body with hoses and showers of different temperatures.[2] The course of treatment advocated by Kniepp were known as a "cure." The "Kniepp cure" became popular in German-speaking countries, northern Italy, and in the bordering countries of Holland and France, and is still used today.[10]

Winterwitz (1834–1912), an Austrian professor and founder of a hydrotherapy school and research center in Vienna, is recognized as devoting most of his professional life to the study of the practice of hydrotherapy (also known as "hydratics"). His institution was known as the "Institute for Hydrotherapy." He was inspired by Priessnitz's and Currie's work to look further at the reaction of tissues to water of various temperatures.[5,9] Winterwitz's studies are recognized as the foundation for the use of hydrotherapy as a treatment regimen, and established an acceptable physiologic basis for hydrotherapy for that time.[1,9]

Some of Winterwitz's students, particularly Kelogg, Buxbaum, and Strasser, made significant contributions to the study of the physiologic effects of the application of heat and cold, thermoregulation of the human body, and clinical hydrotherapy.[2] This early research served as an impetus for the inception of such treatments as whirlpool baths and underwater exercise. These treatment techniques, however, did not come into regular use until the beginning of the 20th century.[2]

One of the first Americans to devote his life to the research of hydrotherapy was Dr. Simon Baruch. He traveled to Europe to study under Dr. Winterwitz and to speak with those who were considered empirics, such as Priessnitz.[3] In his book, *An Epitome of Hydrotherapy*, Baruch[8] discusses the principles and methods of using water to treat such conditions as typhoid fever, influenza, sunstroke, tuberculosis, neurasthenia, chronic rheumatism and gout, and neuritis. Baruch also published two other books in 1893, *The Uses of Water in Modern Medicine*[8] and *The Principles and Practice of Hydrotherapy*.[3] He was the first professor at Columbia University to teach hydrotherapy.[3] Although it was recognized as a therapeutic tool for many other medical conditions much earlier, descriptions of water therapy as a treatment modality for spinal disorders can be found in the literature as early as 1892.[11]

By the mid-1800s, the use of hydrotherapy had taken a downswing in Great Britain. Baruch[8] believed this was because of the lack of medical publications touting its worthiness and sparse documentation of treatment techniques that could be followed by physicians. Baruch[8] also noted a prejudice against the use of "water for curing" on the part of many noted physicians of that time.

Development of Spas in Europe and England

By definition, a *spa* is a resort that is built around a natural spring and usually surrounded by breathtaking natural beauty.[12] Baths of mineral and thermal water can be traced as far back as 500 BC in Greece, and served as precursors to the modern spas of Europe.[2] These Greek baths sprang up around natural hot springs, as did later baths in Roman territories during the time of the Roman Empire. Health resorts surrounding baths were used for treatment of many physical ailments during the Roman era, and some sprang up even in the barbarian territories occupied by the Romans during this time.[10] Military hospitals and even military fortresses were built at several of the Roman baths. These baths served as treatment facilities for many soldiers during war, as well as being used for the long-term care of war injuries.[2] Like the noteworthy Roman public pool and bath system, the bath resorts were also destroyed during the decline of the Roman Empire.[2]

The baths near natural thermal and mineral springs were reestablished during the Middle Ages.[2] These baths were primarily used for soaking for various periods of time in waters of differing temperatures.[2] Many of the baths had a regular spa physician who prescribed the treatment protocols for a client.[2] During this time, the baths were used to treat such ailments as rheumatism, paralysis, and the after-effects of injury.[2] The hygienic conditions of these baths began to deteriorate during the 16th and 17th centuries.[2] There was a sharp decline in the use of the baths after the Thirty Years' War because of the significant spread of disease through them.[2]

Initial documentation of bathing in the sea dates from Roman times.[2] This custom disappeared during the Middle Ages, but began to resurface during the 18th century in England.[2] The popularity of sea bathing spread to France and Germany, and spas were developed around sea bathing resorts; in Germany, a seaside hospital was founded on the North Sea in 1880 by F. W. Beneke.[2]

The water of natural springs has been used for a long time in Europe to treat diseases, even before any scientific evidence indicated the benefits of exercise in water. The hot springs of Carlsbad, Czechoslovakia received a charter as early as 1401.[3] There are several other mineral springs of significant fame in Europe, including the spas in Leukenbad and Bad Ragaz, Switzerland, and Bad Nauheim in Germany.[3] At the beginning of the 20th century, spas in England were staffed with people who had little training in the use of water as a therapeutic modality.[9] These spas were also available only to those who could personally afford it. Physicians in England were not pleased with this system and, in 1930, they insisted that the British Red Cross open and staff a clinic for the treatment of rheumatic diseases with trained health professionals.[9]

The natural spring water at spas was used therapeutically in a variety of ways, including such treatments as bathing, Vichy spray massage, the underwater douche, whirlpool baths, peat and mud baths, the aeration bath, and cold plunges. Some of the European spas incorporated aquatic rehabilitation procedures, performed by health care professionals such as physical therapists, with the more traditional spa treatments.[12] Davis and Harrison[12] note two reputable spas in Europe, Bad Ragaz and Leukenbad, that have achieved international reputations for the rehabilitation component of their spa treatments. The rehabilitation portion of these programs includes both an aquatic and a land component. Drinking the water for medicinal purposes was also encouraged at the spas.[12]

The modern spas in Britain have been around since the 18th century, and have fallen into decline since the end of World War II. This decline in British spas has been attributed to the inception of the National Health Service in 1948 and the lack of qualified and well-trained personnel.[12] The spas of continental Europe and Russia, however, remain vital components of the health care systems of their respective countries.[12] The role of these spas is not only therapeutic but preventative in nature. In addition to the water treatments at spas, there is a strong emphasis on a healthy lifestyle, including engaging in intellectual activities, exercise, and good nutrition.

Development of Spas and Hydrotherapy in the United States

American Spas of the 18th Century

The use of bathing and the forerunners of spas and bathhouses can be traced as far back as the European explorers of the New World who witnessed Native Americans using water and baths at springs for magical, religious, and hygienic purposes.[13] While the settlers were establishing the original British colonies, there was little emphasis on the use of water other than for basic survival needs to sustain human and animal life.[13] During the time of the Revolutionary War and later, some emphasis was placed on the use of water for hygienic purposes in army hospitals and the use of cold baths to decrease a person's elevated temperature from diseases such as yellow fever.[13]

Whites first visited the natural springs of Hot Springs, Virginia in 1720 and White Sulphur Springs, West Virginia in 1764.[13] The oldest spa in the United States is thought to be in Berkeley Springs, Virginia (now in West Virginia), and was known in 1761 as Warm Springs.[13] It has been documented that many people suffering from rheumatism visited what were considered the healing waters of this spa.[13] As early as 1792, the Sweet Springs, as they were called, of Hot Springs, Virginia were known to have a hotel.[13] The founding history of the spa at White Sulphur Springs is not fully known. It has been recorded that the first white women used the spring for medicinal purposes in 1778. By 1859, the spa at White Sulphur Springs was able to accommodate 2000 people.[13] Several other spas sprang up around natural springs in Pennsylvania and New Jersey toward the end of the 18th century. Highly touted professionals of the time wrote about the medicinal values of the waters of these mineral springs to treat several maladies of the day.[13]

The most famous of the original natural springs in America was Saratoga Springs in New York. Early writings, one from 1787 to 1792, discussed the contents and possible medicinal benefits of the spring waters at Saratoga.[13] It was not until 1794 that a permanent structure was built that included bath houses and shower baths for use by disabled patrons.[13]

American Spas and Hydrotherapy of the 19th Century

During the 19th century, more spas began to sprout up along the Appalachians and from Connecticut to Arkansas.[13] Construction of the first bathhouse in Hot Springs, Arkansas took place in 1830.[13] During the first decades of the 19th century, traveling in a touring fashion from spa to spa become a fashionable activity for members of the middle class and wealthy society. The purpose of this touring was more social in nature than therapeutic.

Hydrotherapy was brought to America by many European-trained physicians returning to America with knowledge of the current teachings in Europe. These concepts were taken by these trained physicians to spas throughout America.[13] Medical schools in America also began to teach the concepts of hydrotherapy. Each spa had its own physician, and in many instances it was the physician who owned the spa.[13] In America, the practice of spa therapy was conducted in conjunction with hydrotherapy.

In the 1840s, American patronage of the spas continued to increase, but did not equal in any fashion the degree of visitation by Europeans to their spas.[13] In 1840, the largest spa in the United States attracted about 500 patrons, compared with Baden-Baden, Germany, one of the larger spas of Europe, which accommodated 20,000 visitors that year.[13] Several physicians also opened up what were known as "Water-Cure" establishments in 1847 and 1848 in urban surroundings. These physicians incorporated the practices of Priessnitz, Kniepp, and other well-known European hydrotherapists. The lay people of the time were completely convinced of the extravagant benefits claimed for this type of medical intervention for conditions such as mental illness, epilepsy, and paresis.[13]

After the Civil War, there was a significant increase in the number of spas in the United States, which numbered 632 by 1886. This was accompanied by an increased ability for existing and developing spas to advertise, leading to competition, commercialism, and a search by spa owners for any type of new attraction that would draw patrons.[13] This competition between a large number of spa resorts, in conjunction with the promotion of recreational attractions at seashore resorts, led to a decline in spa visitations as a recreational and social activity throughout the United States.[13] Although the proof of the therapeutic and curative values of the spring waters was scarce, many physicians still maintained an interest in and expressed the value of medical hydrology.[13]

American Spas and Hydrotherapy in the 20th Century

During the 20th century, spas continued to decline in interest to both the physician and the patient, while spas continued to prosper in Europe.[13] It was also noted that the lack of competent medical advisors at spas resulted in their continued decline in the early 1900s. By the turn of the century, Baruch was recognized as the foremost specialist of hydrotherapy in America. In 1907, he was awarded the first chair in hydrotherapy at Columbia University.[13] Although hydrotherapy was viewed with significant skepticism by his peers, Baruch continued to study hydrotherapy into the 1930s.[13]

Baruch[8] criticized the medical community of

his time for contributing to the decline in the use of hydrotherapy as a beneficial modality. His reasons included such factors as faulty installment of hydrotherapy equipment and untrained personnel such as "massage operators," as well as others who failed because they had not received proper instruction in the principles and techniques of this branch of therapeutics. He also attributed the lack of training in curricula such as nursing programs, and the lack of factual and fully informative textbooks for physicians and other health care professionals, as further reasons for the decline in the use of hydrotherapy. In the conclusion of his book,[8] Baruch urged the medical community to "change their preconceived ideas that hydrotherapy is a fad."

In 1937, the president of the American Congress of Physical Therapy appointed a committee to collect data on the spas and health resorts in the United States.[13] This committee was directed to determine some of the causes for the decline of spas in the United States as well as the therapeutic agents used at these facilities.[13] One of the major accomplishments of this committee was the formulation of a list of approved health resorts and standards.[13] This committee later became an advisory committee to the Council on Physical Medicine and Rehabilitation of the American Medical Association.[13]

History of Water Therapy in the Early to Mid-1900s in Europe

During the latter part of the 19th century and in the early years of this century, the property of buoyancy began to be used to exercise patients in the water. Basmajian[14] points out that European spas began to treat "locomotor" and rheumatic disorders. In 1898, the concept of hydrogymnastics was recommended by von Leyden and Goldwater.[1,3] The concept of hydrogymnastics entailed the use of underwater exercise, and it serves as the closest forerunner to the current concept of aquatic rehabilitation.

Hydrogymnastics implies the use of exercise in water rather than passive treatment of the patient by a health care professional. In 1928, the physician Walter Blount described the use of a water tank larger than a whirlpool bath that included a motor-activated whirlpool.[13] This became known as a Hubbard tub (or tank). The designated initial use of the Hubbard tank was

for the performance of exercises in the water by patients.[13] The invention of the Hubbard tank assisted the development of pool exercise programs.

During the early to mid-1900s, emphasis in Europe was placed on the development of two aquatic treatment techniques: the Bad Ragaz ring method and the Halliwick method.

Bad Ragaz Technique

Bad Ragaz is a town in Switzerland built around a natural warm water spa. The thermal springs of this spa feed three modern indoor pools.[15] The spas in Bad Ragaz began to be used for exercising in the 1930s. The techniques used at this time were straight-plane range of motion exercises with the patient positioned horizontally and stabilized in several ways against the wall of the pool.[15]

The Bad Ragaz techniques did not originate in Bad Ragaz, but rather in Germany. The original techniques were developed by Dr. Knupfer and were brought to Bad Ragaz in 1957 by Nele Ipsen.[15] The primary purpose of these exercises was to promote stabilization of the trunk and extremities and to work on resistive exercises. The exercises were still primarily performed in straight-plane patterns. These techniques, like their predecessors, were also performed in the horizontal plane. The patient was supported by inner tubes or "rings" at the neck, pelvis, and ankles, and therefore the technique was also referred to as the "ring method." During the late 1950s, these techniques were passed down from therapist to therapist, but not placed in writing.[15]

In 1967, Bridget Davis incorporated the proprioceptive neuromuscular facilitation techniques into the ring method.[15] It was Beatrice Egger, however, who further developed these techniques and published them in the German language.[15] This became a barrier to many American physical therapists, who began hearing about the ring method in the United States in the 1970s.[15] All of the documentation of the techniques was in German, and the courses taught in Europe were also in German.[15] Today, there are two primary English-language books that document the Bad Ragaz techniques.[9,12]

The modern Bad Ragaz techniques incorporate movement techniques with straight-plane and diagonal patterns with resistance and stabilization provided by the therapist. The patient is still maintained horizontally using various flotation devices in the same anatomic positions mentioned previously. The techniques are used for both orthopedic and neurologically impaired clients. Both active and passive techniques are incorporated with several purposes in mind, including tone reduction, pregait training, trunk stabilization, and active and resistive exercise. Chapter 15 of this book is devoted to a discussion of this form of aquatic rehabilitation.

The Halliwick Method

The Halliwick method was developed by James McMillan in 1949 at the Halliwick School for Girls in Southgate, London.[16] The primary purpose of McMillan's techniques was to help handicapped clients become more independent and safe swimmers.[17] The initial emphasis of the Halliwick method was recreational in nature, with a goal of individual independence in the water.

Over the years, McMillan had maintained his original protocols and had adopted other techniques in addition to his original method. More recently, these techniques have been used therapeutically by many therapists to treat pediatric and adult clients with various developmental and neurologic disabilities in Europe and the United States. The Halliwick method emphasizes the abilities of patients in the water, and not their disabilities on land.[16] McMillan continued to offer educational courses in Europe to those interested in learning the Halliwick method. Chapter 16 of this book is devoted to the current teachings of the Halliwick method.

Arrival of Aquatic Rehabilitation in the United States

As mentioned, Winterwitz founded a teaching institution in Vienna, Austria, in conjunction with his research into the use of hydrotherapy.[3] Similar educational institutions, known as "Institutes for Hydrotherapy," were opened in Boston in 1903 and in Philadelphia in 1909.[3,9] There is some evidence for the use of water in treatment of patients' maladies in the United States during this time. Water treatments were developed by Joel Shew, a physician, in his hydropathic establishment in New York.[1,13] As a general rule, however, use of water as a treatment technique

in the United States lagged behind the European practice throughout the 19th century.

Charles Lowman began using therapeutic exercise in the water in his medical practice in 1911, when he treated children with cerebral palsy in bathtubs.[4] He then visited the Spaulding School for Crippled Children in Chicago in 1924 and witnessed the treatment of patients with paralysis with exercise in a wooden tank.[4] On his return to Los Angeles, Lowman converted a 30 × 15-foot lily pond into two treatment pools; one was used to treat patients with paralysis, including polio, and the other was made into a salt pool to treat infectious diseases.[4]

Lowman touted the positive experience of his hospital's water therapy program in an article he wrote for the December, 1924 issue of *Nation's Health*.[4] Lowman increased the national awareness of the use of therapeutic exercise in a water environment when he presented a paper and film on this topic at the American Orthopedic Society meeting in Atlanta, Georgia in April of 1926.[4] Many facilities began to build specially designed therapeutic pools to use in the treatment of patients, particularly those with paralysis. One such facility was the Orthopedic Hospital in Los Angeles, built in 1924.[4]

Physical therapists began being trained in the use of water exercises for treatment of their patients over the next two decades. The successful results of treatment in the water medium received favorable comment from many leading orthopedic surgeons in the United States,[4] and the method continued in popularity until the middle to late 1950s. Lowman, however, in his 1952 book *Therapeutic Use of Pools and Tanks*, expressed concern about the lack of teachers and physical therapists trained in the use of therapeutic exercises in a water medium.[4]

Promotion of Aquatic Rehabilitation During the Polio Epidemic and After Both World Wars

Medically supervised exercises in water began to gain popularity in the United States in the early 1900s, particularly after the polio epidemic of 1916.[11] The usefulness of aquatic therapy for the patient with poliomyelitis was discovered by chance in Warm Springs, Georgia.[3] A young person with poliomyelitis fell from his wheelchair into a pool. While attempting to keep himself afloat, the young boy discovered that he could move his paralyzed legs. This movement had not been possible on land. He continued with a pool exercise program to strengthen his lower extremities and was able to progress from being wheelchair-bound to ambulating independently without braces, using only a cane.[3]

Basmajian[14] is quick to indicate that because of the successful use of a water medium in the treatment of patients with poliomyelitis after World War I and the treatment of orthopedic conditions after both World Wars, this method of treatment became an accepted part of rehabilitation programs all over the United States. These programs were not necessarily in treatment areas associated only with hot spring spas, but in a therapeutic environment, and did much to enhance and promote a change in emphasis from hydrotherapy as a passive thermal and chemical modality to the use of water as a therapeutic exercise technique.

In 1924, President Franklin D. Roosevelt popularized the use of pool exercises and therapeutic swimming (hydrogymnastics) at Warm Springs, Georgia. The water medium was used to treat his polio.[3,6] Roosevelt was a vital force in organizing treatment of other patients with polio by qualified medical personnel.[3] In 1927, the Georgia Warm Springs Foundation was incorporated to provide physical rehabilitation, including hydrogymnastics.[3]

client populations. Most rehabilitation facilities in Europe possess some type of aquatic therapy facility. Aquatic therapy has been readily incorporated with a land rehabilitation program where appropriate for many years, and the practice continues. Given the strong emphasis in many of these countries on prevention, there are also many aquatic exercise programs geared toward prevention and general health and well-being. Two examples of such prevention and maintenance initiatives are exercise programs for the geriatric population and programs for women during pregnancy and beyond. From Australia, Campion[1] contributed a great deal to the aquatic rehabilitation literature, which has influenced aquatic programs in Europe. She devotes an entire section of her book to the issue of prevention and includes not only the physical aspects of health promotion and exercise in the water medium, but the psychological and sociologic benefits of participation in such programs.

Because of their largely publicly funded health care systems, the European countries do not appear to face many of the problems seen in the United States related to issues such as research to support the efficacy of aquatic rehabilitation, and subsequent reimbursement for such services. Participation in such therapeutic processes appears to be widely accepted for the benefits it provides in the rehabilitation process.

Aquatic Rehabilitation in Europe From the 1960s to Present

Since 1965, aquatic physical therapy and rehabilitation techniques have been included as curricular components for students studying for the membership examination in the Chartered Society of Physiotherapy in England.[9] Before this, the Chartered Society conducted postregistration training in hydrotherapy to ensure that physiotherapists were properly trained in the use of water as a therapeutic medium.[9] This information is included in physical therapy programs in the United Kingdom on a routine basis, and the level of training appears to be well beyond that which is taught in most entry-level physical therapy curricula in the United States.

Aquatic rehabilitation in Europe has long been an integral component of the rehabilitation process, with a wide range of diagnoses and

Decline of Aquatic Rehabilitation in the United States in the 1950s and 1960s

There appear to be several reasons for the decline in use of aquatic therapy in the rehabilitation process during the 1950s and 1960s in the United States. By this time, polio in the United States was virtually controlled, thus eliminating an entire population of clients for whom aquatic exercise was used. Many of the veterans of World War II were no longer receiving rehabilitation for their war injuries. It would also appear that the use of aquatic physical therapy as a component of the rehabilitation process was overtaken by the movement toward highly technical modalities and exercise equipment during the "Age of Technology," which began in the mid-1950s. There was also a concomitant decline in the use of spas throughout the United States, even for purposes of prevention and psychological health.

Two other factors that contributed to the decline in use of aquatic rehabilitation during this time were extensive insurance reimbursement procedures and the lack of educational training in entry-level curricula regarding the use of water as a therapeutic exercise medium. With the inception of Medicare and Medicaid in the 1960s, as well as private health insurances in the 1950s and 1960s, the emphasis in reimbursement for various physical rehabilitation services was geared toward the highly touted technical equipment of the time. Aquatic programming was viewed as being geared more toward recreational, preventative, and maintenance activities, and was not recognized as a skilled service for which a qualified practitioner was needed. In addition, aquatic techniques were not an evident component of entry-level curricula for most rehabilitation disciplines, including physical therapy. Most of the education was done through postgraduate continuing education courses, of which only a limited number of clinicians took advantage. This limited contact with aquatic therapy techniques by a select number of clinicians did not serve to popularize the use of water for client rehabilitation.

Resurgence of Aquatic Rehabilitation in the United States in the 1970s and 1980s

The use of aquatic therapy experienced a resurgence during the 1970s and 1980s. In the third edition (1978) of his textbook, *Therapeutic Exercise*, Basmajian[14] devotes a chapter to the use of exercise in water and the specific benefits obtained by such exercise. In this chapter he also discusses the appropriate selection of clients, some treatment techniques, and the use of equipment to enhance water treatment techniques. The treatments he discusses emphasize the active participation of clients in underwater exercise that was beginning to see a resurgence in the United States. With the Vietnam War, clinicians again returned to the water for the rehabilitation of injured soldiers.

During this time, there was also a movement toward a more healthy lifestyle, with some emphasis on sports participation and other lifelong exercise activities, including swimming. Many people participated in swimming as an excep-

tionally good aerobic activity in the attempt to become more fit and healthy. The water environment began to be viewed favorably as an exercise medium with little chance of injury or harm. During this time, water began to be used for the early rehabilitation of athletic injuries that could not be safely initiated on land. In the mid- to late 1980s, "water aerobics" became popular for participants who were not able to tolerate high-impact aerobics classes on land. Exercise in the water environment for people with arthritis became popular with a program developed in 1974 for community-based exercise entitled "Twinges in the Hinges." This program was developed by Kit Wilson at the Whittier YMCA in California. The popularity of the use of water as a safe activity for people with arthritis was further spurred by the joint effort of the National Arthritis Foundation and the YMCA with the development of the National Arthritis Foundation YMCA Aquatic Program, which began in 1983.[18] These community-based maintenance and aerobic programs appear to have assisted the resurgence of the use of water as a therapeutic medium by health care practitioners.

Since the late 1970s and continuing into the 1990s, there has been a marked increase in research related to the physiologic responses to immersion and to exercise in the water medium. This research needs to be expanded further, but that which has been done so far provides the clinician with a base on which to develop treatment programs.

Present Status of Aquatic Rehabilitation in the United States and Europe

Throughout the 1990s, aquatic rehabilitation has continued to become increasingly popular in many inpatient and outpatient physical rehabilitation facilities that incorporate this form of therapy into the client's treatment regimen. Most of the new rehabilitation and outpatient facilities that have been built since the early 1990s have incorporated some type of pool or aquatic environment for physical therapy within the building plans or equipment budget expenditures. Many existing rehabilitation and outpatient facilities have been upgraded and renovated to include an aquatic component. Other centers use pool facilities in their community when it is not feasible to build an aquatic facility of their own.

Several national organizations have been formed since the late 1980s that address the specific needs of allied health care professionals, physical educators, and fitness instructors who are keenly interested in using rehabilitation, exercise, and recreational activities within a water medium to hasten client progress during the rehabilitation process and to enhance the overall well-being of otherwise healthy clients. The Aquatic Physical Therapy Section of the American Physical Therapy Association was founded in 1992 by two physical therapists, Judy Cirullo and Richard Ruoti. Organizations with a mission of promoting the use of water as a beneficial exercise medium include the American Association of Medical Hydrology; the Aquatic Exercise Association; the Aquatic Council of the American Alliance for Health, Physical Education, Recreation and Dance; the American Lap Swimmers Association; and the United States Water Fitness Association, to name only a few. There are many other national and local organizations that promote the use of recreational water activities for people with disabilities who would like to participate in recreational activities with their able-bodied counterparts, such as Capable Partners, Inc., the National Association of Handicapped Outdoor Sportsman, Inc., Physically Challenged Outdoorsman's Association, and the Committee on Water Skiing for the Disabled of the American Water Ski Association. The reader is encouraged to investigate such organizations or chapters of these national organizations and to use them as referral sources for disabled clients who would like to return to more functional activities on discharge from a rehabilitation program.

A large variety of client populations and diagnoses are being treated today in an aquatic environment in conjunction with other rehabilitation services within individual treatment programs. The benefits of incorporating treatment in the water environment in a client's treatment plan are extensive. Many clinicians throughout the United States and Europe have been incorporating these treatment techniques very successfully in their clients' care plans. This avenue for treatment in many client populations will only continue to grow into the 21st century. The use of aquatic rehabilitation in the United States continues to lag behind the practice of our European counterparts. There appear to be several reasons for this, of which reimbursement issues, efficacy studies, development of treatment protocols, and education of entry-level students are just a few problem areas.

Like many other therapeutic treatment techniques that have withstood the test of time and possibly the scrutiny of efficacy research, aquatic physical therapy and rehabilitation is currently facing this dilemma. Morris[19] points out that there is a shortage of efficacy research in aquatic physical therapy and other disciplines that address patient outcomes. Although there are many reasons why researchers do efficacy studies, one of which is concern for the well-being of patients, the need to legitimize a particular treatment form and the justification of reimbursement are vital to the promulgation of a treatment technique.[20,21] The lack of efficacy research to substantiate the benefits of participation in an aquatic rehabilitation program in conjunction with the unfamiliarity of third-party payers with what actually constitutes aquatic rehabilitation, have led to the present dilemma of difficulty in obtaining reimbursement for skilled aquatic rehabilitation services.

Lewis[22] has noted that the issues of efficacy studies and reimbursement are even more important in light of the changes that are being investigated with regard to health care reform. Most are aware of the transition of many insurance companies toward managed care with limited allotment of funding for physical rehabilitation services. These managed care policies also considerably limit reimbursement for such services as physical and occupational therapy. Providing evidence of enhanced and productive outcomes with regard to patient function will be one of the primary means to legitimize reimbursement of rehabilitation services. This can be accomplished only by reputable research that addresses patient outcomes.

Last, a treatment procedure can be used by only those practicing clinicians familiar with the treatment techniques incorporated within the procedure. In 1993, Morris and Jackson[23] investigated the presence and content of aquatic physical therapy instruction in entry-level physical therapy (PT) and physical therapist assistant (PTA) academic programs. Of those PT and PTA programs that answered the survey (59%), only 62% include specific aquatic physical therapy content in their entry-level curricula. Morris and Jackson[23] also noted that the accreditation standards for PT/PTA programs do not specify aquatic physical therapy as a requirement for curricular content.[24,25] They go on to express concern that exclusion of this material from entry-level curricula would hinder both those interested in conducting aquatic physical therapy and those already using aquatic physical therapy services for their clients.

Although it is evident that aquatic rehabilitation has made great strides and advances since the early 20th century, there is still a great deal of room for further improvement and enhancement of this therapeutic procedure. This can be accomplished only by the continued efforts of health care professionals who believe in the positive benefits of incorporating aquatic rehabilitation in a therapeutic treatment program.

Summary

From its rudimentary beginnings, the use of water as a healing medium and later as a therapeutic procedure has grown tremendously. Historical records demonstrate that the value of the use of water in a treatment program has increased over time to its current status. The dilemmas faced currently by those health care professionals who use the water environment in their therapeutic programs will serve as a testimony to those clinicians who will follow them. These dilemmas will become the history for future clinicians who pursue the use of aquatic rehabilitation as a viable treatment procedure.

REFERENCES

1. Campion MR. *Adult Hydrotherapy: A Practical Approach.* Oxford, England: Heinemann Medical Books; 1990:4, 5, 199–239.
2. Krizek V. History of balneotherapy. In: Licht S, ed. *Medical Hydrology.* Baltimore, Md: Waverly Press; 1963:132, 134–135, 140–145, 147–149.
3. Finnerty GB, Corbitt T. *Hydrotherapy.* New York, NY: Frederick Ungar Publishing Co; 1960:1–4.
4. Lowman C. *Therapeutic Use of Pools and Tanks.* Philadelphia, Pa: WB Saunders; 1952:1, 1x.
5. Roberts P. *Hydrotherapy: Its History, Theory, and Practice in Occupational Health.* May, 1981:235–244.
6. Haralson KM. Therapeutic pool program. *Clinical Management.* 1985;5(2):10–13.
7. Wyman JF, Glazer O, eds. *Hydrotherapy in Medical Physics I.* Chicago, Ill: Year Book Publishers; 1944:619.
8. Baruch S. *An Epitome of Hydrotherapy.* Philadelphia, Pa: WB Saunders; 1920:45–99, 151–198.
9. Skinner AT, Thomson AM. *Duffield's Exercise in Water.* 3rd ed. London, England: Bailliere Tindall; 1983:1–3.
10. Franke K. Kneipp treatment. In: Licht S, ed. *Medical Hydrology.* Baltimore, Md: Waverly Press; 1963:321.
11. Johnson C, Garrett G. Taking the plunge. *Team Rehab Report.* 1994;5(2):15–17.
12. Davis B, Harrison RA. *Hydrotherapy in Practice.* New York, NY: Churchill Livingstone; 1988:171–177.
13. Kamenetz HL. History of American spas and hydrotherapy. In: Licht S, ed. *Medical Hydrology.* Baltimore, Md: Waverly Press; 1963:160–163, 165–167, 169–176, 182–183.
14. Basmajian JV. *Therapeutic Exercise.* 3rd ed. Baltimore, Md: Williams & Wilkins; 1978:275.
15. Cunningham J. Applying Bad Ragaz method to the orthopedic client. *Orthopedic Physical Therapy Clinics in North America.* June 1994:251–260.
16. Martin J. The Halliwick method. *Physiotherapy.* 1981; 67(10):288.
17. Grosse SJ, Gildersleeve LA. The Halliwick Method. Milwaukee Public Schools, 1984:1.
18. Arthritis Foundation. *Arthritis Foundation YMCA Aquatic Program (AFYAP) and AFYAP PLUS: Guidelines and Procedure.* Atlanta, Ga: Arthritis Foundation; 1990:1.
19. Morris DM. Is aquatic therapy effective? *Aquatic Physical Therapy Report* 1993;1(3):4–5.
20. Dumboldt E. *Physical Therapy Research: Principles and Applications.* Philadelphia, Pa: WB Saunders; 1993:6–7.
21. Becker LR. Enthusiastic physical therapists jump feet first into aquatic research. *Advance for Physical Therapists.* 1993;4(22):10.
22. Lewis C. Efficacy studies gain importance in the reform arena. *PT Bulletin.* 1993;8(28):6.
23. Morris DM, Jackson JR. Academic programs survey: aquatic physical therapy content in entry level PT/PTA education. *Aquatic Physical Therapy Report.* 1993;1(4):13–16.
24. Commission on Accreditation in Physical Therapy Education. *Evaluative Criteria for Accreditation of Education Programs for the Preparation of Physical Therapist Assistants.* Alexandria, Va: American Physical Therapy Association; 1993.
25. Commission on Accreditation in Physical Therapy Education. *Evaluative Criteria for Accreditation of Education Programs for the Preparation of Physical Therapists.* Alexandria, Va: American Physical Therapy Association; 1992.

2

Aquatic Physics

Bruce E. Becker

As subsequent chapters will demonstrate, the therapeutic and physiologic effects of water are amazingly broad. This circumstance is the result of a remarkable series of effects of the principles of hydraulic physics, in combination with some powerful but little understood effects of immersion on the human psyche. These physical principles, many known since the advent of science, affect nearly all the physiologic systems of the human organism. Many have suggested that this is because of our ancestral home in the embryonic saline waters of some primordial Earth ocean. The renowned French physician Michel Odent refers to the human as *Homo aquaticus*, the "diving ape," and presents a cogent argument for the multiplicity of physiologic reasons that humans have built their social fabric around water.[1] Indeed, it can scarcely be coincidence that so much of our social, religious, recreational, and medical history involves this element.

Water is a substance composed of two of the most common elements on earth: oxygen and hydrogen. One atom of oxygen bonds with two atoms of hydrogen to form a molecule of water, H_2O, with a molecular weight of 18. The nearest approach of water molecules to each other is in ice, when they are separated by 2.76 Å (angstroms). The radius of the molecule is 1.38 Å. The molecules are bonded triangularly, with the hydrogen atoms separated by an arc of 104°31′, and separated from the oxygen atom by 0.9580 Å. This angle is greater than the expected 90° because of the incomplete sharing of electrons between the oxygen and hydrogen atoms, creating a partially ionized state. The physical configuration of these bonded molecules creates an open electrical field, leading to an affinity for many other chemical substances, and hence water's tremendous capacity as a solvent.[2]

Matter commonly exists at normal earth temperatures in three states: solid, liquid, and gas. A solid maintains a consistent shape and size, which typically does not change without significant force. Liquids, in contrast, readily alter shape, but typically retain volume despite force. Gases are the least fixed, lacking both fixed shape or volume. Both liquids and gases have the ability to flow, and because flow properties are more closely related to density than any other factor, both are referred to as fluids. Water is used in all its forms therapeutically.

Aquatic Physics

Nearly all of the biologic effects of immersion are related to the fundamental principles of hydrodynamics and thermodynamics. An understanding of these principles makes the medical application process more rational. Because aquatic activities take place in a dynamic aquatic environment, it is useful to study the physics of both still and moving water.

Water at Rest

Density and Specific Gravity[3]

Density is defined as mass per unit volume and is designated by the Greek letter ρ (rho). The relation of ρ to mass and volume is characterized by the formula:

$$\rho = \frac{m}{V}$$

where m is the mass of a substance whose volume is V. Density is measured in the international system as kilograms per cubic meter (kg/m^3) and occasionally as grams per cubic centimeter (g/cm^3). A density given in the latter format must be multiplied by 1000 to equal the former. Density is a temperature-dependent variable, although much less so for solids and liquids than for gases.

In addition to density, substances are defined by their *specific gravity*, the ratio of the density of that substance to the density of water. Water has a specific gravity by definition equal to 1 at 4°C. Because this number is a ratio, it has no units. Although the human body is mostly water, the body's density is slightly less than that of water, with an average specific gravity of 0.974, and men averaging a higher density than women. Lean body mass, which includes bone, muscle, connective tissue, and organs, has a typical density of 1.1, whereas fat mass, which includes both essential body fat plus fat in excess of essential needs, has a density of 0.90.[4] Consequently, the human body displaces a volume of water weighing slightly more than the body, forcing the body upward by a force equal to the volume of the water displaced, as is described later.

Hydrostatic Pressure

Pressure is defined as force per unit area, where the force, F, by convention is understood to act perpendicularly to the surface area, A. This relationship is:

$$P = \frac{F}{A}$$

The standard international unit of pressure is called a pascal, abbreviated Pa, after the French scientist Blaise Pascal, and is measured in newtons per square meter (N/m^2). Other common units are dynes per square centimeter (dynes/cm^2), kilograms per square meter (kg/m^2), millimeters of mercury per foot (mm Hg/ft), and pounds per square inch (lb/in^2, abbreviated "psi").

Fluids have been found experimentally to exert pressure in all directions, as the swimmer and diver are already aware. At a theoretic point position immersed in a vessel of water, the pressure exerted on that point is equal from all directions. Obviously, if unequal pressure were being exerted, the point would move until the pressures were equalized on it.

Pressure in a liquid increases with depth, and is directly related to the density of the fluid. If we consider a theoretic point immersed to a distance h below the surface, the force exerted on the point results from the weight of the column of fluid above it. The formula F (force) $= m$ (mass) $\times g$ (the acceleration of gravity) defines the force, and is equal to ρ, the density, times A, the area, times h, the height of the column of fluid. The pressure thus becomes:

$$P = \frac{F}{A} = \frac{\rho A h g}{A}$$

or, cancelling out A (area),

$$P = \rho g h$$

Therefore, pressure is directly proportional to both the liquid density and to the immersion depth, when the fluid is incompressible, as water is at the depths used in therapeutic environments. Sometimes it is useful to know the pressure differential between two immersed points separated by a vertical distance h. This pressure differential may be calculated by the adapted formula:

$$\Delta P = \rho g \Delta h$$

where Δ = the change in pressure and depth. Because P responds not only to the fluid depth, but to any force exerted on an object's surface, the pressure of the Earth's atmosphere is an important contributor to the total force from immersion. Water exerts a pressure of 22.4 mm Hg/ft of water depth, which translates to 1 mm Hg/1.36 cm (0.54 in) H$_2$O depth. Thus, a body immersed to a depth of 48 inches is subjected to a force equal to 88.9 mm Hg, slightly greater than diastolic blood pressure. This is the force that aids the resolution of edema in an injured body part.

Buoyancy

Immersed objects have less apparent weight than the same object on land. There is a force opposite to gravity acting on the object. This force is called *buoyancy*, and equals an upward force generated by the volume of H$_2$O displaced. The force arises from the fact described earlier that pressure in a fluid increases with depth. A cylinder immersed vertically in water has more force exerted on its bottom surface than on its top surface. This cylinder with height h has top and bottom surfaces with area A and is immersed in a liquid with density ρ_f. Because the pressure on the top of the cylinder is equal to $\rho_f g h_1$, where h_1 is the top surface depth, the force developed is $F_1 = P_1 A$, which is equal to $\rho_f g h_1 A$ and is a downward force. There is a force calculated by similar means that acts on the bottom surface of the cylinder in an upward direction. This force can be described as $F_2 = P_2 A = \rho_f g h_1 A$. The net force is called the *buoyant force*, F_B, and acts upward with the magnitude:

$$F_B = F_2 - F_1$$
$$= \rho_f g A (h_2 - h_1)$$
$$= \rho_f g A h$$
$$= \rho_f g V$$

where $V = Ah$ is the volume of the cylinder. Because ρ_f is the density of the liquid,

$$\rho_f g V = m_f g$$

defines the weight of a volume of fluid comparable to the volume of the cylinder. Thus, the buoyant force F_B is equal to the weight of the fluid displaced. This principle, discovered by Archimedes (287?–212 BC) is the reason why we float, why water can be used as a laboratory for weightlessness, and why it can be used to advantage in the management of medical problems requiring weight off-loading. The principle applies equally to floating objects. A human with specific gravity 0.97 will reach floating equilibrium when 97% of his or her volume is submerged[3] (p 193).

The buoyancy factor may be therapeutically altered simply through adjustment of the amount of human body immersed. Should partial weight-load offset be the desired effect, the immersion depth is reduced: with immersion to the xiphoid, most humans are around 75% off-loaded, and with immersion to the umbilicus, around 50%.

Physiologic Effects

Vascular System Effects

The combined effects of water's density, incompressibility, and hydrostatic pressure create significant compression on all the body tissues on immersion. As was mentioned, the compression is depth dependent. On immersion to the neck, approximately 700 cm[3] of blood are displaced from the extremities and abdominal vessels into the great veins of the thorax and into the heart. This causes a significant increase in right atrial pressure, stroke volume, and cardiac output.[5,6] There is an effect on systemic vascular resistance, which drops dramatically,[7] and on muscle circulation, which increases several-fold.[8]

Soft Tissue Effects

All soft tissues are compressed, so that lymphatic return is greatly enhanced. Normal lymphatic pressure is a negative pressure system, so that even minimal water depth immersion exceeds the lymphatic pressure. Even in the case of significant lymphedema, pressures within the lymphatic vessels are only a few millimeters of mercury. Immersion can thus assist the process of edema resolution.

Center of Buoyancy Versus Center of Balance

The fact that the force of buoyancy is an upward force has important consequences in the therapeutic aquatic environment. Although the human center of gravity is located slightly posterior to the midsagittal plane and at the level of the umbilicus, the human center of buoyancy is in the midchest. When both are aligned in a vertical plane, only vertical vector forces are apparent, but when these points are not aligned vertically, rotational forces called *torque* arise. This torque force may assist the floating human in maintaining an upright head-out posture, or, when buoyancy devices are used, torque may tend to float a person face down or supine. These same forces affect a limb and become a vector continuum as the limb moves through water.

Joint Effects

As the body gradually immerses, water is displaced, creating the force of buoyancy. This offloads the immersed joints progressively, and with neck immersion, only about 15 pounds of compressive force is exerted on the spine, hips, and knees. For a body suspended or floating in water, the downward effects of gravity are essentially counterbalanced by the upward force of buoyancy. This effect may be of great therapeutic utility, allowing rehabilitative intervention when gravity-loaded joint movement is prohibited. For example, a fractured pelvis may not become mechanically stable under full body loading for a period of many weeks, but in water immersion, gravitational forces may be partially or completely offset so that only muscle torque forces are present on the fracture site(s), allowing "active-assisted" range of motion activities, gentle strength building, and even gait training.

Refraction

When light passes from one medium to another, it encounters a boundary layer and usually undergoes a transformation at this interface. Part of the incident light is reflected at the boundary, and the portion passing into the new medium may change direction. This bending, or vector change, is referred to as *refraction* and is governed by specific properties of the material, particularly the speed of light in the material, and the angle of incidence of the light beam.

This phenomenon was studied in the early 1600s by Willebrord Snell, who discovered that there was a consistent relation between θ, the angle of incidence, and n, the index of refraction. This relation, called Snell's Law, states

$$n_1 \sin \theta_1 = n_2 \sin \theta_2$$

where θ_1 is the angle of incidence, θ_2 is the angle of refraction, and n_1 and n_2 are the respective indices of refraction in the two media. Thus, if light enters a medium where n is greater (and speed less), the beam of light is bent toward the normal (a perpendicular to the interface), and, conversely, when light exiting from a medium of high n enters a medium of low n, it deviates away from the normal. Because water presents more resistance to the speed of light, light reflected off an immersed person's foot bends away from the imaginary perpendicular when it crosses the water–air boundary. Thus, from the pool edge, a person standing in waist-deep water appears to have foreshortened trunk and legs.

From a pool-edge perspective, monitoring body position of an immersed person requires an understanding of this principle and experience with adjustment for its variance. As the immersed person is placed farther away from the observer into the pool, the angle change is greater and the difference between actual position and visualized position increases. In a therapeutic environment, it requires experience and careful attention to recognize the difference between the "virtual reality" of a body part location and its real position.

Surface Tension

The surfaces of liquids behave in a different fashion than the body of fluid. It has been noted that the surface of a liquid acts like a membrane under tension. Thus, a drop of water may hang on the end of a straw, and a needle heavier than water may float on the surface of a glass of water, suspended on this membrane-like barrier. This is because the attraction between adjacent molecules of water is circumferential everywhere except at the surface, where the attraction bonding is parallel to the surface. Surface tension is defined as the force F per unit length L that acts across any line in a surface and tends to pull the surface open[3] (pp 196–200). It is denoted by the Greek letter γ (gamma), and the force equation is

$$\gamma = \frac{F}{L}$$

Work must be done to increase the surface area of the fluid. Consequently, in the absence of a force input, fluids tend to shape in ways that minimize the surface area. Thus a raindrop assumes a shape that offers the minimum surface area consistent with the drop's volume, speed, and temperature.

The resistive force of surface tension becomes an active variable to the extent that surface area increases. Thus, when a swimmer kicks the water vigorously, breaking the surface into froth and droplets, considerable force has been exerted to overcome surface tension. A diver entering the water "cleanly" creates little spray, and thus has wasted a minimal amount of energy in moving from air to water.

Thermodynamics

Specific Heat

Water is used therapeutically in all its thermal forms: solid, liquid, and gas. A major reason for its usefulness lies in the physics of aquatic thermodynamics. All substances on earth possess energy stored as heat. This energy is measured in a quantity called a *calorie*, abbreviated "cal." A calorie is defined as the heat required to raise the temperature of 1 g of water by 1°C, from 14.5°C to 15.5°C. The energy required to raise the temperature of water varies slightly, even though this difference is less than 1% in the range from 0°C to 100°C. Sometimes, the energy required to raise temperature is defined in kilocalories, the amount required to raise 1 kg of water 1°C. and this unit by convention is termed a *Calorie* (with a capital "C"), abbreviated "Cal." This is the unit in which food energy content is measured. The British system measures heat energy in *British thermal units* (BTU), the amount of energy required to raise 1 pound of water 1°F. A mass of water possesses a definable, measurable amount of stored energy in the form of heat.

The amount of energy stored may be released in change to a lower temperature, or additional energy may be required to raise temperature. The formula defining the quantity of energy required or released is:

$$Q = mc\Delta T°$$

where m equals the mass of water, c equals the specific heat capacity of the fluid, and $\Delta T°$ equals the change in temperature. The work required to produce this energy is called *the mechanical equivalent of heat*, and is measured in *joules* (J). One calorie is equivalent to 4.18 J. A body immersed in a mass of water becomes a dynamic system. If the temperature of the water exceeds the temperature of the submerged body, the system equilibrates to a different level, with the submerged body warming through transference of heat energy from the water, and the water cooling through loss of heat energy to the body. By the first law of thermodynamics, the total heat (and thus energy) content of the system remains the same. Energy applied to this system raises the kinetic energy of some of the molecules, and when high–kinetic-energy molecules collide with lower–kinetic-energy molecules, they transfer some of their energy, raising and equilibrating the total energy of the system.

Again, by the centimeter/gram/second (cgs) system definition, water is defined as having a specific heat capacity equal to 1. Air, in contrast, has a significantly lower specific heat capacity (= 0.001). Water thus retains heat 1000 times more than an equivalent volume of air (Table 2-1).

Thermal Energy Transfer

The therapeutic utility of water depends greatly on both its ability to retain heat and its ability to transfer heat energy. Exchange of energy in the form of heat occurs in three ways: conduction, convection, and radiation. Conduction may be defined as heat transfer through individual molecular collisions occurring over a small distance. Convection transfers heat through the mass movement of large numbers of molecules over a large distance. Liquids and gases in general are poor conductors but good convectors. Radiation transfers heat through the transmission of electromagnetic waves. Conduction and convection require contact between the exchanging energy sources; radiation does not. Conduction occurs in the absence of movement, but convection requires that energy transfer occurs through movement of one source across the other. The rate of radiant energy transfer from a body is proportional to the fourth power of its temperature in degrees Kelvin. It is also proportional to surface area, to the emissivity of the material, and to the distance between the energy-radiating and energy-absorbing bodies.

Heat transfer across a gradient is measured by the amount of heat in calories transferred per second across an imaginary membrane. Substances vary widely in their ability to conduct heat. Water is an efficient conductor of heat and transfers heat 25 times faster than air (Table 2-2).

As can be seen from this table, metals and water tend to conduct heat well, and gas or gas-containing materials (eg, cork and down) conduct heat poorly. The latter are thus good insula-

TABLE 2-1. Various Heat Capacities

Substance	Specific Heat, c_p
Water (15°C)	1.00
Ice (−5°C)	0.50
Steam (110°C)	0.48
Alcohol	0.58
Protein	0.40
Human body	0.83
Mercury	0.03

Data from Giancoli DC. *Physics: Principles With Applications.* 2nd ed. Englewood Cliffs, NJ: Prentice Hall, Inc; 1985:253.

TABLE 2-2. Thermal Conductivity

Substance	Thermal Conductivity, k (kcals/s·m·C°)
Water (15°C)	1.4×10^{-4}
Air	0.055×10^{-4}
Human tissue (bloodless)	0.50×10^{-4}
Glass	2.0×10^{-4}
Silver	10×10^{-2}
Copper	9.2×10^{-2}
Down	0.06×10^{-2}
Cork	0.1×10^{-4}

Data from Giancoli DC. *Physics: Principles With Applications.* 2nd ed. Englewood Cliffs, NJ: Prentice Hall, Inc; 1985:260.

tors, whereas the former are good conductors. Human tissue without blood becomes a rather good insulator.

The human body produces considerable heat through the conversion of food calories into other energy forms. Only about 20% of this converted energy is used to do work, and the rest is converted into thermal energy. Core temperature would rise about 3°C per hour during light activity, if it were not for the body's ability to dissipate heat. This dissipation process relies on all heat transfer mechanisms, but by far the most important is convection, which results from the flow of warm blood from the core to the skin and lungs, where contact with the cooler air occurs. Blood becomes a convective fluid that transfers heat to the surface. Because energy must be dissipated further, the body uses another mechanism, allowing energy loss through the latent heat of evaporation of sweat and respiratory loss, further cooling the skin. This mechanism is remarkably efficient, because the evaporative loss of 2.5 mL of water cools the body 0.94°C (2°F). This fact is of considerable importance in scuba diving, where the humidity of inspired air approaches 0%, and the temperature of surrounding water is usually lower than the diver's body.[9] Thus, even for a diver in tropical waters where the water temperature may be 84°F to 86°F, the heat lost through respiratory water evaporation may cool the diver's core temperature significantly, and require the diver to don a wetsuit to prevent this heat loss.

Heat transfer increases as a function of velocity. Thus, a swimmer loses more heat when swimming rapidly through cold water than a person standing still in the same water. Fortunately for the swimmer, heat is produced through exercise. Heat transfer is achieved through all three mechanisms, conduction, convection, and radiation, with transfer to an immersed human body mostly occurring through conduction and convection, although heat loss from the body to the surrounding water occurs mostly through radiation and convection. This thermal conductive property, in combination with its high specific heat, makes water a versatile medium for rehabilitation because it retains heat or cold while delivering it easily to the immersed body part.

Water in Motion

Water at motion becomes a complex physical substance. In fact, despite centuries of study, many aspects of fluid motion are still incompletely understood. But the major principles of flow are valid and apply to general activities.

Flow Motion

Water may have several characteristics in motion. When water moves smoothly inside a vessel, with all layers moving at the same speed, the water is said to be in *laminar* or *streamline flow*. In this type of movement, all molecules are moving parallel to each other and paths do not cross. Typically, laminar flow rates are slow, because when water moves rapidly even minor oscillations create uneven flow, and parallel paths are knocked out of alignment. When this occurs, another type of pattern occurs called *turbulent flow*. Within the mass of water, flow patterns arise that run dramatically out of parallel, and may even set up paths running in opposite directions. These paths are called eddy currents and appear like whirlpools in response to obstacles in the flow path, or to irregularities in the surface of flow-directing vessels. Examples are the eddy holes that occur in fast-moving streams behind boulders, and eddy currents that form in the bloodstream behind artery walls encrusted with cholesterol plaque. Turbulent flow absorbs energy at a much greater rate than streamline flow, and the rate of energy absorption is determined by the internal friction of the fluid. This internal friction is called *viscosity*. The major determinants of water motion are viscosity, turbulence, and speed.

Viscosity

Water at room temperature, and through most of the range of its common therapeutic uses, is a liquid. Liquids all share a property called viscosity, which refers to the magnitude of internal friction specific to the fluid. Different fluids are characterized by varying amounts of molecular attraction within the fluid, and as layers of fluid are set into motion, this attraction creates resistance to movement, and is detected as friction. Energy must be exerted to create movement, and because in the first law of thermodynamics, energy is never lost but rather transformed and stored as potential or kinetic energy, some energy is transformed into heat, some into kinetic energy, and some may be stored as energy by increasing surface tension. Fluids are in part defined by individual viscosity, expressed quantitatively as the *coefficient of viscosity*, which is designated the Greek letter η

TABLE 2-3. Coefficients of Viscosity for a Variety of Fluids

Fluid	Temperature (°C)	Coefficient of Viscosity (η[Pa·s])
Water	0	1.8×10^{-3}
Whole blood	37	4×10^{-3}
Blood plasma	37	1.5×10^{-3}
Engine oil (SAE 10)	30	200×10^{-3}
Glycerin	20	1500×10^{-3}
Water vapor	100	0.013×10^{-3}

Data from Giancoli DC. *Physics: Principles With Applications*. 2nd ed. Englewood Cliffs, NJ: Prentice Hall, Inc; 1985:208.

(eta). The greater the coefficient, the more viscous the fluid and the greater the force required to create movement within the fluid. This force is proportionate to the number of molecules of fluid set into motion, and the velocity of their movement. Thus, the equation that expresses this relation must define the volume of the fluid in motion, measured as A, the area, and l, the depth, and the velocity v of the motion; the corresponding formula is expressed:

$$F = \eta A \frac{v}{l}$$

Solving this equation for η finds that $\eta = Fl/vA$. The SI unit of measurement of viscosity is measured in newton-seconds/m², equal to a Pascal-second (Pa·s). In the cgs system, the measurement is dyne-seconds/cm². One unit is called a *poise*, after the French scientist J. L. Poiselle (1799–1869), who studied the physics of blood circulation. Often coefficients are stated in *centipoise*, one-hundredth of a poise (Table 2-3).

Laminar Flow

As water moves smoothly within a vessel, the speed of movement changes with the size of the vessel. The flow rate is defined as the mass of water moving past an imaginary point per unit of time t: m/t.

$$\frac{m}{t} = \frac{\rho_1 V_1}{t} = \frac{\rho_1 A_1 l_1}{t} = \rho_1 A_1 v_1$$

where ρ_1 represents fluid density at a point in space 1, V_1 represents the volume of water, v_1 the velocity of flow, and l_1 the length of the

water column of area A_1. As water moves past a subsequent point 2, the same volume of water with area A_2 and length l_2 may need to increase or decrease velocity to adapt to vessel area changes, because water is essentially incompressible.

Poiselle developed an equation that describes the laminar flow of an incompressible fluid through a tube of fixed internal radius and length:

$$Q = \frac{\pi r^4 (P_1 - P_2)}{8 \eta L}$$

As can be seen in the formula, Q (the volume rate of flow) is directly proportional to the pressure gradient and inversely proportional to the viscosity, but it is also proportional to the fourth power of the tube radius. Therefore, if the tube doubles in radius, flow volume increases by a factor of 16. This equation holds true only for laminar flow, however, and provides only an approximation of turbulent flow volumes.

Turbulent Flow

Flow volumes lessen when turbulence occurs, largely because of the significant rise in internal friction in the fluid. The onset of turbulent flow is obviously a function of fluid velocity, but is also related to fluid density and viscosity, and enclosure radius. The transition from laminar flow to turbulent flow often occurs abruptly. This transition point is characterized by a formula incorporating these factors, and is called the *Reynolds number* (Re), after the English physicist Sir Joshua Reynolds. This number is calculated by the formula:

$$Re = \frac{2 \bar{v} r \rho}{\eta}$$

where $\bar{v}$ is the average fluid velocity, ρ its density, and r the radius of the tube in which the fluid is flowing. Typically, Reynolds numbers greater than 2000 produce turbulent flow.

Drag Contribution

When an object moves relative to a fluid, it is subjected to the resistive effects of the fluid. This force is called *drag force* and is caused by fluid viscosity and turbulence, when present. This force is defined by a *second Reynolds number*.

$$Re' = \frac{vL\rho}{\eta}$$

where this v now equals the velocity of the object relative to the fluid. Although the Reynolds formulas are similar, the results produced are different. A 1-mm object moving through water at 1 mm/sec has a Reynolds number of 1. When this formula produces a Reynolds number equal to or less than 1, the flow is usually laminar, and the force needed to move through the fluid is directly proportional to the speed of the object. The viscous force F_v is directly proportional to the object speed:

$$F_v = kv$$

The magnitude of k depends on the size and shape of the object and on the fluid viscosity. If the object is a sphere, this k is equal to

$$k = 6\pi r\rho$$

With faster movement, higher Reynolds numbers are produced, and the drag force begins to increase as the square of the velocity. Streamlining reduces the resultant Reynolds number. The speed needed to produce Reynolds numbers between 1 and 10 produces turbulence behind the object, known as a wake. At these speeds, the force increases with the square of the velocity, $F_v \propto v^2$. As the speed increases yet further, with Reynolds numbers around 10^6, there is an abrupt increase in drag force. This force results from turbulence produced not only behind the moving object but in the layer of fluid passing over the object, known as the boundary layer.

Resistance Effects

Water is intermediate in viscosity as liquids go, but still presents much resistance to movement. As shown in the preceding section, under turbulent flow conditions this resistance increases as a log function of velocity and depends on the shape and size of the object. The source of greatest drag in a swimming human is the head, although the negative pressure following the swimmer causes the greatest force resisting forward movement. There is turbulence produced by the moving body surface areas, and a drag force produced by the turbulence behind. Viscosity, with all its attendant physical properties, is the quality that makes water a useful strengthening medium, because it resists more as more force is exerted against it, although that resistance drops to zero instantly with cessation of force. Thus, when a person rehabilitating feels pain and stops movement, the force drops instantly, allowing great control of strengthening activities within the "envelope" of tolerance.

To use the earlier example of the client with a pelvic fracture, with immersion, movement of the lower extremities may be slow and guided, in which case most of the resistance is from drag force under laminar conditions, and quite predictable. As the client's strength builds and bone integrity increases, movement speed may increase, which raises the drag force and takes resistance from laminar into turbulent flow conditions, with attendant logarithmic increases in resistance, as well as some less predictable forces from the water turbulence. This turbulent movement may facilitate proprioceptive joint feedback, requiring an improved effort at modulation on the client's part to achieve smooth movement through the arc of joint range. Yet, as pain intervenes, the client may cease forceful movement, and the viscous damping of the water will very rapidly stop further limb movement. Thus, all properties of water in motion play a role in this rehabilitative use.

Technologies to Amplify Physical Principles

Almost all of the physical principles described in this chapter are clinically useful without additional modification. Many of these principles, however, may be extended into a broader range of clinical applications through additional technology. For example, buoyancy force may be increased through the use of flotation devices such as belts, tubes, or jackets. Such devices may assist the client in maintaining a desired body position, supporting a particular body part, or adding an additional force to overcome in strengthening activities. Similarly, devices that add surface area, such as finned boots, may be used to increase resistance to movement, requiring the client to exert more strength and motor control to propel the limb through water. Technologies are available that add flow velocity to water, requiring a person to overcome not only normal resistance but added laminar flow resistance. Immersible devices have been designed that guide a limb through a specifically designed movement, such as bicycling or treadmill walking. As more creative energies are applied to the world of aquatic rehabilitation (and its perceived market opportunities), more specific equipment will undoubtedly emerge.

Summary

The many physical principles that govern the behavior of water are complex. The principles that affect the therapeutic process derive from nearly all of them. Water's density, incompressibility, and heat capacity and transmission qualities all are profound forces to contend with. The biologic consequences of these forces can beneficially affect nearly all homeostatic systems, as is shown in subsequent chapters. These physiologic effects start immediately with immersion. Heat transfer begins, and because the specific heat of the human body is lower than that of water, the body loses or gains heat faster than does water. Hydrostatic pressure effects begin immediately, although most of these effects cause plastic deformation of the body, occurring through time. As is demonstrated later in this book, blood displaces cephalad, right atrial pressure begins to rise, pleural surface pressure rises, the chest wall compresses, and the diaphragm is displaced cephalad. The work of breathing is greatly increased in the immersed human. The pressure forces central return of lymph, and pushes out extracellular fluid. There are significant renal responses to these forces, altering blood volume, pressure, and diuresis. Tissue circulation is increased; temperature regulation mechanisms begin to come into play. The human organism is profoundly affected.

It behooves the scientific practitioner of aquatic therapy to understand the complex interplay of these forces in the therapeutic environment. Only through understanding can better methodologies be developed. It is hoped that this chapter has furthered that understanding.

REFERENCES

1. Odent M. Homo aquaticus. In: *Water and Sexuality.* Harmonsdworth, England: Arkana Books; 1990: 84–95.
2. Kuroda PK. What is water? In: Licht S, ed. *Medical Hydrology.* Baltimore, Md: Waverly Press, Inc; 1963: 1–24.
3. Giancoli DC. *Physics: Principles With Applications.* 2nd ed. Englewood Cliffs, NJ: Prentice Hall, Inc; 1985: 184–214.
4. Bloomfield J, Fricker P, Fitch K. *Textbook of Science and Medicine in Sport.* Champaign, Ill: Human Kinetics Books; 1992:5.
5. Arborelius M, Balldin UI, Lilja B, Lundgren CE. Hemodynamic changes in man during immersion with the head above water. *Aerospace Medicine.* 1972;43: 593–599.
6. Risch WD, Koubenec HJ, Beckmann U, Lange S, Gauer OH. The effect of graded immersion on heart volume, central venous pressure, pulmonary blood distribution and heart rate in man. *Pflugers Arch.* 1978;374: 117.
7. McMurray RG, Fieselman CC, Avery KE, Sheps DS. Exercise hemodynamics in water and on land in patients with coronary artery disease. *Cardiopulmonary Rehabilitation.* 1988;8:69–75.
8. Balldin UI, Lundgren CEG, Lundvall J, Mellander S. Changes in the elimination of ^{133}xenon from the anterior tibial muscle in man induced by immersion in water and by shifts in body position. *Aerospace Medicine.* 1971;42:489–493.
9. Somers L. Diving physics. In: Bove AA, Davis JC, eds. *Diving Medicine.* 2nd ed. Philadelphia, Pa: WB Saunders; 1990:9–18.

3 Physiologic Effects of Immersion at Rest

Jolie Bookspan

Physiologic responses to immersion at rest have been described in over 3000 years of medical writings of the Persians, Hindus, Greeks, Egyptians, and Chinese. Modern scientific work details the mechanisms behind the effects. Two systems are described here: the cardiovascular system and the renal system.

Cardiovascular Effects of Immersion

The set of cardiovascular responses to immersion, including bradycardia, peripheral vasoconstriction, and preferential shunting of blood to vital areas, is collectively known as the dive reflex. Extent of bradycardia is used as an index of the depth of the reflex. The dive reflex occurs in response to a variety of immersion conditions: face immersion, as when washing; head-out, full-body immersion, as during water exercise and water therapy; and full immersion during underwater swimming, breath-hold diving, and scuba diving.

> **Manifestations of the Human Dive Reflex**
>
> - Bradycardia
> - Peripheral vasoconstriction

Role in Humans

Bradycardia resulting from the dive reflex does not reduce oxygen demand to protect humans from hypoxia[1-5] or extend breath-holding time,[6,7] and has not been found to contribute to survival after near-drowning in cold water. Once the person is unconscious, lowered metabolism from extreme cold is the likely mechanism in occasional cases of survival.[8] The role of the dive reflex in humans who swim in cool and cold water is primarily heat conservation by means of peripheral vasoconstriction,[9] and secondarily a regulatory maneuver to maintain blood pressure.[10]

Mechanisms

Irving[11] postulated a general vertebrate diving reflex. However, it is likely that multiple and competing mechanical and neural factors are involved in human response to immersion. Interaction among these variables is also important.

Temperature

Cold produces two principal effects to lower heart rate. Trigeminally distributed cold receptors trigger neural reflex bradycardia, and cold-induced vasoconstriction shunts blood to the thorax, increasing venous return. Increased venous return increases atrial filling, contractility by means of the Starling mechanism, and stroke volume. To maintain cardiac output, heart rate reflexively drops.

Most researchers have found that apneic bradycardia, induced by face immersion and full-body immersion, is water temperature dependent in humans,[12-14] with lower temperature potentiating the bradycardic response,[3,14-18] but only to a point. Face immersion in water between 20°C and 10°C produced no difference in heart rate,[19] and there appears to be a lower limit of 10°C before a pressor response raises heart rate.[20] Magnitude of human bradycardia has also been found to be directly proportional to skin temperature of the body.[21] Head-out immersion in warm water (36°C and 37°C) increases heart rate because of heat-induced peripheral vasodilation.[22] Summarizing work by previous researchers, Tuttle and Corleaux[23] stated that immersion in cold water reduces heart rate, immersion in warm and hot water increases heart rate, and water at body temperature was considered to be thermoneutral.

Extent of limb vasoconstriction is inversely proportional to water temperature. Vasoconstriction increases with decreasing temperature.[10,17,24] Water warmer than 20°C but below 40°C may have no effect on peripheral blood flow during immersion.[10] Warmer water increases peripheral vasodilation, which functions in cooling.

Immersion

Gravity operates fully underwater, but its effects are less. Reduced effect of gravity shifts blood and fluid from the dependent limbs to the upper body, beginning immediately on exposure and reaching a maximum in 24 hours.[25] Increased blood and fluid volume centralization increases venous return, which stimulates baroreceptors, increases cardiac filling and stroke volume, and reflexively reduces heart rate.[26]

Immersion bradycardia was found to be unrelated to the level of body immersion without head immersion by some researchers.[14,16,27] However, in the case of Campbell and associates,[27] water temperature was 34°C, too warm to elicit substantial bradycardia. Craig[15] reported that immersion to different body levels altered heart rate because of changes in venous return.

Although headward fluid shifts are popularly attributed to the hydrostatic pressure gradient, with greater pressure with deeper depths squeezing blood from foot to head,[27–29] water pressure does not progressively squeeze blood upward. Increasing water pressure with depth is almost identical to the increase in blood pressure toward the part of the body that is lower (head or feet), regardless of postural orientation. Water pressure does not squeeze blood in any direction. Headward fluid shifts are observed when immersed lying prone, where there is no hydrostatic gradient[30]; when upside down un-

derwater, where the hydrostatic gradient is reversed; and in space, where there is no pressure differential at all[25] (see section on Renal Effects of Immersion).

Full immersion is not required for bradycardia.[15] Facial immersion is sufficient stimulus to elicit bradycardia[12,31,32] and peripheral vasoconstriction.[33] Simply covering the face of an apneic human subject with a wet, cold face cloth induces bradycardia,[34,35] but that effect may be more the result of cold than wetting. The bradycardic effect of immersion is greater when body immersion is combined with face or head immersion than in body immersion alone.[14,16] Evidence is conflicting as to the role immersion plays without apnea.[36,37]

Apneic full-body immersion (including face) reduces forearm[30] and calf blood flow.[27] Apneic body immersion without face immersion may produce a blood flow response intermediate between that of face immersion alone and that of full-body with face immersion,[38] or may have no influence.[33]

Wetting

Whether facial wetting, per se, in humans is a factor that elicits bradycardia is disputed. It is possible that wetting is important only insofar as water is a conductor of heat. Parfrey and Sheehan[17] found face immersion with a plastic film covering produces significantly less bradycardia than face immersion with wetting at every 5°C temperature interval from 5°C to 25°C, but not 30°C. The film prevented wetting but allowed cold transmission. Bradycardic response to face immersion was unrelated to wetting when breath holding was performed in 5°C water with the face covered by a polyvinyl sheet, according to Moore and colleagues.[16] Work by the same authors did not indicate a difference in bradycardic response between diving with or without a face mask. However, wetting may be a factor in warmer-temperature water, according to other work.[39]

Posture

Because of the buoyant effect of immersion countering venous pooling in the limbs, described earlier, fluid centralization responsible for bradycardia occurs to a similar degree regardless of posture—upright or prone—when immersed. Work by Bookspan and colleagues[30] showed that development of bradycardia or limb vasoconstriction does not change with postural change underwater.

In air, by contrast, bradycardia results from a posture change, from standing to lying down.[14] Postural bradycardia in air with head lowering is caused by a baroreceptor response from increased venous return.[14,15] Vascular beds in the forearm vasodilate because of decreased sympathetic outflow.[40,41]

A postural change, in air, from lying to standing or sitting, reverses bradycardia.[42,43] Increasing hydrostatic pressure forces blood to the lower limbs, which decreases venous return[41] and, in turn, stroke volume.[44] Leg blood flow and heart rate both increase. Forearm vasomotor tone increases,[45] decreasing forearm blood flow[40] and thereby increasing central volume to maintain cardiac output,[46] blood pressure,[47] and perfusion.[41]

Apnea

Breath holding (apnea) decreases heart rate.[39] Water immersion with breath holding produces a greater degree of bradycardia than that observed during apnea in air,[19,39,48,49] and speeds development of bradycardia.[10] Nonapneic immersion may reduce the bradycardic effect,[19,48,49] or eliminate it.[36,39]

There has been much investigation into which aspects of apnea contribute to bradycardia: cessation of breathing movements,[38] hypercapnia,[39,50] hypoxia,[51] intrapleural pressure,[14] inspiratory level,[14] and intrathoracic pressure and Valsalva maneuver subsequent to maximal inspiration.[15] Apneic bradycardia may be related to intrathoracic pressure[15] and may be further limited by intrapleural pressure.[14] However, changes in intrathoracic pressure and inadvertent Valsalva maneuver subsequent to maximal inspiration may also be responsible for heart rate changes. Increased intrathoracic pressure stimulates baroreceptors to reduce heart rate; however it also reduces venous return from the periphery, blunting the bradycardic effect.[15] Swallowing or attempts at breathing against a closed glottis blunt the bradycardic effect (yielding higher heart rate values, but still bradycardic compared with control values).[52,53]

The bradycardic effect is intensified with immersion after inspiration,[36] as is the effect on peripheral blood flow,[54] whereas tachycardia results from apneic immersion at end exhalation.[14,49] Tachycardia occurs during apnea after maximal expiration, regardless of intrathoracic pressure.[14] Resumption of breathing increases heart rate even if arterial blood gases are kept constant.[53]

In work investigating the vasoconstrictive effect of apnea, it was shown that both apnea in air and apneic face immersion may reduce peripheral blood flow. Work has been done to identify apnea-induced reduction of blood flow to the forearm,[48,55,56] to the finger,[56] and to the calf,[27,33] although apnea in air produced an increase in forearm blood flow in work by Campbell and associates,[27] and no change in work by Bookspan and colleagues.[30] Reduction in finger blood flow is more marked than reduction in forearm blood flow during apnea, both in air and during face immersion.[56] Greater forearm blood flow reduction occurs with apneic face immersion than nonapneic face immersion[48] or apnea in air.[55] Nonapneic, head-out body immersion increases blood flow in both calf and forearm in 34°C water.[27] Full inspiration before apnea may potentiate peripheral vasoconstriction,[33] and deep inspiration decreases finger blood flow.[57] Valsalva maneuver produces vasoconstriction in both forearm and calf vascular beds,[40] and so must be considered when apnea occurs. Calf and finger blood flow decreases during apnea after deep hyperventilation.[21] Forearm blood flow reaches its lowest value after 30 seconds of apneic immersion.[48] Reduction in forearm blood flow occurs more slowly than heart rate reduction after apneic face immersion.[17]

Other Factors

Other variables affecting heart rate response to immersion are exercise,[39,58] anticholinergic agents such as atropine,[50] increased levels of carbon dioxide,[39,58] and intrapleural pressure.[14,15] Bradycardia elicited by immersion even overrides the tachycardia produced in humans during underwater exercise.[11,39,59] Fitness was found to be related to the magnitude of bradycardic response by Bove and colleagues,[31] but not by Stromme and coworkers[39] or Whayne and Killip.[34] Craig[15] found cardiovascular response independent of depth to 27 m.

Influence of mediation at cortical or supratentorial levels has been demonstrated in both humans and animals. Harassment of human subjects, and subject anxiety immediately before and during immersion, attenuated or eliminated bradycardia in humans.[10,42] Anticipation of face immersion elicited bradycardia.[10,60] Fear potentiated the bradycardic response.[60,61]

The Dive Reflex is Different in Humans and Marine Animals

Human cardiovascular response to immersion differs in several ways from that of diving animals. The extent of the difference between human and animal response led Paulev[54] to believe it may be inappropriate to extend the term "dive reflex" to the human cardiovascular response to immersion.

Not Protective in Humans

The dive reflex appears to be a phylogenetically ancient protective mechanism in animals. When they are removed from water, bradycardia is found in fish.[62] In aquatic mammals like whales and seals, the dive reflex plays a major role in conserving oxygen. Unlike marine mammals, humans do not retain an oxygen-conserving benefit.[1–5] In cold water, although heart rate decreases in humans, there is no concurrent reduction in metabolism or oxygen demands of the body's vital organs. Conversely, an immediate response to cold immersion is increased metabolism, evidenced by increased oxygen consumption. Metabolism increases as an immediate adaptation to dealing with the work of staying warm in the cold. In the conscious breath-hold diver, exaggerated cardiovascular response in people sensitive to apnea or immersion can result in blackout or death, a link first described in 1942.[63] Subsequent work has been substantiating.[21,47,64]

Heart Rate

Marine mammals display heart rate reductions of up to 90%. Bradycardia appears to a lesser degree in humans, with maximal reduction to 50% of predive control values.[14]

Temperature Dependence

Cardiovascular response in animals is independent of water temperature.[58,65] Unlike animals, human change in heart rate and peripheral blood flow is temperature sensitive,[14–18,66] with lower temperatures potentiating bradycardia[18,34,67] and peripheral vasoconstriction[68] (see earlier section on Temperature).

Arrhythmias

Unlike diving mammals, humans often exhibit arrhythmias during diving bradycardia,[47,62] particularly after underwater exercise. Olson and colleagues observed arrhythmias in over 75% of their subjects.[37] Incidence of arrhythmia is temperature dependent, with lower temperature associated with higher incidence of arrhythmia.[34,69] The frequency of cardiac arrhythmia in the Ama (Korean women divers) was found to be 43% in summer water of 27°C and 72% in winter water of 10°C.[69] Arrhythmias were documented during apnea in air,[70] particularly while maintaining maximal inspiration and after release of a prolonged breath hold. However, tendency to arrhythmia is greater during apneic immersion than during apnea in air, and tends to occur late in a breath-hold dive and during recovery.[21]

Breath Holding

Breath-holding time during submersion has been documented up to 120 minutes in whales,[65] and longer in elephant seals. Human submersions are usually short, averaging up to 2.5 minutes.[65] Even record-breaking breath holds by highly trained humans are short compared to average breath holds of diving mammals. The dive reflex does not increase underwater breath-holding time compared to breath-holding time in the air.[6] Cold water shortens breath-hold duration compared to warmer water.[7]

Marine mammals like whales, seals, dolphins, and sea otters also have the anatomic ability to collapse their lungs on submersion, displacing air away from pulmonary blood to reinforced upper airway passages. This protects from various ill effects of exposure to air under pressure, including oxygen toxicity, nitrogen narcosis, and decompression sickness ("the bends").[71] Humans typically inspire deeply before submersion, holding air volume in the lung at near maximal inspiratory capacity. Pulmonary gases continue to exchange at depth, resulting in the occasional case of decompression sickness among breath-hold divers making repeated, deep dives. This is not part of the dive reflex, but is another example of the diving dimorphism between humans and marine mammals.

Limb Blood Flow

Arterial limb blood pressure in the diving seal falls as low as venous pressure.[26] Strauss observed that no bleeding occurred in incisions

TABLE 3-1. Dive Reflex Comparison Between Marine Mammals and Humans

Marine Mammals	Humans
Major oxygen conservation and protection from hypoxia	No reduction in oxygen demand; cold immersion raises oxygen consumption in conscious humans
Major bradycardia and peripheral vasoconstriction	Variable bradycardia and peripheral vasoconstriction
Independent of water temperature	Acutely temperature sensitive
No great tendency to cardiac arrhythmias	Increased arrhythmias
High breath-hold ability during immersion	Decreased breath-holding time in cold water compared to nonimmersion and warm water conditions; breath-hold time decreases because of increased oxygen demands of cold immersion

made in the hind flipper of a seal during the dive.[72] Human peripheral blood flow reduction is more moderate and variable (Table 3-1).[30]

Individual Variation

Human cardiovascular adjustment to diving varies among individuals and conditions.[11,21] Some subjects demonstrate profound response, others no change. Those unfamiliar with the water may override vagal response with sympathetic stimulation, resulting in heart rate increase,[1] although considerable bradycardia has been observed in untrained subjects as well as those who are trained,[15,21] and similar degrees of bradycardia have been demonstrated in good and poor swimmers.[73]

Anatomy and Physiology

The inverse relation between water temperature and magnitude of human immersion bradycardia suggests cold-fiber receptors as an important afferent component in humans.[3,54] Magnitude of bradycardia seems to depend on amount of exposed trigeminal skin over certain facial areas,[17,39] although the role is sometimes disputed.[22,48,49] The efferent limb is the vagus nerve.[37] The carotid sinus is the end of the efferent pathway.[15]

Increased venous return with immersion increases carotid sinus pressure, slowing heart rate.[15] Atrial wall stretch receptors distend secondary to blood shifting from limbs to thorax, because of peripheral vasoconstriction from cold[74] and the buoyant effect of immersion. An inverse relationship between lung volume

and heart rate suggests a neural reflex initiated by stretch receptors sites in the lung or thorax.[75]

Increased carbon dioxide levels stimulate chemoreceptors to lower heart rate in ducks[58] and humans.[39] Decreased arterial oxygen tensions may increase the bradycardic effect in humans by stimulating carotid body chemoreceptors.[51]

Peripheral vasoconstriction is governed by increased sympathetic vasoconstrictor outflow to resistance vessels.[27,38,55] Although atropine blocks bradycardia in response to diving,[50] its administration has no significant effect on vasoconstrictor response, suggesting the response is not affected by cholinergic sympathetic vasodilator fibers.[56] α-Excitatory receptors provide primary control of limb vasoconstriction, nullifying vasodilation by β-inhibitory receptors.[3] Finger vasoconstriction may result from a neural reflex. It is absent in denervated or sympathectomized limbs.[57]

Components in peripheral blood flow change include apnea,[17,27,33,48] deep inspiration,[57] esophageal pressures,[54] temperature,[3] hydrostatic pressure of the water,[27] and lung volume at the initiation of apnea.[33,54]

Clinical Application of the Dive Reflex

The major clinical application of the bradycardic effect of the dive reflex is treatment of paroxysmal tachycardias. Apneic face immersion in cold water has been found, in some cases, to convert supraventricular tachycardia to sinus rhythm in adult cardiac patients without complications within 15 to 35 seconds.[76,77] It has been found to be effective in junctional tachycardia in adults,[78] and in supraventricular tachycardias in infants.[79,80] However, there are also reports of the face immersion maneuver exacerbating cardiac dysfunction in those with ventricular sympathetic irritability.[81]

Practical Lessons for the Practitioner

Sudden vasoconstriction, decrease in heart rate, increase in heart volume from increased venous return, and incidence of abnormal heart rhythms are not well tolerated by everyone's cardiac system, particularly for older men and in colder water.

> **Suggestions to Minimize Adverse Effects**
>
> - Avoid diving in "all at once"—get in slowly.
> - Have participants wet their faces and hands.
> - Avoid very cold immersions.

Renal Effects of Immersion

Renal response to immersion includes increased urine output, called "diuresis,"[82–86] with attendant plasma volume loss[87]; sodium loss, called "natriuresis"[86,88]; potassium loss, called "kaliuresis"; and suppression of arginine vasopressin[89,90] and plasma renin and aldosterone.[91] Cold water potentiates the response.[83,92] The collected effects occur with head-out body immersion,[86,93] as during water exercise and rehabilitation, and with full immersion, as during underwater swimming, breath-hold diving, and scuba diving. Renal effects also occur with non-immersed exposure to cool water, readily apparent in showers.

Immersion diuresis has been intensely studied in several areas—renal and cardiovascular volume homeostasis in normal and disease states, effects of extended commercial and underwater scientific diving missions, and effects of microgravity during space travel. It is also a topic of intrigue to swimmers and aquatic in-

structors who want to know why immersion makes a person have to "go."

> **Renal Response to Immersion**
>
> - Diuresis—increased urine excretion
> - Natriuresis—increased sodium excretion
> - Kaliuresis—increased potassium excretion

Role in Humans

Several effects of immersion, coupled with peripheral vasoconstriction with cold immersion, shift blood away from the limbs, producing central hypervolemia. The role of immersion diuresis is usually explained as a strong homeostatic compensatory mechanism to counter distended cardiac receptors,[94] thereby reducing atrial distention.[95] It has been postulated as a possible protective response of the heart against volume or pressure overload.[96]

Mechanisms

Buoyancy

The buoyant effect of immersion to counter venous pooling was described earlier in the section on Cardiovascular Effects. To recap, when at rest on land, venous blood pools in the dependent limbs because of gravity, vessel elasticity and distensibility, and lack of countering ambient pressure. Were veins iron pipes, there would be no distention and no pooling on land, no matter how great the gravity. Forces opposing vessel stretching are the elastic restoring force of the vessels and ambient pressure.

In air, ambient pressure is small, allowing pooling. With microgravity in space, there is no pooling. During immersion, water pressure counters limb pooling. Water pressure increases with depth at the same rate that venous blood pressure, on land, increases toward the feet (or head, if a person stands on it). Because of gravity, the fluid at any level bears the weight of all the fluid above it. Increase in water pressure with depth is almost identical to the increase in blood pressure toward the lower body part (head or feet), regardless of postural orientation, "canceling" venous pooling. Without pooling, more blood returns to the thorax. Centralizing blood volume is a trigger for both the dive reflex and diuresis.

Removal of venous pooling and central blood shifting is sometimes mistakenly attributed to the hydrostatic gradient squeezing blood from foot to head.[28] However, countering water pressure does not progressively squeeze blood upward; rather, it matches the increasing venous pressure with distance down the vessels, and operates equally on a person in any posture. Similar volume shifting occurs during immersion, whether head-up or prone.[30] Diuresis also occurs in any position in a space vehicle after transition from eugravity to microgravity in absence of any hydrostatic pressure gradient, because of this same removal of pooling.[25]

Negative-Pressure Breathing

During head-out immersion, air pressure at the mouth is approximately 20 cm H_2O less than hydrostatic pressure on the chest. This lower pressure is transmitted through the airways to the lung. Lower pressure of the interior lung than on the chest wall creates a negative pressure during inspiration. The feeling is like trying to drink through a straw. Negative-pressure breathing increases blood volume in the intrathoracic compartment,[28] and this central blood shift results in volume-compensatory diuresis. Conversely, positive-pressure breathing decreases intrathoracic blood volume, and depending on pressure used, blunts or eliminates diuresis.[97,98]

Temperature

Lower temperature potentiates the renal response to immersion. Cold-induced peripheral vasoconstriction shifts blood centrally,[9] increasing thoracic blood volume and the cascade of regulatory renal responses. Heat-induced limb vasodilation shifts blood peripherally, reducing thoracic blood volume and subsequent diuretic effect.[99] The temperature effect is apparent even without immersion. Exposure to cold air alone triggers diuresis and plasma volume loss.[87]

Time of Day

Magnitude of diuresis during head-out immersion is greater during the day than at night. The mechanisms are not fully defined. A study by Miki and colleagues[100] indicated that circadian variation in atrial natriuretic factor (ANF) response to immersion could not account fully for nocturnal inhibition of the renal response to head-out immersion. Circadian variation in renal response to immersion is probably a minor factor in aquatic rehabilitation.

Fluid Density

Salt water, denser than fresh water, slightly increases buoyancy and the diuretic effect of fluid shifting.[99] Density, like time of day, is a minor determinant of the magnitude of renal response to immersion.

Hydration

The diuretic response to head-out immersion in hydrated subjects is greater than that in dehydrated subjects.[101,102] The main diuresis-inducing factor during water immersion in dehydrated subjects may be suppression of antidiuretic hormone (ADH), not increased ANF.[103]

Age

Aging increases secretion of ANF in response to immersion.[96] Work by Tajima and associates[104] found that plasma ANF and diuretic response to head-out immersion is greater in elderly[11,12,26,94,103,105–112] than younger[2,15,22,71,82,83,88,99] experimental subjects, and plasma aldosterone, vasodilative reaction to ANF, and ADH were attenuated, although there was the same central blood shift.

Emotion

Fear, apprehension, or other emotional stress from difficult or unknown conditions during immersion increases diuresis.[102]

Exercise

Exercise in the cold reduces diuresis.[102]

Mechanisms of Immersion Diuresis

- **Buoyancy.** Central hemodynamic shifts due to buoyancy during immersion, increasing output. A major factor in diuresis.

- **Negative-pressure breathing.** This increases output. A minor contribution.
- **Temperature.** Colder temperature increases output. A major factor.
- **Time of day.** Diuresis is higher during the day than at night. A minor factor.
- **Fluid density.** Higher density of salt water than fresh water slightly increases buoyancy and the diuretic effect of fluid shifting. A minuscule factor.
- **Hydration.** Dehydration increases conservation and decreases output.
- **Age.** More and faster diuresis in older compared with younger subjects, even with the same headward blood shift.
- **Emotion.** Emotional stress from difficult or unknown conditions increases output.
- **Exercise.** Exercise in the cold reduced output.

Anatomy and Physiology

Immersion shifts blood centrally. Central blood volume overload suppresses ADH and the renin–angiotensin–aldosterone system, and stimulates ANF.

Antidiuretic Hormone

Antidiuretic hormone (vasopressin) suppression acutely increases diuresis. It is a major regulator of fluid output volume.[113] ADH is a cyclic peptide hormone with a large ring structure. ADH is produced in the hypothalamus and secreted by the posterior lobe of the pituitary gland. In contrast to ANF secretion, arterial baroreceptors rather than cardiopulmonary mechanoreceptors are the major receptors in ADH regulation.[114]

Antidiuretic hormone is released into the bloodstream with decreases in plasma osmotic pressure and extracellular fluid volume. ADH normally works to produce vasoconstriction, raise blood pressure, and concentrate and decrease fluid output, inhibiting diuresis.[113] It does this by increasing permeability of the collecting ducts of the kidney, so that urine becomes more concentrated and smaller in volume.

Immersion increases central venous pressure.

A small negative correlation exists between central venous pressure and ADH.[89] In this manner, immersion suppresses ADH, increasing diuresis.

Atrial Natriuretic Factor

Of greater consequence than ADH to the renal effects of immersion is ANF. ANF is a propeptide; its major source is the atrial myocytes. Its second messenger is cyclic guanosine monophosphate. Because this peptide is secreted in the atria, and is a major factor in natriuresis, it is sometimes called atrial natriuretic peptide.

Several influences stimulate release of ANF, including sodium loading, increased blood pressure, exercise, and atrial distention or pressure secondary to acute central hypervolemia from immersion.[115,116] ANF contributes to diuresis,[117,118] natriuresis,[117–119] vasodilation,[116] and the suppression of aldosterone, ADH, and thirst,[96,105] and reduces plasma volume through extravascular shift.[96] It is uncertain if increased ANF contributes directly to these renal responses or works through other factors.[118]

Cardiac receptor activation is an important determinant of renal response to immersion.[120] However, cardiopulmonary mechanoreceptors by themselves may not constitute the sole afferent limb.[94] Arterial baroreceptors also contribute to the ANF response.[90]

Renin–Angiotensin–Aldosterone System

The renin–angiotensin–aldosterone system counterbalances and fine-tunes the ANF–ADH system in regulation of fluid balance.[121] Decreased renal blood flow from fluid loss, reduced blood pressure, or volume shifts triggers a cascade beginning with renin.

Renin is a kidney enzyme. It breaks off part of the 14-amino-acid (tetradecapeptide) molecule angiotensinogen, made in the liver, to make the decapeptide hormone angiotensin I. Angiotensin-converting enzyme removes two more amino acids from angiotensin I to make the octapeptide angiotensin II. Angiotensin II, a potent vasoconstrictor, acutely raises blood pressure. Angiotensin II also acts on the adrenal glands to cause them to synthesize and release aldosterone, which increases sodium retention, and so, water retention. These combined effects counterbalance low blood volume.

Plasma levels of angiotensin II change inversely with plasma ANF in several situations such as postural change on land, volume expansion, high altitude, and immersion.[105] Angiotensin II suppression secondary to immersion increases diuresis.

Circulating angiotensin also stimulates production of aldosterone, as does increased blood pressure, and sodium clearance from diuresis and natriuresis. Aldosterone is a steroid hormone secreted by the adrenal cortex and regulated by the kidney. Aldosterone regulates water, sodium ion, and potassium ion balance by increasing potassium ion excretion in place of sodium ions, so that the body retains more sodium ions and water.

Neurohormonal Factors

- **Antidiuretic hormone (ADH).** Immersion suppresses ADH secretion, increasing diuresis.
- **Atrial natriuretic factor (ANF).** Immersion shifts blood centrally, distending the atria, stimulating ANF release, and increasing diuresis.
- **Renin–angiotensin–aldosterone system.** Counterbalances the ANF–ADH system. Suppression during immersion increases diuresis.

Clinical Application

A major clinical application of immersion is to reduce edema.[109] Immersion-induced central volume expansion and subsequent diuresis mobilizes extravascular fluid, reducing fluid volume retained. Bed rest is often used to treat edema because of its fluid centralization effect from hydrostatic forces with head-down posture (discussed in the section on Cardiovascular Effects). Immersion reduces edema more rapidly than bed rest, with high safety and the additional benefits of active exercise. Immersion activities as an exercise modality for pregnancy offer several advantages over land-based exercise.[107]

Practical Lessons for the Practitioner

Because of the real physiologic effect of immersion to induce diuresis, participants should shower before entering the pool to take care of "clearance" ahead of time.

Summary

From the literature, it is clear that cardiovascular and renal responses to immersion are multidimensional responses that remain to be defined entirely. Immersion is not a single condition. Therefore, the cardiovascular and renal response have several underlying mechanisms.

The human cardiovascular response of bradycardia and limb vasoconstriction does not protect from hypoxia, as it does in marine mammals. Face or head immersion is sufficient stimulus to evoke bradycardia, and enhances bradycardia in combination with body immersion. Whether wetting with water, per se, is a factor in eliciting a maximal bradycardic effect is undetermined; it may be that cold, more than the wetting itself, is the important trigger. Bradycardic response to body and face immersion is temperature dependent, with colder temperatures potentiating the response.

Like heart rate, limb blood flow changes in response to the multiple influences of immersion. Peripheral vasoconstriction occurs in response to apnea and submersion. Vasoconstriction conserves heat during cold immersion, and may help to raise central venous pressure. Immersion in cold water ($>20°C$) increases peripheral vasoconstriction. Immersion in warm ($>34°C$) water increases peripheral blood flow.

As with cardiovascular response, the renal response is multifactorial in mechanism and effect. Fluid centralization from immersion suppresses ADH and increases ANF secretion to normalize volume by increasing diuresis. The renin–angiotensin–aldosterone system normally counterbalances the ANF–ADH system to restrict excess sodium and water loss. Immersion suppresses the renin–angiotensin–aldosterone system and ADH, and increases secretion of ANF. The combined effects increase diuresis, plasma volume loss, natriuresis, and kaliuresis.

Immersion has several components that shift blood and fluids centrally. Buoyancy from water pressure is a major contributor. Negative-pressure breathing is a small factor. Hydrostatic gradient does not squeeze blood upward, as is sometimes thought; rather, it negates venous pooling by matching venous blood pressure. Fluid shifts occur regardless of postural orientation underwater. Diuresis increases in cold water, and decreases with exercise. It is influenced to a large extent by state of hydration, and to a small extent by the time of day, density of the water, age, emotional state, and other factors.

Varying combinations of mechanical, neurohormonal, and environmental factors influence the magnitude and time course of hemodynamic control. Intricate feedback loops constitute a continually changing set of interlaced influences. On the other hand, sometimes it's no more than "When you gotta go, you gotta go."

REFERENCES

1. Bove AA. Cardiovascular response to the environment. *Undersea Hyperb Med.* 1979;1(8):1–7).
2. Craig AB, Medd WL. Man's response to breath-hold exercise in air and in water. *J Appl Physiol.* 1968;24:773–777.
3. Furedy JJ, Morrison JW, Heslegrave RJ, Arabian JM. Effects of water temperature on some noninvasively measured components of the human dive reflex: an experimental response-topography analysis. *Psychophysiology.* 1983;20:569–578.
4. Heistad DD, Wheeler RC. Simulated diving during hypoxia in man. *J Appl Physiol.* 1970;28:652–656.
5. Raper AJ, Richardson DW, Kontos HA, Patterson JL. Circulatory responses to breath holding in man. *J Appl Physiol.* 1967;22:201–206.
6. Pierce AL. The relationship between bradycardia from face submersion and breath holding ability in skin divers. Unpublished master's thesis. Philadelphia, Pa: Temple University, 1969.
7. Sterba JA, Lundgren CE. Diving bradycardia and breath-holding time in man. *Undersea Biomedical Research.* 1985;12(2):139–150.
8. Hayward JS, Hay C, Matthews BR, Overweel CH, Radford DD. Temperature effect on the human dive response in relation to cold water near-drowning. *J Appl Physiol.* 1984;56:202–206.
9. Granberg PO. Human physiology under cold exposure. *Arctic Med Res.* 1991;50(Suppl 6):23–27.
10. Wolf S. The bradycardia of the dive reflex: a possible mechanism of sudden death. *Trans Am Clin Climatol Assoc.* 1965;76:192–200.
11. Irving L. Bradycardia in human divers. *J Appl Physiol.* 1963;18:489–491.
12. Kawakami Y, Natelson BH, DuBois AB. Cardiovascular effects of face immersion and factors affecting diving reflex in man. *J Appl Physiol.* 1967;23:964–970.
13. Moore TO, Morlock JF, Lally DA, Hong SK. Thermal cost of saturation diving: respiratory and whole body heat loss at 16.1 ata. In: Lambertsen CJ, ed. *Proceedings of the Fifth Symposium on Underwater Physiology.* Bethesda, Md: Federation of American Societies for Experimental Biology; 1976:741–754.
14. Song SH, Lee WK, Chung YA, Hong SK. Mechanism of apneic bradycardia in man. *J Appl Physiol.* 1969;27:323–327.
15. Craig AB. Heart rate response to apneic underwater diving and to breath holding in man. *J Appl Physiol.* 1963;18:854–862.
16. Moore TO, Lin YC, Lally DA, Hong SK. Effects of temperature, immersion and ambient pressure on human apneic bradycardia. *J Appl Physiol.* 1972;33:36–41.
17. Parfrey P, Sheehan JD. Individual facial areas in the human circulatory response to immersion. *Ir J Med Sci.* 1975;144:335–342.
18. Paulev PE. Cardiac rhythm during breath holding and water immersion in man. *Acta Physiol Scand.* 1968;73:139–150.
19. Folgering H, Wijnheymer P, Geeraedts L. Diving bradycardia is not correlated to the oculocardiac reflex. *Int J Sports Med.* 1983;4:166–169.
20. Greene MA, Boltax AJ, Lustig GA, Rogow E. Circulatory dynamics during the cold pressor test. *Am J Cardiol.* 1965;16:54–62.
21. Thornton RH, Rohter FD, Michael ED. Circulatory adjustments to training for apneic diving. *Research Quarterly.* 1964;35:205–212.
22. Craig AB, Dvorak M. Thermal regulation during immersion. *J Appl Physiol.* 1966;21:1577–1585.
23. Tuttle WW, Corleaux JF. The response of the heart to water of swimming pool temperature. *Research Quarterly.* 1935;6:24–26.
24. Burch GE, Giles TD. A digital rheoplethysmographic study of the vasomotor response to "simulated diving" in man. *Cardiology.* 1970;55:257–271.
25. National Aeronautics and Space Administration. The cardiovascular/cardiopulmonary system: heart, lungs, and blood vessels. National Aeronautics and Space Administration, Spacelab Life Sciences 1 First Space Laboratory Dedicated to Life Sciences Research. Houston, Tex: Lyndon B. Johnson Space Center, 1989.
26. Irving L, Scholander PF, Grinnell SW. Significance of the heart rate to the ability of diving seals. *Journal of Cellular and Comparative Physiology.* 1941;18:283–297.
27. Campbell LB, Gooden BA, Lehman RG, Pym J. Simultaneous calf and forearm blood flow during immersion in man. *Australian Journal of Experimental Biology Medical Science.* 1969;47:747–754.
28. Gauer OH, Henry JP, Behn C. The regulation of extracellular blood volume. *Ann Rev Physiol.* 1970;32:547–595.
29. Wolf JP, Nguyen NU, Baulay A, Dumoulin G, Berthelay S. The role of posture on the changes in plasma atrial natriuretic factor and arginine vasopressin levels during immersion. *Eur J Appl Physiol.* 1990;61:284–288.
30. Bookspan J, Paolone AM. Posture apnea interaction during total body cold water immersion. *Undersea Biomedical Research.* 1991;18(Suppl):66. Abstract.
31. Bove AA, Lynch P, Connell J, Harding J. Diving reflex after physical training. *J Appl Physiol.* 1968;25:70–72.
32. Elsner RW, Franklin DL, Van Citters RL, Kenny DW. Cardiovascular defense against asphyxia. *Science.* 1966;153:941–949.
33. Folinsbee L. Cardiovascular response to apneic immersion in cool and warm water. *J Appl Physiol.* 1974;36:226–232.
34. Whayne TF, Killip T. Simulated diving in man: comparison of facial stimuli and response in arrhythmia. *J Appl Physiol.* 1967;22:800–807.
35. Whayne TF, Smith TY, Eger EI, Stoelting RK, Whitcher CE. Reflex cardiovascular responses to simulated diving. *Angiology.* 1972;23:500–508.
36. Blix AS, Krog J, Myhre HO. The effect of breathing

on the cardiovascular adjustments induced by face immersion in man. *Acta Physiol Scand*. 1971;82: 143–144.

37. Olsen C, Fanestil D, Scholander P. Some effects of breath holding and apneic underwater diving on cardiac rhythm in man. *J Appl Physiol*. 1962;17: 932–938.

38. Campbell LB, Gooden BA, Horowitz JD. Cardiovascular responses to partial and total immersion in man. *J Physiol*. 1969;202:239–245.

39. Stromme SB, Kerem D, Elsner R. Diving bradycardia during rest and exercise and its relation to physical fitness. *J Appl Physiol*. 1970;28:614–621.

40. Essandoh LK, Duprez DA, Shepherd JT. Postural cardiovascular reflexes: comparison of responses of forearm and calf resistance vessels. *J Appl Physiol*. 1987;63:1801–1805.

41. Menagesha YA, Bell GH. Forearm and finger blood flow responses to passive body tilts. *J Appl Physiol*. 1979;46:288–292.

42. Borst C, Weiling W, Van Brederode JFM, Hond A, De Rijk LG, Dunning AJ. Mechanisms of initial heart rate response to postural change. *Am J Physiol*. 1982;243:H676–H681.

43. Ward RJ, Danziger F, Bonica JJ, Allen GD, Tolas AG. Cardiovascular effects of change of posture. *Aerospace Medicine*. 1966;37:257–259.

44. Sapova NI. Rheographic indicators of blood circulation in the brain and limbs during active orthostatic test. *Kosmoloskaia Biologiia Aviakosmoloskaia Meditsina*. 1983;17:36–39.

45. Paterson NAM. The effects of increased vasomotor tone on reactive hyperemia in the human forearm. *Australian Journal of Experimental Biology Medical Science*. 1967;45:651–660.

46. Lind AR, Leithead CS, McNicol GW. Cardiovascular changes during syncope induced by tilting men in the heat. *J Appl Physiol*. 1968;25:268–276.

47. Landsberg PG. Bradycardia during human diving. *South Afr Med J*. 1975;49:626–630.

48. Brick I. Circulatory responses to immersing the face in water. *J Appl Physiol*. 1966;21:33–36.

49. Speck DF, Bruce DS. Effects of varying thermal and apneic conditions on the human dive reflex. *Undersea Biomedical Research*. 1978;5:9–14.

50. Andersen H. The reflex nature of physiologic adjustments to diving and their afferent pathway. *Acta Physiol Scand*. 1961;58:263–273.

51. Moore TO, Elsner R, Lin YC, Lally DA, Hong SK. Effects of alveolar PO_2 and PCO_2 on apneic bradycardia in man. *J Appl Physiol*. 1973;34:795–806.

52. Gandevia SC, McCloskey DI, Potter EK. Reflex bradycardia occurring in response to diving, nasopharyngeal stimulation and ocular pressure, and its modification by respiration and swallowing. *J Physiol (Lond)*. 1978;276:383–394.

53. Gooden BA. The diving response in clinical medicine. *Aviat Space Environ Med*. 1982;53:273–276.

54. Paulev PE. Respiratory and cardiovascular effects of breath holding. *Acta Physiol Scand*. 1969;76(Suppl 324):7–116.

55. Elsner RW, Gooden BA. Reduction of reactive hyperemia in the human forearm by face immersion. *J Appl Physiol*. 1970;29:627–630.

56. Heistad DD, Abboud FM, Eckstein JW. Vasoconstrictor response to simulated diving in man. *J Appl Physiol*. 1968;25:542–549.

57. Bolton B, Carmichael EA, Stürup G. Vasoconstriction following deep inspiration. *J Physiol*. 1936;86: 83–94.

58. Andersen H. Factors affecting the circulatory adjustments to diving. *Acta Physiol Scand*. 1963;58: 173–185.

59. Butler PJ, Woakes AJ. Heart rate in humans during underwater swimming with and without breathhold. *Respir Physiol*. 1987;69:387–399.

60. Scholander PF, Elsner RW. A comparative view of cardiovascular defense against acute asphyxia. *Acta Anaesthesiol Scand Suppl*. 1968;29:15–33.

61. Wolf S, Schneider RA, Groover ME. Further studies in the circulatory and metabolic alterations of the oxygen conserving (diving) reflex in man. *Trans Assoc Am Physicians*. 1965;78:242–254.

62. Scholander PF, Hammel HT, LeMessurier H, Hemmingsen E, Garey W. Circulatory adjustment in pearl divers. *J Appl Physiol*. 1962;17:154–190.

63. Tuttle WW, Templin JL. A study of normal cardiac response to water below body temperature with special reference to a submersion syndrome. *J Lab Clin Med*. 1942;28:271–276.

64. Bove AA, Pierce AL, Barrera F, Amsbaugh GA, Lynch PR. Diving bradycardia as a factor in underwater blackout. *Aerospace Medicine*. 1973;44: 245–248.

65. Strauss MB. Physiologic aspects of mammalian breath-hold diving: a review. *Aerospace Medicine*. 1970;41:12.

66. Shilling CW, Werts MF, Schandelmeier NR. *The Underwater Handbook: Guide to Physiology and Performance for the Engineer*. New York, NY: Plenum Press; 1976.

67. LeBlanc JB. *Man in the Cold*. Springfield, Ill: Charles C Thomas; 1975.

68. Sondeen JL, Hong SK, Claybaugh JR, Krasney JA. Effect of hydration state on renal responses to head-out water immersion in conscious dogs. *Undersea Biomedical Research*. 1990;17:395–411.

69. Hong SK, Song SH, Kim PK, Suh CS. Seasonal observations on the cardiac rhythm during diving in the Korean Ama. *J Appl Physiol*. 1967;23:18–22.

70. Lamb LE, Dermksian G, Sarnoff CA. Significant cardiac arrhythmias induced by common respiratory maneuvers. *Am J Cardiol*. 1958;2:563–574.

71. Denison DM, Kooyman GL. The structure and function of the small airways in pinniped and sea otter lungs. *Respir Physiol*. 1973;17:1–10

72. Strauss MB. *Marine Adaptations to Diving*. Report No. 562. Groton, Conn: U.S. Naval Submarine Medical Center Submarine Base; 1969.

73. Elsner RW. Cardiovascular adjustments to diving. *Fed Proc*. 1963;22:179–198.

74. Harding PE, Roman D, Wheelan RF. Diving bradycardia in man. *J Physiol (Lond)*. 1965;181:401–409.

75. Angelone A, Coulter NA. Heart rate response to held lung volume. *J Appl Physiol*. 1965;20:464–468.

76. Wayne MA. Conversion of paroxysmal atrial tachycardia by facial immersion in ice water. *JACEP*. 1976; 5:434–435.

77. Wildenthal K, Leshin SJ, Atkins JM, Skelton CL. The diving reflex used to treat paroxysmal atrial tachycardia. *Lancet*. 1975;1:12–14.

78. Mehta D, Wafa S, Ward DE, Camm AJ. Relative efficacy of various physical manoeuvres in the termina-

tion of junctional tachycardia. *Lancet.* 1988;1: 1181–1185.

79. Hamilton J, Moodie D, Levy J. The use of the diving reflex to terminate supraventricular tachycardia in a 2-week-old infant. *Am Heart J.* 1979;97:371–374.

80. Sperandeo V, Pieri D, Palazzolo P, Donzelli M, Spataro G. Supraventricular tachycardia in infants: use of the "diving reflex." *Am J Cardiol.* 1983;51: 286–287.

81. Arabian JM, Furedy JJ, Morrison J, Szalai JP. Treatment of PAT: bradycardiac reflexes induced by dive vs. body-tilt. *Pavlovian Journal of Biological Science.* 1983;18(2):88–93.

82. Claybaugh JR, Pendergast DR, Davis JE, Akiba C, Pazik M, Hong SK. Fluid conservation in athletes: responses to water intake, supine posture, and immersion. *J Appl Physiol.* 1986;61:7–15.

83. Deuster PA, Smith DJ, Smoak BL, Montgomery LC, Singh A, Doubt TJ. Prolonged whole-body cold water immersion: fluid and ion shifts. *J Appl Physiol.* 1989;66:34–41.

84. Harrison MH, Keil LC, Wade CA, Silver JE, Geelen G, Greenleaf JE. Effect of hydration on plasma volume and endocrine responses to water immersion. *J Appl Physiol.* 1986;61:1410–1417.

85. Rochelle RD, Horvath SM. Thermoregulation in surfers and nonsurfers immersed in cold water. *Undersea Biomedical Research.* 1978;5:377–390.

86. Fyhrquist F, Tikkanen I, Tötterman KJ, Hynynen M, Tikkanen T, Andersson S. Plasma atrial natriuretic peptide in health and disease. *Eur Heart J.* 1987; 8(Suppl B):117–122.

87. Young AJ, Muza SR, Sawka MN, Pandolf KB. Human vascular fluid responses to cold stress are not altered by cold acclimation. *Undersea Biomedical Research.* 1987;14:215–228.

88. Coruzzi P, Biggi A, Musiari L, Ravanetti C, Vescovi PP, Novarini A. Dopamine blockade and natriuresis during water immersion in normal man. *Clin Sci.* 1986;70:523–526.

89. Norsk P, Bonde-Petersen F, Warberg J. Central venous pressure and plasma arginine vasopressin in man during water immersion combined with changes in blood volume. *Eur J Appl Physiol.* 1986; 54:608–616.

90. Norsk P, Epstein M. Effects of water immersion on arginine vasopressin release in humans. *J Appl Physiol.* 1988;64:1–10.

91. O'Hare P, Bhoola K, Chapman I, Roland J, Corrall R. Importance of circulating and urinary tissue kallikrein in the control of acute natriuresis and diuresis evoked by water immersion in man. *Adv Exp Med Biol.* 1986;198(Pt B):225–232.

92. Trippodo NC, MacPhee AA, Cole FE. Partially purified human and rat atrial natriuretic factor. *Hypertension.* 1983;5(Suppl 1):81–88.

93. O'Hare JP, Dalton N, Roland JM, et al. Plasma catecholamine levels during water immersion in man. *Horm Metab Res.* 1986;18:713–716.

94. Kinney EL, Cortada X, Ventura R. Cardiac size and motion during water immersion: implications for volume homeostasis. *Am Heart J.* 1987;113(2 Pt 1): 345–349.

95. Epstein M, Norsk P, Loutzenhiser R, Sonke P. Detailed characterization of a tank used for head-out water immersion in humans. *J Appl Physiol.* 1987; 63:869–871.

96. Weidmann P, Saxenhofer H, Shaw SG, Ferrier C. Atrial natriuretic peptide in man. *J Steroid Biochem.* 1989;32:229–241.

97. Fenn WO, Otis AB, Rahn H, Chadwick LE, Hegnauer AH. Displacement of blood from the lungs by pressure breathing. *Am J Physiol.* 1947;151:258–269.

98. Hunt NC. Positive pressure breathing during water immersion *Aerospace Medicine.* 1967;38:176–180.

99. Edgecombe W, Bain W. An abstract of observations on the effect of baths, massage, and exercise on the blood pressure. *J Physiol (Lond).* 1952;24:48–50.

100. Miki K, Shiraki K, Sagawa S, de Bold AJ, Hong SK. Atrial natriuretic factor during head-out immersion at night. *Am J Physiol.* 1988;254(2 Pt 2):R235–R241.

101. Behn C, Gauer OH, Kirsch K, Eckert P. Effects of sustained intrathoracic vascular distention on body fluid distribution and renal excretion in man. *Pflugers Arch.* 1969;313:123–135.

102. Epstein M, Duncan DC, Fishman LM. Characterization of natriuresis caused in normal man by immersion in water. *Clin Sci.* 1972;43:275–287.

103. Kurosawa T, Sakamoto H, Katoh Y, Marumo F. Atrial natriuretic peptide is only a minor diuretic factor in dehydrated subjects immersed to the neck in water. *Eur J Appl Physiol.* 1988;57:10–14.

104. Tajima F, Sagawa S, Iwamoto J, Miki K, Claybaugh JR, Shiraki K. Renal and endocrine responses in the elderly during head-out water immersion. *Am J Physiol.* 1988;254(6 Pt 2):R977–R983.

105. Johnston CI, Hodsman PG, Kohzuki M, Casley DJ, Fabris B, Phillips PA. Interaction between atrial natriuretic peptide and the renin-angiotensin aldosterone system: endogenous antagonists. *Am J Med.* 1989;87(6B):24S–28S.

106. Katz VL, McMurray R, Berry MJ, Cefalo RC, Bowman C. Renal responses to immersion and exercise in pregnancy. *Am J Perinatol.* 1990;7:118–121.

107. Katz VL, McMurray R, Goodwin WE, Cefalo RC. Nonweightbearing exercise during pregnancy on land and during immersion: a comparative study. *Am J Perinatol.* 1990;7:281–284.

108. Katz VL, Rozas L, Ryder R, Cefalo RC. Effect of daily immersion on the edema of pregnancy. *Am J Perinatol.* 1992;9:225–227.

109. Katz VL, Ryder RM, Cefalo RC, Carmichael SC, Goolsby R. A comparison of bed rest and immersion for treating the edema of pregnancy. *Obstet Gynecol.* 1990;75:147–151.

110. Knight DR, Horvath SM. Immersion diuresis occurs independently of water temperatures in the range 25 degrees–35 degrees C. *Undersea Biomedical Research.* 1990;17:255–256. Letter. Comment on: *Undersea Biomedical Research.* 1989;16:427–437.

111. Kokot F, Grzeszczak W, Wiecek A. Water immersion induced alterations of atrial natriuretic peptide in patients with noninflammatory acute renal failure. *Mater Med Pol.* 1989;21:155–159.

112. Kokot F, Grzeszczak W, Wiecek A, Zukowska-Szczechowska E. Water immersion induced alterations of plasma atrial natriuretic peptide (ANP), diuresis and natriuresis in kidney transplant patients. *Mater Med Pol.* 1990;22:304–307.

113. Farrow S, Banta G, Schallhorn S, et al. Vasopressin inhibits diuresis induced by water immersion in humans. *J Appl Physiol.* 1992;73:932–936.

114. Norsk P, Bonde-Petersen F, Warberg J. Arginine vasopressin, circulation, and kidney during graded

water immersion in humans. *J Appl Physiol.* 1986; 61:565–574.

115. Ogihara T, Shima J, Hara H, et al. Significant increase in plasma immunoreactive atrial natriuretic polypeptide concentration during head-out water immersion. *Life Sci.* 1986;38:2413–2418.

116. Ruskoaho H, Lang RE, Toth M, Ganten D, Unger T. Release and regulation of atrial natriuretic peptide (ANP). *Eur Heart J.* 1987;8(Suppl B):99–109.

117. Leung WM, Logan AG, Campbell PJ, et al. Role of atrial natriuretic peptide and urinary cGMP in the natriuretic and diuretic response to central hypervolemia in normal human subjects. *Can J Physiol Pharmacol.* 1987;65:2076–2080.

118. Pendergast DR, de Bold AJ, Pazik M, Hong SK. Effect of head-out immersion on plasma atrial natriuretic factor in man. *Proc Soc Exp Biol Med.* 1987;184: 429–435.

119. Epstein M, Loutzenhiser R, Friedland E, Aceto RM, Camargo MJ, Atlas SA. Relationship of increased plasma atrial natriuretic factor and renal sodium handling during immersion-induced central hypervolemia in normal humans. *J Clin Invest.* 1987;79: 738–745.

120. Hajduczok G, Miki K, Hong SK, Claybaugh JR, Krasney JA. Role of cardiac nerves in response to head-out water immersion in conscious dogs. *Am J Physiol.* 1987;253(2 Pt 2):R242–R253.

121. Gerbes AL, Arendt RM, Gerzer R, et al. Role of atrial natriuretic factor, cyclic GMP and the renin-aldosterone system in acute volume regulation of healthy human subjects. *Eur J Clin Invest.* 1988;18:425–429.

CHAPTER

4

Physiologic Responses to Water Exercise

Kirk J. Cureton

The physiologic responses to exercise on land have been studied extensively, and are described in detail in textbooks of exercise physiology.[1-3] Water presents a unique medium in which to exercise, and some responses to exercise in the water are different from those on land. Considerable information is available on the physiologic responses and adaptations to swimming,[4,5] but less information is available on nonswimming exercise performed in water. The aim of this chapter is to summarize the physiologic responses to acute exercise and adaptations to chronic exercise training in water. Emphasis is placed on differences between exercise in water and on land and on nonswimming exercise, which is more likely to be used in rehabilitation and therapy.

Responses During Exercise

Aerobic Energy Metabolism

The aerobic and anaerobic mechanisms through which energy is supplied for physical activity are discussed in detail in exercise physiology textbooks.[1-3] During dynamic light and moderate exercise used in water exercise programs, most of the energy used to support physical activity is supplied through aerobic metabolism (oxidative phosphorylation). The rate of oxygen uptake ($\dot{V}o_2$) measured with respiratory spirometry is used to quantify the rate of aerobic metabolism. The maximal rate of aerobic metabolism possible during exercise is called the maximal oxygen uptake ($\dot{V}o_2$max). Because aerobic me-

tabolism depends on the processes of respiration and circulation, the $\dot{V}o_2$max is often used as a measure of overall cardiovascular–respiratory capacity or fitness.[6,7]

Another measure often used to express the rate of aerobic metabolism during exercise is the MET (metabolic equivalent of the resting metabolic rate). Energy expenditure during submaximal and maximal exercise expressed in METs refers to multiples of the resting metabolic rate. Intensity of exercise is often expressed in units of energy expenditure as $\dot{V}o_2$, as a percentage of the maximal rate of oxygen uptake (%$\dot{V}o_2$max), or in METs.

Because of the different physical properties of water, the factors that determine the energy cost of exercise in water are different from those for exercise on land. For weight-bearing exercise on land such as walking, jogging, bench stepping, and aerobic dance, the rate of energy expenditure is determined primarily by the intensity of exercise (movement speed and force development), body weight, and skill in performing the activity. In nonweight-bearing types of exercise, such as stationary cycling and rowing, body weight is much less of a factor. For the same movement pattern, energy expenditure in the water may be different than on land because (1) the buoyant force of water reduces the body weight in water and, therefore, reduces the energy required to lift the body against the force of gravity; and (2) the greater viscosity of water increases the energy required to overcome the resistance to movement through the water (drag). Thus, energy expenditure in water depends less on energy expended to move the body weight and more on energy expended to overcome drag compared with exercise on land. Resistance to movement through the water is related to body size, shape, and position and movement speed.[8] In addition, in cool water, greater energy may be required to maintain body temperature than at the same temperature on land because of the greater heat conductivity of water, which causes heat to be removed from the body more rapidly through conduction and convection.[9] A number of studies have directly compared the energy expenditure of nonswimming exercise in water with the same activity performed on land, and found that the energy expenditure may be greater, the same, or less, depending on the activity, water depth, and speed at which the activity is carried out.

Cycling

Several studies have measured $\dot{V}O_2$ during cycling in water on a modified ergometer. These studies have been useful because the work rate can be systematically varied and the extra energy expenditure associated with the increased viscosity of water quantified. During cycling with the legs or arms and legs, $\dot{V}O_2$ increases linearly as a function with work rate in water and on land.[10–12]. Costill[11] found that supine or prone head-out cycling on a modified ergometer at 50 revolutions/min in water 25°C required 33% to 42% more energy than cycling at the same work rate sitting upright or prone on land in air 24°C. The extra energy required was attributed to the added resistance of movement through water. Craig and Dvorak,[10] however, found no difference in the $\dot{V}O_2$ during cycling with the arms and legs at 30 revolutions/min at different submaximal work rates in water 30°C and 35°C than in air. In water 25°C, $\dot{V}O_2$ was higher than in air. The lack of a difference in $\dot{V}O_2$ due to movement of the limbs through a more viscous medium in warmer water was attributed to the slow pedal rate. Although cycling in water is unlikely to be used for rehabilitative or therapeutic exercise, these studies suggest that energy expenditure of nonweight-bearing exercise such as cycling in water is increased because of the increased viscosity of water if movements are rapid. The additional effect of water temperature evident in these studies is discussed later in the chapter.

Walking and Jogging

Water walking and jogging have become popular nonswimming aerobic activities. These activities have been used as part of rehabilitative, therapeutic, and general conditioning programs, and are thought to be particularly useful for people with lower extremity injuries. Because of the unpredictable offsetting metabolic effects of reduced body weight and increased resistance to movement in water, the rate of energy expenditure during walking and jogging in water has provoked interest.[13] In particular, there has been interest in determining whether the intensity is sufficient to improve cardiorespiratory function and physical work capacity.[14]

Evans and colleagues[15] studied the energy expenditure during walking at two speeds and during jogging at three speeds across a pool in waist-deep water (31°C). They found that $\dot{V}O_2$ increased nearly linearly with increasing speed. $\dot{V}O_2$ at all speeds was greater in water than during treadmill exercise on land. Approximately one half to one third of the speed (1.6 to 3.5 miles/h) was needed to walk or jog across a pool through waist-deep water at the same level of energy expenditure as during treadmill walking and jogging (3.4 to 8.3 miles/h) on land. At the highest speed, the $\dot{V}O_2$ was above 3.0 L/min, indicating that jogging in water can be very strenuous. This study showed that during walking and jogging across a pool in waist-deep water, resistance to movement has a bigger effect on energy expenditure than does reduced body weight.

Gleim and Nicholas[16] compared the energy expended during walking on a dry treadmill on land with walking at various speeds on an underwater treadmill at different water depths. They found that $\dot{V}O_2$ during water walking was increased in ankle- (25% to 55%), knee- (26% to 67%), thigh- (34% to 72%), and waist-deep (14% to 67%) water at moderate walking speeds (2 to 4.5 miles/h; Fig. 4-1). At these speeds, $\dot{V}O_2$ increased curvilinearly with speed for both dry and water walking. At speeds above 5 miles/h, $\dot{V}O_2$ during jogging in ankle-, knee-, and thigh-deep water was higher than jogging in air, but by a lesser amount than at lower speeds (20% to 24%, 35% to 37%, and 40% to 45%, respectively). In waist-deep water at speeds above 5 miles/h, there was no difference in the $\dot{V}O_2$ compared with jogging in air. These comprehensive data illustrate the complex opposing effects of buoyancy and water resistance on energy ex-

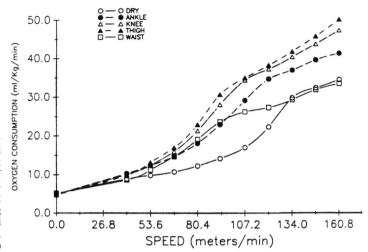

FIGURE 4-1. Oxygen consumption (uptake) during walking and jogging on a treadmill at different speeds in air (dry) and in water of different depths. (Gleim GW, Nicholas JA. Metabolic costs and heart rate responses to treadmill walking in water at different depths and temperatures. *Am J Sports Med.* 1989;17:248–252, with permission.)

penditure in the water. Apparently, in waist-deep water, the effect of buoyancy on energy expenditure offset the effect of water resistance so that energy expended in water and dry treadmill walking was the same. When compared with the data of Evans and colleagues,[15] these data suggest that the energy expenditure of jogging on a treadmill in waist-deep water is considerably less than that of jogging across a pool.

Several studies have evaluated metabolic, cardiovascular, and perceptual responses to deep-water running. Bishop and others[17] compared physiologic responses to deep water running with a buoyant vest with responses to running on a treadmill at the same perceived level of exertion. Subjects exercised at an intensity they preferred for a 45-minute training run. Ratings of perceived exertion (RPE) did not differ between the two exercise modes (RPE = 11 to 12). Average $\dot{V}O_2$ (1.97 vs. 2.68 L/min) and heart rate (122 vs. 157 beats/min) were significantly lower during the water running. The authors concluded that the metabolic cost for deep-water running with a buoyant vest at a preferred intensity of exertion is less than that for treadmill running.

Ritchie and Hopkins[18] compared the energy expenditure during deep-water running without a flotation device and treadmill running during 30-minute runs at a "hard" pace in trained male runners. The mean $\dot{V}O_2$ expressed relative to body weight was 49 mL/kg·min during the water running and 53 mL/kg·min during the treadmill run. The authors concluded that the intensity was sufficient to improve $\dot{V}O_2$max, and, there-

fore, that water running was an effective training technique.

Gehring and coworkers[19] compared the energy expenditure during deep-water running with and without a buoyant vest and treadmill running on land in competitive and noncompetitive female runners. A 20-minute bout of exercise at a self-selected pace, typical of a 45-minute training run, was performed under each condition. In the competitive runners, energy expenditure was the same under the three conditions. In the noncompetitive runners, energy expenditure during water running with and without a vest was lower than during treadmill running, and energy expenditure during water running with a vest was lower than without a vest. It is clear that energy expenditure at a given level of perceived effort is not the same during deep-water running and running on land.

Intensity of deep-water running increases directly with cadence.[20] Establishing the relation between cadence and energy expenditure or other related measures (heart rate, perceived exertion) provides a means for individually prescribing exercise intensity during water running.

Bench Stepping

Traditional bench stepping in water 42 inches deep requires less energy (17% to 20%) than bench stepping on land.[21] Heart rate and ratings of perceived exertion are also lower. These data show that the effect of buoyancy on energy expenditure is more important when exercise involves considerable movement against gravity and limited movement of the limbs through the water.

Calisthenics

Several other studies have reported rates of energy expenditure for different types of aerobic exercise or calisthenics performed in the water. Kirby and associates[22] studied the energy expenditure of pool walking and running in chest-deep water, horizontal abduction and adduction with paddles in chin-deep water, and pool running in place using the arms in shoulder-deep water. Water temperature was 36°C. They found these activities required approximately 2, 6, 4.5, and 7 METs, respectively.

Johnson and colleagues[23] studied the energy expenditure of four men and four women performing arm (shoulder abduction–adduction and flexion–extension) and leg (flexion–extension) exercises standing in water and on land. $\dot{V}O_2$ expressed relative to body weight was greater during the arm and leg exercise performed in the water than on land. During leg exercise, energy expenditure was 7 to 10 METs in the water, compared with 6 to 8 METs on land. During arm exercise, energy expenditure was 3 to 4 METs in water, compared with 2.5 to 3 METs on land. The authors concluded that water exercises should be particularly useful in therapeutic, rehabilitative, and recreational conditioning programs in which exercises of moderate intensity are desired.

Cassaday and Nielsen[24] compared the energy expenditure for arm and leg calisthenics performed in the water and on land at three cadences. Energy expenditure for bilateral shoulder abduction–adduction movements and hip flexion–extension movements were higher in water than on land. Values for upper extremity exercise ranged from 3 to 6 METs in water and 2 to 3.5 METs on land, whereas values for the lower extremity exercise ranged from 4 to 9 METs in water and 4 to 6.5 METs on land. Energy expenditure increased linearly with cadence for both land and water exercise. The authors concluded that the exercises performed in water would be of sufficient intensity to elicit aerobic training adaptations in cardiac patients.

Vickery and colleagues[25] studied the 20-minute low-gear, 30-minute middle-gear, and 60-minute high-gear aqua dynamics water exercise programs promoted by the President's Council on Physical Fitness and Sports. The programs consisted of exercises performed in water and

lap swimming. The average $\dot{V}O_2$ was 1.2 to 1.3 L/min or 51% to 57% of $\dot{V}O_2$max. The results suggested that aqua dynamics had sufficient intensity to improve the physical work capacity of sedentary people with low physical work capacity.

Swimming

Energy expenditure during swimming has been extensively studied.[5,26] $\dot{V}O_2$ increases linearly as a function of speed, despite the fact that resistance to movement through the water (drag) increases as the square of speed.[8] There are dramatic differences in energy cost, depending on the stroke used and the skill level of the swimmer. These differences make it difficult to predict accurately the energy cost of swimming, and tabled values[2] must be considered only rough approximations. In general, the energy cost of swimming a given distance is about four times the cost of running the same distance.[2]

The absolute $\dot{V}O_2$ required to swim at a given speed or to swim a given distance is lower in women than in men.[5,27–32] This difference has been attributed to smaller body size, which reduces body drag and the energy required to move the body through the water; lower body density, which increases buoyancy and decreases the energy required to keep the body on the surface; and less torque about the center of the body volume (buoyancy), which reduces the energy needed to maintain a horizontal position.[5] Most of the reported gender difference appears to be related to body size and swimming skill, because in equally trained male and female competitive swimmers, there is no difference when $\dot{V}O_2$ is expressed relative to body weight.[5,29,30,32,33]

Effect of Water Temperature

Oxygen uptake during exercise in water may be increased in cold water because of the added effect of shivering. The magnitude of the effect is a function of the degree of fatness of the subjects, exercise intensity and duration, and water temperature. At rest, shivering occurs when water temperature is below approximately 28 °C to 34°C, depending on the duration of the immersion and the degree of body fatness.[34] During light to moderately heavy submaximal exercise, $\dot{V}O_2$ is increased when water temperature is below approximately 26°C,[35–38] with the increase in $\dot{V}O_2$ proportional to the fall in body

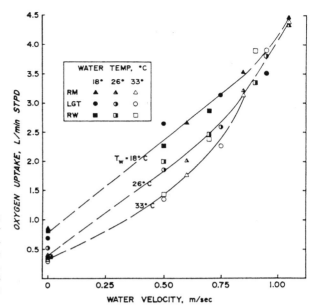

FIGURE 4-2. Oxygen uptake of three subjects during swimming at different velocities in water of different temperatures. Oxygen uptake during submaximal swimming is elevated because of shivering in cool and cold water. (Nadel ER, Holmer I, Bergh U, et al. Energy exchanges of swimming man. *J Appl Physiol*. 1974;36: 465–471, with permission.)

core temperature below 37°C. The effect can be large, with the difference between swimming in cold (18°C) and warm (33°C) water being over 0.5 L/min (Fig. 4-2).

Maximal Oxygen Uptake

Maximal oxygen uptake is not altered by water immersion per se, because under thermoneutral conditions it is similar during upright head-out cycling in the water and cycling on land.[39,40] This means that the higher preload (end-diastolic volume) and stroke volume observed during submaximal exercise in water either do not extend to maximal exercise, or that they are compensated for by lower arteriovenous difference.

Maximal oxygen uptake is lower during most other forms of water exercise than during exercise on land. Compared with $\dot{V}O_2$max measured during treadmill running on land, $\dot{V}O_2$max is lower during shallow-water (90%) and deep-water running with and without a buoyant vest (74% to 87%) in trained runners.[41–43] Maximal heart rate and blood lactate are also lower during maximal water running, suggesting the work rate achieved at exhaustion is less in the water. The lower maximal responses suggest that exercise prescriptions for water running should not be based on maximal heart rates or oxygen uptakes measured on land.

Maximal oxygen uptake and work capacity are reduced up to 5% during cycling[44–46] and swimming[37,38] by cold water that reduces body core temperature. This reduction is associated with a reduction in maximal heart rate. Maximal arteriovenous oxygen content difference may also be reduced because of a shift to the left in the oxygen–hemoglobin dissociation curve with a decrease in blood temperature,[44] but this has not been measured.

Maximal oxygen uptake is lower during swimming than during treadmill running by approximately 15% in untrained recreational swimmers,[47–50] but less or no different in highly trained competitive swimmers.[51,52] Reduced maximal heart rate accounts for much of the $\dot{V}O_2$max difference, when observed. A number of factors, including body position, face immersion, thermal stress, muscle mass activated, and state of training of the muscles involved, could contribute to this difference.

Two tests for predicting $\dot{V}O_2$max from water exercise performance have been proposed. Conley and others[47,48] presented regression equations for predicting swimming and running $\dot{V}O_2$max from 12-minute swim performance in recreational male and female swimmers. The accuracy of these equations is poorer than that provided by prediction of $\dot{V}O_2$max from 12-minute run performance, but similar to the accuracy of many other field tests for predicting $\dot{V}O_2$max. Kaminsky and coworkers[53] showed that the distance run on a 500-yard shallow-water run test also provides a reasonably accurate estimate of $\dot{V}O_2max$ determined on the treadmill in young men and women.

Anaerobic Energy Metabolism

Anaerobic metabolism in active skeletal muscles occurs when the demand for energy exceeds the rate of supply through aerobic metabolism. This usually occurs at the onset of exercise and throughout higher-intensity bouts of exercise. The metabolic end-product of anaerobic glycolysis is lactic acid (lactate), and accumulation of lactic acid in the blood is often used as an indicator of the amount of anaerobic metabolism that has occurred during exercise. Lactic acid dissociates into lactate and hydrogen ions, with the hydrogen ions increasing the acidity of the muscle cells and blood, causing hyperventilation and, at high levels, fatigue.[54,55] During exercise on land, little lactic acid accumulates in the blood up to intensities corresponding to approximately 50% $\dot{V}O_2max$ in sedentary people and 70% $\dot{V}O_2max$ in endurance-trained people. The intensity at which lactic acid begins to accumulate in the blood is called the lactate threshold. At intensities above the lactate threshold, lactate accumulates exponentially as a function of increasing intensity.[54]

Blood lactate accumulations at submaximal intensities between approximately 40% and 80% $\dot{V}O_2max$ are not different during cycling in water and on land[56] (see Fig. 4-7). However, at maximal exercise, blood lactate is lower in the water. The pattern of accumulation for plasma epinephrine parallels that of lactate. Epinephrine is known to stimulate glycogenolysis, and it is possible that reduced blood epinephrine results in less glycogen breakdown and glycolysis during maximal cycling in water.

Several studies have compared accumulation of lactic acid in the blood during deep-water running and treadmill running. In one study,[42] trained male runners completed 4 minutes of deep-water running and treadmill running at four submaximal intensities that elicited the same range of $\dot{V}O_2$ values. At different $\dot{V}O_2$ values and different percentages of $\dot{V}O_2max$, blood lactate accumulation was considerably greater during water running than during treadmill running on land. For example, at a $\dot{V}O_2$ of 3.0 L/min, blood lactate concentrations were 5.0 and 1.3 mmol/L, and at 70% $\dot{V}O_2max$, 4.6 and 1.5

mmol/L (see Fig. 4-6). The authors speculated that the higher lactate concentrations in the water may have been caused by reduced muscle blood flow, altered muscle fiber activation pattern, greater involvement of the arms, or a lower state of training for water than land running. Blood lactate after maximal exercise was lower in the water than on land (10.0 vs. 12.4 mmol/L). Town and Bradley[57] also observed that blood lactate after maximal shallow-water or deep-water running in trained runners averaged only 81% of that after maximal treadmill running on land. This may be because less muscle is recruited and a lower rate of work performed as a result of the lack of weight bearing, as reflected by the lower $\dot{V}O_2max$ in both studies.

Frangolias and colleagues[58] compared blood lactate responses during 42 minutes of deep-water running and treadmill running at an intensity equal to the ventilatory threshold. For the first 14 minutes of exercise, blood lactate responses were the same. Between minutes 21 and 42, blood lactate decreased more during exercise in the water (25%) than on land (12%). The greater change during exercise in the water indicates that lactate entry into the blood was less or its rate of removal was greater during the latter stages of the water runs than treadmill runs. Blood lactate accumulation appears to be similar in swimming and running.[37]

Circulation

The effects of immersion in water on the cardiovascular responses at rest and to cycling at submaximal and maximal intensities have been studied extensively with a variety of sophisticated methods. These studies clearly indicate that the cardiovascular response to exercise in water is different than on land. During upright, head-out immersion in water, there is a shift in blood volume from the lower limbs and abdomen to the thorax.[59] This translocation of blood increases central venous pressure, left ventricular end-diastolic volume, stroke volume, and cardiac output, and decreases systemic vascular resistance at rest and during submaximal exercise.[39,40,60,61] Systolic and diastolic blood pressures are unchanged or slightly higher. Contractility as measured by ejection fraction is unchanged. Heart rate tends to be unchanged at rest and at lower intensities of exercise, but is decreased at higher intensities of submaximal exercise and at maximal exercise compared with

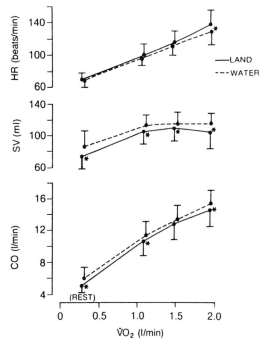

FIGURE 4-3. Relation of heart rate (HR), stroke volume (SV), and cardiac output (CO) to oxygen uptake ($\dot{V}O_2$) during cycling of progressively increasing intensity on land and immersed to the neck in water. (Sheldahl LM, Tristani FE, Clifford PS, et al. Effect of head-out water immersion on cardiorespiratory response to dynamic exercise. *J Am Coll Cardiol.* 1987;10:1254–1258, with permission.)

exercise on land (Fig. 4-3). The changes in exercise responses due to water immersion are larger than those due to changing from upright to supine posture.[40]

Stroke volume and cardiac output are increased by increased preload through the Frank-Starling mechanism. The fact that the left ventricular end-diastolic volume and stroke volume are larger during upright exercise in water than during exercise on land in the supine posture indicates the heart is not functioning at its maximal volume in the supine posture on land, as sometimes hypothesized. Thus, the preload reserve does not appear to be fully used during upright exercise on land.

The stroke volume and cardiac output during submaximal swimming are not greater than during running at the same $\dot{V}O_2$.[49] This is surprising, because the supine posture and water immersion increase venous return and end-diastolic filling, and it would be expected that stroke volume would be higher during swimming than during upright exercise on land. Use of the arms

or perhaps a smaller active muscle mass in swimming may explain the unexpected response.

The relation of heart rate to $\dot{V}O_2$ during exercise in water compared to exercise on land is of particular importance, because heart rate is commonly used to prescribe and regulate the metabolic intensity of exercise. It is a common observation that heart rate is sometimes, but not always, lower during exercise in the water compared with exercise at the same $\dot{V}O_2$ on land. The response is, in part, dependent on the water temperature. During light and moderate upright head-out exercise such as cycling or walking/jogging in water of thermoneutral temperature (~31°C to 33°C), heart rate is not different from that during the same exercise performed on land at the same $\dot{V}O_2$,[10,12,15,39,40,56,61] but during moderately heavy, strenuous, and maximal exercise, heart rate is usually,[39,40,56,61,62] but not always,[12,15] lower by approximately 10 beats/min. Exercise in water colder than approximately 30°C reduces the heart rate at all intensities[10,12,36,63] (Fig. 4-4). Data for swimming are similar.[37,38,64]

The reason for the lower heart rate during higher-intensity exercise in water of thermoneutral temperature is uncertain. It seems reasonable that it is linked to reduced sympathetic nervous activity to the heart, which is responsible for the increase in heart rate during higher intensities of exercise.[65] Reduced sympathetic nervous system activity could be caused by reduced neural stimuli from higher brain centers, the active muscles, or baroreceptors.[66,67] Connelly and associates[68] found plasma norepinephrine at 80% and 100% $\dot{V}O_2$max and plasma epinephrine at 100% $\dot{V}O_2$max were reduced during cycling in water compared with the same activity performed on land, supporting this hypothesis (see Fig. 4-7). The reason for lower plasma catecholamine concentrations only at the higher work intensities is unknown. It would be expected that the increase in central blood volume and stroke volume would stimulate baroreceptor activity and thereby lower sympathetic nervous system activity. However, systolic blood pressure is not different during exercise in the water compared with land, and the role of the cardiopulmonary baroreceptors on sympathetic nervous system activation in unknown. Sympathetic activity could be reduced if muscle blood flow and oxygen delivery were increased in proportion to the increased cardiac output, thereby

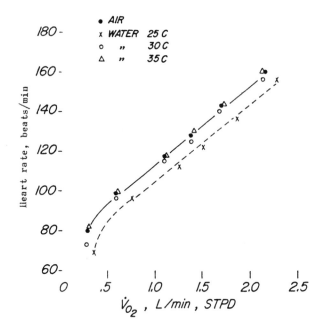

FIGURE 4-4. Relation of heart rate to oxygen uptake ($\dot{V}O_2$) during arm and leg cycling on an ergometer in air and in water at different temperatures. Heart rate at rest and during submaximal exercise is reduced in cool water. (Craig AB, Dvorak M. Comparison of exercise in air and in water of different temperatures. *Med Sci Sports.* 1969;1:124–130, with permission.)

reducing metabolic activation of chemoreceptors in the active muscles.

With decreasing water temperature, heart rate decreases and stroke volume increases during exercise.[12] It is likely that in cool or cold water, a peripheral vasoconstriction increases total peripheral resistance and augments central blood volume, which increases stroke volume and provides a strong stimulus mediated through the baroreceptors to slow the heart rate reflexly. Lower heart rates during swimming than during treadmill work on land could also be affected by posture, a difference in the muscle mass activated, and the reflex bradycardia elicited by face immersion.[69]

Water depth also affects heart rate during upright shallow-water exercise, because it affects the energy requirement of exercise and the extent of increase in the central blood volume. During water aerobics, heart rate is 8 to 11 beats/min lower in chest-deep water than in waist-deep water.[70]

It is clear that the relation of heart rate to $\dot{V}O_2$ during exercise in the water compared with that on land is variable and depends on the exercise intensity, exercise mode and muscle mass activated, and water and temperature. Therefore, caution must be exercised in using heart rate to prescribe and regulate exercise intensity during water exercise. In particular, the use of a measured maximal heart rate derived from a treadmill-graded exercise test on land to prescribe

exercise intensity for swimming or for any form of exercise in cool or cold water will result in a prescription that is too high.[71,72]

Ventilation

The hydrostatic pressure of water immersion causes inward movement of the rib cage, upward movement of the diaphragm, and a shift of blood into the thorax from the limbs and abdomen that reduces lung volumes; vital capacity and total lung capacity are reduced about 5% to 10%, and functional residual capacity is reduced approximately 1 L (60% to 70%). The reduced lung volume causes increased resistance to air flow.[73–75] Despite these changes, resting ventilation, tidal volume, and respiratory rate are unaltered.[10,61] During submaximal cycling,[10,12,61] leg extension exercise,[63] jogging in deep water with a buoyant vest,[42] and swimming,[49,64] ventilation is the same as in exercise on land at the same $\dot{V}O_2$ (Fig. 4-5). Different water temperatures between 18°C and 33°C have little effect.[10,12,35,63] During maximal exercise in water compared with on land, ventilation is the same in cycling,[40] but tends to be reduced in other forms of exercise in proportion to the reduction in $\dot{V}O_2$max.[42,64,76] In trained swimmers in whom $\dot{V}O_2$max is the same during swimming and running, maximal ventilation is still reduced during swimming.[51] Although during swimming the

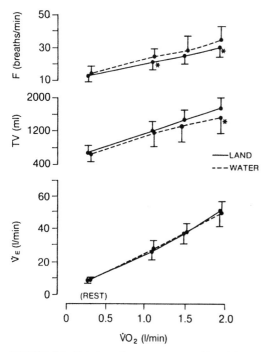

FIGURE 4-5. Relation of respiratory rate (F), tidal volume (TV), and ventilation (V̇E) to oxygen uptake (V̇O₂) during cycling of progressively increasing intensities on land and immersed to the neck in water. (Sheldahl LM, Tristani FE, Clifford PS, et al. Effect of head-out water immersion on cardiorespiratory response to dynamic exercise. *J Am Coll Cardiol.* 1987;10:1254–1258, with permission.)

maximal ventilation is less than during treadmill running, blood gases and the percentage saturation of hemoglobin with oxygen are similar.[49] Therefore, in spite of the effect of hydrostatic pressure on lung volumes and the restriction in breathing that may occur with swimming, ventilation during exercise in the water is similar to that during exercise on land.

Thermoregulation

The regulation of body temperature during exercise in water is different than in air because evaporation of sweat, the primary means of heat dissipation during exercise in air, does not occur in water, and because heat loss or gain through convection and conduction is much greater in the water.[9] Heat exchange through conduction and convection is greater because the heat conductance and specific heat of water are about 25 and 1000 times greater, respectively, than those of air. Thus, when water temperature is

above skin temperature, heat gain is greater in the water, whereas when water temperature is less than skin temperature, heat loss occurs more readily.

During exercise in air, core body temperature increases in direct proportion to the relative intensity of exercise (%V̇O₂max), but is independent of environmental temperature between approximately 5°C and 30°C to 35°C.[77] During exercise in water, the effect of exercise intensity on core temperature is the same, but there is a much narrower range of environmental temperatures for which core temperature is not affected by environmental temperature. Depending on water temperature, core body temperature may rise, remain the same, or decrease (Fig. 4-6). During exercise, the water temperature needed to prevent a rise in core temperature during prolonged exercise varies from 34°C to 17°C, depending on the intensity of exercise and the person's amount of body fat.[35,36]

Costill and coworkers[35] measured body skin and rectal temperatures during 20-minute strenuous swims that required a V̇O₂ of approximately 3.0 L/min in water 17°C, 27°C, and 33°C. With immersion, skin temperatures rapidly changed to within 2°C of water temperature. Mean rectal temperatures increased in direct proportion to water temperature (0.2°C to 0.6°C). In four subjects, the rectal temperature at the end of the swim in 17°C water was the same as at the beginning of the swim, indicating heat dissipation had occurred at a very high rate.

Nadel and colleagues[38] measured skin and esophageal temperatures in men who swam 20 minutes of breast stroke in a flume at two speeds and three water temperatures (18°C, 26°C, and 34°C). Core temperature changes were related to water temperature, swim speed, and body fatness. After 20 minutes of swimming at the slow speed (0.5 m/sec), esophageal temperatures decreased in water 18°C and 26°C and increased at 34°C. The decrease in core temperature at the two lower temperatures was inversely related to body fatness. At the faster speed, core temperature increased at 26°C and 34°C in all subjects, increased at 18°C in the fatter subject, but decreased at 18°C in the two leaner subjects. V̇O₂ was elevated during swimming at 18°C and 26°C because of shivering.

Sheldahl and associates[78] found that obese women who cycled at 40% V̇O₂max had no change in rectal temperature during 90 minutes of cycling in water 20°C, 24°C, and 28°C. Lean women had a progressive fall in rectal tempera-

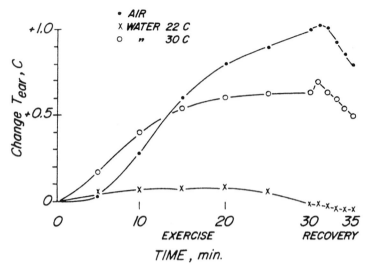

FIGURE 4-6. Change in core (tympanic membrane) temperature during 30 minutes of continuous arm and leg cycling and during recovery by a lean man in air and in water of different temperatures. (Craig AB, Dvorak M. Comparison of exercise in air and in water of different temperatures. *Med Sci Sports.* 1969; 1:124–130, with permission.)

ture at the two lower temperatures and no change at the highest temperature. In the lean women, energy expenditure was elevated at the two lower temperatures because of shivering.

Endocrine

Immersion to the neck in water of thermoneutral temperature (34°C to 35°C) causes several hormonal alterations that may affect metabolic, cardiovascular, and renal function. Plasma norepinephrine, renin, aldosterone, and antidiuretic hormone concentrations are suppressed; plasma atrial natriuretic peptide concentration is increased; and urinary excretion of sodium and urine flow are increased.[79–81] These changes are thought to be caused directly or indirectly by the baroreceptors through the shift in blood volume to the thorax; increased central venous pressure, venous return, and stretch of the atria; and increased stroke volume and pulse pressure.

These hormonal alterations appear to persist during exercise. Connelly and coworkers[56] found epinephrine and norepinephrine concentrations were lower during strenuous and maximal upright head-out cycling in water compared with cycling on land (Fig. 4-7). Decreased norepinephrine and epinephrine concentrations during exercise in water are thought to reflect, at least in part, decreased sympathetic nervous activity caused by reduced afferent input to the hypothalamus from cardiopulmonary and perhaps arterial baroreceptors. The lower sympa-

thetic nervous and catecholamine responses could have contributed to the lower heart rate and blood lactate responses observed. The sympathoadrenal and fluid-regulating hormone responses to water immersion exercise appear to be similar to those in exercise in the supine posture, in which there is also a redistribution of the blood volume to the thorax. Perrault and colleagues[82] observed that plasma atrial natriuretic peptide concentration was greater and epinephrine, norepinephrine, vasopressin, renin, and aldosterone concentrations were lower in supine compared with upright graded cycling. Although data comparing fluid-regulating hormones during exercise in water and on land are not available, it is likely that a similar pattern exists.

Adaptations to Training

Metabolism and Circulation

The different physiologic responses to acute exercise in water and on land could result in different degrees of adaptations to repeated bouts of exercise (training). For example, the larger left ventricular dimensions, stroke volume, and cardiac output at the same level of $\dot{V}O_2$ during upright head-out submaximal exercise in water provide a greater volume overload on the heart, which might lead to greater changes in $\dot{V}O_2$max and circulatory responses to submaximal exercise compared with exercise on land. Blood volume adaptations might also be different after

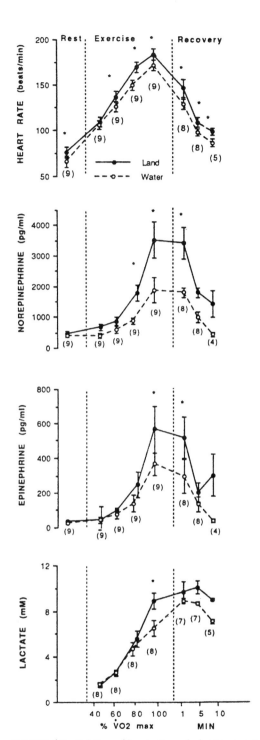

FIGURE 4-7. Relation of heart rate and plasma norepinephrine, epinephrine, and lactate to %$\dot{V}O_2$ max during cycling at progressively increasing intensities on land and immersed to the neck in water. (Connelly TP, Sheldahl LM, Tristani FE, et al. Effect of increased blood volume with water immersion on plasma catecholamines during exercise. *J Appl Physiol.* 1990;69:651–656, with permission.)

training in the water if the release of fluid-conserving hormones (vasopressin, renin, aldosterone, and antidiuretic hormone) is altered by the central shift in blood volume, as it is during supine exercise.[82] The different amounts of muscle recruited with altered patterns of movement might result in adaptations in the active muscle that are specific to a given mode of exercise performed in the water.

Water temperature may have independent effects on training adaptations. The physiologic responses to exercise in hot water differ from those in cold water; there is a greater rise in body core temperature, more muscle metabolite accumulation and disruption in intracellular homeostasis, higher stroke volume, and lower heart rate. Thus, the different volume overload on the heart, and stimuli for hypervolemic and cellular adaptations caused by training in hot water compared with cold water, might affect metabolic and cardiovascular adaptations to training. Finally, in cool water, the blunted rise in core body temperature and reduced skin blood flow could alter metabolic, thermoregulatory, and cardiovascular adaptations that may be responding, in part, to the thermal load. The method used for equating exercise intensity is important in research in this area, because the $\dot{V}O_2$max and the relation of heart rate to $\dot{V}O_2$ may be different in the water.

Several well-designed studies have directly compared the metabolic and cardiovascular adaptations to stationary cycling training on land and in water of different temperatures. Avellini and colleagues[83] compared the responses to cycling on land (22°C), cycling in water at a thermoneutral temperature (32°C), and cycling in water at a cold temperature (20°C). All groups trained 1 hour per day, 5 days per week at the same absolute and relative intensity (75% of land cycling $\dot{V}O_2$max), for 4 weeks (Fig. 4-8). During training, the heart rates of the two groups that trained in the water were considerably lower (160 and 150 beats/min) than in the group that trained on land (170 beats/min), but the absolute and relative $\dot{V}O_2$ (%$\dot{V}O_2$max) were the same. The increase in land-cycling $\dot{V}O_2$max was similar in the three groups (13% to 15%). It was concluded that the adaptation in $\dot{V}O_2$max to training in the water and on land at the same metabolic intensity was the same, even though the training heart rate differed by as much as 20 beats/min. Improvements in $\dot{V}O_2$max measured on the treadmill were less than improvements measured on the cycle ergometer, indicating the ad-

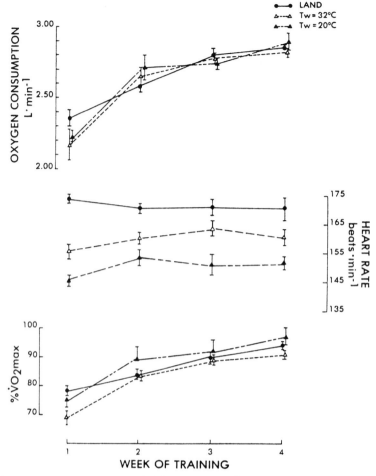

FIGURE 4-8. Oxygen consumption (uptake), heart rate and %$\dot{V}O_2$max during 4 weeks of cycling training on land and in water at two temperatures. Changes in $\dot{V}O_2$max after training were the same (13% to 16%) despite large differences in training heart rates. (Avellini BA, Shapiro V, Pandolf KB. Cardiorespiratory physical training in water and on land. *Eur J Appl Physiol.* 1983;50:255–263, with permission.)

aptations were, in part, specific to cycling exercise. Because the heart rates were different in the three groups, but the adaptation in $\dot{V}O_2$max was the same, the results imply that heart rate is a poor guide to the training stimulus provided by exercise.

Sheldahl and associates[84] compared metabolic and circulatory adaptations to upright cycling training in air and in water of thermoneutral temperature in middle-aged men. Training was 30 minutes, 3 days per week for 12 weeks at 60% to 80% of cycling $\dot{V}O_2$max. Increases in $\dot{V}O_2$max for the two training groups were similar (14% to 16%). Cardiovascular adaptations measured during submaximal exercise at 40%, 60%, and 80% of $\dot{V}O_2$max were also the same. Stroke volume increased; heart rate and systolic and diastolic blood pressure decreased; and cardiac output remained the same after training in both groups (Fig. 4-9). It was concluded that despite a greater stroke volume during training in the water, the adaptations in $\dot{V}O_2$max and in circulatory responses to submaximal exercise were the same as for men who trained on land.

Young and coworkers[85] studied the effect of training in hot (35°C) and cold (20°C) water on improvement in $\dot{V}O_2$max in young men. Subjects trained by cycling on a stationary ergometer in neck-deep water 60 minutes, 5 days per week for 8 weeks at the same absolute $\dot{V}O_2$ (~60% of cycling $\dot{V}O_2$max). During the training, the heart rate and core (rectal) temperature, respectively, of the group that trained in hot water averaged 27 beats/min and 1.5°C higher than the group

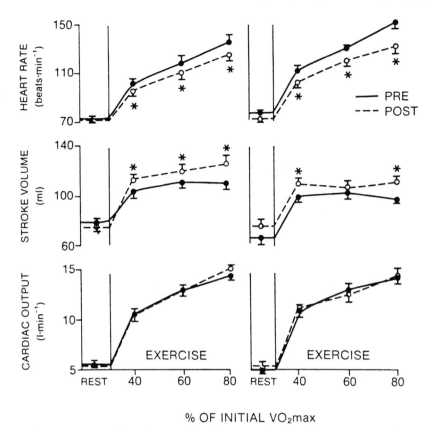

FIGURE 4-9. Heart rate, stroke volume, and cardiac output during cycling at progressively increasing intensities on land and immersed to the neck in water before and after 12 weeks of cycling training on land and in water. (Sheldahl LM, Tristani FE, Clifford PS, et al. Effect of head-out water immersion on response to exercise training. *J Appl Physiol.* 1986;60:1878–1881, with permission.)

that trained in cold water. $\dot{V}O_2$max increased 13% in both groups. Training increased muscle oxidative capacity to a similar degree in both groups, and blood volume did not change significantly in either group. The results of the study suggest that skin and body core temperature do not affect the metabolic and cardiovascular adaptation to training. The lack of a change in plasma and blood volume may have been because the release of vasopressin, renin, and aldosterone is suppressed during water exercise, as in supine exercise, because of the greater venous return and larger end-diastolic and stroke volumes. Because the heart rates of the two groups during training differed by more than 25 beats/min, results of the study reinforce the conclusion that training heart rates are a poor indicator of the metabolic adaptations to training.

A disadvantage of training in cool water is that it does not improve heat tolerance. Avellini and

colleagues[86] compared the effects of cycling training in 20°C and 32°C water and on land on heat tolerance in unconditioned and unacclimatized men. Training consisted of pedaling for 1 hour per day, 5 days per week for 1 month. Before and after training, subjects completed a heat stress test that involved walking for 3 hours at about 30% $\dot{V}O_2$max at 49°C, 20% relative humidity. Training in water at the two different temperatures and on land improved $\dot{V}O_2$max about 15%. Training on land and in 32°C water improved heat tolerance as measured by decreased core temperature, skin temperature, and heart rate during the heat tolerance test. Subjects who trained in 20°C water did not show improved heat tolerance, although heart rate was significantly lower. Training in water appears to enhance heat tolerance only if body core temperature is permitted to rise during exercise.

Swim training improves $\dot{V}O_2$max, but the intensity of training apparently determines whether the effects generalize to running. Magel and associates[87] investigated the effect of 10 weeks of interval swim training, 1 hour per day, 3 days per week on $\dot{V}O_2$max measured during tethered swimming and treadmill running in young men. $\dot{V}O_2$max increased significantly (11%) when measured during tethered swimming, but did not increase when measured during treadmill running. Although these data suggest that adaptations to swim training are specific to the muscles and movement patterns used in the exercise, other studies[88,89] indicate that adaptations to more intense swim training and other forms of aerobic exercise performed in water[90,91] do generalize. However, the findings indicate that when assessing the effects of low- or moderate-intensity water exercise programs, it may be important to employ tests that use the same muscles and movement patterns as those used in training.

Martin and coworkers[89] reported that strenuous swim training (30 to 45 minutes, 6 days per week for 12 weeks) and weight training on land increased $\dot{V}O_2$max by 15% when measured during upright cycling on land and by 10% when measured during supine cycling on land in sedentary middle-aged men and women. The improvement in $\dot{V}O_2$max during upright cycling resulted from equal increases in maximal cardiac output and maximal arteriovenous oxygen content difference, whereas the increase measured during supine cycling was caused by increased maximal cardiac output. Maximal stroke volume was increased 10% and 18% during the upright and supine tests, and left ventricular end-diastolic volume index was increased 18% on both tests. Indices of cardiac contractility (ejection fraction and end-systolic volume index) were unchanged by the swim training. These results suggest that metabolic and cardiovascular training adaptations resulting from chronic swimming generalize to upright and supine cycling exercise on land. How exercise posture affects adaptations to nonswimming water exercise training is unknown. Ray and Cureton[92] found a postural specificity to the effects of supine and upright cycling training on land on $\dot{V}O_2$max, which suggests that posture may play a role in adaptations to water exercise as well.

Lieber and colleagues[88] directly compared the effects of swim training and run training on $\dot{V}O_2$max measured during running in sedentary young and middle-aged men. The unique aspect of the study was that the groups trained at the same absolute intensity (heart rate equal to 75% of treadmill $\dot{V}O_2$max). This design feature is important because maximal heart rate and $\dot{V}O_2$max are lower when assessed during swimming than during running on the treadmill, which means the swimmers trained at a higher mode-specific relative exercise intensity (%$\dot{V}O_2$max) than runners. $\dot{V}O_2$max measured on the treadmill increased the same amount after run training (28%) and swim training (24%). The results suggest that there is no specificity of swim training when the absolute intensity of the training is held constant and when sufficient muscle mass is engaged in the training to cause central adaptations. These findings are important for interpreting the results of studies involving all forms of water exercise, because the intensity of training is often adjusted to compensate for differences in mode-specific $\dot{V}O_2$max.

Deep-water run training has been shown to be effective in increasing and maintaining $\dot{V}O_2$max and running performance. Untrained subjects who performed 16 to 36 minutes of deep-water interval-type running at 63% to 82% of maximal heart rate, 3 days per week for 8 weeks, increased treadmill and water-running $\dot{V}O_2$max 10.7% and 19.6%, respectively.[93,94] Eyestone and colleagues[95] found that 6 weeks of deep-water running, cycling on land, or running on land for 20 to 30 minutes, 3 to 5 days per week at 70% to 80% of maximal heart rate were equally effective in maintaining $\dot{V}O_2$max and 2-mile run time that had been developed with previous run training. Although these studies did not have control groups, they strongly suggest that deep-water running is an effective mode of training for increasing or maintaining $\dot{V}O_2$max and running performance.

Two studies have evaluated the effects of water calisthenics and aerobics. Minor and coworkers[90] compared the effects of water aerobics, walking on land, and range of motion exercises (control) on land in patients with rheumatoid arthritis or osteoarthritis. All groups met for 1 hour, 3 days per week for 12 weeks. Exercise sessions for the aerobic training groups included a warm-up, 30 minutes of continuous activity, and a cool-down. The water exercise group jogged in shallow and deep water and performed calisthenics in chest-deep water. During the period of continuous activity, heart rate was 60% to 80% of maximum heart rate. The water exercisers and walkers increased $\dot{V}O_2$max by 20% and 19%, respectively, whereas no change occurred in the control group.

Ruoti and colleagues[91] studied the effect of a water exercise program on muscular endurance, body composition, and aerobic work capacity in 12 elderly (59 to 75 years of age) men and women. Treadmill-walking $\dot{V}O_2$max, percentage of body fat estimated using hydrostatic weighing, resting heart rate, heart rate during water walking at a standard speed, and muscular endurance of the arms and shoulder muscles were measured before and after a 12-week water exercise program involving calisthenics and aerobic exercise. A 10-minute warm-up, 40 minutes of sustained exercise at approximately 80% of maximal heart rate, and a 10-minute cool-down were performed three times per week. $\dot{V}O_2$max increased 15%, resting heart rate decreased 7%, heart rate at a standard speed of walking in the pool decreased 20%, and muscular endurance of the arms increased 11% to 35%. Body fatness did not change significantly. It was concluded that nonswimming water exercise is an effective means to improve cardiorespiratory function and physical work capacity in the elderly.

Body Composition

In theory, water exercise should be an effective means of increasing energy expenditure to promote weight and fat reduction, particularly for the obese, because the risk of weight-bearing injuries and heat stress is less. However, several research studies have suggested that water exercise may not be effective in producing weight loss. Gwinup[96] compared the effects of swimming, stationary cycling, and walking 1 hour daily for at least 6 months, without dieting, on weight loss in overweight women. Women who walked or cycled lost 10% to 12% of their weight, whereas women who swam did not lose weight. Weight changes were paralleled by changes in triceps skinfold. There was no quantification of the work performed or body composition changes, and neither caloric intake nor components of energy expenditure were measured. Therefore, the reason for the differential weight loss was not explained. It was reasoned that the swimmers must have compensated for increased energy expenditure through increased caloric intake. He concluded that although swimming is an enjoyable form of exercise that promotes fitness, it does not produce body weight or fat loss.

In other studies, cycling in cold (20°C) water at 30% to 40% $\dot{V}O_2$max for 90 minutes, 5 days per week for 8 weeks by obese women,[78] and performing nonswimming water exercises for 40 minutes at 80% maximum heart rate, 3 days per week for 12 weeks by the elderly[91] also failed to reduce body weight or fat. In contrast, Lieber and associates[88] found that intense swim training at 75% of treadmill $\dot{V}O_2$max for 60 minutes, 3 days per week for 11.5 weeks significantly reduced body fat (-2.4%) in young sedentary men. The change was not significantly different from that (-1.8%) in a group who did a comparable amount of run training on land. A relatively large amount of strenuous water exercise may be needed to modify body composition.

Summary

Although most responses and adaptations to exercise in water are qualitatively similar to those resulting from exercise performed on land, important quantitative differences exist that may affect exercise prescription for water recreational, therapeutic, and rehabilitative activity programs. The buoyant force, greater viscosity, and increased heat conductivity of water compared to air usually alter aerobic energy expenditure during submaximal exercise in water so that it may be greater, the same, or less than during the same activity performed on land, depending on the activity, water depth, water temperature, and speed at which the activity is carried out. $\dot{V}O_2$max is often lower in many forms of water exercise than during uphill treadmill running on land because of lower maximal heart rate, and perhaps decreased active muscle mass and state of training of the muscles involved. Blood lactate accumulation during submaximal exercise in water may be less, the same, or greater than during comparable exercise on land at the same absolute or relative intensity. During maximal exercise, blood lactate accumulation is less during water exercise. The hydrostatic pressure of water immersion increases venous return to the heart and alters the cardiovascular response to exercise. During submaximal upright exercise, stroke volume and cardiac output are greater, and, at higher intensities, heart rate is lower than during exercise on land at the same $\dot{V}O_2$. The relation of heart rate to $\dot{V}O_2$ is variable and depends on the exercise intensity, exercise mode, and water depth and temperature. The heart rate for a certain $\dot{V}O_2$ is often lower during water exercise, so caution must be used in using heart rate to prescribe and regulate the intensity of water exercise. Although lung volumes are altered by the increased hydrostatic pressure of water, the ventilatory response to submaximal exercise is essentially the same as during exercise on land. Maximal ventilation may be reduced in proportion to the reduction in $\dot{V}O_2$max. Evaporation of sweat does not occur in water, and the higher heat conductivity and specific heat of water cause heat to be gained and lost more readily from the body through conduction and convection. Depending on water temperature, core body temperature may increase, stay the same, or decrease. Sympathoadrenal and fluid-regulating hormone responses are suppressed during upright exercise in the water because of redistribution of the blood volume to the thorax. Reduced sympathetic nervous system activity and blood epinephrine levels may account for the lower heart rate and blood lactate accumulation during strenuous submaximal and maximal exercise.

Despite a number of important differences between physiologic responses to exercise in the water and on land, metabolic, muscular, cardiovascular, and body composition adaptations to dynamic, submaximal exercise training are the same if training is performed at the same $\dot{V}O_2$. An exception is the blood volume adaptation to training, which appears to be absent after training in the water. Because of the decreased weight-bearing stress on the lower extremities and the increased resistance afforded by water, water exercise programs have clear advantages for therapeutic and rehabilitative conditioning programs.

REFERENCES

1. Astrand PO, Rodahl K. *Textbook of Work Physiology.* New York, NY: McGraw-Hill; 1986.
2. McArdle WD, Katch FI, Katch VL. *Exercise Physiology: Energy, Nutrition and Human Performance.* Philadelphia, Pa: Lea & Febiger; 1991.
3. Wilmore JH, Costill DL. *Physiology of Sport and Exercise.* Champaign, Ill: Human Kinetics; 1994.
4. Holmer I. Physiology of swimming man. *Exerc Sport Sci Rev.* 1979;7:87–123.
5. Lavoie JM, Montpetit RR. Applied physiology of swimming. *Sports Med.* 1986;3:165–189.
6. Mitchell JH, Sproule BJ, Chapman CB. The physiological meaning of the maximal oxygen intake test. *J Clin Invest.* 1958;37:538–547.
7. Taylor HL, Buskirk E, Henschel A. Maximal oxygen uptake as an objective measure of cardiorespiratory performance. *J Appl Physiol.* 1955;8:73–80.
8. Clarys JP. Human morphology and hydrodynamics. In: Terauds J, Bedingfield EW, eds. *Swimming III.* Baltimore, Md: University Park Press; 1979:3–41.
9. Nielsen B. Physiology of thermoregulation during swimming. In: Eriksson B, Furberg B, eds. *Swimming Medicine IV.* Baltimore, Md: University Park Press; 1978:297–304.
10. Craig AB, Dvorak M. Comparison of exercise in air and in water of different temperatures. *Med Sci Sports.* 1969;1:124–130.
11. Costill DL. Energy requirements during exercise in the water. *J Sports Med Phys Fitness.* 1971;11:87–92.
12. McArdle WD, Magel JR, Lesmes GR, et al. Metabolic and cardiovascular adjustment to work in air and water at 18, 25 and 33 degrees C. *J Appl Physiol.* 1976; 40:85–90.
13. Wilder RP, Brennan DK. Physiological responses to deep water running in athletes. *Sports Med.* 1993;16: 374–380.
14. American College of Sports Medicine. Position stand on the recommended quantity and quality of exercise for developing and maintaining cardiorespiratory and muscular fitness in adults. *Med Sci Sports Exerc.* 1990;22:265–274.
15. Evans BW, Cureton KJ, Purvis JW. Metabolic and circulatory responses to walking and jogging in water. *Res Q.* 1978;49:442–449.
16. Gleim GW, Nicholas JA. Metabolic costs and heart rate responses to treadmill walking in water at different depths and temperatures. *Am J Sports Med.* 1989; 17:248–252.
17. Bishop PA, Frazier S, Smith J, et al. Physiologic responses to treadmill and water running. *Physician Sportsmedicine* 1989;17:87–94.
18. Ritchie SE, Hopkins WG. The intensity of exercise in deep-water running. *Int J Sports Med.* 1991;12:27–29.
19. Gehring M, Keller B, Brehm B. Physiological responses to deep water running in competitive and non-competitive runners. *Med Sci Sports Exerc.* 1992; 24:S23.
20. Wilder RP, Brennan D, Schotte DE. A standard measure for exercise prescription for aqua running. *Am J Sports Med.* 1993;21:45–48.
21. Bufalino KD, Moore AF, Sloniger EL, et al. Physiological and perceptual responses to bench stepping in water and on land. *Med Sci Sports Exerc.* 1992;24: S183.
22. Kirby L, Sacamano JT, Balch DE, et al. Oxygen consumption during exercise in a heated pool. *Arch Phys Med Rehabil.* 1984;65:21–23.
23. Johnson BL, Stromme SB, Adamczyk JW, et al. Comparison of oxygen uptake and heart rate during exercises on land and in water. *Phys Ther.* 1977;57: 273–278.
24. Cassady SL, Nielsen DH. Cardiorespiratory responses of healthy subjects to calisthenics performed on land versus in water. *Phys Ther.* 1992;72:532–538.
25. Vickery SR, Cureton KJ, Langstaff JL. Heart rate and energy expenditure during aqua dynamics. *Physician Sportsmedicine* 1983;11:67–72.
26. Holmer I. Oxygen uptake during swimming in man. *J Appl Physiol.* 1972;33:502–509.
27. Costill DL, Kovaleski J, Porter D, et al. Energy expenditure during front crawl swimming: predicting success in middle-distance events. *Int J Sports Med.* 1985;6:266–270.
28. Pendergast DR, DiPrampero PE, Craig AB, et al.

Quantitative analysis of the front crawl in men and women. *J Appl Physiol.* 1977;43:475–479.

29. Montpetit R, Lavoie JM, Cazorla G. Energy expenditure during front crawl swimming: a comparison between males and females. In: Ungerechts BE, Wilke K, Reischle K, eds. *Swimming Science V.* Champaign, Ill: Human Kinetics; 1988:229–236.

30. Montpetit R, Lavoie JM, Cazorla G. Aerobic energy cost of the front crawl at high velocity in international class and adolescent swimmers. In: Hollander AP, Huijing PA, de Groot, eds. *Biomechanics and Medicine in Swimming.* Champaign, Ill: Human Kinetics; 1983:228–234.

31. Rennie DW, Pendergast DR, Di Prampero PE. Energetics of swimming man. In: Clarys JP, Lewillie L, eds. *Swimming II.* Baltimore, Md: University Park Press; 1991:97–104.

32. Van Handel PJ, Katz A, Morrow JR, et al. Aerobic economy and competitive performance of U.S. elite swimmers. In: Ungerechts BE, Wilke K, Reischle K, eds. *Swimming Science V.* Champaign, Ill: Human Kinetics; 1988:219–220.

33. Smith HK, Montpetit RR, Perrault H. The aerobic demand of backstroke swimming, and its relation to body size, stroke technique, and performance. *Eur J Appl Physiol.* 1988;58:182–188.

34. Craig AB, Dvorak M. Thermal regulation during water immersion. *J Appl Physiol.* 1966;21:1577–1585.

35. Costill DL, Cahill PJ, Eddy D. Metabolic responses to submaximal exercise in three water temperatures. *J Appl Physiol.* 1967;22:628–632.

36. Craig AB, Dvorak M. Thermal regulation of man exercising during water immersion. *J Appl Physiol.* 1968;25:28–35.

37. Holmer I, Bergh U. Metabolic and thermal response to swimming in water at varying temperatures. *J Appl Physiol.* 1974;37:702–705.

38. Nadel ER, Holmer I, Bergh U, et al. Energy exchanges of swimming man. *J Appl Physiol.* 1974;36:465–471.

39. Christie JL, Sheldahl LM, Tristani FE, et al. Cardiovascular regulation during head-out water immersion exercise. *J Appl Physiol.* 1990;69:657–654.

40. Sheldahl LM, Wann LS, Clifford PS, et al. Effect of central hypervolemia on cardiac performance during exercise. *J Appl Physiol.* 1984;57:1662–1667.

41. Butts NK, Tucker M, Smith R. Maximal responses to treadmill and deep water running in high school female cross country runners. *Res Q Exerc Sport.* 1991;62:236–239.

42. Svedenhag J, Seger J. Running on land and in water: comparative exercise physiology. *Med Sci Sports Exerc.* 1992;24:1155–1160.

43. Krahenbuhl GS, Pangrazi RP, Burkett LN, et al. Field estimation of VO2max in children eight years of age. *Med Sci Sports.* 1977;9:37–40.

44. Bergh U, Ekblom B. Physical performance and peak aerobic power at different body temperatures. *J Appl Physiol.* 1979;46:885–889.

45. Davies M, Ekblom B, Bergh U, et al. The effects of hypothermia on submaximal and maximal work performance. *Acta Physiol Scand.* 1975;95:201–202.

46. Pirnay F, Deroanne R, Petit JM. Influence of water temperature on thermal, circulatory and respiratory responses to muscular work. *Eur J Appl Physiol.* 1977;37:129–136.

47. Conley DS, Cureton KJ, Dengel DR, et al. Validation of the 12-minute swim as a field test of peak aerobic

power in young men. *Med Sci Sports Exerc.* 1991;23:766–773.

48. Conley DS, Cureton KJ, Hinson BT, et al. Validation of the 12-minute swim as a field test of peak aerobic power in young women. *Res Q Exerc Sport.* 1992;63:153–161.

49. Holmer I, Stein EM, Saltin B, et al. Hemodynamic and respiratory responses compared in swimming and running. *J Appl Physiol.* 1974;37:49–54.

50. McArdle WD, Magel JR, Delio DJ, et al. Specificity of run training on VO2max and heart rate changes during running and swimming. *Med Sci Sports.* 1978;10:16–20.

51. Magel JR, Faulkner JA. Maximum oxygen uptakes of college swimmers. *J Appl Physiol.* 1967;22:929–938.

52. Holmer I, Lundin A, Eriksson BO. Maximum oxygen uptake during swimming and running by elite swimmers. *J Appl Physiol.* 1974;36:711–714.

53. Kaminsky LA, Wehrli KW, Mahon AD, et al. Evaluation of a shallow water running test for the estimation of peak aerobic power. *Med Sci Sports Exerc.* 1993;25:1287–1292.

54. Jones NL, Ehrsam RE. The anaerobic threshold. *Exerc Sport Sci Rev.* 1982;10:49–83.

55. MacLaren DP, Gibson H, Parry-Billings M, et al. A review of metabolic and physiological factors in fatigue. *Exerc Sport Sci Rev.* 1989;17:29–66.

56. Connelly TP, Sheldahl LM, Tristani FE, et al. Effect of increased central blood volume with water immersion on plasma catecholamines during exercise. *J Appl Physiol.* 1990;69:651–656.

57. Town GP, Bradley SS. Maximal metabolic responses of deep and shallow water running in trained runners. *Med Sci Sports Exerc.* 1991;23:238–241.

58. Frangolias DD, Rhodes EC, Belcastro AN. Comparison of metabolic responses to prolonged work at tvent during treadmill and water immersion running. *Med Sci Sports Exerc.* 1994;26:S10.

59. Aborelius M, Balldin UI, Lilja B, et al. Hemodynamic changes in man during immersion with the head above water. *Aerospace Medicine.* 1972;43:592–598.

60. Bonde-Petersen G, Christensen NJ, Henriksen O, et al. Aspects of cardiovascular adaptation to gravitational stresses. *Physiologist.* 1980;23:S7–S10.

61. Sheldahl LM, Tristani FE, Clifford PS, et al. Effect of head-out water immersion on cardiorespiratory response to dynamic exercise. *J Am Coll Cardiol.* 1987;10:1254–1258.

62. Yamaji K, Greenley M, Northey DR, et al. Oxygen uptake and heart rate responses to treadmill and water running. *Canadian Journal of Applied Sports Science.* 1990;15:96–98.

63. Moore TO, Bernauer EM, Seto G, et al. Effect of immersion at different water temperatures on graded exercise performance in man. *Aerospace Medicine.* 1970;41:1404–1408.

64. McArdle WD, Glaser RM, Magel JR. Metabolic and cardiorespiratory responses during free swimming and treadmill walking. *J Appl Physiol.* 1971;30:733–738.

65. Rowell LB. *Human Circulation: Regulation During Physical Stress.* New York, NY: Oxford University Press; 1986.

66. Mitchell JH. Cardiovascular control during exercise: central and reflex neural mechanisms. *Am J Cardiol.* 1985;55:34D–41D.

67. Rowell LB. What signals govern the cardiovascular

responses to exercise?. *Med Sci Sports Exerc*. 1980; 12:307–315.

68. Connelly TP, Sheldahl LM, Tristani FE, et al. Effect of increased blood volume with water immersion on plasma catecholamines during exercise. *J Appl Physiol*. 1990;69:651–656.

69. Oldridge NB, Heigenhauser GJF, Sutton JR, et al. Resting and exercise heart rate with apnea and facial immersion in female swimmers. *J Appl Physiol*. 1978; 45:875–879.

70. Kennedy CA, Foster VL, Sockler JM, et al. The influence of water depth and music tempo on heart rate response to aqua aerobics. In: *Proceedings of the International Symposium on the Scientific and Medical Aspects of Aerobic Dance Exercise*. 1989:96–104.

71. Fernhall B, Manfredi TG, Congdon K. Prescribing water-based exercise from treadmill and arm ergometry in cardiac patients. *Med Sci Sports Exerc*. 1992; 24:139–143.

72. Mercer JA, Jensen RL, Fromme CF. Prediction of exercise prescription for deep water running (DWR) based on treadmill running (TM). *Med Sci Sports Exerc*. 1994;26:S10.

73. Agostoni E, Gurtner G, Torri G, et al. Respiratory mechanics during submersion and negative pressure breathing. *J Appl Physiol*. 1966;21:251–258.

74. Farhi LE, Linnarsson D. Cardiopulmonary readjustments during graded immersion in water at 35 degrees C. *Respir Physiol*. 1977;30:35–50.

75. von Dobeln W, Holmer I. Body composition, sinking force, and oxygen uptake of man treading water. *J Appl Physiol*. 1974;37:55–59.

76. Butts NK, Tucher M, Greening C. Physiologic responses to maximal treadmill and deep water running in men and women. *Am J Sports Med*. 1991;19: 612–614.

77. Sawka MN, Wenger CB. Physiological responses to acute exercise–heat stress. In: Pandolf KB, Sawka MN, Gonzalez RR, eds. *Human Performance Physiology and Environmental Medicine at Terrestrial Extremes*. Indianapolis, Ind: Benchmark; 1988:97–151.

78. Sheldahl EM, Buskirk ER, Loomis JL, et al. Effects of exercise in cool water on body weight loss. *Int J Obes*. 1982;6:29–42.

79. Norsk P, Bonde-Petersen F, Warberg J. Arginine vasopressin, circulation, and kidney during graded water immersion in humans. *J Appl Physiol*. 1986;61: 565–574.

80. Epstein M, Pins DS, Sancho J, et al. Suppression of plasma renin and plasma aldosterone during water immersion in normal man. *J Clin Endocrinol Metab*. 1975;41:618–625.

81. Epstein M, Loutzenhiser R, Friedland E, et al. Relationship of increased plasma atrial natriuretic factor and renal sodium handling during immersion-in-

duced central hypervolemia in normal humans. *J Clin Invest*. 1987;79:738–745.

82. Perrault H, Cantin M, Thirault G, et al. Plasma atrial natriuretic peptide during brief upright and supine exercise in humans. *J Appl Physiol*. 1989;66: 2159–2167.

83. Avellini BA, Shapiro Y, Pandolf KB. Cardiorespiratory physical training in water and on land. *Eur J Appl Physiol*. 1983;50:255–263.

84. Sheldahl LM, Tristani FE, Clifford PS, et al. Effect of head-out water immersion on response to exercise training. *J Appl Physiol*. 1986;60:1878–1881.

85. Young AJ, Sawka MN, Quigley MD, et al. Role of thermal factors on aerobic capacity improvements with endurance training. *J Appl Physiol*. 1993;75: 49–54.

86. Avellini BA, Shapiro Y, Fortney SM, et al. Effects of heat tolerance and physical training in water and on land. *J Appl Physiol*. 1982;53:1291–1298.

87. Magel JR, Foglia GF, McArdel WD, et al. Specificity of swim training on maximum oxygen uptake. *J Appl Physiol*. 1975;38:151–155.

88. Lieber DC, Lieber RL, Adams WC. Effects of run-training and swim-training at similar absolute intensities on treadmill VO_2max. *Med Sci Sports Exerc*. 1989;21: 655–661.

89. Martin WH III, Montgomery J, Snell PG, et al. Cardiovascular adaptations to intense swim training in sedentary middle-aged men and women. *Circulation*. 1987;75:323–330.

90. Minor MA, Hewett JE, Webel RR, et al. Efficacy of physical conditioning exercise in patients with rheumatoid arthritis and osteoarthritis. *Arthritis Rheum*. 1989;32:1396–1405.

91. Ruoti RG, Troup JT, Berger RA. The effects of non-swimming water exercises on older adults. *Journal of Orthopaedic and Sports Physical Therapy*. 1994; 19:140–145.

92. Ray CA, Cureton KJ. Interactive effects of body posture and exercise training on maximal oxygen uptake. *J Appl Physiol*. 1991;71:596–600.

93. Michaud TJ, Brennan DK, Wilder RP, et al. Aquarun training and changes in treadmill running maximal oxygen consumption. *Med Sci Sports Exerc*. 1992;24: S24.

94. Brennan DK, Michaud TJ, Wilder RP, et al. Gains in aquarunning peak oxygen consumption after eight weeks of aquarun training. *Med Sci Sports Exerc*. 1992;24:S23.

95. Eyestone ED, Fellingham G, George J, et al. Effect of water running and cycling on maximum oxygen consumption and 2-mile run performance. *Am J Sports Med*. 1993;21:41–44.

96. Gwinup G. Weight loss without dietary restriction: efficacy of different forms of aerobic exercise. *Am J Sports Med*. 1987;15:275–279.

APPLICATIONS OF AQUATIC REHABILITATION

5
Aquatic Rehabilitation of Clients With Musculoskeletal Conditions of the Extremities

Lori Thein

Christine McNamara

Physical therapists and aquatic exercise specialists have been using water to treat conditions of the extremities for many years. However, the routine use of aquatic physical therapy in rehabilitation after an extremity injury did not become widespread until the early 1970s. Pool training has become a regular component of many athletic team practice sessions, and many athletes routinely exercise in the pool when recovering from injury. This training and the regular aquatic fitness classes provided by many organizations have stimulated an increased interest in aquatic physical therapy for extremity rehabilitation and training.

A wide variety of people can benefit from aquatic physical therapy for extremity injuries. Any person with limitations or restrictions of weight bearing can use progressively deep to shallow water to advance weight bearing. Progressive resistive exercise can be performed throughout the entire available range of motion (ROM) in the lower extremity when using the turbulence provided by the water. Movement patterns that are normally gravity resisted in standing become buoyancy assisted when standing in the pool. This property can provide assistance with normally painful movements, thereby facilitating motion. Buoyancy-assisted exercises can be performed to assist ROM of the shoulder, hip, and knee joints. The pool provides a medium in which the client with extremity injuries can perform continuous, repetitive movement patterns in a variety of directions.

These movements can enhance joint mobility, joint nutrition, muscular control, and endurance.[1,2]

This chapter focuses on the treatment of a variety of musculoskeletal conditions in the general orthopedic client. These principles can be applied to the treatment of musculoskeletal problems in a variety of populations. Treatment is goal oriented and includes activities of daily living, work, or sports. The information is not all-inclusive, but rather demonstrates how the physical principles of water can be applied to the rehabilitation of clients with musculoskeletal problems. The goal-oriented section is followed by an impairment-specific section that demonstrates how the goal-specific activities may be implemented in the treatment of specific musculoskeletal conditions. The combination of land-based and aquatic-based rehabilitation techniques is also discussed.

Goal-Oriented Rehabilitation

Activities to Increase Mobility

Range of motion activities are well suited to the medium of water. The combination of buoyancy-induced skeletal unloading and muscular relaxation can enhance ROM and flexibility. The therapist must be aware of the differences between performing mobility exercises in the water and on land. The most notable of these

BOX 5-1. Buoyancy-Assisted Range of Motion Exercises in Standing Position*

Hip: flexion, extension, abduction, internal/external rotation
Knee: flexion, extension
Ankle: dorsiflexion, plantarflexion
Shoulder: flexion, extension, abduction
Elbow: flexion
Wrist: flexion, extension
Forearm: supination

---

* All exercises may be supplemented with a flotation device.

TABLE 5-1. Buoyancy-Supported Range of Motion Exercises*

Side-Lying Position	Supine Position
Hip: flexion, extension	Hip: abduction, adduction, internal external rotation
Knee: flexion, extension	
Ankle: dorsiflexion, plantarflexion	Ankle: inversion, eversion
Shoulder: flexion, extension	Shoulder: abduction, adduction, internal external rotation
Elbow: flexion, extension	
Wrist: flexion, extension	Forearm: pronation, supination

* All exercises may be supplemented with a flotation device.

differences is the potential for inadvertent overexertion or overstretching in the pool. Clients should avoid pushing their exercises into the painful range when performing ROM exercises in the water, and they should not be sore after the aquatic therapy session.

In fully using the water as an ROM tool, the therapist needs to consider several factors: (1) the force of buoyancy and its effect on the desired motion, (2) the position of the extremity and available ROM at the joint, (3) the direction of the desired motion, and (4) the use of any flotation device.

Buoyancy is the most valuable tool in mobility activity design. The force of buoyancy can be used differently in various phases of rehabilitation. Early-phase ROM exercises are performed using buoyancy in an assistive role, similar to gravity-assisted activities on land. Buoyancy-assisted ROM exercises are performed in a plane that directs the force of buoyancy in an upward direction. For example, shoulder flexion in a buoyancy-assisted position is performed standing or sitting, with the client moving the arm toward the surface of the water (Box 5-1). As the client progresses, buoyancy is used in a supportive role in a side-lying position, with the arm moving across the surface of the water. Maintaining this position may require assistance from the therapist. Additional support can be achieved by using flotation devices on the exercising extremity (Table 5-1). Finally, the exercise is progressed to the use of buoyancy as resistance. A prone position may be used, with the motion directed toward the bottom of the pool.

Examples

Shoulder Abduction

Early-phase shoulder abduction is performed with the client in sitting or standing, using a float to assist motion toward the surface. A float may be placed in the client's hand or around the elbow to provide additional support. As the arm approaches the water's surface, the client can squat to increase the amount of abduction (Fig. 5-1). This exercise is progressed to the next level by positioning the client in supine, with or without assistance from the therapist. The abduction motion occurs along the surface of the water with the support of buoyancy throughout the entire ROM. Each exercise is controlled by the client, who can progress the exercise in a pain-free manner.

Hip Flexion

Early-phase hip flexion is performed in the standing position, and can be performed with the knee flexed or extended, with or without a float. In deep water, hip flexion ROM can be performed in a variety of ways with the assistance of a deep-water belt. Straight sagittal plane hip flexion can be performed with a high knee marching step. The exercise may be progressed to the side-lying position, with motion occurring along the surface of the water. Assistance by the therapist or with flotation devices should be provided at the knee or ankle if necessary. The amount of client effort dictates resistance to the hip flexion motion. Other, more challenging exercises such as proprioceptive neuromuscular facilitation (PNF) patterns, bicycling, walking, jogging, and knee-to-chest stretches can be per-

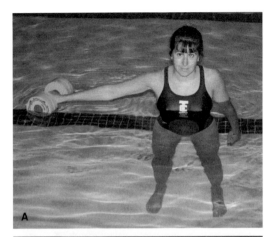

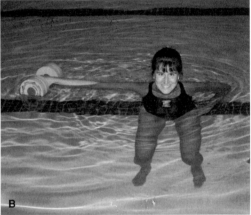

FIGURE 5-1. (***A***), Buoyancy-assisted shoulder abduction. Using a float at the end of the long lever arm increases the effect of buoyancy. (***B***) Squatting can increase the abduction range of motion. Caution must be used to avoid an impingement from excessive abduction.

Activities to Maximize Muscle Function

Strength training principles used in land-based activities are also used when performing strengthening exercises in the water. Whereas resistance on land is provided by weight and gravity, the resistance in water is provided by turbulence and buoyancy, and is influenced by the surface area, the speed of motion, and drag. The training principles and progressions are the same as those used on land. Calisthenics, PNF strengthening, and motor control exercise, open and closed kinetic chain activities, gait training, and functional activities are all easily adapted to the water. If reduced weight bearing is a consideration, strengthening exercises can be performed in deep water or in shallow water with a buoyant vest.

The aquatic environment can be used in circumstances in which resistive exercise on land is contraindicated. For example, a client with a lower extremity stress fracture has the entire spectrum of strengthening exercises available in the pool's deep end. The client with recent surgery or injury can safely perform gait training exercises in chest-deep water during the early rehabilitation phase. The client accomplishes several goals with this simple exercise, including weight bearing on the affected limb, facilitation of healing and more normal sensory feedback

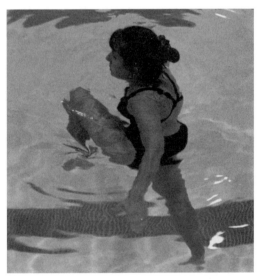

FIGURE 5-2. Buoyancy-assisted hip range of motion using a marching motion in deep water. This activity can be performed with the knee flexed to facilitate knee flexion range of motion.

formed in the standing position, using viscosity as resistance (Fig. 5-2).

Knee Flexion

Range of motion exercises of the knee can be performed in either shallow or deep water, and can be isolated or addressed as a component of a more complex motion. Shallow-water knee flexion ROM is achieved by walking forward, backward, and laterally, emphasizing knee flexion with each step. Squats, static, and dynamic forward lunges, high-step marching, standing hurdler's motion, and wall push-offs can effectively increase knee flexion motion. All of these activities can be performed in deep water with or without the assistance of a deep-water belt (see Fig. 5-2).

through that limb, functional and strength training for the lower quarter, improved mobility of the knee joint, and articular cartilage nutrition.

Strengthening exercises in the water are progressed in a variety of ways, including increasing repetitions or sets, adding equipment (increasing the surface area), increasing the speed of the exercise, changing the client's position, or changing the depth of exercise. Buoyancy and surface area can both be used as tools to achieve strength goals. Buoyancy-assisted exercises are used when the client is incapable of generating torque against the force of buoyancy. The inability to produce torque may result from several factors, including pain, muscular problems, neurologic injury, inert tissue compression, or psychological factors. Muscular endurance is addressed effectively in deep-water exercises such as jogging, vertical kicking, and cross-country skiing.

Strengthening exercises for the upper extremity include specific isolated muscular actions to functional movement patterns. Normal upper quarter movement patterns may be introduced early in the rehabilitation process because of the water's support. In addition, upper extremity strengthening can be encouraged during gait activities such as forward, backward, and lateral walking, with cueing from the therapist for the appropriate upper extremity component.

Addition of equipment (paddles, aqua gloves, weights, and buoys) increases the surface area and turbulence, making the exercise more difficult. Equipment may also change the quality of the exercise. The additional resistance of the equipment can alter normal movement patterns. Monitoring the client ensures that the exercise is being performed properly, without substitution.

Lower extremity strengthening in the pool can begin early in the rehabilitation process, taking advantage of both the reduced-gravity environment and the availability of resistance throughout the ROM. As with any strengthening program, a warm-up should proceed any vigorous activity. Pool warm-up activities such as forward, backward, and lateral walking are easily progressed to strengthening and endurance activities for the trunk and lower extremities by increasing the speed of motion or by adding resistance to the motion with equipment. Changing the focus of the exercise is an effective means of progressing strengthening. For example, a left quadriceps weakness can be addressed as an isolated muscular weakness, or as a weak component of a functional skill. Different cueing and emphasis by the therapist allows

one exercise to facilitate both types of strengthening. This client may begin the aquatic program with 3 to 5 minutes of forward walking, with cueing for a normal gait pattern. Besides serving as a lower extremity warm-up, this exercise also provides the left lower extremity with sensory feedback from a normal gait cycle, facilitated by buoyancy assisting the weak quadriceps during the early stance phase. With the support of the water, the client is able to practice a functional skill. Alternatively, cueing for emphasis on knee extension in this same forward-walking activity shifts the focus to the isolated strength deficit.

Examples

Closed-Chain Lower Extremity Training

Weight bearing, task complexity, repetitions, resistance, ROM, and depth of water must be carefully considered when progressing the pool program. Depth can be used to make an exercise easier or harder. The lower extremity challenge is increased as the depth of the water is decreased. Stabilization or balance exercises can be more difficult in deeper water owing to greater buoyancy. Early-phase closed-chain exercises begin with simple weight shifts forward, backward, and laterally, performed in an appropriate depth based on the client's condition. These shifts can be progressed to brief single-leg stance, and then to a full step with return to the starting position (lunge). This activity increases the challenge by prolonging single-leg stance time. One- and two-legged squats are progressed by increasing the repetitions or by adding weight (two- to one-legged, or decreasing the depth). The single-leg stance position can also be used to progress stabilization and balance by performing small-amplitude hip flexion, extension, and abduction–adduction motions with the contralateral leg (Fig. 5-3). The focus of this activity is easily altered, such as bending the knee to emphasize quadriceps work, or balancing on the toes for increased plantarflexor work. Progression of single-leg stance activities might include performing PNF patterns with the contralateral leg, or adding resistive equipment. In addition, resistive exercises performed with the upper extremity while balancing on a single leg further increase the balance challenge (Fig. 5-4). Forward and diagonal lunges and upper extremity functional movements with a plow are examples of these exercises (Figs. 5-5 and 5-6).

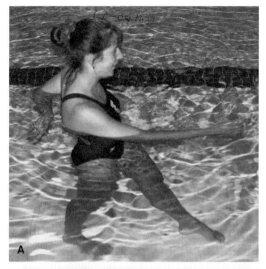

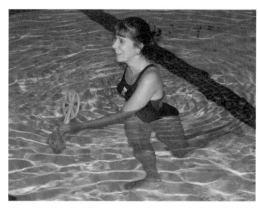

FIGURE 5-4. Adding resistive equipment to upper extremity movement patterns increases the challenge to balance.

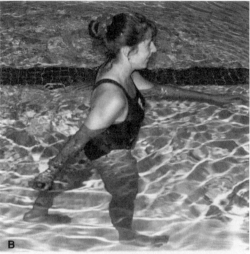

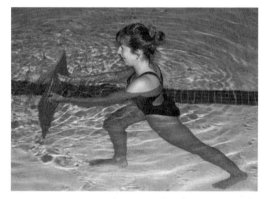

FIGURE 5-5. Resistive lunging with a plow trains coordination and balance in a functional movement pattern.

FIGURE 5-3. Single-leg stance with contralateral leg extension (*A*) and flexion (*B*) challenges balance.

Upper Extremity Stabilization Exercises

Shoulder stabilization exercises should be initiated early in the aquatic exercise program. Low-level stabilization exercises are performed with the client leaning against the side of the pool with both shoulders under water. This position assists in stabilizing the scapulae on the trunk. From this position the client can perform a variety of strengthening exercises. With the elbows and wrists extended and in various degrees of shoulder flexion, the client can resist an anterior–posterior force applied by the therapist. A small playground ball can be used unilaterally, with the client attempting to push it toward the bottom of the pool and then resisting and con-

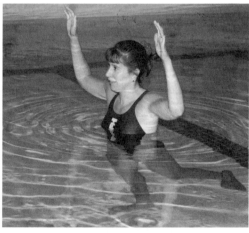

FIGURE 5-6. Contralateral leg patterns without assistance from the upper extremities challenge postural stabilizing musculature.

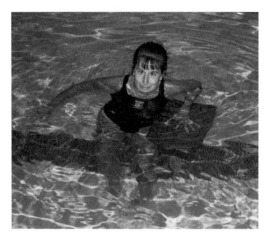

FIGURE 5-7. Submerging a kickboard and controlling it while moving it in several directions requires stabilization of the shoulder girdle musculature.

trolling it as it comes back toward the surface. Facing the side of the pool, the client can execute small-amplitude (allowing minimal elbow flexion) and large-amplitude (allowing maximum elbow flexion) push-ups or let-downs (client falls toward the wall). These exercises can be performed bilaterally or unilaterally. A variation of this exercise is performed unilaterally with the body perpendicular to the side of the pool.

Intermediate-level stabilization exercises are performed away from the edge of the pool, requiring a more dynamic stabilization effort. Standing in chest-deep water with the arms at the side, small-amplitude, rapid movements in flexion and extension, abduction and adduc-

tion, and internal and external rotation can produce dynamic cocontraction around the joint. Proper postural alignment should be maintained, with minimal trunk motion. Scapular protraction and retraction can be performed in standing posture using gloves or paddles to increase resistance.

Advanced stabilization exercise can be performed in either shallow or deep water, either unilaterally or bilaterally. The client is required to submerge a kickboard or ball, and using one or both shoulders, keep the device as motionless as possible (Fig. 5-7). This task requires stabilization in all directions. Other variations of this exercise include a variety of shoulder and elbow positions and board positions (anterior, posterior, lateral), in standing or in prone in the deep water (Fig. 5-8). The challenge can be progressed by asking the client to move the board slightly in all directions while keeping it submerged. This task requires a constant downward force in combination with the forces required to move the board in a controlled manner. Other stabilization exercises using a kickboard include small-amplitude pushing and pulling motions with the board submerged anteriorly, posteriorly, and laterally. In deep water, shoulder stabilization exercises can be combined with lower extremity strengthening. For example, in a vertical kicking exercise, the client uses the upper extremities to keep the trunk as still as possible. This task is most effectively accomplished using small sculling motions of the hands with a minimal amount of motion at the glenohumeral and scapulohumeral joints.

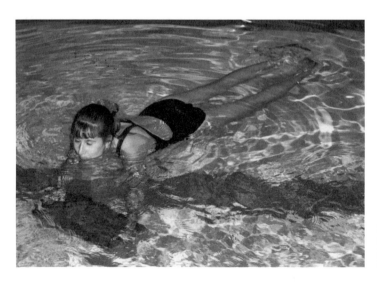

FIGURE 5-8. Stabilizing exercises can be progressed to more challenging positions, such as 90° of shoulder flexion.

Rotator Cuff Training

Early-phase rotator cuff strengthening in the pool is performed with the arms at the side and elbows extended. Small-amplitude rotations and pendulum exercises, with or without a weight, are effective methods of introducing rotator cuff action. Flexing the elbows to 90° increases the resistance to internal and external rotation. Pronating the forearm reduces this resistance, and positioning the forearm in neutral increases the resistance. The use of aqua gloves or paddles increases the surface area, thereby increasing resistance. As strength of the rotator cuff increases, the position of abduction should be gradually increased to provide an additional challenge. Abduction–rotation isometrics or resistance through a very small ROM progresses both motions simultaneously and safely. As the client gets stronger, abduction strengthening in the frontal plane can be performed with the elbow flexed and then extended. PNF exercises are effective methods of improving rotator cuff strength in a functional movement pattern. These patterns can be performed in sitting, standing, or prone (with a snorkel), using gloves or weights, or simply using the open hand as resistance. Once a strength base has been established, functional activity simulation should be incorporated. Sport-specific activities such as throwing or tennis serving can be performed entirely under water. Work tasks involving the shoulder can also be simulated. The assembly-line worker who must perform through the full range of external rotation and abduction to internal rotation and adduction can train this motion in the pool. Correct posture and biomechanical principles should be emphasized by the therapist.

Activities to Progress Weight Bearing

The pool is an ideal environment for the rehabilitation of injuries that limit weight bearing. A clear understanding of the effect of buoyancy on weight bearing and body type, and their relation to land-based activities (rehabilitative and functional), is imperative to remain within weight-bearing restrictions. ROM, strength, or functional activities performed in deep water are used to prepare the limb and trunk for weight bearing.

Progression of weight bearing is accomplished primarily by decreasing the water depth at which an exercise is performed. Performing an exercise with increased speed can be used to progress weight bearing in shallow water. Harrison and colleagues found walking at a fast pace to increase the loads over static stance by as much as 76%.[3] Land-based tasks should be initiated before the water program is discontinued to facilitate a smooth transition from pool to land. Weight bearing as tolerated is allowed in the early healing phase of some lower extremity dysfunctions, although the total *quantity* of weight bearing may need to be controlled. Alternating between deep- and shallow-water activities may be well tolerated by these clients. For example, Zelko and DePalma describe a protocol for rehabilitation of a person with a lower extremity stress fracture that is based on the relation between the resorptive process (osteoclast activity) and the reparative process (osteoblast activity).[4] This cyclic training program includes a 2-week period of training at an exertion/impact level that is pain free and produces limited fatigue. A 1-week period of "active" rest follows, in which exertion and impact are reduced but not eliminated. The active rest period enables the resorptive process to slow as the reparative process continues. Finally, some clients may bypass the deep-water program completely, participating only in shallow-water weight-bearing activities.

Example: Impact Loading and Plyometrics

After progression to full weight bearing, some clients may require impact or plyometric training to facilitate return to their previous activity level. Impact loading and plyometric training can be performed in the water without the deleterious effects of impact in a gravity environment. Plyometric training can be defined as quick, powerful movements involving a prestretching of the muscle–tendon unit that activates the stretch–shorten cycle.[5] Plyometrics challenge the client to respond quickly, and to change the direction of motion with speed and force. Early-phase impact activities for the lower extremities can be performed in neck-deep water, where the forces of buoyancy support the take-off phase and cushion the landing phase. However, this depth inhibits the speed of the exercise, minimizing any eccentric component of the activity. As such, the water depth should be progressively decreased until the exercises are performed in waist-deep water. For example, performing a tuck jump is easiest in neck-deep water, and emphasis should be on proper technique at this depth. Decreasing the depth of water during this jump increases both the difficulty and the impact. If the water is shallow enough, an impact activity can become plyometric. Caution must be observed when performing impact activities with bare feet on a tile surface in shallow water owing to the possibility of impact-related injuries. A shock-absorptive shoe should be used when performing repetitive impact exercises in shallow water.

Activities for Cardiovascular Training

Cardiovascular training in the water is a component of many rehabilitation programs. The positive effects of hydrostatic pressure on the heart and the unloading effect of buoyancy on the musculoskeletal system make the water an ideal training environment. Most aquatic cardiovascular training begins in the deep end, taking full advantage of nonimpact conditioning. Progression from the deep to the shallow end allows for graded and controlled increases of gravitational loads.

Monitoring exercise intensity in the water is most easily accomplished using the Borg perceived exertion scale. Aquatic specialists may find this method more effective than using heart rate because the effects of exercise and immersion on heart rate are still unclear. Wilder and colleagues, however, found a correlation between cadence and heart rate in a group of deep-water runners.[6] As such, cadence may be an indicator of exercise intensity. A learning curve exists for deep-water training, and the rate of perceived exertion may change as the person becomes more accustomed to the water.[7]

Examples

Water Walking and Jogging

The primary difference between water walking and jogging is the pace. Generally speaking, the technique is the same, making an easy transition from walking to jogging. The exercises may be performed with or without a deep-water belt, depending on the skill and fitness of the client. For most people, proper technique is easier with a belt and may allow the completion of a lengthy workout without substitution.

When first instructing a client in deep-water walking, it is best to provide as few directions

as possible. For example, the therapist may simply tell the client to begin walking, and then correct the technique. An upright, fully erect posture with minimal forward lean is the appropriate position for water walking. Lower extremity motion is similar to that when walking on land, and should be directed by the therapist. Exaggerated range or normal range can be performed, depending on the client's goals. Lower extremity motion is accompanied by a reciprocal arm swing, which should be exaggerated at both the shoulder and elbow. The hand should be kept loose at the start, and progressed to cupping or gloving the hands to increase the resistance. Weights added to the upper or lower extremities, or increasing the speed or duration of the activity, increase the exercise difficulty. The position and progression of the upper and lower extremities and spine should be based on the client's needs, goals, and abilities.

Deep-water jogging should also be initiated with as little instruction as possible. A portion of the first few deep-water jogging sessions should be devoted to learning pace and control, thereby improving the effectiveness of further water- and land-based training sessions. Starting the jog in the shallow end and jogging "off the bottom" into the deep end is an effective teaching method. The person should maintain an erect or nearly erect posture when running (Fig. 5-9). As the speed and duration of the activity increase, the client will tend to assume a more horizontal position, simulating swimming. As such, close monitoring of technique is critical. Lower extremity motion during deep-water jogging requires less hip flexion than water walk-

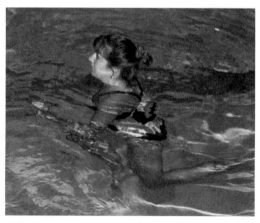

FIGURE 5-9. Proper deep water running technique requires nearly erect posture.

ing, and the legs should remain underneath or slightly behind the hips, with the ankles in neutral. Some modifications of technique may be impairment specific, such as the client with sacroiliac pain who needs a technique emphasizing hip and lumbar flexion. The arm motion is similar to water walking. Deep-water jogging requires a higher cadence than water walking, and the exercise is progressed by increasing the cadence or adding resistive equipment.

The amount of forward propulsion achieved with deep-water jogging is highly technique dependent, and varies from person to person. In general, those clients who jog with an open or gloved hand and a degree of forward lean experience more propulsion, whereas the person jogging with an erect posture and a closed fist may move very little. The specific posture chosen should depend on the needs of the client. If pool space is a concern, most deep-water belts have a loop to allow tethering to the side of the pool.

Deep-water walking and jogging training sessions can be structured as any land-based cardiovascular program. Interval training, pyramids (increasing or decreasing variables), fartleks (speed play), sprints, and distance workouts are all possible in the water.[8] Land-based jogging or running programs are easily converted to water workouts by using estimated time as the training parameter.

Cross-Country Skiing

Cross-country skiing is a total-body fitness exercise that can be modified to isolate either upper or lower extremities. Deep-water skiing also may be used as a stabilization exercise, a postural exercise, or abdominal-strengthening exercise. The technique requires a vertical position in the deep end with reciprocal flexion and extension motions of the upper and lower extremities in varying degrees of elbow and knee extension. Initially, a deep-water belt may be necessary to assist the client in maintaining the vertical position. The objective of the exercise is to move the arms and legs as quickly as possible while still maintaining an erect posture.

The difficulty of this exercise can be modified in several ways. Keeping the elbows and knees fully extended is very difficult, requiring the client to maintain an erect posture and to push and pull primarily with the shoulders, hips, hands, and feet. Allowing various degrees of elbow and knee flexion and extension reduces the power requirement. Variations of this exer-

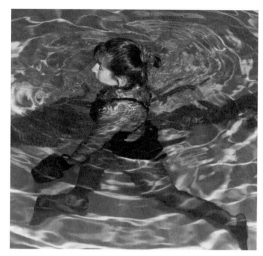

FIGURE 5-10. Deep water cross-country skiing technique using gloves and fins.

cise include the addition of aqua gloves or paddles for the upper extremities, and fins for the lower extremities (Fig. 5-10).

Vertical Kicking

Vertical kicking is one of the most challenging cardiovascular training exercises, requiring abdominal, paraspinal, and lower extremity strength. This activity should be reserved for the later stages of training and for those demonstrating good postural control.

Vertical kicking is performed in the deep water with the client floating in a vertical position. A flotation belt may be used early in the rehabilitation program to help maintain this position. However, this significantly reduces the exercise difficulty, and should be discontinued as soon as possible. The person must maintain an erect posture throughout the activity, and should be watched for proper technique. Substitution, such as flexing at the hip, can significantly reduce the difficulty of the exercise and can place an additional strain on the lumbar spine. Initially, the client should perform small flutter kicks, with the hands performing a sculling motion by the hips. As the client's strength and skill progress, the hands should be moved toward the surface of the water, and eventually out of the water.

Safe and correct execution of vertical kicking requires quick, forceful, small flutter kicks and an erect posture. The therapist may find it useful to review flutter kicking technique before initiation of vertical kicking, emphasizing the following points: (1) force should initiate at the hip and not the knee, (2) only slight knee flexion and extension should occur, (3) the foot should be plantarflexed, and (4) no back strain should be observed or felt.

Several methods exist to alter the difficulty of vertical kicking. Adding small fins makes it easier for the client to stay afloat, but more muscular strength is required with each kick. Holding small weights or raising the hands out of the water increases the difficulty. As with all turbulent activities, increasing the speed of the exercise also increases the difficulty. Modifying the technique can also change the emphasis of the activity. Kicking with more knee flexion and extension increases the focus on the quadriceps and hamstrings. For the advanced client, vertical kicking using the breaststroke (whip) or butterfly (dolphin) significantly increases the challenge.

Vertical kicking may be introduced into the cardiovascular training regimen and structured in a variety of different ways. Interval training is extremely effective owing to the rigorousness of vertical kicking. This activity should be monitored by the therapist to ensure proper technique and to prevent additional injury.

Impairment-Oriented Rehabilitation: Upper Extremity

Hypomobility: Adhesive Capsulitis

Adhesive capsulitis of the shoulder primarily involves the glenohumeral joint and alters normal scapulohumeral rhythm. Loss of glenohumeral mobility often results from immobilization, whether imposed by something external (eg, a sling) or internal (eg, the person's unwillingness to move). Immobilization after fractures can produce fibrosis, shortening, and weakening of the associated soft tissues. An acute injury such as a fall or an overuse injury can start the cycle of increased pain and self-imposed immobilization. The immobilization initiates a self-perpetuating cycle that can worsen if no intervention occurs. It is not uncommon for a person to present several months after the original injury and after a progressive deterioration in motion and function.

Physical therapy treatment must address the pain, loss of mobility, and loss of strength associated with this condition. The joint capsule is very pain sensitive, which contributes to the pain associated with adhesive capsulitis. The hypomobility and diminished accessory motion of the glenohumeral joint place the capsule on stretch well before the end of the "normal" ROM. As such, the limited ROM and pain work in concert to prevent use the of extremity. In addition, weakness develops secondary to disuse and changes in the length–tension ratios of the surrounding musculature. The pain, loss of mobility, and weakness combine to cause loss of function of the limb. Clients can often accomplish simple tasks with the elbow held close to the side. However, any tasks requiring strength with the arm away from the body are nearly impossible.

The goal of physical therapy intervention in adhesive capsulitis is to increase the client's function. This can be accomplished by addressing the pain, loss of mobility, and weakness. Hydrotherapy has been used in the past to assist in decreasing pain. The laminar flow of water and the warmth and support of the aquatic environment can relax the client and decrease pain. The decrease in pain allows completion of mobility and strengthening exercises that may be too painful to perform on land. Activities should be performed in neck-deep water to obtain the water's full pain-minimizing benefits.

The person with adhesive capsulitis should perform exercises several times per day, thereby accomplishing a greater volume of activity spread over the course of a day. The relative percentages of land- and water-based exercise vary depending on access to the pool, the client's schedule, and the degree of impairment. As the client progresses, the amount of time in aquatic rehabilitation decreases and the time spent in land-based exercise increases. Cardiovascular training can also be performed in the pool throughout each phase.

Early Phase

Activities that increase the mobility of the shoulder girdle can be performed in a number of positions. Choice of position depends on which direction is most limited, and the degree of limitation. In addition to using buoyancy to facilitate stretching, physiologic stretching can be performed using the side of the pool or a ballet bar. Placing a hand on the wall increases shoulder flexion, abduction, or external rotation. Bad Ragaz activities can also be incorporated to facil-

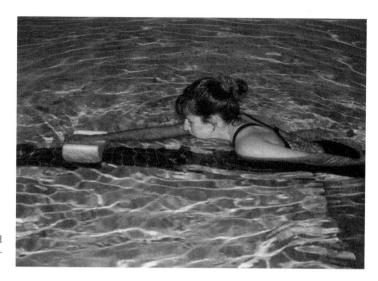

FIGURE 5-11. Buoyancy-assisted range of motion for shoulder flexion using a pull buoy in prone.

itate mobility. Increases in motion are of little use if the person is unable to function within the new range. This population often achieves shoulder elevation in the frontal and sagittal planes with scapular elevation rather than using normal scapulohumeral rhythm. Normalization of movement about the shoulder girdle can be easily reinforced in the pool owing to the water's support. Stabilization exercises for the scapulothoracic articulation should be included in the program concurrent with mobility activities. Simply walking through the water using a normal or exaggerated arm swing can increase mobility and normalize movement.

Clients with adhesive capsulitis often have good strength within their available range. They often lack endurance, however, and pool activities should focus on high-repetition, low-resistance strengthening exercises, using normal movement patterns. Isometrics can be performed by walking against the resistance of the water, or by using Bad Ragaz techniques. As range increases, isotonic exercises can be performed in a variety of positions using buoyancy and turbulence to increase resistance.

Intermediate Phase

Rehabilitation activities in the pool progress as the client's range, strength, and function progress. As the range of elevation increases to 0 to 150 degrees, prolonged passive stretch can be performed in the pool in prone for flexion and side lying for abduction (Figs. 5-11 and 5-12). The therapist must ensure that the client has adequate external rotation range to prevent impingement when stretching into abduction above 90 degrees. Passive stretch for external

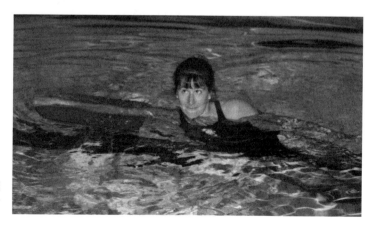

FIGURE 5-12. Buoyancy-assisted range of motion for shoulder abduction using a kickboard.

rotation can also be performed in prone in varying degrees of shoulder abduction.

The person should have enough range at this stage to generate torque through an ROM. As such, isotonic strengthening can be performed through the available range using buoyancy and turbulence. Cardinal plane exercises isolating specific muscles should be progressed to functional movement patterns once adequate strength and normal movement patterns have been established. Visualization of the movement pattern in the pool is often difficult owing to refraction. As such, the therapist should observe the client performing specific exercises on land to ensure that proper movement patterns are being reinforced.

Exercises should continue to focus on high-repetition, low-resistance activity until fatigue or substitution occurs. Land-based exercises in this stage may include physiologic stretching, joint mobilization, upper body ergometry, and progressive resistive exercise. An appropriate balance between the pool- and land-based exercises is necessary to maintain a constant quantity of exercise without overexertion.

Late Phase

The late phase of rehabilitation is used to "fine tune" and prepare the client to return to activity. Most of the stretching and strengthening exercises are performed on land during this phase. The pool can be used as an adjunct to the land-based program. Swimming activities can be performed to increase upper extremity endurance within a large ROM. The pool can be an adjunct to the exercise program by providing the opportunity for vigorous exercise on alternate days when not in therapy, or half-days for people participating in work-hardening programs. Exercises can be designed to simulate work activities such as pushing, pulling, and lifting. Clients returning to sports can reproduce many of these movement patterns in the pool. A circuit training program should be established to provide diversity and to achieve various client goals.

Hypomobility: Other Upper Extremity Joints

Hypomobility can occur in other joints and articulations throughout the upper extremity. Immobilization of the elbow or wrist can follow frac-

tures, dislocations, or surgery. Hypomobility secondary to fibrosis in the joint capsule, ligaments, and other soft tissues results. Shifts in the length–tension ratios of the surrounding musculature give rise to muscle weakness throughout the extremity.

Pool exercises are based on the same principles and progressed in the same manner as activities to treat adhesive capsulitis about the shoulder. When immersion is permitted, pool activities may be initiated using buoyancy to facilitate motion. Owing to the short lever arm at the wrist, additional flotation equipment is particularly helpful in stretching and mobilization exercises at the wrist, and the wall may be used for traditional physiologic stretching. Active, active assisted, and passive exercises can be combined to enhance mobilization and articular cartilage nutrition in the supported pool environment. Bad Ragaz techniques allow the therapist to control the mobilization/resistive force and range.

Resistive exercises should be initiated as soon as tolerated by the client. Isometric exercises may be performed in many positions using the wall or the contralateral extremity. Isometrics may also be performed by holding the arm in a static position and walking into the resistance of the water. Exercises should be progressed from isometric to isotonic when enough range is available to generate a torque. Increasing the moving object's surface area with gloves or other pool equipment enhances torque produc-

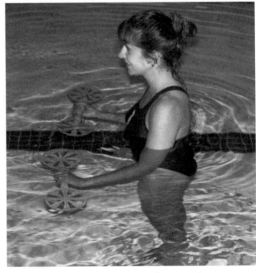

FIGURE 5-13. Resistive range of motion for pronation and supination using paddles.

tion, particularly if ROM is limited. Elbow and wrist flexion and extension exercises should be progressed to multijoint, multiplane activities. The use of resistive paddles increases the lever arm for pronation and supination, facilitating both resistance and range (Fig. 5-13).

The pool program parallels activities on land, and should progress to patterns involving the entire upper extremity as mobility, strength, and pain permit. The client progresses to spending more of his or her rehabilitation time on land, owing to the need for more eccentric activity later in the rehabilitation program. The pool can be used as an adjunct to traditional land-based activities, incorporating swimming or other general exercise patterns into the client's return-to-activity plan.

Hypermobility: Shoulder Instability

Glenohumeral instability is a common problem in younger people, but is relatively uncommon in middle-aged and elderly populations. Instability can occur in one direction or in more than one direction. The most common types of instability seen are anterior, posterior, and multidirectional. Instability in those younger than 25 years of age has a significant rate of reoccurrence and, as such, should be treated aggressively. The acronym TUBS is used to describe the *T*raumatic dislocation, which is usually *U*nilateral, includes a *B*ankart lesion, and eventually requires *S*urgery for treatment. In contrast, the acronym AMBRI is used to describe the *A*traumatic, *M*ultidirectional, *B*ilateral instability that responds best to *R*ehabilitation, but occasionally requires a surgical *I*nferior capsular shift.[9]

Rehabilitation goals in the client with glenohumeral instability include restoration of normal mobility, increased muscular strength and endurance, improved proprioception and motor control, and return to previous level of function. Muscular strength and endurance training should include the scapular stabilizing muscles because of their role in providing a solid base of support for the glenohumeral joint. Moreover, people with glenohumeral instability must retrain dynamic muscular control in the provocative position of external rotation and abduction for anterior instability, and forward flexion and horizontal adduction for posterior instability. When appropriate levels of strength in a neutral

position have been attained, the client should begin training in a more provocative position.

Rehabilitation of the client with instability follows the same process and moves toward the same goals regardless of surgical stabilization. Differences in protocol depend on several factors, including the person's age, direction of instability, number of previous dislocations (if any), and activity type and level (work and sport), and the philosophy of the treating physician. Restoration of ROM, maintenance and progression of muscular strength and endurance, and return to full function are the guiding goals. A sample program following a Bankart reconstruction can be found in Table 5-2.

Early Phase

Therapeutic goals in the early phase are to normalize movement patterns in the upper extremity, while dynamically maintaining the humeral head within the glenoid. The person with clinical or subclinical subluxation who presents primarily with secondary impingement likely has no measurable ROM deficit. A thorough evaluation is necessary to ensure that imbalances in muscle length (and resultant length–tension ratios) are not contributing to the problem.

Those clients sustaining a frank dislocation or presenting after a surgical stabilization procedure have decreased mobility throughout the shoulder girdle. Mobility exercises should follow the guidelines established for the surgical procedure and the direction of instability. In general, elevation to 90 degrees is allowed passively or with some assistance in the early phase. External rotation (anterior instability) or internal rotation (posterior instability) ROM progresses more slowly than elevation. Mobility exercises in standing or sitting and progressing to prone can use buoyancy to facilitate ROM in elevation. Pendulum exercises can be performed in the traditional position with the face in or out of the water. Waterproof wrist weights can gently increase traction on the shoulder as well as provide additional momentum.

Isometric strengthening can be performed by holding the arm still while walking against the resistance of the water, and isotonic strengthening can be performed through an ROM when the client is ready for this activity. All major muscle groups should be trained with constant reinforcement of proper firing sequences. Scapular stabilizing muscles should be trained in the pool or on land to provide a solid base of support

TABLE 5-2. Example of Rehabilitation Program After a Bankart Capsulolabral Reconstruction Using Pool- and Land-Based Exercises

Pool Activities	Land Activities
Early Phase	
Pendulum exercises	Pendulum exercises
Buoyancy-assisted shoulder flexion	Passive ROM 0°–90° flexion/abduction
Buoyancy-assisted shoulder abduction	Passive ROM 0°–90° internal rotation
Passive ROM for extension and internal rotation	Resisted scapular protraction/retraction
Turbulence-resisted scapular protraction/retraction	Active scapular elevation/depression
Resisted shoulder shrugs	Bicycling for CV conditioning
Resisted scapular depression	Isometrics to all shoulder girdle muscles
Resisted elbow flexion/extension	Closed-chain weight shifts in neutral
Ambulation with arm swing	
Active shoulder internal/external rotation in position of internal rotation	
Scapular stabilization against wall	
Intermediate Phase	
Buoyancy-assisted ROM to full elevation in prone	Passive/active ROM to full
Passive ROM for external rotation against wall	Upper-body ergometer
Isotonic exercise for shoulder flexion/extention, abduction/adduction, internal/external rotation	Shoulder stabilization against wall
Shoulder stabilization using ball or board in vertical	Stairmaster on knees for upper extremity endurance
Rapid alternating movements in neutral	Proprioceptive neuromuscular facilitation techniques
Cross-country skiing or deep-water running for CV conditioning	PRE for scapular and shoulder girdle muscles
Late Phase	
Provocative exercises in prone	Continued PRE exercises in increasingly provocative
Rapid alternating movement in provocative positions	positions
Plyometric exercises such as ball tosses, chest passes	Plyometrics
Swimming	Functional progression
Functional progression	

ROM, range of motion; CV, cardiovascular; PRE, progressive resistance exercises.

for the glenohumeral joint. Pool exercises should be coupled with manually resisted exercises on land that provide the client with an understanding of the proper level of resistance. Moreover, the land-based exercises provide an opportunity to reinforce proper muscle-firing patterns and prevention of substitution, as well as to conduct an ongoing assessment of the client's progress.

Intermediate Phase

The mobility goal in the intermediate phase is the achievement of full active ROM. Passive stretching in the pool parallels physiologic stretching on land and progresses to the end range. As mobility continues to progress, changes in the pool position can facilitate gaining the full ROM. Stretching in prone and supine

using the pool wall or buoyant equipment can increase motion in full elevation.

The strength goal in this phase is the development of a core of strength using normal movement patterns in proper postural positions. Strengthening exercises should be progressed from resistance through an ROM in neutral abduction to exercises in positions of increasing abduction. Buoyant and resistive equipment may be used to increase the resistance; increasing the speed of movement creates turbulence and, likewise, enhances the resistance. Bad Ragaz techniques provide another method for controlling the range, quality, and quantity of resistance in the pool. Resisted abduction techniques in supine and resisted flexion exercises in prone provide an opportunity for the therapist to control forces in provocative positions in the pool. Proprioceptive activities such as alternating isometrics in progressively provocative positions can be incorporated toward the end of this phase. Brisk rhythmic stabilization activities in an open chain or closed chain using a kickboard or ball can begin to train cocontraction and dynamic stabilization about the shoulder.

Late Phase

The primary goal in the late phase is to prepare the client to return to his or her prior level of activity. This may be limited to activities of daily living, or more vigorous work-related activities or sports. Pool exercises should be progressed to positions and patterns that replicate on-land demands. Overhead demands can be resisted in prone, supine, or side lying in the pool, using the properties of buoyancy, surface tension, or viscosity to increase resistance. Bad Ragaz techniques should be progressed to increasingly provocative positions, and resistance and repetitions should mimic the functional demands of the client's activity choices. Rhythmic stabilization/alternating isometric exercises should be performed in increasingly provocative positions.

Pool exercises should be paralleled with provocative exercises on land. Multidirectional resistive exercises in the provocative position, alternating isometrics, and closed-chain exercises can facilitate dynamic stabilization about the shoulder. Plyometrics can be performed on land or in the pool, depending on the postural challenge desired. Swimming can be used as an adjunct to increase muscle endurance and train the shoulder with the arm in an overhead position. Work activities can be replicated in the pool and should be used as a component of a work-hardening program.

Other Movement Dysfunctions

Movement dysfunctions about the shoulder girdle can occur as a result of acromioclavicular joint or rotator cuff injuries. Acromioclavicular joint problems may be the result of a traumatic injury (macrotrauma) causing a separation, or of an overuse injury (microtrauma) with ensuing degenerative joint disease. Most acromioclavicular joint problems can be treated conservatively with appropriate anti-inflammatory measures and rehabilitation. Occasionally, surgery is necessary to relieve symptoms, and may include a Neer-Mumford procedure or subacro-

mial decompression.[10] After injury or surgery, clients usually present with limited ROM, a painful arc of motion, pain-limited strength, point tenderness, and loss of upper extremity function.

Rehabilitation activities focus on goals of increased mobility and strength throughout the shoulder girdle without irritating the acromioclavicular joint. The proximity of the subacromial soft tissues (subacromial bursa, rotator cuff tendon, and long head of the biceps tendon) necessitates care to avoid creating a secondary impingement. The rotator cuff should be specifically strengthened to prevent this complication.

Rotator cuff injuries range from impingement of the subacromial bursa, rotator cuff tendon, and long head of the biceps tendon, to partial or complete tears of the rotator cuff. Partial and complete tears usually occur approximately 1 cm from the insertion into the greater tuberosity, and involve the supraspinatus and infraspinatus tendons primarily.[11] Chronic rotator cuff tendinitis or impingement syndrome requires prolonged conservative treatment, including the judicious use of anti-inflammatory measures, and a program of kinesthetic training and progressive resistive exercise for the entire shoulder girdle. A minimum of several months of conservative care is the general rule before any surgical procedure is considered.[10] Strengthening exercises should focus on the external rotators, the supraspinatus, and the scapular stabilizers.

Early Phase

Goals in the early phase focus on the restoration of normal mobility, normalization of movement patterns, and maintenance of strength. The relative emphasis of these goals depends on the specific lesion and its resultant movement dysfunction. Initiation of resistive exercises is of little use if substitution occurs, reinforcing abnormal postures and movement patterns.

Mobilization activities should be performed for all joints and articulations throughout the upper quarter. A thorough evaluation may uncover muscle imbalances requiring specific stretching techniques. Passive physiologic stretching may be performed in a variety of positions in the pool and on land. The stretching should be progressed slowly into the overhead or across-chest positions because these tend to be the most painful. Buoyancy-supported stretching can be performed in prone using buoyant equipment to facilitate the stretch.

The vertical support of the pool can be effectively used to reinforce normal movement patterns. Clients with movement dysfunctions often achieve elevation of the arm by excessive scapular elevation. Active-assisted shoulder abduction performed in vertical can be used to reinforce normal scapulohumeral rhythm. The support of the water often decreases pain enough to prevent excessive scapular elevation during abduction and flexion. Rhythmic mobility through walking with an arm swing or repeated movements in a pain-free range can facilitate mobility and normal arthrokinematics. Normalization of movement patterns is essential before progressing to resistive exercises.

Strength deterioration due to pain can be minimized by isometric or isotonic exercise in the pool. Immersion in a resistive medium allows for resistive exercise in nearly any direction at any position. These exercises maintain strength and prevent reinforcement of abnormal movement patterns or postures. All shoulder girdle muscles, including the scapular stabilizing muscles, should be trained.

Intermediate Phase

The person should have achieved nearly full pain-free ROM by the beginning of the intermediate phase. The focus in this phase is the development of muscular strength and endurance throughout the upper quarter, while maintaining proper posture and movement patterns. Resistive exercises should be performed in a variety of positions in the pool, including vertical, prone, and supine. Activities should be progressed from a neutral position of abduction to increasing positions of elevation, and from single-plane patterns to multiplane, multijoint patterns. The client should attempt to increase the speed of movement to replicate land-based activities. Exercises should be performed to fatigue and should be based on a low-resistance, high-repetition program.

Pool exercises should parallel land-based activities. The rotator cuff should be specifically trained both concentrically and eccentrically, while the scapular stabilizers function to provide a solid base of support. As a baseline of strength is developed, the musculature should be trained in a manner simulating the person's functional activities. The relative percentage of land- or water-based activities depends on the exercise tolerance, pool availability, and the client's goals.

Late Phase

The late phase is used to prepare the person for return to his or her previous level of activity, whether activities of daily living, work, or sport. The baseline of strength obtained in the intermediate phase should be converted to endurance and function in the late phase. Pool activities should replicate activities performed at work or in sport, and traditional lap swimming can be used for additional endurance training. Deep-water running, cycling, or cross-country skiing also use repetitive, resistive arm movements. The principles of progressive, resistive exercise and functional progressions for these injuries are the same as those for hypermobility or hypomobility.

Impairment-Oriented Rehabilitation: Lower Extremity

Ligament Injuries

A variety of soft tissue injuries in the lower extremity can be successfully treated in the pool. Clients with ligament injuries at the knee and ankle enjoy early weight-bearing and proprioceptive activities in the pool, while minimizing weight bearing. If seen acutely, these people can be started in the pool immediately to prevent loss of proprioception and strength. The anterior cruciate ligament (ACL) and medial collateral ligament are two of the more commonly injured ligaments in the knee, whereas the anterior talofibular ligament is commonly sprained at the ankle. Because of its role as a primary stabilizer of the knee during rotational movements, people with ACL injuries often complain of instability episodes. Repeated episodes of instability often lead to secondary medial meniscal tears owing to the posterior horn's role in providing secondary stability.[12] As such, many active people choose ACL reconstruction to stabilize the knee.[13] Rehabilitation of these clients should progress in an orderly and well thought-out course, with the biomechanics of the ligaments and muscular forces as the scientific basis.

Medial collateral ligament injuries result from a valgus stress to the knee. The medial collateral ligament and middle third of the medial capsule comprise the primary restraint to valgus stress at 30 degrees of flexion. Studies evaluating the outcome of surgical versus conservative management of medial collateral ligament injuries demonstrate successful results with nonoperative treatment.[14–16] Regardless of surgical or conservative treatment, rehabilitation should progress through an orderly and planned progression, gradually increasing the forces on the static and dynamic stabilizers of the lower extremity.

Rehabilitation goals after a lower extremity muscle injury include the restoration of normal muscle length, increasing the muscle's ability to produce torque around a joint, and improving the muscle's ability to function in a variety of roles, such as prime mover, static stabilizer, or agonist. These goals should be coordinated to improve the client's functional abilities. Static physiologic stretching, progressive resistive exercises, muscular endurance activities, and functional movement patterns can be initiated and progressed in the pool. Because the person is immersed in a resistive medium, movement in any direction can be resistive, and the resistance is proportional to the surface area and speed of movement.

Clients with ligament injuries, either acutely or postreconstruction, can begin working toward their physical therapy goals earlier in the pool. ACL or posterior cruciate ligament injuries, medial or lateral collateral ligament injuries, and ankle sprains all result in limitations of motion, strength, proprioception, and function that are amenable to exercise in the pool. Goals after ligament injuries include the restoration or normal mobility, control of joint effusion, recovery of muscle function, and return to the previous level of activity. Early weight bearing can be initiated to normalize the gait pattern, to facilitate joint mobility and muscle action, and to train proprioception. Specific restrictions on amount and direction of resistance, appropriate planes of movement, and range of stretching and resistance are determined by the extent and degree of injury or surgery. Other issues, such as the presence of degenerative joint disease, meniscectomy or meniscus repair, varus alignment, or osteochondral lesion, also influence the rehabilitation program.

Tovin and colleagues have compared two groups of people after ACL reconstruction.[17] During postoperative weeks 2 through 8, groups performed a similar set of exercises either on land or in the water. Testing at 8 weeks after surgery demonstrated higher outcomes scores (Lysholm scales) and less effusion in the water group. No differences were noted between groups in passive ROM, thigh girth, or isokinetic/isometric muscle function. As such, the pool may be an effective medium for rehabilitating clients after ACL reconstruction.

Two other factors are important in therapeutic pool exercise for the person with a lower extremity injury. First, the hydrostatic pressure of the water can minimize swelling in an acutely injured lower extremity, thereby allowing the person to exercise while some compression is applied to the joint. The deeper the limb immersion, the greater this benefit.[18] Second, eccentric muscle action is minimized in the pool secondary to the water's buoyancy. As such, the therapist must create exercise programs to enhance eccentric training in the pool. As the rehabilitation program progresses, more time is spent in land-based activities to emphasize eccentric muscle training. The specific types of activities are dictated by the injury, surgery, and stage of healing. Pool exercises throughout the stages of healing should mirror activities on land in terms of kinetics and kinematics. Progression from exercises in one plane should progress to more challenging planes and to multiplane activities. A sample program after ACL reconstruction can be found in Table 5-3.

Early Phase

Rehabilitation goals in the early phase focus on the restoration of normal ROM, normalizing gait, decreasing pain, decreasing effusion, and maintaining strength and proprioception. Simple immersion assists in controlling the lower extremity swelling because of the hydrostatic pressure. The client should be placed in the deep end of the pool with a flotation vest to perform nonweight-bearing exercises. Weight-bearing exercises should be performed in chest-deep water, unless progression of weight bearing is the primary goal, or if the person is fearful of deeper water. Weight bearing in the early phase can enhance proprioceptive ability as well as minimize swelling through muscle contraction. Simple movement through the water along with the relief of weight bearing often decreases pain enough to progress other aspects of the rehabilitation program.

Restoration of ROM is often a goal in the early rehabilitation phase. Increased mobility at the hip, knee, or ankle can be accomplished in the pool in a nonweight-bearing, limited weight-bearing, or full weight-bearing position. A standing squat or lunge can facilitate increases

TABLE 5-3. Example of Pool- and Land-Based Exercise Program After Anterior Cruciate Ligament Reconstruction

Pool Activities	Land Activities
Early Phase	
Ambulation forward/backward in chest-deep water	Weight bearing as tolerated
Seated buoyancy-assisted knee extension	Active/passive ROM
Buoyancy/turbulence-resisted knee flexion	Wall slides
Squats	Toe raises
ROM/physiologic stretching	Bike
Straight leg raising four ways	Balance board
Lateral step-up	
Cross-country skiing in deep end	
Single-leg balance	
Intermediate Phase	
Deep-water running/biking	Squats
Lunges	Lunges
Advanced single-leg balance	Leg press
Prone and supine kicking	Isokinetic exercise
Lap swimming	LE PRE
Resisted knee and hip exercises	
Vertical kicking	
Late Phase	
Impact activities	Continued LE PRE
Continued PRE and cardiovascular conditioning	Running
	Functional progression

ROM, range of motion; LE, lower extremity; PRE, progressive resistance exercises.

in flexion at all lower extremity joints. Flotation devices on the foot can facilitate mobility using buoyancy. For example, sitting with the knee extended and a flotation device on the foot assists knee extension, whereas the opposing knee flexion motion is buoyancy resisted (Fig. 5-14). Flotation devices can also be used in a vertical position, either weight-bearing in the shallow end or nonweight-bearing in the deep end, to facilitate hip mobility in a variety of directions. Standing or sitting knee-to-chest movements can increase flexion of the hip and knee. The steps can be used for sitting stretching activities while still immersed and supported by the water.

Mobility exercises should be combined with activities to maintain or increase the client's proprioceptive abilities. Limited or full weight-bearing exercises such as ambulation, active motion, lunges, single- and double-foot squats, and step-ups assist in the development of proprioception after a soft tissue injury. If full weight bearing is allowed, balance can be challenged by provocative activities in single-leg stance such as contralateral leg swings while weight bearing on the involved extremity.

An essential goal in the early phase is the restoration of normal gait mechanics and movement patterns. People often develop compensatory gait patterns secondary to pain, effusion, or lower extremity strength or motion limitations. Normal gait mechanics can be reinforced in the pool because of the water's physical properties. The chosen water depth should demonstrate a balance between the amount of weight bearing permitted and the resistance from increased surface area when in a deeper immersion. Proper posture should always be emphasized as a component of the gait program to ensure reinforcement of proper movement patterns.

Activities to maintain muscle function should be initiated in the pool in this phase. The therapist must bear in mind the multiple functions of muscle in normal lower extremity activities. Muscles do not exclusively act concentrically as prime movers, but also eccentrically as decelerators and isometrically as stabilizers. Many of the functions can be initiated early in the pool, although eccentric muscle action is difficult to reproduce in deeper water. Resistance to move-

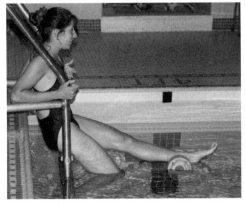

FIGURE 5-14. Buoyancy-assisted knee extension can be performed sitting on a step. This same position can be used for hamstring muscle stretching. Flexion of the knee in this position is buoyancy resisted.

ment is proportional to the surface area and to client effort. The therapist therefore should provide guidance to the person to ensure that safe limits are not exceeded by strength activities that are too vigorous.

Intermediate Phase

Once the acute phase has passed, physical therapy goals emphasize obtaining the final degrees of mobility, increasing the muscle's ability to produce torque, advancing proprioception and balance, and progressing weight bearing. Continued stretching both in the pool and on land is an important activity until full motion is achieved. Progressive resistive exercise for all lower extremity muscle groups should be incorporated into the pool program. The fundamental principles of overload, specificity, exercise to fatigue, and observation for substitution should guide the volume and intensity of exercise.

Determination of which muscle groups should be exercised or emphasized should be based on the injury or surgical procedure and the results of the physical therapy evaluation. Dynamic cocontraction of the hip muscles and the quadriceps and hamstrings across the knee is an important goal in rehabilitation after ligament injuries to the knee, and cocontraction of the invertors and evertors at the ankle is emphasized after ankle ligament injuries. This cocontraction is achieved by closed kinetic chain activities, or by rapid alternating movements in an open chain. Both of these activities can be performed in the pool.

The client should be spending increasing time in land-based, gravity-resisted exercises as the intermediate phase progresses. Emphasis should be on providing progressively difficult activities that challenge the body in areas of deficits. These deficits may be muscular, proprioceptive, or kinesthetic, and many deficits can be addressed with the same activity. New activities can be initiated in the pool before attempting them on land.

Late Phase

The late phase is considered the "fine-tuning" phase, preparing the client for return to full activity. Full motion and nearly full strength are prerequisites for this phase of rehabilitation. The exercise program should progress from single-plane to multiplane activities, with emphasis on the most challenging plane. For the person with

knee or ankle instability, frontal plane or transverse plane movement patterns are more difficult than sagittal plane patterns. A longer lever arm increases the moment arm, allowing additional torque imposition on the static and dynamic joint structures. The lever arm can be lengthened by using a straight leg or by adding fins or other resistive equipment to the foot or to the arms during stabilization exercises.

Impact loading and functional movement patterns can be initiated in the pool during this phase. If shallow water (waist-deep or lower) is used to initiate impact loading, support must be provided for the foot to prevent impact-related injuries. Multiple planes and speeds should be incorporated, including forward and backward walking and running, sidestepping, karioka, and lateral bounding. Plyometric-type activities can also be initiated in the pool, minimizing the amount of impact. Single-leg balance activities can be performed at increasing speed progressively to challenge coordination and balance (see Figs. 5-4 through 5-6).

Most of the rehabilitation program should be performed on land in this phase. However, new activities such as functional work-hardening or sport movement patterns can be initiated and trained in the pool (Fig. 5-15). Often the client participates in a supervised, land-based exercise program 3 days per week, and perform an independent exercise program in the pool on alternate days. A circuit program should be established, incorporating cardiovascular exercise, progressive resistive exercise, proprioceptive challenges, and functional activities.

Other Soft Tissue Dysfunctions

Clients with quadriceps, hamstring, and calf strains or quadriceps contusions can begin rehabilitation acutely in the pool. Buoyancy can be used effectively, first in an assistive role, and progressed to supportive and resistive roles. People with movement dysfunctions such as anterior knee pain, tendinitis, and patellofemoral dysfunction can begin muscular retraining exercises in the pool.

These clients benefit from muscle retraining exercises while minimizing weight bearing. Hip rotation exercises, vastus medialis obliques training, and normalization of movement patterns can be incorporated into exercises at varying water depths. Stretching of shortened tissues in combination with strengthening of length-

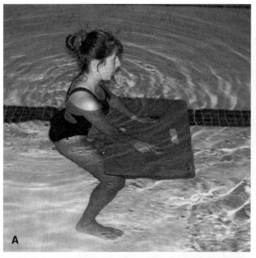
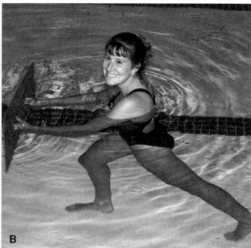
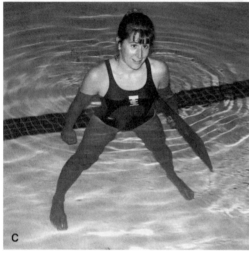

FIGURE 5-15. Functional activities simulated in the pool using a plow. (**A**), Squatting and lifting. (**B**) Pushing and pulling. (**C**) Sidestepping.

ened, weakened muscles while maintaining proper postural alignment can be initiated in the pool while the compressive forces of gravity are minimized.

Treatment of patellofemoral dysfunction requires a thorough evaluation of lower extremity soft tissue and bony relationships, with emphasis on restoration of normal arthrokinematics. Rehabilitation goals include decreased inflammation; restoration of muscular strength, power, endurance, and flexibility; development of proprioceptive abilities; and normalization of patellar mechanics.[19] Taping is often used in the early phase to decrease the client's pain and to assist in further assessment. Subsequently, retraining of the vastus medialis obliques is incorporated to provide medial patellar stabilization. Stretch-

ing of the lateral patellar structures diminishes the lateral patellar compression that is often a component of patellofemoral pain.[20] Most patellofemoral dysfunctions can be treated conservatively, although clients who fail conservative treatment, or who have patellar instability, may qualify for a realignment or stabilization procedure, respectively.[21–23]

Return of muscle function in the lower extremity should begin with normalization of movement patterns, which can be facilitated by limited weight bearing in the pool. However, visualization of mechanics can be inhibited by the refraction in the pool, and the therapist should pay particular attention to proper movement patterns. Demonstration of exercises on land ensures proper mechanics.

Early Phase

The early phase of rehabilitation should focus on restoring any motion loss, maintaining strength and proprioception, and normalization of movement patterns. Activities on land include physiologic stretching, limited weight-bearing proprioceptive activities, isometric muscle exercises, and gait training. Exercises in the pool should include forward walking in chest-deep water, single-leg balance, and physiologic stretching. Muscle training exercises may be incorporated using buoyancy-assisted, supported, or resisted exercises. The exercise planes, ranges, and muscle groups trained are determined by the specific tissue injured and the stage of healing. Active mobility exercises can lubricate articular surfaces and decrease pain. Cardiovascular training may be incorporated, using limited or nonweight-bearing exercises in a variety of directions.

Intermediate Phase

Once nearly full motion has been achieved and movement patterns normalized, the client may be progressed to the intermediate phase. This phase focuses on development of muscle strength and endurance, while continuing to attain the last degrees of motion. Progressive resistive exercises can be performed using buoyancy or turbulence as resistance. Single-plane exercises should be progressed to multiplane, multijoint activities, with increasing resistance and balance challenges. Floats and fins can increase resistance, although increasing the speed of movement is both more challenging and more functional.

Land exercises should progress to full weight-bearing activities as tolerated, with the focus on activities that stress the muscle(s) involved in the injury. Single-plane exercises should be progressed to multiplane activities, and increasing challenge presented to the neuromuscular system. The bicycle, stair-stepper, or cross-country ski machine may be used for cardiovascular and lower extremity endurance training. The therapist should continuously monitor the client for normal posture, including the low back, hip, knee, and foot.

Late Phase

The final rehabilitation phase should fine-tune the person for return to their work, sport, or other leisure activity. Increasing time is spent in land-based exercises owing to limited eccentric work in the pool. Impact exercises may be initiated in the pool and progressed to impact exercises on land, first on a minitramp, and progressing to traditional flooring. The pool makes a good alternate-day exercise medium that may minimize swelling because of hydrostatic pressure, and decrease joint stressing because of buoyancy.

Conditions Associated With Weight-Bearing Limitations

Several conditions throughout the lower extremity result in restrictions in weight bearing. Stress fractures, acute fractures, or the aftermath of total hip, total knee, or tibial osteotomy surgeries are all situations that often result in some period of restricted weight bearing. Degenerative joint disease, osteochondral lesions, meniscectomy, and rheumatoid arthritis are all conditions that can benefit from exercise with reduced weight bearing. Limited weight bearing using buoyancy can be initiated early to prevent atrophy and motion loss, and abnormal movement pattern development. Harrison and coworkers studied the amount of weight bearing that occurred during static stance and slow and fast walking, and found that fast walking can increase weight bearing in the pool by as much as 76%.[3] Static immersion to the anterior-superior iliac spine results in approximately 50% to 75% weight bearing, whereas immersion to the xiphoid process and C7 limits weight bearing to 25% to 50% and 0% to 25%, respectively.[3] The appropriate level of weight bearing is determined by the specific condition and medical considerations.

Early Phase

When initiating weight bearing, the water depth is determined by the percentage of weight bearing allowed, the anticipated speed of ambulation, and the client's comfort in the water. If the client is uncomfortable in deeper water, shallow water in combination with a flotation belt can be used to limit weight bearing. If no weight bearing is allowed, the deep end can be used to exercise the lower extremity and cardiovascular system. Deep-water striding, bicycling, cross-country skiing, or resistive exercises can be incorporated into a circuit training program to provide a balanced strength, ROM, and cardiovascular conditioning program.

The primary goal in this phase is to restore normal gait mechanics, including proper heelstrike, weight transfer, knee and hip flexion, and knee extension. Gait mechanics are often altered because of pain, muscle tightness or weakness, joint effusion, or habit. Proper posture along with appropriate mechanics reinforce correct movement patterns, and make the transition to land-based gait activities easier. As such, activities used to train gait and posture on land can be incorporated into the pool. A ballet bar along the side of the pool can be used for balance. The use of aqua socks or shoes diminishes irritation on the plantar surface of the foot. Ambulation using varying stride lengths should be alternated with activities to restore ROM throughout the lower extremity joints.

Mobility exercises should emphasize the ROM necessary to achieve normal gait and to facilitate normal arthrokinematics. Passive physiologic stretching can be performed in standing or sitting on steps or a bench. Active mobility exercises should be incorporated using the principle of buoyancy and increasing lever arms. For example, a buoyant ankle cuff used in a vertical or sitting position with the hip at 90° facilitates passive knee extension and hip flexion.

Intermediate Phase

The primary goal in the intermediate phase is increased endurance in gait. Once the client has been progressed to full weight bearing and can demonstrate proper gait mechanics, increasing the time of ambulation facilitates increases in endurance. Walking exercises can be performed in varying water depths depending on the client's tolerance to weight bearing. Ambulation at faster speeds can be alternated with side-stepping, crossovers, and backward walking. As always, normal gait patterns and proper posture should be emphasized. If jogging is a goal for the client, this activity should be initiated in the pool during this phase. Pool activities at the end of the intermediate phase should begin to resemble the activity to which the client will be returning; the time, repetitions, distance, and movement patterns should resemble those appropriate to the client's recreational, work, or sport activities.

Other goals in the intermediate phase are the restoration of full motion and return of muscle function. The multiple functions of muscle throughout the gait cycle and during other functional activities, such as stair climbing, form the basis for conditioning exercises. Concentric, eccentric, and isometric functions should be trained in various ranges, joint positions, and movement patterns. Increasing the length of the lever arm, the surface area, and speed of movement can increase the exercise challenge. Resistive exercises for the hip musculature, quadriceps, hamstrings, and calf muscles should be progressed from single-plane to multiplane movement patterns.

Rehabilitation exercises on land should mirror those exercises performed in the pool. Physiologic stretching, open kinetic chain strengthening, and closed kinetic chain (partial weight-bearing) exercises should be performed on a daily basis. The therapist must bear in mind the effects of exercise on the involved tissues. Shear forces across the joint surfaces, meniscal loading, and articular cartilage loading result from both open and closed kinetic chain exercises. Judgments about which exercises are appropriate given the location and extent of injury must be made about exercises in the pool as well as on land.

Late Phase

The late phase of weight bearing is a progression to full weight bearing on land. The amount of time spent in land-based activities should increase as this phase progresses. The pool provides an adjunct to land-based activities, and the principles of rehabilitation follow those in the late phase of soft tissue injuries. Impact loading, plyometric-type exercises, and functional activities can be initiated in the pool. The hydrostatic pressure of the water can control swelling as these activities are initiated. The person with a weight-bearing injury should complete a functional progression before returning to full activity, whether it is work or sport.

❑ CASE STUDY 5-1

TD is a 17-year-old, right-hand dominant football player who sustained two left shoulder anterior and inferior glenohumeral dislocations. He underwent a capsulolabral reconstruction and presented 2 weeks after surgery for initiation on a rehabilitation program. Passive ROM was from 0 to 50 degrees flexion, 0 to 64 degrees abduction, 0 to 23 degrees internal rotation, and 0 degrees of external rotation in neutral abduction. Strength was grossly diminished throughout. Rehabilitation goals for motion in the early phase consisted of increasing shoulder flexion and abduction from 0° to 90°, and internal rotation motion from 0 to 80 degrees. Strength goals included increased isometric strength in all directions in neutral position to 70% maximum voluntary contraction without pain. The proprioceptive goal was the ability to elevate the humerus within the available range using normal scapulohumeral rhythm. TD was initiated on buoyancy-assisted shoulder flexion and abduction in a vertical position. As he tolerated, the assistance was increased by use of a buoyant bell. Internal rotation mobility was increased by passively attempting to reach behind his back while in the pool. Supine Bad Ragaz techniques were used to increase mobility in shoulder abduction. TD was then required to contract his shoulder adductors to prevent abduction beyond 90 degrees. These mobility exercises were paralleled by passive and active-assisted mobilization exercises on land. Isometric strengthening was accomplished by walking against the resistance of the water with the arm in varying positions of flexion and abduction, and by moving in different planes. The wall of the pool was also used for isometric resistance. Normalization of scapulohumeral rhythm was accomplished by using buoyancy-assisted elevation to reduce the amount of muscle force necessary to achieve elevation. This resulted in normal elevation without pain.

Motion goals in the intermediate phase included the restoration of full motion, with flexion, abduction, and internal rotation as the primary goals, and the return of external rotation progressing last.

Strength goals included the development of a strength base and ability to produce pain-free torque about the shoulder joint in all directions, using normal movement patterns. Buoyancy-assisted exercises progressed to the prone position with a flotation bell to facilitate full overhead flexion and abduction as well as external rotation in varying degrees of abduction. These exercises paralleled land-based stretching exercises in supine. Strength exercises were performed with buoyancy as resistance in standing for shoulder extension and in prone for shoulder internal rotation at 90 degrees abduction. Resistive exercises for the entire shoulder girdle, including the scapular stabilizers, were incorporated using turbulence as resistance. Gloves and paddles were the primary means of increasing surface area and turbulence. Emphasis was placed on the rotator cuff and scapular stabilizers. Closed-chain exercises were initiated against the side of the pool. Progressive resistive exercises on land emphasized the same goals, and were accomplished with light weights, exercising in nonprovocative positions.

The final phase focused on increasing strength, dynamic cocontraction, and motor control in increasingly provocative positions. Rapid alternating movements in the pool in provocative positions

gave TD the opportunity to control the force loads. As he became increasingly comfortable with training in overhead positions (primarily in prone), he increased the speed of movement, thereby increasing the turbulence and force production. Additional closed-chain exercises were incorporated in prone, using the side of the pool for resistance. These activities paralleled provocative and plyometric activities on land, including ball tosses and push-up exercises. Caution must be exercised when training a person in a provocative position in the pool, owing to the relaxation and risk of dislocation in the pool. At postoperative week 24, TD was discharged to full activity.

❏ CASE STUDY 5-2

PG is a 35-year-old truck driver who slipped while at work, sustaining a hyperextension injury to his right knee. The hyperextension resulted in a complete ACL tear, posterior horn of the medial meniscus tear, and a large osteochondral lesion on the medial femoral condyle. He underwent an initial arthroscopic partial meniscectomy and debridement. He was not referred to physical therapy and contracted a secondary arthrofibrosis requiring another surgical procedure. He was then referred to physical therapy for ROM and strengthening activities. On exam, PG had motion from 0° to 120° of flexion, poor quadriceps tone, a flexed knee gait, and a positive Lachman's test. Physical therapy goals were the normalization of gait, increased mobility of the knee joint, and increased strength throughout the lower extremity.

The early phase of rehabilitation consisted nearly exclusively of exercises in the pool. Passive stretching to increase ROM was paralleled with stretching exercises on land. A great deal of time was spent trying to normalize gait and to decrease pain with weight bearing. Gait activities included walking at differing stride lengths, in different directions, at varying depths, and at different speeds. Lunges, bilateral squats, and stepping-in-place exercises were incorporated to facilitate proper mechanics. Strengthening exercises in the early phase were primarily open kinetic chain owing to the pain and substitution that occurred with closed kinetic chain activities.

The intermediate phase focused on increasing endurance in gait. The two components of this were PG's muscle endurance as well as the joint surface's tolerance to loading. As fibrocartilage developed at the osteochondral lesion, progressive loading was incorporated to assist in the remodeling of the newly formed tissue. PG was still unable fully to weight-bear normally in a gravity environment, although his range of weight bearing was improved and progressing. Full passive ROM had been achieved, but episodes of instability, both weight bearing and shifting while nonweight bearing, hindered progress. Multiplane, closed-chain stability exercises were initiated in the pool in gradually decreasing depths of water. Land-based exercises consisted of controlled closed-chain and open-chain progressive resistive exercises. The addition of a functional knee brace diminished the number of instability episodes, allowing increased activity with less pain.

The final phase of PG's program focused on decreasing the amount of time spent in the pool and increasing the amount of land-based exercise time. He experienced many setbacks resulting from too much activity producing a knee effusion. Pool activities were increased and land-based activities decreased during these times to minimize weight bearing and to use the hydrostatic pressure in the control of swelling. Currently PG is participating in an independent pool program on a maintenance basis and a maintenance progressive resistive exercise program at a health club, and has regular follow-ups for reevaluation and progression. He may be undergoing an ACL reconstruction in the future if episodes of instability continue at the present rate.

Summary

Aquatic rehabilitative exercises provide an opportunity to train in a gravity-minimized environment while being immersed in a resistive medium. Any motion can be resistive given adequate surface area and speed of movement. Movements can also be supported, assisted, or resisted by buoyancy. The choice of specific exercises is based on the injury or disease, the physical evaluation, and the client's goals. Exercises should be coordinated with the land-based program and should be progressed simultaneously. Weight bearing, resistance, repetitions, and pattern complexity can all be increased easily in the pool. The pool provides a rich environment both for primary rehabilitation techniques and as an adjunct to a land-based exercise program.

REFERENCES

1. Arnoczky S, Adams M, DeHaven K, et al. Meniscus. In: Woo SLY, Buckwalter JA, eds. *Injury and Repair of the Musculoskeletal Soft Tissues*. Rosemont, Ill: American Academy of Orthopaedic Surgeons; 1988: 487–538.
2. Mow V, Rosewasser M. Articular cartilage: biomechanics. In: Woo SLY, Buckwalter JA, eds. Injury and

Repair of the Musculoskeletal Soft Tissues. Rosemont, Ill: American Academy of Orthopaedic Surgeons; 1988:427–464.
3. Harrison RA, Hillman M, Bulstrode S. Loading of the lower limb when walking partially immersed. *Physiotherapy*. 1992;78:164–166.
4. Zelko RR, DePalma BF. Stress fractures in athletes: diagnosis and treatment. *Forum Medicus*. 1986:3–15.
5. Voight ML, Draovitch P. Plyometrics. In: Albert M, ed. *Eccentric Muscle Training in Sports and Orthopaedics*. New York, NY: Churchill Livingstone; 1991: 45–74.
6. Wilder RP, Brennan D, Schotte DE. A standard measure for exercise prescription for aqua running. *Am J Sports Med*. 1993;21:45–47.
7. Yamaji K, Greenley M, Northey DR, Hughson RL. Oxygen uptake and heart rate responses to treadmill and water running. *Can J Spts Sci*. 1990;15(2):96–98.
8. Mathews DK, Fox EL. *The Physiological Basis of Physical Education and Athletics*. Philadelphia, Pa: WB Saunders; 1976.
9. Matsen FA, Thomas SC, Rockwood CA. Anterior glenohumeral instability. In: Rockwood CA, Matsen FA, eds. *The Shoulder*. Philadelphia, Pa: WB Saunders; 1990:526–622.
10. Rockwood CA, Young DC. Disorders of the acromioclavicular joint. In: Rockwood CA, Matsen FA, eds. The Shoulder. Philadelphia: WB Saunders; 1990: 413–476.
11. Neer CS. Anterior acromioplasty for the chronic impingement syndrome in the shoulder. *J Bone Joint Surg [Am]*. 1972;54:41–50.
12. Fu FH, Thompson WO. Biomechanics and kinematics of meniscus. In: Finerman GAM, Noyes FR, eds. *Biology and Biomechanics of the Traumatized Synovial Joint: The Knee as a Model*. Rosemont, Ill: American Academy of Orthopaedic Surgeons; 1992: 153–184.
13. Buckley SL, Barrack RL, Alexander AH. The natural history of conservatively treated partial anterior cruciate ligament tears. *Am J Sports Med*. 1989;17: 221–225.
14. Burroughs P, Dahners LE. The effect of enforced exercise on the healing of ligament injuries. *Am J Sports Med*. 1990;18:376–378.
15. Vailas AC, Tipton CM, Matthes RD, et al. Physical activity and its influence on the repair process of medial collateral ligaments. *Connect Tissue Res*. 1981;9: 25–31.
16. Woo SL, Inoue M, McGurk-Burleson E, et al. Treatment of the medial collateral ligament injury: II. structure and function of canine knees in response to differing treatment regimens. *Am J Sports Med*. 1987;15: 22–29.
17. Tovin BJ, Wolf SL, Greenfield BH, et al. Comparison of the effects of exercise in water and on land on the rehabilitation of patients with intra-articular anterior cruciate ligament reconstructions. *Phys Ther*. 1994; 74:710–719.
18. Risch WD, Koubenec HJ, Beckmann U, Lange S, Gauer OH. The effect of graded immersion on heart volume, central venous pressure, pulmonary blood distribution, and heart rate in man. *Pflugers Arch*. 1978;374:115–118.
19. Griffin LY. Rehabilitation of the knee extensor mechanism. In: Fox JM, Del Pizzo W, eds. *The Patellofemoral Joint*. New York, NY: McGraw-Hill, Inc; 1993: 279–290.

20. Merchant AC. The lateral patellar compression syndrome. In: Fox JM, Del Pizzo W, eds. *The Patellofemoral Joint*. New York, NY: McGraw-Hill, Inc; 1993: 157–168.

21. Ferkel RD. Lateral retinacular release. In: Fox JM, Del Pizzo W, eds. *The Patellofemoral Joint*. New York, NY: McGraw-Hill, Inc; 1993:309–324.

22. Friedman MJ. Tibial tubercle transfer technique. In: Fox JM, Del Pizzo W, eds. *The Patellofemoral Joint*. New York, NY: McGraw-Hill, Inc; 1993:325–332.

23. Singer KM, Isham M, Helpenstell T. Tibial tubercle elevation. In: Fox JM, Del Pizzo W, eds. *The Patellofemoral Joint*. New York, NY: McGraw-Hill, Inc; 1993:333–334.

6

Aquatic Rehabilitation of Clients With Musculoskeletal Conditions of the Spine

Christine McNamara and Lori Thein

Rehabilitation of spinal injuries is a constantly progressing area of physical therapy. Postural dysfunctions, chronic pain from sprain and strain, and discogenic pain are just a few of the most commonly reported spinal injuries. With 8 of every 10 people experiencing some form of back pain in their lifetime,[1] the focus on recovery from a spinal injury is expanding to include prevention as well as improved levels of physical fitness. Aquatic exercise allows for strengthening of the trunk and supporting musculature without the potentially harmful effects of impact. Cardiovascular training can be carried out in deep water virtually impact free.

This chapter discusses the implications of using aquatic exercise in the treatment of various spinal injuries and provides guidelines for the integration of these exercises into the total rehabilitation program. Included in these guidelines is the transition from aquatic to land-based activity, as the client progresses through the rehabilitation program.

This chapter is divided into goal-oriented and impairment-oriented sections. The goal-oriented section provides information regarding sample aquatic exercises and techniques to achieve goals in the areas of posture, flexibility, strength, endurance, and function. These exercises and techniques are meant to be guidelines only, and are therefore self-limiting. Information in the impairment-oriented section includes a brief discussion of pathologic processes, and the specific needs of the client and how they will be addressed by aquatic therapy. Reference

from the goal-oriented to the impairment-oriented section will be helpful in completing a sample aquatic program for a client.

As with all physical therapy treatment options, proper client selection for the aquatic program is critical. The client's willingness to participate in and remain committed to the aquatic program is as crucial as proper exercise prescription and program use. Because many clients with spinal injuries have ongoing pain, client education is critical. This fosters independence because it ensures that the client not only performs exercises correctly, but understands why each exercise is beneficial. Return to normal function and prevention of further incidence of pain are ultimately the goals for all clients. Where aquatic exercise falls in the total rehabilitation process in achieving these goals is determined by the therapist and is based on the client's needs and abilities. Aquatic exercise can also be incorporated into the daily fitness program of the client who has completed the rehabilitation process, providing an alternative to impact activities.

Goal-Oriented Rehabilitation

Activities to Improve Posture

Kendall and associates state that "ideal skeletal alignment . . . is consistent with sound scientific principles, involves a minimal amount of stress and strain, and is conducive to maximal efficiency of the body."[2] All spinal injuries, therefore, have a postural or alignment component. Many injuries of the upper and lower extremities can be attributed in part to postural problems as well. Postural education should begin with the first visit to the pool and should be reviewed and progressed regularly. Any postural education and strengthening program, aquatic or land based, should include total spinal alignment and proper posture. An understanding of the normal curvature of the spine and the function that it serves is the basis from which all future postural education is built. Basic instruction in the normal cervical and lumbar lordosis and thoracic kyphosis is the cornerstone of this knowledge. Initially, the aquatic specialist may find it useful to assist the client, with instruction and physical cueing if necessary, in performing total spinal alignment on the deck, before getting into the water (Fig. 6-1). As the client becomes more skilled in establishing proper posture, this quick alignment check at the beginning of each aquatic session reinforces movement from a

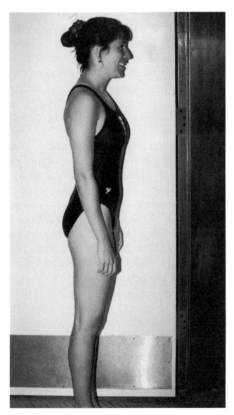

FIGURE 6-1. Practicing total spinal alignment on the deck as a precursor to aquatic activities that will challenge proper posture.

proper postural base. In addition, total spinal alignment is a prerequisite skill for lumbar stabilization and abdominal and other postural muscle strengthening.

The unique properties of the water produce a *reduced gravity environment* that provides the *opportunity* for resistance at any point in the range of motion (ROM), and in all directions of movement. A clear understanding of proper posture and its importance in prevention and recovery is the most valuable tool for the therapist teaching and treating the spine-injured client.

Postural strengthening activities performed in the water are subtle. Rarely do they involve large-amplitude motion or exertion of maximal force. Most often, postural strengthening exercises emphasize control, technique, and proper postural alignment. The therapist designing and implementing a postural education and strengthening program needs to ensure that the client understands that postural changes will not be achieved quickly, nor will they remain without consistent work. These basic principles of postural training are no different when applied to aquatic exercise.

The following section includes a progression of postural strengthening exercises. This progression should serve as a model from which the reader can develop other postural exercises and progressions. In designing and implementing such programs, the aquatic specialist should remember that although they are common, it is not only lumbar spine injuries or dysfunctions that require postural training as part of the rehabilitation process. Any *functional activity* that is more effectively performed from a sound postural base is enhanced also.

With a clear understanding of proper postural alignment, the client may now move on to pelvic control. Kendall and associates describe the neutral position of the pelvis in proper posture as a position in which the anterior–superior iliac spines are in the same horizontal plane, and the anterior–superior iliac spines and the symphysis pubis are in the same vertical plane.[2] Proper spinal alignment, or neutral spine, provides greater stability to the spine,[2,3] while using the ligamentous and muscular systems to stabilize and control it.[2,3] Kendall and associates further state that the "position of the pelvis is the key to good or faulty postural alignment." For many clients, pelvic control begins with instruction in a posterior pelvic tilt. Initially, this is most easily performed with the client leaning back against the side of the pool, knees forward and slightly bent. Cueing from the therapist can be provided by palpating the lower rectus abdominis. The purpose of this portion of the exercise is for the client to "locate" and facilitate contraction of the lower abdominal musculature. Once the client can consistently control a posterior pelvic tilt against the wall, the exercise is moved to a free-standing position. Repeated pelvic tilts are then performed in the standing position with the knees slightly bent. Execution of this motion in the standing position should be accomplished with as little trunk motion as is necessary. Pelvic tilts can initially be used as an isolated lower abdominal strengthening exercise, as described earlier. Further along in the postural strengthening program, however, a posterior pelvic tilt can be used by the client as part of a spinal alignment check between bouts of more aggressive exercise. Conversely, for the client who enters the aquatic program with a flattened lumbar lordosis, instruction and practice in an anterior pelvic tilt is necessary. This client should be positioned perpendicular to the side of the pool so the therapist can physically cue anteriorly and posteriorly as necessary. During this exercise, it is important for the therapist to monitor (1) motion occurring at the pelvis and lumbar spine, and not the hip or knees; and (2) maintenance of proper postural alignment in the other segments of the spine. Once the client has consistently demonstrated the ability to move the pelvis into the desired (deficient) direction, smooth, full ROM from the anterior to posterior position and back again should be practiced. This provides the basis for learning neutral spine.

Achieving and maintaining a neutral spine is not only a strengthening activity for abdominal musculature, but a prerequisite skill for all movement and position changes. Early efforts at achieving a neutral spine are most successful with the client in chest-deep water and receiving physical cueing from the therapist at the lumbosacral junction posteriorly and the lower abdominals anteriorly. The therapist can use a variety of methods of instruction in achieving neutral spine with supplemental verbal and physical cueing. One effective method is to instruct the client to begin in a full posterior pelvic tilt position, move to a full anterior pelvic tilt position, and then select a position of comfort between those two as neutral spine. This activity is progressed from having the client *hold* the therapist-assisted neutral spine position, to the client

achieving neutral spine and holding it unassisted. From here, the client is instructed to maintain neutral spine while executing other exercises such as squats, toe raises, and upper extremity and trunk strengthening. Practicing neutral spine consistently throughout the aquatic exercise program both reinforces total spinal alignment and strengthens the muscles needed to achieve it.

Proper posture is reinforced through all warm-up, strengthening, and cool-down activities, as well as in all functional activities. Simple forward walking in the water allows the client ample opportunity to practice proper posture. For the client just learning total spinal alignment and performing a walking exercise, it may be necessary to stop every 20 to 30 feet to perform a realignment check. Again, physical cueing from the therapist may be necessary at each of these breaks. Normal gait is essential in this type of activity; because walking in water feels very different from walking on land, "normal" gait itself may require additional instruction from the therapist. For example, the most common mistake in a forward-walking exercise is for the client to allow the arms to float on the surface of the water, rather than in a reciprocal arm swing, as they do on land. In learning, practicing, and strengthening total spinal alignment, the client learns to move, change positions, and alter effort while maintaining proper posture.

Stabilization exercises are of significant importance to the spine-injured client. These exercises, also referred to as dynamic stabilization exercises, are designed to develop muscle patterns that stabilize the spine in the neutral position.[4] In their 1989 study on nonoperative treatment of herniated intervertebral discs, Saal and Saal identified the need for stabilization training to achieve adequate dynamic control of lumbar spine forces to eliminate repetitive injury to the intervertebral discs, facet joints, and related structures.[4] Furthermore, proper stabilization of the spine provides the necessary support for more complex and challenging activities. Whether the existing injury is muscular or bony, postural or traumatic, strengthening of the proximal musculature improves the overall quality and effectiveness of the total rehabilitation program. It also serves to reduce the chance of reinjury. Stabilization exercises of the spine may be introduced earlier in the treatment plan when performed in the water, because of the unloading effect buoyancy has on the spine.[5] These types of exercises can be performed statically or dynamically, with or without equipment. The range of exercises that facilitate stabilization of the spine is broad. Some stabilization exercises have been previously discussed in this section: pelvic tilts and neutral spine, for example. Abdominal strengthening exercises, discussed later in this chapter, are stabilization exercises as well. Any activity or exercise that challenges proper spinal alignment or strengthens the muscles that promote this alignment are considered stabilization exercises.

Forward, backward, and sideways walking become spinal stabilization exercises when the client is asked to maintain correct posture while executing them. Increasing the speed of these exercises increases the stabilization effort required. Adding equipment, such as a resistance board or aqua gloves, to a walking exercise (in any direction) further increases the difficulty. Equipment selection should be goal specific. For example, aqua gloves may be used to challenge thoracic and lower cervical paraspinal and trunk musculature by increasing the load placed on these muscles, as well as adding an additional challenge to maintaining proper posture. Using a resistance board when walking focuses strengthening on the abdominals, lower extremities, and lower trunk musculature (Fig. 6-2). For the client working on strengthening spinal musculature, both of these exercises and pieces of equipment may be appropriate. Exercises that challenge the trunk to remain motionless and the spine in proper alignment while the extremi-

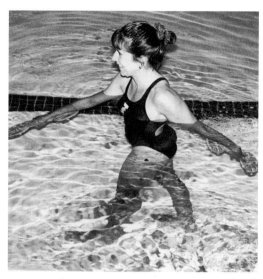

FIGURE 6-3. Spinal stabilization exercises: trunk strengthening with paddles.

ties are moving are effective in improving skill and strength in stabilization. In chest-deep water, an exercise of this type is performed with the client standing with good posture, one foot comfortably in front of the other, and knees slightly bent. From this position, the client performs reciprocal shoulder flexion and extension, with as much speed or force as possible, while continuing to maintain proper posture. To make this exercise more difficult, the client may wear gloves or use paddles (Fig. 6-3). In deep water, a similar goal is accomplished with a cross-country skiing-type exercise in which a reciprocal leg swing is added to the arm swing. In this instance, equipment can be added to the upper or lower extremities, or both.

Unilateral strengthening activities are also beneficial in improving stabilization of the spine. A unilateral hip abduction–adduction exercise strengthens the abductors–adductors on the moving side, as well as the hip flexors, extensors, and abductors–adductors on the standing side. In addition, the trunk musculature in general undergoes a strengthening activity in resisting lateral flexion. Exercises that require single-leg stance are ideal stabilization exercises for the lower extremity required to bear the weight. Unilateral shoulder abduction through full ROM requires stabilization of the trunk in resisting lateral flexion. Early in this exercise, the trunk is supported by buoyancy; as resistance is added to the motion, the trunk must work more independently. As each example, upper and lower

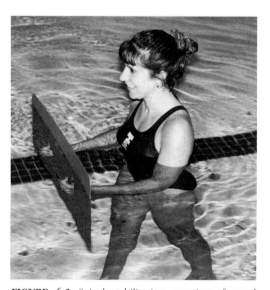

FIGURE 6-2. Spinal stabilization exercises: forward walking with a resistance board.

extremity, demonstrates, these types of exercises strengthen both the moving and the stationary sides. Proprioceptive neuromuscular facilitation (PNF) patterns of the upper and lower extremities require motion of the extremity and support for the motion by the trunk and proximal musculature. PNF exercises add further challenge because they cross planes of motion and include rotations.

Morgan states that dynamic spinal stabilization, or maintaining a neutral position, is a complex neuromuscular skill requiring fine adjustments in muscle tension in response to fluctuating loads.[6] Advanced stabilization exercises provide a more dynamic challenge. An efficient method of achieving this with variety is to begin with the client sitting on a kickboard (Fig. 6-4). The initial skill required of this activity is the ability to balance while sitting on the kickboard with good upright posture. Increasing the length of time balancing in this position is the first progression of the challenge. As the client progresses in strength, skill, and balance, additional challenges may be attempted: small anterior and posterior pelvic tilts, gentle flexion and extension of one leg, then reciprocally with both legs, movement of the arms in any direction or pattern away from the trunk, rotation and sidebending motions of the trunk, and combination upper and lower extremity movements. The variety in this type of activity makes it an effective and enjoyable strengthening exercise.

As with any type of goal-oriented rehabilita-

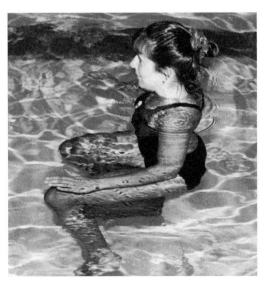

FIGURE 6-4. Advanced spinal stabilization exercises: balancing on a kickboard.

tion, the therapist may also find it useful to focus on particular muscle groups in achieving proper spinal stabilization. The trunk muscles function to stabilize the thorax, pelvis, and spine for movements of the head and extremities, to maintain posture, and to provide dynamic control against the force of gravity as movement shifts away from the base of support.[3] Some of the more important muscle groups are highlighted here. The *thoracolumbar fascia* covers the deep muscles of the back of the trunk, dividing the muscles of the back and posterior abdominal region. It passes anterior to the serratus posterior superior and is continuous with the superficial lamina of the deep cervical fascia on the back of the neck.[7,8] In the thoracic region, the thoracolumbar fascia is a thin, fibrous lamina covering the extensor muscles of the vertebral column and separating them from the muscles connecting the vertebral column to the upper extremity.[8] In the lumbar region it is found in three layers: (1) attached posteriorly to the spines of the lumbar and sacral vertebrae and to the supraspinous ligaments; (2) attached in the middle to the transverse processes of the lumbar vertebrae, the iliac crest, and the lower border of the 12th rib; and (3) attached anteriorly to the transverse process of the lumbar vertebrae and the iliolumbar ligament.[7,8] This diamond-shaped fascial network is a large stabilizing structure of the spine, providing support for the translation of forces from the lower extremities to the spine (and vice versa) and, when tightened, prevents a flexion moment.[3] Strengthening of the internal and external obliques and hip extensors and abductors, as well as the lumbar extensors, supplements the support of the thoracolumbar fascia.

The *erector spinae*, or sacrospinalis, form a longitudinal series, extending from the sacrum to the skull.[9] This strong stabilizing muscle group begins at the sacrum and thickens as it ascends along the lumbar spine.[8,9] At approximately the level of the last rib, it separates into three columns that ascend the back of the chest, inserting into the ribs and vertebrae.[9] The medial column of the three consists of slips extending between the upper lumbar and upper thoracic spines, continuing with extensions into the neck.[8–10] The large, long, intermediate group comprises the bulk of the erector spinae.[9] It extends from the upper lumbar vertebrae to the transverse processes of the thoracic and cervical vertebrae (C3–C6). An additional portion of the longissimus has been described, extending from the ilium to the transverse processes of the lumbar vertebrae.[9] The direction of the erector spinae and its subdivisions is chiefly upward, with the longissimus and the splenius also extending laterally.[9] This muscular network is primarily responsible for postural support, and eccentric trunk flexion[3] provides the trunk with a posterior strut of stability to work with the anterior strut provided by the abdominals. Maintaining proper posture is an early form of erector spinae strengthening. Advanced strengthening is addressed efficiently with deep-water exercise such as vertical kicking and cross-country skiing. The *psoas*, which extends from the transverse processes of the lumbar vertebrae to the lesser trochanter of the femur, provides additional support in the translation of forces from the lower extremities to the spine, and is easily incorporated into the aquatic strengthening program. Shallow-water activities such as forward walking, high-step marching, and forward and lateral lunges all work the hip flexors. Deep-water walking, jogging, and cycling work the hip flexors in an unloaded fashion. Because of its lumbar spine attachments, the psoas also increases the flexion forces on the lumbar spine (A. Cole, MD, personal communication, June, 1995).[3] Therefore, caution should be exercised when having the client with acute low back pain work hip flexion (A. Cole, MD, personal communication, June, 1995). The *trapezius* (*upper, middle*, and *lower fibers*) extends from the ligamentum nuchae and spinous processes of C7 and T1 to the acromion process and spine of the scapula, and provides postural support to the cervical and thoracic spine, as well as the scapulae.[10] As with other postural muscles, strength of the trapezius is first facilitated through proper posture. Further strengthening of the trapezius is performed with the client in neck-deep water, sitting or standing. Shoulder shrugs, shoulder circles, and scapular retraction all work the various fibers of the trapezius; each of these exercises can be increased in difficulty by adding aqua gloves, paddles, or weights.

Abdominal strengthening should begin early in the aquatic exercise experience. Having the client perform pelvic tilts and maintain neutral spine while working in the water promotes early-phase lower abdominal strengthening. Once the client can control neutral spine, it is safe to progress to more aggressive abdominal strengthening. It is important, however, that the client not deviate from neutral spine as the abdominal strengthening process progresses. Awareness of spinal position and proper posture needs to be an ongoing, *active* component

of the aquatic program. The next phase of strengthening exercises for lower abdominals consists of one- and two-legged bent-knee lifts to 90 degrees of hip flexion. The starting point for each exercise should be neutral spine; if necessary, the progression described in neutral spine should be reviewed. The mechanism for strengthening is that of the abdominals resisting anterior pelvic tilt as the hip flexes.[11] Therefore, the exercise is useful as an abdominal strengthening exercise only if the client can maintain a posterior pelvic tilt.[11] The client is progressed in this exercise from shallow to deep water, and from bent-knee lifts to single and double straight leg lifts. Other methods of progressing abdominal strengthening exercises are (1) adding weight to the lower extremity, first proximally (just above the knee) and moving it distally (to the ankle); (2) adding resistance to motion in any direction through use of a resistance board while continuing to require the client to maintain neutral spine; and (3) from a vertical flotation position in neutral spine (with or without the assistance of flotation dumbbells) in deep water, performing any or all of a series of exercises: single- and double-leg bent-knee lifts (as described earlier), single and double straight leg raises (to 90 degrees hip flexion), and a straight leg scissoring motion performed in the sagittal and coronal planes.

Internal and external oblique strengthening is achieved by performing a bent-knee lift to 90 degrees of hip flexion and rotating the legs right and left in the transverse plane. The neutral spine position is a requirement throughout this exercise as well. In shallow water, this exercise is progressed by adding weight or surface area to the moving leg, or by having the client perform the exercise free standing as opposed to leaning against the side of the pool. In deep water, the exercise begins with the client's back against the side of the pool, legs fully extended, and spine in neutral. The exercise is then progressed from single to double leg, as described earlier. In deep water, it may also be progressed to a free-floating execution with the assistance of flotation dumbbells.

Upper abdominal strengthening can also be performed in a variety of ways, but is most effectively addressed by instructing the client in proper trunk control and spinal alignment, as described earlier. Increasing and adding resistance to upper extremity motion while walking in any direction challenges the upper abdominals to maintain trunk alignment and control. The use of aqua gloves, paddles, and the like

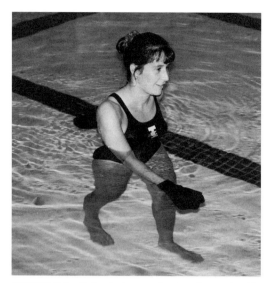

FIGURE 6-5. Abdominal strengthening: forward walking with upper extremity resistance.

adds resistance but still allows normal motion to occur (Fig. 6-5). The popular abdominal exercise known as "crunches" is performed in the water by having the client float supine with flotation dumbbells under the knees or feet, and curling forward, clearing the upper portion of the scapulae. The arms can be placed at the side for balance or across the chest as strength improves. This activity requires more trunk control when performed in water compared with land because the water does not provide a firm surface to return to after each repetition. Upper abdominal strengthening is achieved in deep water by adding a resistive component to the upper extremity motion of any cardiovascular activity.

Some pointers for the therapist to bear in mind when instructing and checking technique of abdominal strengthening are (1) monitor speed of movement; do not allow quick motion unless the exercise is designed as such; (2) check for compensation by low back musculature or Valsalva maneuver; and (3) neutral spine/total spinal alignment should be carried over to land-based activity—abdominal and otherwise.

Activities to Increase Range of Motion and Flexibility

Range of motion and flexibility exercises are performed safely and easily in the water. The unloading effect provided by buoyancy and the

increase in superficial circulation through water temperature, laminal flow, and hydrostatic pressure combine to provide an environment of support and general muscular relaxation.[5] This support also helps to decrease potential for muscle guarding. For the spine-injured client, the increased mobility afforded by the properties of water increases the likelihood for pain-free movement into ROMs that on land would likely be painful. Consid[...] specialist designing ROM [...] cises for these clients shou[...] they do not overstretch [...] should rarely push into p[...] ROM and flexibility exerci[...] should they be extremely so[...] is completed. All of the basic [...] proper land-based ROM and flexibility exercises should be followed when performing them in the water.

As part of the postural education program, both ROM and flexibility exercises are addressed at each session. Although the ultimate goal of these exercises is improved posture, many clients need to achieve sufficient ROM or flexibility first. The client with a reduced lumbar lordosis, for example, is not able to achieve neutral spine properly until lumbar extension ROM and hamstring flexibility are improved first. In this case, hamstring stretches and anterior pelvic tilts may be components of the warm-up activities (Fig. 6-6). Because proper posture is a goal for most spine-injured clients, a complete ROM and flexibility program should address all relevant structures. This list can range from appropriate gastrocnemius/soleus and hamstring flexibility to adequate segmental motion of the spine. As often as possible, ROM and flexibility exercises should be incorporated into other aquatic activities. A forward-walking exercise, for example, with focus on proper posture, can also include emphasis on proper extension at the lumbar spine, improving segmental motion as well as postural muscle strength. A paraspinal stretching exercise can be used as a rest period between different, more active exercises. Any appropriate combination of strengthening and ROM/flexibility exercises can be implemented to achieve the desired goals.

Traditional stretching exercises such as a hip flexor or gastrocnemius stretch require little or no modification of technique. Other exercises such as a piriformis or iliotibial band stretch are executed more easily and require less balance when performed in the water. As outlined in

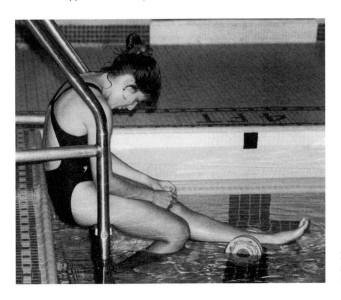

FIGURE 6-6. Hamstring stretch with use of a flotation buoy; the same position can be used for a slump stretch.

Chapter 5, buoyancy can be used in a variety of ways to achieve ROM or flexibility changes. Refer to Chapter 5 for a discussion of buoyancy-supported, -assisted, and -resisted exercises.

Activities to Increase Muscular Strength and Endurance

Increasing the strength and endurance of the paraspinal and abdominal musculature is of primary importance in the rehabilitation of a spinal injury or dysfunction because these are supportive structures of the spine.[1] To be thorough in the rehabilitation process, however, strength of all the structures providing additional support to the spine must also be addressed: the hip and lower extremity musculature, the upper extremity, shoulder girdle, and musculature of the trunk. With representation of all of these major muscle groups, it is not feasible or time efficient to address each of them individually in a strengthening program. The aquatic specialist is required to develop strengthening activities for movement *patterns*, functional tasks, and for muscle groups acting not only as movers but as stabilizers. Guidelines and sample progressions for strengthening of the upper and lower extremities are covered in Chapter 5; please refer to that chapter for further detail. Likewise, abdominal strengthening is addressed in the posture section of this chapter. The following section outlines additional activities to strengthen the trunk and supporting musculature.

Strengthening and endurance activities for the musculature supporting the spine should be incorporated into as many different types of activities in as many different combinations as possible: ROM, resistive, postural, and functional. PNF strengthening exercises are ideal in strengthening movement patterns. Because PNF patterns incorporate multiplane movement, they are ultimately more efficient and functional as strengthening exercises. Rotation of the extremities and the trunk is easily introduced into the rehabilitation program through these types of exercises. PNF patterns can be performed with or without resistive equipment, in shallow or deep water, and for the upper or lower extremities and the trunk. With proper client positioning, the aquatic specialist may assist the acute client through partial or complete PNF patterns as tolerated. The advanced client can perform PNF patterns aggressively in deep water, first without, then with resistive equipment. As guided by the aquatic specialist, deep-water PNF exercises can be structured to be strengthening or cardiovascular training activities.

Incorporating trunk rotation into the spinal rehabilitation program is essential for complete strengthening and stabilization. Trunk rotation is often problematic for the spine-injured client, and therefore should be introduced cautiously. Emphasis should be placed on strengthening the multifidii, rotatores, internal and external obliques, and hip medial and lateral rotators. Strengthening of the obliques has been covered previously in the section on abdominal strengthening. In planning comprehensive trunk strengthening and stabilization activities, remember that besides rotating the trunk slightly to the opposite side,[2] the multifidii also function as a flexion restraint (A. Cole, MD, personal communication, June, 1995), allowing the obliques to rotate the trunk. Rotational strengthening may begin in deep water with the assistance of a deep-water belt. From the vertical position, the client performs gentle, large-amplitude trunk rotations, right and left, leading slightly with the shoulders and allowing the lower extremities to follow. As tolerated, this motion is made smaller and smaller, initiated less with the shoulders and more with the trunk. The deep-water belt may be tethered to the side of the pool to add resistance to the motion. As the client progresses, the depth of water is decreased, reducing the supportive role of buoyancy and increasing the control required of the client. In chest-deep water the progression is similar, with early motion initiated gently by the shoulders. As strength and tolerance to rotation increases, the lower extremities remain more fixed. Tethering to the side of the pool or using paddles or a resistance board all add resistance to the motion. Rotational strengthening can also be incorporated into moving exercises such as forward and sideways walking. This is accomplished by elongating stride length and emphasizing trunk rotation with each step.

Cardiovascular Training

Cardiovascular training is important in completing the rehabilitation process and facilitating the transition to a regular fitness regime. Perhaps more than any other, the cardiovascular phase of rehabilitation is frequently ignored. Once a person has had an episode of back pain, he or she is four times more likely to have a recurrence than the general population.[12] Conditioning and fitness activities in the end-phase of rehabilitation from a spinal injury therefore serve as significant preventive measures. In deep water, the client can engage in cardiovascular training activities that in any other medium would involve deleterious levels of impact on the spine.

The pool offers the spine-injured client a full spectrum of rehabilitative activities. As outlined in previous sections, ROM, postural, and calisthenic exercises can be performed virtually impact free in deep water. As appropriate, the depth of water is decreased, providing progres-

sive loading to facilitate the transition to land-based activities. Abdominal strengthening can be progressed from assisted to resisted levels, all in deep water. Perhaps the most effective training that occurs in the water, however, is cardiovascular training. By paying close attention to spinal position and technique, cardiovascular training activities also address trunk strength and spinal stability. For example, a cross-country skiing exercise is modified by decreasing the total ROM executed by the extremities, and maintaining a vertical trunk position. The paraspinals, abdominals, and other supportive musculature of the spine are facilitated in maintaining a stable base from which the extremities can move. Deep-water jogging in an upright posture also challenges trunk strength and endurance. Deep-water jogging without a flotation belt increases the role of the upper body. With appropriate client selection, this is an excellent method of challenging upper trunk and abdominal strength. In deep water, with the assistance of a flotation belt, a client can perform a variety of strengthening exercises in a circuit training structure. A sample circuit for a client in the final phase of rehabilitation from a back injury is outlined in Table 6-1.

Monitoring intensity of exercise is essential to proper cardiovascular training. Patients may be instructed in monitoring heart rate, using Karvonen's formula, and adjusted for exercise in the water.[13] This adjustment is necessary because of the influence of hydrostatic pressure on hemodynamics. For further discussion of hydrostatic pressure and the other physical principles of water, refer to Chapter 2. For the client unfamiliar with monitoring heart rate and exercise intensity, instruction in use of the Borg scale of perceived exertion is useful. This method of monitoring exercise intensity is quick, efficient, and effective and can be carried over to other mediums of exercise. Finally, every client should be guided toward and encouraged to maintain a postrehabilitation fitness program. Cardiovascular training in deep water is an excellent alternative to land-based activities of the same type. Lap swimming is also an appropriate and recommended fitness activity. The basic swimming strokes may require modification to ensure safe and proper positioning for the client. Swim stroke analysis and modification are covered in more detail in the chapter on Adapted Swimming.

TABLE 6-1. Sample Circuit Training Program

Station	Exercise/Repetitions	Comment
1. Proprioceptive neuromuscular facilitation	20 reps. each LE	
2. Deep-water marching	30 cycles	1 cycle = 1 rep. with each LE
3. Cross-country skiing	20 cycles	1 cycle = 1 swing with each UE/LE; use short, quick swings
4. Hurdler's step	20 reps. each LE	
5. Shuttle run	6 min	Alternate slow/fast by 30-sec intervals
6. Deep-water walking	6 min	Emphasis on lumbar/hip extension

Each station may increased in duration as the patient progresses. This is approximately a 20-minute workout, after which the patient should perform an appropriate cool-down sequence.
LE, lower extremity; UE, upper extremity; rep., repetition.

Impairment-Oriented Rehabilitation

Mechanical Back Pain

Mechanical back pain includes such conditions as discogenic pain, facet syndrome, and degenerative joint disease.[14,15] The specific physical limitations found in people with mechanical back pain respond well to early therapeutic exercise.[16] Early movement and exercise can help deter the development of secondary problems, such as decreased strength and flexibility, that often result with persistent pain and lack of movement.[17–19] Moreover, the pool can be used throughout the course of rehabilitation, for training posture (neuromuscular training), mobility, strength and endurance, and functional tasks.[20]

A thorough understanding of the soft tissue and bony structure, function, responses to stress, and normal stages of healing is necessary when treating the client with mechanical back pain.[15,21] This allows the therapist to control the loads and forces in both the land-based and aquatic rehabilitation programs. The relations between hypomobile and hypermobile segments and the implications for movement patterns provide the framework for the evaluation and rehabilitation program.[20] As the therapist evaluates motion in the spine, the relative contributions to that motion from the individual segments must be noted. Failure to recognize a compensatory hypermobility can result in exaggeration of a dysfunction. Hypomobility of one segment, for example, can create a hypermobility of adjacent segments as the spine works for normal motion. The client must understand proper posture and movement patterns before

advancing in the rehabilitation program, which will challenge said postures and movement patterns. This prevents the reinforcement of incorrect postures or faulty movement patterns.[20] It is often difficult to visualize the client's posture and movement patterns in the pool because of refraction,[22] and the therapist must observe the exercise closely from the deck, in the pool, and underwater.

One of the first goals in treating the client with mechanical low back pain is the reduction of pain.[23] Unloading the spine by means of immersion into the shallow or deep end of the pool, along with sensory input from flow along the body and the water's warmth, can contribute to pain reduction.[24] Once pain is reduced, simple movements can be initiated to increase mobility in a pain-free range. These can be performed in shallow or deep water, and in the position of greatest comfort relative to buoyancy. Dynamic lumbar stabilization techniques, described earlier in this chapter, can be performed in shallow water and progressed to deep water as control is demonstrated.

As mobility is increased and pain diminishes, progressive resistive exercises can be initiated through a pain-free ROM. The client should be able to demonstrate proper posture and control of his or her body position before beginning any resistive exercises. These activities should be progressed to functional movement patterns and activities that simulate the activities of interest to the client.

The pool rehabilitative exercises should complement the land-based exercises providing a comprehensive program for each client. Initially, for example, because of pain or lack of motion, it may be necessary for the client to execute most of the prescribed exercise program in the water. As the client progresses, a larger percentage of the exercise program should be performed on land so the person learns to function easily in a gravity environment. However, the pool is a comfortable, safe environment to initiate new activities and use as an independent adjunct to the land-based exercise program.

Early Phase

The primary goals in the early rehabilitation phase for people with mechanical back pain are the reduction of pain, correction of any postural faults (eg, lateral shift, lumbar spine flexion), and the establishment of normal movement patterns. Simply immersing the client reduces the compressive forces at the spine,[17] and support of the body diminishes protective splinting. However, the decreased pain associated with immersion also places the person at risk for overwork. Guidelines must be provided for the client to prevent an increase in symptoms on leaving the pool.[25]

A variety of positions relative to buoyancy can be used, depending on the position of greatest comfort for the client. The supine buoyancy-supported position, stabilized with flotation devices, can produce relaxation. Bad Ragaz techniques for passive lateral trunk flexion are conveniently performed in this position. Passive trunk flexion and extension can be performed by passively flexing the hips and knees in supine. Gentle traction for the lumbar or cervical spine can be accomplished in supine by stabilizing distally or proximally at the trunk and then providing a traction force at the head or hips. Activities in the vertical position can be weight bearing in shallow water or nonweight bearing in deep water. Vertical traction can also be accomplished in the deep water by using ankle weights and flotation vests (Fig. 6-7). Dynamic lumbar stabilization may be initiated in supine or vertical and is a prerequisite for moving on to more advanced activities. Traditional physiologic stretching, including slump stretching and hamstring stretching, can be comfortably performed in the pool using a step or railing.

Gentle, active mobilization can be initiated through a pain-free range. This can be accomplished in prone or supine by Bad Ragaz techniques, or by active movements supported or assisted by buoyancy. Gentle trunk rotations or flexion and extension activities in the shallow or deep end provide controlled forces through-

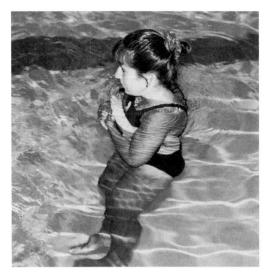

FIGURE 6-7. Deep-water vertical traction with support of flotation belt.

out the spine. Functional movement patterns such as marching in place, stepping, striding, or cross-country ski motions produce normal loads and stresses on the tissues, provided they are performed correctly. Any exercise the therapist wishes to initiate on land can usually be initiated in the pool first. The early phase continues until pain is diminished and movement patterns are normalized.

Intermediate Phase

Rehabilitation goals in the intermediate phase focus on increasing the pain-free ROM, improving the client's ability to generate torque in the trunk musculature for extended periods of time, and increasing the number of activities that can be performed without pain. The client usually can demonstrate proper posture when cued, but has difficulty maintaining the posture for any length of time or during any functional activities. Endurance can be progressed by increasing the volume of activity, both in the pool and on land. In general, these clients tolerate increased volume by minimizing the exercise intensity and by performing exercises several times over the course of the day. The key for the therapist and client is finding a balance of activity that results in improvement in function without an increase in symptoms. Exercise in the pool allows the person to increase the exercise time and repetitions without increasing joint compression.

Resistive trunk rotations can be performed by

stabilizing the feet on the bottom of the pool and rotating the trunk, or by stabilizing the trunk by holding on to a stationary object with the arms and rotating the legs. The resistive force can be increased by lengthening the lever arm or by the addition of resistive gloves, paddles, or fins. Bad Ragaz techniques can provide resistive forces to the trunk in a variety of patterns and positions. As always, proper posture and movement patterns must be reinforced. A variety of exercises should be incorporated to provide diverse loads and stresses on the tissues.

A circuit program of exercise, described earlier in this chapter, can be incorporated and performed independently once the therapist has ensured that the exercises are being performed correctly. This provides an adjunct to the land-based program. As the intermediate phase progresses, activities should begin to resemble the activities to which the client will be returning.

Late Phase

As pain-free ROM, dynamic control of posture, and muscular endurance are increased, the exercise program begins to focus on the client's functional needs. Work and sport activities can be simulated in the pool, and aquatic rehabilitation can provide variety to the work-hardening program. Proper movement patterns in work, sport, or daily activity can be initiated in the pool at a reduced speed with lowered compressive forces, providing an opportunity to train the correct postures. Resistive equipment or equipment used at work or sport (eg, crates, boards, bats, racquets) can be incorporated into the pool program and function well in a circuit training routine. The time, resistance, and repetitions should simulate the functional demands of the client's activities. As the client progresses, increased time should be spent in land-based activities, although the pool remains a sound extension of the land program. For those clients with degenerative joint disease, the pool may become the primary form of exercise to maintain fitness and condition owing to the unloading benefits.

Soft Tissue Injuries

Acute soft tissue injuries of the spine include muscular strains and ligament sprains. These may occur as a result of work, sports, or accidents. If the injury is muscular, pain is reproducible by passive stretch, active contraction, and palpation of the muscle. Ligamentous sprains are unaffected by resistive tests, although passive stretching may be painful because of stretching the ligament. Muscular strains and ligamentous sprains can occur simultaneously. In either case, the rehabilitation protocol proceeds based on the specific findings on examination. As with all rehabilitation programs, the stages of healing form the scientific basis for exercise prescription.

The person presenting with a soft tissue injury complains of pain as well as a loss of mobility, and demonstrates a decrease in the ability to produce torque. The extent of symptoms varies with the degree of injury, the stage of healing, and the secondary compensations that have developed. Loss of mobility may be unidirectional or multidirectional, and strength is limited by pain. Rehabilitation goals parallel the stages of healing and address the specific deficits found on examination. Initially, pain reduction is important because this allows the person to begin therapeutic exercises. Active and passive mobility exercises maintain the normal relations between the soft tissues and bony structures. These exercises prevent excessive scar formation and subsequent mobility loss. Appropriate exercises also provide a stimulus for the healing response. Movement patterns should be taught and reinforced early to prevent substitution and secondary postural problems.

As healing progresses, loading of the spinal soft tissues should advance in an orderly manner, applying gradually increasing loads on the injured and supporting tissues. The principle of specific adaptations to imposed demands and the plastic nature of soft tissues provide the foundation for exercise progression. Specific loads must be placed on the healing tissue to provide a stimulus for remodeling. The therapist must be able to visualize the loads placed on the injured tissues relative to the stages of healing and to the demands that will be placed on the client when returning to activity. Increased loads include exercise through a greater ROM, and increased resistance or repetitions. Exercise progresses to increasing time spent in land-based activities as healing progresses.

Early Phase

Physical therapy goals in the early phase focus on decreasing pain, normalizing movement patterns, and initiating mobility activities. Immersion alone decreases pain because of the warmth of the water, laminal flow, and un-weighting. The stabilizing muscles obtain some external support from the hydrostatic pressure of the water. Immersion should be to a depth that provides enough unweighting of the spine to decrease pain. Sound movement patterns should be reviewed, including gait and flex-ion–extension, side bending, and rotation movements in pain-free ranges. Activities can be performed in supine, prone, or vertical, using the support or assistance of buoyancy. Preven-tion of overwork is critical for the client with a soft tissue injury. Frequently, no discomfort is noticed until leaving the pool, and the pain often progresses over the next 24 hours. This situation can be avoided by minimizing the amount of exercise performed in this phase. Passive physi-ologic stretching should be performed in all di-rections, and can be performed in the pool with the support of buoyancy. The volume of activity can be gradually increased as the person's toler-ance is determined.

As with all pool exercise, the therapist must ensure that proper postures and movement pat-terns are being reinforced. Mobility at one seg-ment obtained at the expense of an adjacent seg-ment can create more problems than it helps. These movement patterns are carried over into land-based exercises and, as such, should be executed properly without requiring a great deal of cognition on the client's part. Once the acute pain has subsided and movement patterns have been normalized, the client may progress to more advanced activities.

Intermediate Phase

The goals in the intermediate phase include in-creasing the range of mobility to full range with-out pain, and increasing the muscles' ability to produce torque. The multiple roles of various muscles should be recognized, and training should include these roles. For example, the trunk muscles can function concentrically as pri-mary movers, eccentrically as decelerators or antagonists, or isometrically as stabilizers. The pool provides a rich environment for training these functions. Gait activities in shallow water normalize movement patterns and increase the strength and endurance of the trunk muscula-ture. Walking forward, backward, and laterally with varying stride lengths and varying speeds alters the loads on the spine. Increasing the sur-face area by use of a plow or increasing the

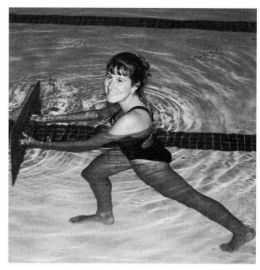

FIGURE 6-8. Altering loads on the spine: forward walk-ing with resistance board and increased stride length.

speed of activity increases the resistance (Fig. 6-8).

The arms can be extended and gloves or pad-dles added to increase the lever arm. Trunk rota-tion and trunk flexion–extension and lateral flexion exercises can be performed in a variety of positions and should be progressed from sin-gle-plane motions to multiplane activities. Re-sisted shoulder and leg exercises in a sagittal and frontal plane challenge the spinal musculature both statically and dynamically.

The client should continue movement and stretching exercises as necessary to produce a flexible scar. Overstretching should be avoided because this can produce a chronic inflamma-tory situation. The rehabilitation program should include increasing land-based exercises during this phase, progressing impact as toler-ated. As control is demonstrated during simple, single-plane exercise, the activities should be-come more vigorous in the attempt to train through a greater ROM for a longer time. When a solid base of strength and endurance using proper mechanics is established, the client should progress to the late rehabilitation phase.

Late Phase

The goals in the late rehabilitation phase focus on preparing the client for return to the previous level of activity. The strength and endurance base established in the intermediate phase is now used during function. If return to a physical

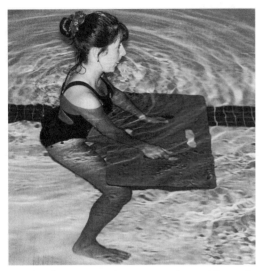

FIGURE 6-9. Functional activity simulation: lifting task.

job is the goal, specific work-hardening activities should be incorporated into the pool program. Lifting, pushing, and pulling tasks can all be simulated in the pool (Fig. 6-9). Sports activities can also be incorporated. Running, throwing, lifting, and pushing skills can be incorporated into a circuit training program. The specific musculoskeletal and cardiovascular demands of the job should be analyzed and reproduced in the pool.

The greatest percentage of the rehabilitation program should be performed on land during this phase. This ensures proper antigravity muscle function while performing specific tasks. However, the pool program is a good place to initiate any new activity, and provides a different training environment on alternate days. As always, the client should demonstrate proper performance of any skill before placement in an independent pool rehabilitation program.

Postural Dysfunction

Postural dysfunctions of the cervical, thoracic, or lumbar spine are seen with increasing frequency as the population becomes more sedentary. People who sit or stand in a single position for most of the day often present with intermittent back or neck pain. Prolonged stress on soft tissues such as the joint capsules and ligaments results in a diffuse, aching pain. Symptoms are produced by positioning and not movement. Frequently, the only objective finding is poor

posture that reproduces pain. If the person is left untreated, secondary dysfunction syndromes develop, characterized by adaptive shortening in some soft tissues and lengthening and weakness in others.

Rehabilitation activities for the client with postural dysfunctions focus on attaining and maintaining proper posture. In addition to postural retraining exercises, activities to stretch shortened tissues and strengthen lengthened and weakened tissues should be initiated.

Early Phase

The physical therapy goals in the early phase focus on correcting posture and gently mobilizing the shortened tissue. The specific exercises depend on the direction of dysfunction and the stiffness of the tissue. Mobilization activities should be gentle to prevent an inflammatory reaction. Shortened, stiff tissues respond best to gentle oscillations and a light, passive, prolonged stretch. These activities can be performed in the pool in a variety of positions. Traction for the cervical or lumbar spine can be performed in supine with the support of buoyancy and flotation devices. Bad Ragaz techniques can be used to mobilize into lateral flexion while in supine, and trunk flexion and extension can be performed in side lying, supine, or vertical. Stepping exercises in deep or shallow water as well as ambulation in a variety of planes facilitate varying degrees of trunk flexion–extension and rotation. The amount of rotation can be exaggerated by a using large arm swing.

While gentle mobilization exercises are initiated, the client should be introduced to proper posture and the proper knee, hip, lumbar, scapular, and head positions to minimize the dysfunction. The client must be reminded that the spine is a series of joints, and that the position of one segment is compensated by another segment. This concept can be extended to contributing joints and articulations such as the knee and scapula. Excessive hyperextension of the knee contributes to anterior pelvic tilt, whereas increased scapular protraction and medial humeral rotation contribute to an increased kyphosis. These postures are compensated at the cervical spine by increased cervical lordosis and capital extension. As such, each exercise, whether for mobility or strengthening, must be performed in proper mechanical alignment. Specific postural retraining exercises are detailed in the Goal-Oriented Rehabilitation section of this chapter.

Intermediate Phase

The intermediate phase focuses on increasing the client's strength in the new ROM as it is obtained. Muscles that have been in a lengthened or shortened position for a prolonged period of time become weakened. As new range is obtained, the client must train the muscles at their new resting length. The proper posture must be maintained during the training exercise to ensure that muscles are being trained at the appropriate length. Resistive exercises focus on increasing both the strength and the endurance of these muscles in a variety of positions and functions.

Activities in this phase include resistive walking in a variety of directions, shallow- or deepwater jogging, cross-country skiing, bicycling, and marching (Fig. 6-10). Bad Ragaz techniques can facilitate and reinforce stabilizing mechanisms during movement in varying patterns. Fins, resistive equipment, gloves, or paddles can be used to increase the resistance of the exercise. Increasing the lever arm also adds an additional challenge to the exercise. Movements should progress from single-plane patterns to multiplane activities. Resistive exercises for the upper and lower extremities can be used to challenge the balance and postural mechanisms.

For clients with thoracic and cervical spine

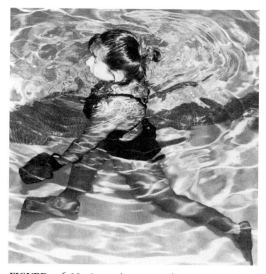

FIGURE 6-10. Strengthening–endurance exercise: cross-country skiing with fins and gloves.

postural dysfunctions, increasing emphasis should be placed on strengthening the scapular stabilizing muscles. The rhomboids, middle and lower trapezius, serratus anterior, and lateral shoulder rotators should be specifically strengthened, whereas the pectoral muscles, levator scapula, upper trapezius, and other internal rotators should be stretched. Scapular stabilization exercises should be incorporated and can be performed against the wall, on a step, or with a kickboard. These activities are described in detail in Chapter 5. These muscles have a postural stabilizing function and, as such, should be trained for endurance rather than maximum torque generation.

As the shortened tissue becomes increasingly mobile and strong, the percentage of time in pool exercise should decrease and the amount of time spent exercising in the gravity environment increased. Land-based exercise should also include postural retraining exercise, physiologic stretching, and mobilization, as well as strengthening exercises for the lengthened, weak musculature. The pool program should support the exercises performed on land, and often precedes performance of a specific skill on land.

Late Phase

The last phase of rehabilitation emphasizes return to full activity in the client's normal environment. The pool program becomes a complement to the land-based exercise program. Traditional lap swimming helps to maintain mobility and muscular endurance throughout the trunk; for further discussion of swim stroke modification, refer to Chapter 14. A circuit training program including mobility exercises, postural retraining, cardiovascular training, and progressive resistive exercise can be performed on alternate days. The ranges and postures used for training should simulate those required of the person when he or she returns to work, sport, or activities of daily living. Any specific implements or tools used should be incorporated into the pool program.

Other Impairment-Oriented Considerations

Instability in the spine can result from acute fracture, stress fractures, spondylolysis, or from hormonal changes associated with pregnancy. In addition, hypermobility at a segment or series of segments can result from hypomobility in adjacent areas. These problems should be treated with dynamic stabilization exercises as well as specific strengthening or stretching exercises, as indicated. People with spondylolysis or spondylolisthesis usually present with pain during extension or rotation of the lumbar spine. The degree of immobility or pain depends on the degree of slippage, if any, and any underlying postural dysfunctions. Exercises for this person focus on dynamic cocontraction in gradually increasing positions of extension. Despite the pain and instability with spinal extension, there may be an underlying mobility loss contributing to the problem. The opposite may also be true, as seen in young female gymnasts. These athletes often present with increased mobility throughout their spines. The specifics of the rehabilitation program vary from individual to individual.

Pregnant women often complain of low back pain, particularly as pregnancy progresses. This complaint is often the result of a change in the center of gravity with increased weight anteriorly, increasing the moment arm. This places additional strain on the low back musculature, and, when combined with increased ligamentous laxity secondary to hormonal changes, predisposes the woman to low back pain. In addition to the use of braces to support the increased mass, dynamic stabilization exercises can assist in providing stability to the area.

Early Phase

The pool provides an ideal exercise environment for the client with spinal instability. The hydrostatic pressure of the water provides additional external support to the trunk. Dynamic lumbar stabilization exercises can be initiated in chest-deep water and parallel the stabilization exercises performed on land. The exercises can be performed in shallow water, standing against the side of the pool, and progressed to deep water with no support. The arms and legs should be used initially to assist in maintaining a neutral spine. As the client demonstrates control over the spinal position, control should be maintained solely with the trunk musculature.

When control of posture can be demonstrated, simple challenges may be initiated. These may be as simple as single-plane arm or leg motions while maintaining the spine in neutral. The number and variety of exercises should be increased before the complexity of the task.

Any flexibility deficits also should be addressed in this phase. Physiologic stretching can be performed in the pool or as part of the land-based program. The client should be performing simple lumbar stabilization exercises in supine in the land-based program at this time.

Intermediate Phase

The client should be able to demonstrate good control of the spine in a variety of movement patterns and for moderate lengths of time as criteria for progression to the intermediate phase. The primary goals in this phase are to increase the complexity of movement patterns, increase muscle endurance and strength, and progress the lumbar stabilization sequence. Lumbar stabilization exercises should be progressed to include simultaneous movement of the arms and legs. Movement patterns should be progressed from single-plane, single-joint to multijoint, multiplane exercises. Exercises in chest-deep water should be progressed to waist-deep to increase the postural challenge. Cardiovascular training exercises requiring postural stabilization, such as deep-water bicycling, cross-country skiing, walking, and jogging, should be incorporated.

Strength and endurance can be increased by increasing the intensity and volume of exercise. Exercises should remain in the pain-free range, but the quantity, resistance, and duration should be increased. The person with spondylolysis should be able to stabilize the lumbar spine while performing hip extension exercises actively and with resistance. Pregnant women should be able to perform a variety of lower extremity and trunk strengthening exercises while preventing excessive lumbar lordosis.

As progression toward the late phase occurs, the client with spondylolysis should begin training in increased positions of lumbar extension. This allows controlled loads to be placed on the spine in a safe, progressive manner. Initially, loads should be passive, in the form of passive extension exercises. These can be performed buoyancy supported in side lying, or buoyancy assisted in prone.

Late Phase

For the pregnant woman, the late phase is likely a maintenance phase until hormone levels stabilize and ligamentous stability is achieved. For many, this may be several months, until lactation is completed. The pool will likely become the primary exercise medium for this population. The pregnant woman is able to increase or maintain her cardiovascular fitness while minimizing heat production and lower extremity edema. The program should consist of activities the woman enjoys, and may include lap swimming, postural exercises, abdominal strengthening exercises, lower extremity toning exercises, and physiologic stretching. Specific activities depend on the individual woman's goals.

Late-phase rehabilitation for the client with spondylolysis focuses on preparations to return to activity. Progressive loading in increasing positions of extension along with continued reinforcement of proper body mechanics are the foundation of the program. These activities should be performed in the vertical position if this is the primary posture to which the person will be returning. Some workers may be returning to work in prone or supine; if so, the program should emphasize these postures. In contrast to the pregnant woman, the client with spondylolysis spends progressively less time in the pool for his or her rehabilitation program. A progressive resistive exercise program for the abdominal muscles, low back musculature, and associated musculature should always emphasize exercise with a neutral spine. The volume and intensity of exercise should mimic the client's work, daily activities, or sport.

Case Studies

The following case studies illustrate the use of aquatic physical therapy, including progression from aquatic to land-based programs, in treatment of a spine-related injury.

❏ CASE STUDY 6-1

LL is a 47-year-old woman with an 8-year history of low back pain with posterior unilateral radiating symptoms to the popliteal fossa. Plain radiographs and magnetic resonance imaging revealed moderate degenerative changes of the facet joints of L2 through L5, and moderate bulging discs at L4–L5 and L5–S1. Previous physical therapy consisting of extension exercises, mechanical lumbar traction, and modalities was successful in relieving symptoms for short periods of time only. Since the onset of symptoms 8 years ago, LL has been unable to resume the full, active lifestyle she previously had. On initial evaluation, LL demonstrated limitations in lumbar extension greater than lumbar flexion,

poor paraspinal, abdominal, and lower extremity strength, and an intolerance to sitting for longer than 5 to 6 minutes. Extension in lying would consistently relieve symptoms of pain and numbness in the leg, but with minimal carry-over once out of the extended position. LL was referred to the aquatic therapy program for ROM and strengthening exercises as tolerated.

The early phase of rehabilitation consisted of triweekly 20- to 30-minute sessions in the pool. Each session included gentle walking exercises, forward, backward, and sideways, in chest-deep water. Every 5 minutes of exercise in shallow water was interrupted with a 2-minute period of traction in deep water. Traction was accomplished by having LL support herself in deep water, in a vertical position, with a deep-water belt. Relaxation of the trunk and lower extremities was reinforced to assist in increasing the distraction of the lumbar spine. Instruction and practice in proper posture, neutral spine, and total spinal alignment were implemented at each session, progressively. Strengthening exercises in this phase were in the form of postural and positional exercises. Land-based exercises consisted of practice in proper posture in a variety of positions—sitting, standing, bending—and practice in achieving and maintaining neutral spine.

Intermediate-phase rehabilitation focused on continuing to increase strength and tolerance to exercise, as well as ROM. By this time, LL was tolerating 40-minute sessions in the pool triweekly. Speed and stride length were increased in all walking activities, as the depth of water in which they were performed was decreased to waist deep. To increase lumbar extension, several activities were added: backward walking, standing extension, and isolated hip extension in standing. Deep-water walking, with the assistance of a deep-water belt, was introduced and tolerated well in bouts of 7 to 12 minutes, progressively. Vertical traction in deep water was continued, with the frequency decreased to three 3-minute periods, at the beginning, middle, and end of each session. Gentle abdominal strengthening was initiated in the form of posterior pelvic tilts and unilateral knee lifts performed in waist-deep water. Land-based exercises in this phase were in the form of anterior pelvic tilts (now attainable in increased lumbar extension ROM), standing hip extension, lateral flexion stretches, and progressive extension in lying exercises.

The late phase of rehabilitation for LL was multifaceted and included the following components: (1) a limited land-based walking program, initially 5 to 10 minutes, performed on days opposite aquatic therapy, and designed to begin the transition from aquatic to land-based activities; (2) land-based standing and prone extension exercises; (3) a flexibility program, initiated in the water, for hamstrings, hip flexors, and lumbar paraspinal musculature; and (4) cardiovascular activities (deep water jogging and cross-country skiing). Postural, stabilization, and abdominal strengthening exercises continued throughout this phase of rehabilitation. By the middle portion of this final phase of rehabilitation, LL had increased her aquatic therapy sessions to 50 to 60 minutes triweekly and reported significant increases in her tolerance of functional activities. As she progressed, aquatic activities were progressively decreased as land-based activities were increased. LL is now a member of her company's Wellness program, participating in fitness activities 4 days per week. She has also continued deep-water walking and running as part of her fitness routine.

❏ CASE STUDY 6-2

DG is a 36-year-old male English literature professor with a magnetic resonance imaging-confirmed L4–L5 herniated disc, for which he underwent microdiscectomy. Postsurgically, DG was placed on flexion restriction for 4 weeks. At postsurgical week 5, he was referred to physical therapy for progressive ROM, flexibility, and strengthening exercises. At this time the flexion restriction was reduced to include sitting and end-range flexion only. On initial evaluation, DG demonstrated decreased strength of the lower extremities and abdominal and paraspinal musculature, decreased lumbar extension, and decreased hamstring flexibility. He also walked with a slight right-sided limp. Sensation appeared intact, although he did report occasional tingling bilaterally in the posterior thigh. All dural tension tests were negative; reflexes tested normal at the patellar and Achilles tendons.

Early-phase rehabilitation consisted of aquatic exercise to increase mobility and begin ROM and strengthening activities. ROM activities were performed in deep water with a flotation belt; emphasis was placed on lumbar extension and hip flexion and extension. Deep-water walking was initiated to use ROM gains as well as to strengthen the hip and lower extremities. In shallow water, DG performed gait training activities with emphasis on equal weight bearing and increased stride length. Forward, backward, and sideways walking exercises were performed in chest-deep water, with speed and stride length increased as tolerated. Postural education, in the form of instruction in neutral spine and total spinal alignment, was introduced in this phase of rehabilitation as well. DG participated in aquatic therapy sessions 3 days per week for 20 to 25 minutes per session. Land-based exercise consisted of extension exercises, practice in achieving neutral spine in the standing position, weight shifts anteriorly and posteriorly leading with the right leg, and gastrocnemius and soleus stretches in standing.

The intermediate phase of rehabilitation began at postsurgical week 8, at which point DG was tolerating four 30-minute aquatic therapy sessions weekly. All mobility and gait training activities were continued and progressed as tolerated. Walking activities were moved to mid-trunk depth and were performed with resistive equipment. Deep-water walking was increased from 6 to 12 minutes gradually. Isolated upper and lower extremity multiplane strengthening exercises were started, first in shallow, then deep water. Trunk rotation and extremes of trunk flexion were avoided per physician direction. Postural exercises were advanced in the form of resistance to walking activities. At home, DG continued to perform extension exercises pain free. He also began a daily walking program: 10 to 15 minutes on aquatic therapy days, and 20 to 30 minutes on days opposite aquatic therapy.

The late phase of rehabilitation saw DG progress into cardiovascular training activities in the pool, and gradual flexion exercises to full ROM as tolerated. These flexion exercises were performed first in the pool, and then on land. General strengthening exercises for the extremities and the abdominal and paraspinal musculature were continued in both deep and shallow water with several additions. Upper and lower extremity PNF strengthening exercises were initiated, introducing a rotational component to motion. Rotational strengthening was incorporated progressively through small trunk rotations without and then with resistive equipment. Abdominal strengthening was progressed to focus on lower abdominals and obliques. In the prone floating position, gentle unilateral and bilateral knee-to-chest stretches were combined with trunk curls. Land-based flexion exercises were introduced after DG demonstrated tolerance of flexion exercises in the water. During the final phase of rehabilitation, DG was exercising five times weekly—three aquatic and two land-based sessions. As he gained in strength and endurance, the number of land-based sessions was increased as aquatic sessions were decreased. DG made a successful transition to a land-based fitness routine performed three to four times weekly and using such cardiovascular equipment as the Nordic track, Stairmaster, Gravitron, and treadmill. He is also participating in an outdoor walking program.

Summary

Aquatic exercise can be safely implemented as a rehabilitation tool for recovery from spinal injuries. The properties of water provide an environment that is safe for exercise, conducive to early movement, and free of the potentially harmful effects of impact. In effectively using aquatic exercise as a treatment tool for the spine-injured client, the aquatic specialist must identify the advantages afforded by these properties of the aquatic environment. Unloading spinal structures, minimizing postexercise soft tissue edema, and simulating functional activities earlier than on land are just a few of these advantages.[17]

Postural education and strengthening are essential to rehabilitation from a spinal injury, and are integral to the prevention of future injuries. The supportive and resistive properties of water make it an ideal environment in which to pursue postural strengthening.

Finally, aquatic exercise may also be implemented as an effective activity for those clients performing maintenance or general fitness programs.

REFERENCES

1. Saunders HD. *Evaluation, Treatment and Prevention of Musculoskeletal Disorders*. Minneapolis, Minn: Viking Press; 1985.
2. Kendall F, McCreary E, Provance P. *Muscles: Testing and Function with Posture and Pain*. 4th ed. Baltimore, Md: Williams & Wilkins; 1985.
3. Kisner C, Colby L. *Therapeutic Exercise: Foundation and Techniques*. 2nd ed. Philadelphia, Pa: FA Davis; 1990.
4. Saal J, Saal J. Nonoperative treatment of herniated lumbar intervertebral disc with radiculopathy. *Spine*. 1989;14:431–437.
5. Skinner AT, Thomson AM, eds. *Duffield's Exercise in Water*. 3rd ed. London: Balliere Tindall; 1983.
6. Morgan D. Concepts in functional training and postural stabilization for the low back injured. *Topics in Acute Care Trauma Rehabilitation*. 1988;2(4):8–17.
7. Moore K. *Clinically Oriented Anatomy*. 2nd ed. Baltimore, Md: Williams & Wilkins; 1985.
8. Williams P, Warwick R, eds. *Gray's Anatomy*. 36th ed. Philadelphia, Pa: WB Saunders; 1980.
9. Gardner E, Gray D, O'Rahilly R. *Anatomy: A Regional Study of Human Structure*. 2nd ed. Philadelphia, Pa: WB Saunders; 1963.
10. Daniels L, Worthingham C. *Muscle Testing: Techniques of Manual Examination*. 5th ed. Philadelphia, Pa: WB Saunders; 1986.
11. Sahrmann S. *Diagnosis and Treatment of Muscle Imbalances Associated With Regional Pain Syndromes*. Ithaca, NY: 1990.
12. Porter RW, Adams MA, Hutton WC. Physical activity and the strength of the lumbar spine. *Spine*. 1989;14: 201–203.
13. Sheldahl LM, Tristani E, Clifford PS, et al. Effect of head-out water immersion on response to exercise training. *J Appl Physiol*. 1986;60:1878–1881.
14. Magee DJ. *Orthopedic Physical Assessment*. 2nd ed. Philadelphia, Pa: WB Saunders; 1992.
15. Porterfield JA, DeRosa C. *Mechanical Low Back Pain*. Philadelphia, Pa: WB Saunders; 1991.
16. Mayer TG, Gatchel RS, Mayer H, et al. A prospective two year study of functional restoration in industrial low back injury: an objective assessment procedure. *JAMA*. 1987;258:1763–1767.
17. Cirullo JA. Aquatic physical therapy approaches for the spine. *Orthopaedic Physical Therapy Clinics of North America*. 1994;3:179–208.
18. Janda V. Muscles, central nervous motor regulation and back problems. In: Korr IM, ed. *The Neurological Mechanism in Manipulative Therapy*. New York, NY: Plenum; 1978:253–254.
19. Kirkaldy-Willis WH. The pathology and pathogenesis of low back pain. In: Kirkaldy-Willis WH, ed. *Managing Low Back Pain*. 2nd ed. New York, NY: Churchill-Livingstone; 1988:153.
20. DeRosa CP, Porterfield JA. A physical therapy model for the treatment of low back pain. *Phys Ther*. 1993; 72:261–272.
21. Hooker D. Back rehabilitation. In: Prentice WE, ed. *Rehabilitation Techniques in Sports Medicine*. 2nd ed. St. Louis, Mo: CV Mosby; 1994:101.
22. Moschetti M. *Aquaphysics*. Aptos, CA: Aquatechnics; 1990.
23. Hellsing AL, Linton SJ, Kalvemark M. A prospective study of patients with acute back and neck pain in Sweden. *Phys Ther*. 1994;72:116–128.
24. Blades K. Hydrotherapy in orthopedics. In: Campion MR, ed. *Adult Hydrotherapy*. London: Heinemann Medical Books; 1990:156–157.
25. Bates A, Hanson N. *Aquatic Exercise Therapy*. Kelowna, Westbank, British Columbia, Canada: Online Graphics; 1992.

7 Aquatic Rehabilitation of the Neurologically Impaired Client

David M. Morris

Rehabilitating clients with brain injuries presents many complex challenges to medical professionals. The need for neurorehabilitation strategies has steadily increased as improved technology and medical management has allowed more people to survive brain injuries such as head trauma, cerebrovascular accidents, brain tumors, and premature births.[1,2] In addition, longer life expectancies could account for the increased incidence of neurologic disorders such as Parkinson's disease. The direct and indirect costs of these disorders can be staggering. For example, the annual cost of care and loss of earning as a result of cerebrovascular accidents was estimated to be between 7.5 and 11.2 billion dollars in 1979. Also, in 1981, more than 500,000 head injuries were significant enough to require hospitalization.[3,4] These figures become most significant when converted to 1995 dollars. The current health care climate requires increased cost effectiveness for all medical services. Neurorehabilitation professionals, like other health professionals, must constantly seek to develop programs that are cost effective and produce long-term, positive outcomes.

Aquatic neurorehabilitation has been described as a useful adjunct to traditional brain injury rehabilitation programs.[5–12] All of the authors using that description agree that the aquatic environment can benefit clients with brain damage, but there are differences as to the specific approach to be used and its scientific rationale. For example, some advocate aquatic rehabilitation for the treatment of problems commonly associated with brain injuries (ie, weakness, hypertonicity, limited range of mo-

tion), but do not advocate functional activity training in the water.[6,8] They believe that the aquatic environment fails to provide adequate stability, leading to the facilitation of associated reactions that interfere with purposeful movement. However, others believe that the aquatic environment, if properly used, can provide a stable environment for active client participation in functional skill improvement.[9–12] There is similar controversy with regard to aquatic neurorehabilitation for the treatment of ataxia. Some authors consider ataxic conditions to be absolute contraindications to aquatic rehabilitation because clients with these problems become confused with the altered sensory input induced by immersion in the water.[6,8] Others believe that although ataxia is seldom improved in the water, aquatic neurorehabilitation can positively influence ataxia-associated problems like weakness of proximal muscle groups.[9] This author believes that aquatic neurorehabilitation can be used as a treatment for ataxia itself. Some believe that the pool water's warmth leads to tone reduction in clients with brain damage.[7,9] Others credit the supportive nature of water with producing relaxation and therefore reducing the effort necessary to perform movement against a hypertonic antagonistic muscle[6,8,12]; consequently, less "spastic" movement patterns are exhibited. Despite differences of opinion regarding preferred approaches and underlying mechanisms, commonly expressed benefits of aquatic rehabilitation for brain-injured adults include tone reduction, contracture prevention, assistance with static and dynamic balance, earlier and more effective strengthening, cardiovascular benefits, motivation, recreation, and socialization.

This chapter explores contemporary and traditional aquatic neurorehabilitation strategies. Motor control and neurorehabilitation concepts that influence both land and aquatic treatment are emphasized. Client problems resulting from brain injury are addressed from the standpoint of underlying causes and aquatic neurorehabilitation solutions available. Aquatic rehabilitation community programs also are discussed. Before they can understand the rationale behind aquatic neurorehabilitation, therapists must first become familiar with basic concepts related to neurorehabilitation in water and on land.

Rehabilitation of Clients With Neurologic Disorders

Problems encountered during the treatment of brain injury can be classified according to the International Classification of Impairments, Disabilities, and Handicap (ICIDH).[13] According to the ICIDH, an impairment is any loss of or abnormality of an organ, structure, or function. Typical brain injury impairments include weakness, hypertonicity, voluntary movement deficits, limited range of motion, sensory loss, incoordination, and postural instability. A disability is any reduction, partial or total, in the capacity to carry out any functional activity within the range considered "normal" for the average human being. Typical brain injury disabilities include those affecting walking, transferring, and reaching. A handicap is an externally imposed disadvantage that limits or prevents the fulfillment of usual social roles depending on age, gender, and culture for the person. Typical brain injury handicaps include physical barriers, attitudinal barriers, lowered expectations of the client, and fear of the client. The application of rehabilitation approaches, both land-based and aquatic, may influence neurologic disorders at any or all of these levels.

Our assumptions about how humans create and control movement profoundly influence the way rehabilitation professionals evaluate and treat their clients. A thorough understanding of normal movement is prerequisite for developing rehabilitation programs, in any environment, to influence pathologic movement. Theories describing how human movement is produced have been proposed.[1,2,14] Traditionally, the reflex and hierarchical models of motor control have been used by therapists to explain their

evaluation and treatment strategies. In more recent years, however, rehabilitation professionals have been exploring a greater number of motor control theories, including the systems model, motor programming theories, and dynamical action theory.[1,2,14] No one model of motor control is believed fully to explain normal and pathologic movement production. Therapists may find one model most useful in guiding evaluation and treatment for one client, and another model most useful for another client's program. Therefore, neurorehabilitation therapists become more effective in conducting evaluations and providing treatment if they are familiar with several models of motor control. For a concise, yet thorough discussion of these motor control models, readers are advised to read the works of Gordon, Horak, and Schumway-Cook and Woolacott.[1,2,14]

Neurorehabilitation Models

As with theories of motor control, treatment approaches have undergone several paradigm shifts through the history of neurorehabilitation. These changes occurred in response to societal and technologic advances, and have been outlined by Gordon[1] and Horak.[2] The more popular treatment approaches for clients with neurologic deficits can be aligned with three models of neurorehabilitation.

In earlier days of physical rehabilitation, many of the clients served by therapists had poliomyelitis. At that time, the prevalent rehabilitation model was a muscle reeducation model in which therapists identified weak musculature, strengthened those found, and provided orthopedic support or bracing for those body segments where strength would not return. Clients with neurologic disorders were treated in a similar fashion. One source of dissatisfaction with this model was that it did not include consideration for the plasticity of the central nervous system (CNS), that is, the ability for recovery. In addition, clients with neurologic disorders often had more difficulty with patterns of movement and could not isolate specific muscle actions. Such dissatisfaction led to a paradigm shift to the neurotherapeutic facilitation approach.

Developed in the 1950s, the neurotherapeutic facilitation model approach provided the basic philosophy followed by many theorists, including the Bobaths, Knott and Voss, Ayres, Rood, Stockmeyer, and others. Treatment approaches developed from this model dominated the field of neurorehabilitation for the next 30 years and still have a strong influence on rehabilitation practices. With this approach, therapists facilitate normal (or desirable) movement patterns by providing sensory input. Careful steps are taken to avoid abnormal movement patterns, inhibit abnormal muscle tone, and avoid primitive reflexes. Dissatisfaction with this model arose from the lack of functional carry-over; the avoidance of primitive, abnormal movement patterns did not necessarily produce normal functional movement. Also, the client's role in treatment was passive, responding only to the therapist's sensory input. Finally, the approach explained neurologic movement disorders as the result of an aberrant CNS and failed to consider musculoskeletal and environmental influences on movement.

During the 1980s, another paradigm shift occurred. Contemporary movement science research suggests that more functionally oriented neurotreatment, in which clients are more active problem solvers, may be a preferred approach. Such beliefs have led many rehabilitation experts to endorse a task-oriented approach to neurorehabilitation that emphasizes setting specific functional goals for clients. Clients learn to develop effective, efficient compensatory strategies to carry out tasks. They also learn adaptability to perform these tasks under a variety of musculoskeletal and environmental constraints (eg, on different surfaces, with different obstacles to avoid, in different lighting). More emphasis is placed on the client's ability to perform a task rather than specific movement patterns. Like the other neurorehabilitation models, a task-oriented one has dissatisfying aspects. Many clients receiving neurotreatment have a limited ability to participate as active problem solvers because of major physical or mental impairments. Also, it is difficult to retrain the client's ability to anticipate the need for a particular motor strategy.

Rehabilitation therapists may follow one neurorehabilitation model or may use a more eclectic approach. The therapist must, however, understand the rationale for each treatment used. The three models of motor control suffice to explain aquatic neurorehabilitation approaches. Such references are included throughout the remainder of this chapter.

Motor Learning

Motor learning is a field of study that explores the cognitive processes associated with the practice or experience leading to improved

motor skill.[15,16] Rehabilitation professionals have increased their awareness of motor learning principles and, as a result, have modified the way they structure client practice and provide feedback.

Motor learning literature differentiates performance from learning. Motor performance relates to skill demonstrated during the practice session. Skill observed at this time may or may not be incorporated into long-lasting functional skill. Motor learning, in contrast, refers to skill observed after the passing of a significant period of time between the practice session and the skill observation. Motor learning, therefore, is more indicative of permanent functional change. Variables influencing both motor learning and motor performance include the practice session structure (blocked, random, massed, or distributed) and the type and frequency of feedback provided to the client. Traditionally, rehabilitation therapists have often assumed that more consistent practice in identical environmental contexts (eg, practicing the same skill in the same way for long periods of time), and richer, more immediate feedback (eg, giving a wealth of detail on the client's performance immediately after, or often during the execution of the skill) enhanced functional change in client skill. Motor learning research indicates that, in many cases, these variables do enhance motor performance, but are detrimental to motor learning or more permanent skill change. Therefore, more varied practice, multiple environmental contexts, and limited feedback may be more effective when more permanent functional change is desired. Motor learning experts suggest that rehabilitation therapists should encourage their clients to analyze more actively their own movement and problem-solve for skill improvement. A more in-depth discussion of these issues can be found in the writings of Winstein, Schmidt and others.[15–17]

Enhancing Motor Skill Through Task Analysis

Successful motor skill acquisition can occur only if motor tasks with reasonable demands are selected for a client. When planning treatment activities, the neurorehabilitation professional must select tasks that are sufficiently challenging yet involve variables that make the skill accomplishable for that particular client.[18] Traditionally, therapists have not recognized all of the variables influencing the difficulty of tasks. Understanding these variables assists the therapist in analyzing functional skills and modifying treatment activities to increase or decrease difficulty levels as needed. Gentile provides a "taxonomy of tasks" that analyzes motor skills with regard to the motion of the performer, the performance environment, and the role of the performer's upper extremities.[18] For example, a task becomes more difficult to accomplish when the client must interact with a moving environment (eg, walking in a room where others are walking). Another significant variable involves manipulation requirements when the hands are engaged in a task (eg, holding a cane, passing a ball). In this situation, the arms cannot be used to stabilize the body, which leads to greater task complexity. When a task changes from one trial to the next, intertrial variability is said to exist. Such a condition forces the client to modify his or her movement response on an ongoing basis—increasing the skill requirements. The ability to analyze tasks and modify them, when needed, is crucial for the neurotherapist. For a more detailed discussion of the taxonomy of tasks, readers are referred to the more comprehensive work by Gentile.[18]

Motor skill learning is believed to take place in stages.[18,19] The early stage of skill acquisition is characterized by exploration of possible movements in search of a successful strategy. Through trial and error, the learner discards unsuccessful strategies and retains successful ones. At the end of the initial stage, the learner is not consistent in his or her performance, but has developed a general strategy for completing a task. The later stages of skill acquisition work to refine skill by improving consistency in and efficiency of the movement strategy.

Guidelines for Aquatic Neurotreatment

Benefits of the Aquatic Environment for Neurotreatment

The aquatic environment provides multiple benefits for physical rehabilitation programs.[6–8,11,12] The benefits may differ from one diagnostic group to another. In general, the benefits of using water for neurotreatment involve the property of buoyancy.

Buoyant support from water provides weight relief, allowing clients with weakness to assume upright postures at an earlier time in their rehabilitation process. This support becomes increasingly effective with increasing depth of water. This weight relief allows for dramatic leaps in functional ability while in the water. For example, clients who require moderate assistance to stand in parallel bars on land can often ambulate in the pool.

Therapists should be aware, however, that this buoyant support may also lead to movement difficulty. When the client's physical characteristics are conducive to floating (ie, increased adipose tissue, hypotonicity), he or she may become unstable, leading to hypertonicity and associated stereotypic movement patterns. In addition, decreased weight bearing through the joints may further diminish sensory input for clients with sensory deficits. These problems can be avoided through proper handling and use of appropriate water depths for treatment.

Buoyancy assistance can also permit decreased effort to be used with movements of the extremities toward the water's surface. This assistance can be used with the client in a variety of positions (ie, sitting, standing, supine). In water, clients can move the extremities through significantly greater ranges of motion, providing a strengthening, stretching, and muscle re-education benefit. Buoyancy assistance is particularly helpful in assisting clients to regain control of quick, reciprocal movement patterns. Such activities are rarely possible on land until late in the rehabilitation program.

Because clients are so well supported in the water, they are easily handled and guarded by the accompanying therapist. This allows the client to move in a more independent manner with less therapist support. The client is also allowed to attempt higher-level skills in a more aggressive fashion (ie, through greater excursions of movement, at faster speeds). Because the therapist is able to reduce the amount of physical support provided, the client can become more independent in movement problem solving.

The ability to perform more advanced functional skills and move more independently provides psychological benefits, including motivation and self-confidence. Anecdotal experience suggests that this benefit dramatically influences positive rehabilitation outcomes.

Other water properties are of benefit for neurotreatment programs. When faster movement occurs in the water, the turbulent drag provides resistance that is proportional to the speed of movement. In addition to strengthening weak muscles, this resistance may also heighten sensory input, leading to facilitation of the movement pattern.

Providing for Client Stability in the Water

Perhaps the most critical skill for therapists is the ability to instill confidence and a sense of security in their clients—a complex task requiring consideration of multiple factors.[20] Appealing to the client's emotional state (mental adjustment), maximizing buoyant support for assisting or challenging clients' abilities (positioning), using hand placement to provide assistance or allow more independence (handling), and educating clients about how the water influences their stability (understanding), are steps for ensuring client comfort during therapeutic pool treatment. Attention to these four steps improves the therapist's ability to assert control over client movement in the water.

Mental Adjustment

When first approached about the aquatic rehabilitation option, clients often conjure many visions about how the service will be delivered. Many have never been comfortable in water, a fear that is heightened when physical injury or disability are also factors. Some clients believe that they are being referred for swimming lessons when, in fact, neither the therapist nor the client have such intentions. An orientation to aquatic rehabilitation can dispel faulty notions of what will be expected and likewise dramatically reduce client anxieties about treatment. The orientation can include the following:

1. A brief tour of the pool and surrounding area. Areas of varying depth should be pointed out, especially if abrupt changes occur (ie, steep slopes or steps).
2. Methods of entry and exit from the pool. Such activities should be described and demonstrated.
3. The purposes of and general aims for the client's referral to the therapeutic pool. This can include an explanation of why the pool can benefit clients with physical therapy needs. Although they may not be determined before treatment, the therapist could de-

scribe activities the client will likely be performing.
4. Factors that allow the therapist to provide support to the client. Statements like "the buoyancy of the water will make you very light," and "I can lift and carry you very easily in the water," assist in convincing clients that the therapist can manage them safely in the water. Emphasize the fact that most clients truly enjoy their pool treatments.

These activities only require a few minutes to execute and can determine the success of the client's aquatic experience.

Positioning

As on land, certain body positions assumed in the water are easier to control than others. Unfortunately, many clients automatically assume the least stable positions when allowed to do so. Campion describes four positions commonly assumed during therapeutic pool activities.[8] They are the ball, cube, triangle, and stick positions, listed from the most to least stable. Although the ball position is the most stable, it is probably the least used during client care. Instead, the cube is the most practical for use with clients. By submerging the body, assuming a sitting position, and extending the arms, the client positions the trunk and extremities in a manner that maximizes the buoyant support provided by the water (Fig. 7-1). As clients gain more skill and independence, they can assume positions like the triangle (Fig. 7-2) and stick (Fig. 7-3), in which less of the body is submerged and supported by buoyant forces. In an effort to keep their mouths and noses away from the water, many clients assume a stick position when first entering the therapeutic pool. An explanation, and sometimes even persuasion, is required before these clients will try a more stable position.

Handling

As on land, following certain handling principles can dramatically influence the therapist's control over a client's movement. Placing a hand on proximal portions of the body (eg, the trunk) provides more control than more distal positions (eg, hands). Campion[7] describes handling techniques for aquatic therapists. For example, a Bell's hold places the client in a ball (Fig. 7-4) position. The therapist assumes a cube position to improve his or her stability. This hold is commonly used with very dependent clients and is

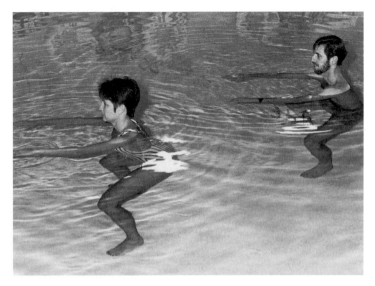

FIGURE 7-1. The cube position.

often used to transport clients from one area in the pool to another. Another frequently used technique is the horizontal backing hold. Using this technique, the therapist asks the client to lie back in the water while resting his or her head on the therapist's shoulder. The therapist then supports the client by holding the posterolateral portions of the client's trunk. This technique is particularly useful when promoting relaxation and when clients are performing lower limb exercises (eg, pedalling, flutterkicks). For further descriptions, readers are advised to refer to the works of Campion.[7]

Understanding

People with many years' experience in the water intuitively understand how water influences stability. Many clients, however, do not share this insight and require explanations to achieve such understanding. Therapists should educate their clients about how buoyant support can be controlled (ie, blowing air out to sink and holding air in to float, holding the arms out to float and bringing the arms in to sink). In addition, therapists and clients should discuss how turbulent drag influences movement through the water.

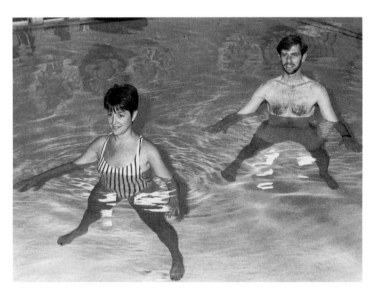

FIGURE 7-2. The triangle position.

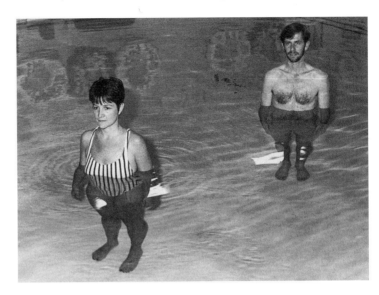

FIGURE 7-3. The stick position.

Aquatic Treatment Design

Therapists should consider factors that influence the difficulty of movement in the water when designing aquatic rehabilitation programs. The following factors are most influential in aquatic treatment design for neurologically involved clients.[12]

Depth of the Water

Because buoyant support increases as more of the body is submerged, clients who have difficulty standing perform exercises easier in deeper water. Therefore, exercises should be first performed in deeper water, with a progressive movement to more shallow depths as the client improves. One exception to this guideline is with arm exercises. Performing such activities in shallow water may prevent clients from submerging the entire upper extremity to maximize buoyancy assistance to movement or resistance from the water's drag.

Unilateral Versus Bilateral Movements

The resistant drag produced with movement in the water increases the effort the client must make. When a submerged extremity is moved, the increased effort challenges the stability provided by the moving person's trunk and proximal segments. This increased effort can be minimized if the client moves only one extremity, particularly if the other extremity is used to provide additional stability (eg, holding onto the side of the pool, standing on the pool floor). As the client's ability to stabilize improves, bilateral movements should be attempted. With regard to resistive force produced and challenging proximal stability, asymmetric bilateral movements (ie, moving the right shoulder into flexion while simultaneously moving the left shoulder into extension) are usually easier than symmetric bilateral movements (ie, both shoulders moving into flexion simultaneously).

Distal Stabilization

When the distal end of a moving body segment is in contact with an object with stable properties (eg, a buoyant support like a float, or a fixed

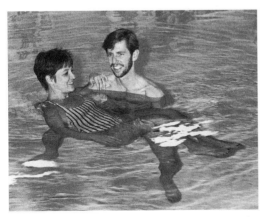

FIGURE 7-4. Using Bell's hold, the therapist places the client in a ball position and assumes the cube position himself for maximal stability.

object like a handle attached to the side of the pool), the client performing the activity can use this support assist in stabilization. Therefore, these "distal end stable" activities are in general easier to accomplish than when the distal end of a moving body segment moves free of any stabilizing influence ("distal end free"). Examples of distal end stable aquatic activities include resting one's hand on a kickboard and moving across the surface of the water in shoulder horizontal abduction/adduction, or performing most Bad Ragaz ring method (BRRM) activities. Distal end free aquatic activities include performing a swimming stroke or deep-water running.

Speed/Excursion of Movement

As a person immersed in water slightly increases the speed of his or her movement, the resistance encountered dramatically increases. Similarly, as clients move through greater ranges of motion, the activity difficulty also increases. Therefore, clients should begin activities slowly and through small ranges of motion and gradually increase both as skill allows. A general guideline for clients is to instruct them to "move as quickly and as far as you can and still do the activity in a comfortable, correct manner." Improper movement patterns are an indication that the client is exceeding his or her abilities regarding speed and excursion.

Specific Aquatic Rehabilitation Approaches Used With Clients Recovering From Brain Injury

Many aquatic rehabilitation approaches can be used in the treatment of clients with brain injury. Four specific approaches are mentioned frequently as being particularly useful with this population. These approaches may influence clients at the impairment level, disability level, or both. Each approach can also be described in terms of traditional neurorehabilitation models.

WATSU

WATSU (Water Shiatsu) was developed by Harold Dull at Harbin Hot Springs, California.[21] Dull describes the technique as Zen Shiatsu principles applied to people floating in the water.

WATSU was created as a wellness technique and was not necessarily intended for use with clients with brain injury. However, rehabilitation therapists who have applied the approach to clients with a variety of physical disorders have reported clinical success. WATSU can be best described as a muscle re-education approach, because specific impairments (usually tight muscles and joints) are targeted for treatment with little regard to the models of motor control. Chapter 17 of this book is devoted entirely to WATSU. Based on an Eastern medicine philosophy, the approach is concerned with stretching the body's meridians (pathways of energy). Through stretching, these pathways are brought closer to the body's surface, allowing the energy to be released. Rotational movements that release blocked energy from joint articulations enhance these effects. As totally passive recipients, clients experience profound relaxation from the water's support and the continual rhythmic movement that flows gracefully from one position to the next. Stretches are composed of transitions and sequences. In general, the therapist stabilizes or moves one segment of the body while movement through the water results in a drag effect, thus stretching another segment. Therapists are encouraged to vary the transitions and sequences according to the needs and limitations of the client. Clients with brain injury often exhibit range of motion limitations secondary to soft tissue restrictions.[22–24] These restrictions can impede functional recovery by preventing movement and the positioning that is most biomechanically efficient. Tone and voluntary movement disorders can further magnify these biomechanical deficits.[23,24] WATSU is particularly helpful when used at the beginning of a treatment session. Pretreatment with WATSU can improve motion during subsequent treatment. Maneuvers that may have specific applications to clients with neurologic impairments include the leg push (promoting hip extension), the hip rock (promoting lateral trunk shortening and elongating), and the rotating accordion (promoting trunk and hip rotation).[21]

The Bad Ragaz Ring Method

The BRRM was developed in the 1930s in Bad Ragaz, Switzerland.[6,25,26] A detailed description of this technique can be found in Chapter 15. The approach was later modified to incorporate certain principles of proprioceptive neuromuscular facilitation (PNF), a therapeutic exercise technique used on land. Both the BRRM and PNF use specific movement patterns to increase strength and range of motion by using arm, leg, and trunk movements in unilateral or bilateral patterns. Bilateral motion may be symmetric (both sides moving in the same direction) or asymmetric (both sides of the body moving in different directions). Patterns may encourage isotonic or isometric muscle contractions. Precise movement instructions are part of both the BRRM and PNF (eg, "bring your right knee to your left shoulder"). However, differences exist between the two techniques. The BRRM requires the therapist to place his or her hands on specific locations while the client is instructed to move in a specific direction. The therapist then becomes a point of stability from which the client moves. Resistance to the client's movement is created by turbulent drag. Proprioceptive neuromuscular facilitation requires the therapist manually to apply graded resistance to movement. The BRRM, on the other hand, usually allows the client to determine the amount of resistance based on his or her speed of movement. Occasionally, however, BRRM patterns incorporate therapist-applied manual resistance. The BRRM allows the therapist to increase the difficulty of the activity by placing the stabilizing hold more distally. Such strategies do not necessarily increase the resistance to movement, but do increase the complexity of the activity by requiring the client to control larger segments of his or her body during the movement. At times, the therapist may use an overflow principle with the BRRM by stabilizing and resisting one portion of the body to facilitate activity in another. The BRRM was principally designed to treat a variety of musculoskeletal movement disorders, but the technique can also be used to treat disorders such as voluntary movement deficit, weakness, and decreased range of motion associated with brain injury. Many of these clients lack the ability to stabilize multiple segments of their body, even when horizontally supported in the water. These clients often require additional trunk flotation support to ensure safety and security. Treatment of voluntary movement deficits should emphasize techniques that promote smooth, slow, rhythmic motion rather than irregular, fast, jerky movement. Postcontraction muscle relaxation is difficult for clients with voluntary movement disorders.[22–24] This problem limits reciprocal motion because of poor activation of antagonistic muscle groups. The result is

muscular cocontraction that severely limits joint motion. The BRRM can be modified by passively moving the client in directions in which this prolonged contraction occurs, allowing voluntary contraction of the antagonistic muscle. Less therapist assistance is required as the client gains better control of reciprocal inhibition (ie, voluntary relaxation of an antagonistic muscle group). Many clients develop the skill to move smoothly and reciprocally. The BRRM has the characteristics of a neurotherapeutic facilitation approach because it encourages improved skill in specific patterns of movement. Results are usually seen at an impairment level.

The Halliwick Method

Developed by James McMillan in the 1930s at the Halliwick School for Girls, the Halliwick method is based on principles of hydrodynamics and human development.[7,8,27,28] The approach is intended as a swimming instruction technique. Many of its activities and principles may also be used for specific therapeutic intervention. The Halliwick method is a neurotherapeutic facilitation rehabilitation technique that follows a disengagement principle. According to this principle, therapists use activities to facilitate movement patterns by varying the activity's level of difficulty and the amount of manual guidance provided. Therapists begin with less difficult activities and manually guide the client to make sure the movement is performed correctly. As the client becomes more skilled, the therapist reduces the amount of assistance provided (disengaging) and increases the level of difficulty of the exercise. Finally, when the client masters the activity, the therapist creates turbulence around the client's body to challenge the skill and reinforce learning. A 10-point program is used to design the exercises. Using the Halliwick method for swimming instruction is ultimately therapeutic for all people because of the conditioning effects inherent in this form of exercise. This is particularly true for people with impairment and disability secondary to brain injury. Application for more specific therapeutic effects includes work to become skillful in vertical rotation control in an anterior direction. Such a movement would help the client actively control flexor musculature and inhibit extensor musculature—a task that is frequently difficult for clients with brain injury. Also, skill gained through balance-instilling activities may carry over and influence postural stability during functional activities. Chapter 16 describes the Halliwick method in greater detail.

Task Type Training Approach

A task type training approach (TTTA), formerly referred to as a functional training approach, is an aquatic rehabilitation program for clients who have had a stroke.[11,12] The guidelines and principles of the TTTA can be extended to include the treatment of all clients with brain injury. The TTTA is best described as a task-oriented approach because emphasis is placed on improving the client's functional skill by working in functional positions with functional activities. In addition, clients are encouraged to become active problem solvers with regard to their movement difficulties, as opposed to passive recipients of manual or verbal input from the therapist. Notably, the TTTA is not a treatment technique, but a set of principles that guide therapists as they design treatment programs for their clients' disabilities. The general principles include:

1. *Work in the most shallow water tolerated.* The buoyant support of the water allows many clients to stand and move independently in a functional manner for the first time. This assistance allows the client to participate actively and aggressively in improving his or her functional disabilities. This practice is conducive to the type of skill achieved during the initial stages of acquisition; developing a general movement strategy. Refinement of skill, however, may require practice in a gravity environment because the ultimate goal is for functional improvement to carry over to land activities. Therefore, the effect of buoyant support should be diminished in a graded manner as clients demonstrate improved skill with functional activities. Performance indicators, such as the inability to maintain an erect trunk in standing or the inability to maintain knee extension to support lower extremities, may indicate that deeper water should be used.

2. *Functional activities should be practiced as a whole.* Although some treatment programs address strengthening or stretching of specific body segments or facilitating specific movement patterns, the TTTA encourages practice of activities that are identical to or closely approximate land-based functional activities. This principle is based on a belief in specificity of training: to influence a functional skill, that particular skill needs to be practiced.[18,19] When performed as a whole, the entire functional skill must be mastered, including control of moving body segments and appropriately graded contraction of stabilizing body segments.

3. *Systematically remove external stabilization provided for clients.* Support provided by holding onto the pool wall or by the therapist's manual assistance may be necessary in the earlier stages of a TTTA. This externally applied stabilization should be sequentially removed as client's develop increased independent control over the functional activity. By doing so, the therapist minimizes the client's dependence on outside support for functional skills.

4. *Encourage stabilizing contractions in upright positions with movement of selected body segments.* Vertical or upright positions (eg, sitting, standing) are positions of function and should be used as much as possible. Stereotypic strategies for the maintenance of postural stability in upright positions have been identified.[29] Clients with neurologic disorders typically have difficulty using these strategies to maintain their balance. Therefore, clients should be encouraged to relearn these maneuvers in a safe but challenging environment—the water. As clients move their extremities in or above the water, their center of balance is challenged. Preventing a fall requires use of effective postural stabilization. The client is forced to problem-solve actively to redevelop these strategies, with attention given to sequential contraction of the appropriate muscles with an appropriate force.

5. *Encourage quick, reciprocal movement.* After many types of neurologic insults, neural shock produces a period of muscle inactivity during which deconditioning occurs. Studies indicate that many clients with neurologic disorders have a predominance of slow-twitch muscle fibers in their skeletal muscles, indicating that a conversion from fast- to slow-twitch fibers has occurred.[22–24] Some believe that this muscle fiber change contributes to the slow, labored movement typically seen in these disorders.[22–24] Many functional activities require rhythmic, reciprocal movements along with quick movement changes

to maximize the use of inertial forces. Movement in this manner ensures smooth and efficient execution of functional activities. The presence of weakness, range of motion limitations, and other voluntary movement deficits prevents clients with neurologic disorders from moving in an effective manner in a gravity environment. The supportive and assistive properties of water dramatically increase the likelihood of these clients performing such activities. Therefore, whenever possible, quick, reciprocal movements should be practiced (eg, marching in place, pedalling the legs while supine). Such practice may produce a conditioning effect that positively influences the impairments constraining clients with neurologic disorders to slow, labored movements.

6. *Encourage active movement problem solving.* Motor learning research suggests that healthy humans learn movement skills better when they actively participate in the learning process.[15-17] For example, when subjects are given less feedback on their performance and are required to practice many and varied activities, they must become more reliant on their own ability to critique and modify their performance, leading to more active participation. Studies of subjects with neurologic disorders have rendered similar conclusions. For this reason, clients should be encouraged to critique their performance and propose movement solutions. Open-ended questions, like "How did you do that time?" and "How can you improve your next attempt?" should be used whenever possible. When working in the pool with clients with neurologic disorders, several factors may make using such principles difficult. Many clients with neurologic disorders have difficulty critiquing their performance because of physical (ie, sensory) and cognitive (ie, perceptual) impairments. In this case, the therapist must provide minimal guiding feedback regarding the client's performance.

7. *Gradually increase the difficulty of the task.* Activities used should be challenging yet accomplishable by the client. Therapists can adjust the task's level of difficulty by using Gentile's taxonomy of tasks. For example, tasks attempted by less skilled clients would likely involve stationary environments, lack intertrial variability, and have few manipulation requirements.

Common Problems Associated With Brain Injury

Therapists must understand the pathophysiology of brain injury to develop effective rehabilitation programs for such clients. Common problems associated with brain injury include voluntary movement deficit, balance dysfunction, and gait dysfunction. All three problem areas may influence each other and may have similar contributing factors.

Voluntary Movement Deficit

Giuliani[24] describes functional movements as "composed of a series of events involving several joints and using many muscles that are activated at the appropriate time and which produce the correct amount of force so that smooth, coordinated movement occurs." Voluntary movement deficit (VMD) is the inability to perform functional movement and is often present after brain injury.[22-24] VMD can range from mild to severe and can be the result of many underlying causes. Traditional assumptions regarding VMD adduce a lack of inhibitory control by the CNS from supraspinal centers over lower centers as the cause of hyperactive stretch reflexes.[1,2] The more recent literature, however, has taken an expanded view of VMD and describes different underlying causes that are both neural and nonneural.[22-24] Giuliani[24] describes the contributing factors to VMD as originating centrally, peripherally, or both. People who demonstrate VMD may have different mechanisms contributing to their movement. Therapists should examine the characteristics of VMD in each client and approach his or her treatment to resolve the specific underlying causes. The following sections describe some common contributing factors considered in evaluation and treatment of VMD.

Central Mechanism Dysfunction

Examples of central factors may include damage to the neural circuitry that generates movement patterns, aberrant input (inhibition or facilitation) to that circuitry, or abnormal motoneuron recruitment.[22-24] Hyperactive stretch reflexes may result from hypertonic muscles supplied by motoneurons that are closer to their discharge thresholds. Such a resting state allows reflex activity to be initiated by even a slight stretch. An imbalance of tonic excitation and inhibition from supraspinal sources acting on the impaired motoneurons is thought to be responsible for the lowered threshold.

Alterations in reciprocal innervation can result in an inability to perform alternating movement patterns. Sahrmann and Norton[30] attributed such movement deficits to prolonged recruitment of hypertonic muscles, resulting in an inability of that muscle to cease contracting voluntarily. The hyperexcitable agonist excessively reciprocally inhibits the antagonistic muscle, putting it at a disadvantage for recruiting sufficient motor units when contraction is required. Movement can occur in one direction but cannot be reversed. This reciprocal movement deficit limits functional skill.

Peripheral Mechanism Dysfunction

After CNS dysfunction, changes in the compliance of muscle and other connective tissues (ie, tendons, ligaments, joint structures) occur.[22-24] An actual reduction in muscle sarcomeres may be responsible for an increase in passive mechanical resistance. Studies link reduced tissue compliance with abnormal movement patterns.[31]

McComas and colleagues[32] found that subjects with CNS dysfunction have a dramatic reduction in the number of functioning motor units. The remaining motor units have slower contraction times, longer conduction latencies, and decremental responses to repetitive discharges. These findings agree with other research that suggests that surviving motoneurons tend to innervate type I slow-twitch muscle fibers, with a progressive reduction of fast-twitch type II muscle fibers. Such a condition may contribute to the slow, labored quality of movement seen in these subjects.

Aquatic Solution for Voluntary Movement Deficit

Water's neutral warmth is thought to be effective in reducing hypertonicity and improving movement quality.[5-8] The need for warm water to treat hypertonicity may not be as great as the need to avoid cold water, because cold water aggravates hypertonic states.

When clients exhibit decreased compliance in muscle and other connective tissues, WATSU and other stretching activities may prove effective because they prepare the client to move

more freely during more active portions of the treatment session.

The BRRM techniques may be used to treat reciprocal innervation dysfunction by emphasizing slow, controlled movement through the range of motion and subsequently increasing the speed of movement to challenge reciprocal innervation control. In cases of severe reciprocal innervation dysfunction, the therapist may choose to encourage active movement by the weak, inhibited muscle groups and passively create movement of the antagonistic muscle through its range of motion (eg, when clients have difficulty relaxing the quadriceps; using the BRRM pattern of hip and knee flexion with ankle dorsiflexion, followed by a gentle push on the lower leg to return the leg passively into an extended position, can allow successive flexion).

The disengagement principle of the Halliwick method suggests that therapists assist their clients' movements to ensure smooth patterns of movement. Therapists assist client movements by using more stable positions for activities (eg, a cube position), using proximal hand holds, and limiting the amount of turbulence created around the client. The low-effort movement reduces the need for excessive motoneuron recruitment and allows isolated movement of specific body segments. For example, shoulder flexion or abduction can occur without developing a shoulder flexor synergy pattern (ie, including forearm pronation and elbow, wrist, and finger flexion).

The TTTA supports the most independent practice of functional skills by the client. The aquatic environment may be one of the few places where quick reciprocal movements can be performed safely. This is important for rehabilitating clients with brain injury because encouraging such activities (eg, pedalling the legs, walking quickly) may decrease the atrophy of fast-twitch muscle fibers and possibly reverse deconditioning effects. Quick, reciprocal activities may need to be performed in an active-assist manner if severe voluntary movement deficits are present. In addition to the pattern and speed of movement, the initiation and cessation of movement should be evaluated and treated because they relate to functional movement.

Balance Dysfunction

Balance is a complex motor task that requires integration of sensory information, motor coordination, and biomechanical control.[14,32,33] The basic task of balance is to position the body's center of gravity over some portion of its base of support (ie, the feet in standing, the buttocks in sitting). When the center of gravity extends beyond the base of support, stability is challenged. Normally, an adult's limits of stability (the maximum angle from the vertical that can be tolerated without a loss of balance) are 12° in an anteroposterior direction and 16° in a lateral direction. People with balance dysfunction have greatly reduced limits of stability. Nashner[29] described automatic, stereotypic postural reactions used by humans to respond to balance disturbances. These reactions include ankle, hip, and stepping strategies. Different strategies are used to maintain balance based on the characteristics of the external balance disturbance and the support surface available. To be effective, the postural reactions must provide proper environmental context, force, and muscle activity. The treatment of balance dysfunction requires a thorough evaluation of the three aspects of normal balance function: biomechanical aspects, motor coordination, and sensory integration.[14,32,33]

Biomechanical Aspects

Biomechanical factors that contribute to poor balance include limited range of motion and muscle weakness.[14,32,33] These factors, often nonneural in nature, prevent movement into biomechanically stable positions. Clients with CNS dysfunction may have longstanding biomechanical problems (eg, limited ankle dorsiflexion) but may have only recently experienced balance problems. These balance problems most likely occurred when the client became unable to compensate for a combination of biomechanical and neurologic deficits. Each biomechanical limitation should be addressed to improve the client's postural stability.

Motor Coordination

Strategies used to maintain balance (ie, ankle, hip, stepping strategies) must be performed in a coordinated and appropriate fashion.[14,32,33] Motor coordination may be reduced to timing problems, including delayed onset of motor activity and improper sequencing of motor activity (eg, an ankle strategy that does not follow a distal-to-proximal progression of muscle contractions). Scaling problems also may interfere with motor coordination when the force of a motor response is either too great or too small. Finally, clients with poor motor coordination may use a motor strategy that is inappropriate for the motor challenge (eg, using a hip strategy when standing on a large, firm surface area and challenged by a small force—a condition usually requiring an ankle strategy). When motor coordination problems exist, clients should be challenged to practice functional skills using the uncoordinated motor strategies until more effective motor patterns are developed. Therapists are challenged to develop treatment activities that facilitate or inhibit certain aspects of the responses to promote effective and appropriate postural reactions.

Sensory Integration

Balance requires awareness of the body's position in space and interaction with the environment regarding movement. Three sensory systems provide this type of information to humans: visual, vestibular, and somatosensory.[14,33,34] Interaction between these systems allows an appropriate postural response to be selected for any given condition. Somatosensation and vision are used most in balance maintenance; however, both can provide conflicting information. For example, when standing beside a large bus, a person may experience a moving sensation from visual input when the bus moves forward; somatosensation, however, indicates that the person is standing still. The vestibular system, although less sensitive than the other two sensory systems, is often critical to proper integration of conflicting sensory input so that an appropriate musculoskeletal response occurs. When sensory integration contributes to balance problems, several treatment approaches may be useful. Therapists may choose to (1) facilitate use of the dysfunctional system to improve its function; (2) encourage compensation from a more efficient sensory system; (3) adapt the client's environment to minimize risk of falling; and (4) repeatedly stimulate a hyperfunctioning vestibular system to habituate the exaggerated response. The most appropriate treatment approach can be selected by examining each sensory system's effectiveness and integrative abilities. Horak and Shumway-Cook[14,34,35] have proposed a Clinical Test for Sensory Interaction in Balance to assist with this process.

Aquatic Solution for Balance Dysfunction

Use of WATSU, the BRRM, the Halliwick method, and other aquatic stretching/strengthening activities can have a positive influence on biomechanical factors associated with balance dysfunction. The aquatic environment is particularly well suited for these activities because the physical properties of water allow easy handling by therapists and effective progressive resistance qualities for clients who have the necessary range of strength capabilities. The principles set forth in the Halliwick method with regard to positioning and handling can be particularly helpful when designing activities that are progressively difficult.

The buoyant support provided by the water allows the person with impairments to assume upright postures in a more independent manner. Clients often can relearn postural synergy mechanisms that have been disrupted after brain injury. Some authors discourage the use of the aquatic environment when sensory disturbances contribute to movement problems.[6,7] The decreased weight bearing and subsequent reduced proprioceptive/sensory input through joint receptors is said to make movement more difficult. This author disagrees with these notions because, first, although decreased compared with standing on land, weight bearing while standing in the water still occurs, and this may be the only situation that provides such an approximation during activities in which clients have sufficient skill or strength to participate actively; and second, other forms of afferent input may be increased in the pool, including cutaneous input from water on the skin, afferent input from muscle receptors of freely moving body parts, and vestibular input as the result of increased activity. This heightened sensory input should compensate for reduced input from joint receptors.

When sensory loss is present, clients should work in the shallowest water possible. The added weight bearing may provide useful input. Protective footwear should be encouraged. Treatment activities should emphasize use of the remaining sensory systems to compensate for the more permanent sensory loss. When sensory integration dysfunction is present, therapists should challenge clients by using multiple sensory inputs during treatments (eg, passing a ball with the client as they are walking across the pool). Activities that encourage movement toward a client's limits of stability can safely be used with little fear of falling. For example, clients are challenged when asked to place a ball in a basket on the side of the therapeutic pool. The therapist can increase the difficulty of this activity by moving into more shallow water, moving the basket farther away, or reducing any manual assistance.

Gait Dysfunction

Esquenazi and Hirai[36] describe the three functional goals of ambulation as (1) to move from one place to another, (2) to move safely, and (3) to move efficiently. The sequelae of brain injury frequently compromise all three goals. Winter[37] outlined three "necessary" tasks for safe ambulation: (1) upward support of the body, (2) maintenance of upright posture and balance, and (3) control of foot movement to provide toe clearance and gentle foot contact. Brain-injured clients often demonstrate significantly reduced walking speed, stride length, and cycle duration compared to normal subjects.[36–39] Although characteristic gait patterns have been described for clients with different types of brain injury, clients do not always present with the typical neurologic gait deviations associated with their diagnosis (eg, hemiplegic gait, Parkinson's gait). Therefore, no matter what their diagnosis, each client should be individually evaluated and treated according to the specific gait abnormalities observed. The following are some of the more commonly seen gait problems associated with brain injury.

Stance Phase

The stance phase of gait must provide adequate support for the weight-bearing extremity and adequate force to propel the body forward during push-off. The gait of clients with brain injury commonly is characterized by poor hip and knee extensor force, inadequate ankle plantar flexor force, and limited hip extension range of motion. All three gait deviations reduce the amount of time spent in single limb stance of the affected extremities. During terminal swing, clients with brain injury often recruit muscles in an extensor synergy pattern. The resulting rigid limb prevents the normal limb loading and weight acceptance seen in normal gait. Force control difficulty also is observed during the push-off phase of stance when these clients fail to exert adequate plantar flexion force. As a result, brain-injured clients fail to transfer weight to the contralateral limb.

Swing Phase

A successful swing phase provides safe foot clearance, foot advancement, and controlled transfer of momentum. Clients with brain injury often exhibit swing phase deviations such as poor foot clearance, excessive cocontraction of the moving leg, abrupt knee and ankle extension in late swing, and inadequate weight shift. Electromyographic studies indicate that during the swing phase of normal subjects, the lower extremity is shortened by active hip flexion accompanied by passive knee flexion. Poor soft tissue compliance in the knee extensors can prevent lower limb shortening in the typical manner. In addition, ankle weakness and limited range of motion may contribute to poor foot clearance.

Other forms of VMD can contribute to an abnormal swing phase. Active hip flexion during the initial swing can elicit a massed flexion pattern in the lower limb. Prolonged recruitment of these muscles prevents the lower limb extension needed during terminal swing.

Aquatic Solution to Gait Dysfunction

The stance phase of a client's gait pattern can be improved by increasing range of motion in the stance limb, particularly in hip extension and ankle dorsiflexion. WATSU can be effective in stretching more proximal regions of the client's lower quarter. Specifically, the spine stretch and leg push increase trunk and hip extension. However, stretching for more distal portions of the lower limb requires stretching methods similar to those used on land (eg, standing calf stretches). Performing such a stretch is advantageous in that buoyant support allows the activity to take place in a more independent and effective manner, especially for clients with standing difficulty. WATSU also can influence the swing phase of gait by improving soft tissue compliance. The reduced stiffness allows passive knee flexion in early swing, ensuring better lower limb clearance.

Isometric and isotonic BRRM activities can improve lower limb stance. Isometric hip and knee extension patterns promote cocontraction of these muscles. Isotonic hip–knee extension with plantar flexion can reduce knee buckling

in midstance and improve push-off. BRRM activities also can be used to improve the swing phase of gait by reducing massed flexion or extension in the lower limb. Therapists may need to assist clients by using more proximal hand holds, reducing the excursion of movement, and assisting through difficult positions in the range of movement. These forms of assistance should be removed as reciprocal motion improves.

A client's ability to control stance can be challenged using the Balance Instillness principle of the Halliwick method. To do so, clients are placed first in the position desired (ie, sitting or standing). The therapist creates turbulence around the client, requiring him or her to contract the appropriate stabilizing muscles. As previously stated, the disengagement principle can be used with all activities aimed at improving stance and swing.

A TTTA can be used to influence gait at the disability level. Activities are performed in upright positions closely approximating those used during ambulation. Stability can be applied externally by the therapist holding the client or by allowing the client to hold onto the side of the pool or a flotation device. This external stabilization is kept to a minimum because the goal for treatment is to reduce such assistance. Activities like the one leg up can allow practice of both stance (ie, holding the lower limb in hip and knee extension) and swing (ie, moving the contralateral limb through reciprocal active hip flexion with passive knee flexion). TTTA principles can be applied to many activities, ranging from low-level, static exercises to high-level, dynamic ones. Descriptions of such activities are provided in Box 7-1.

Buoyancy may prevent sufficient pressure on the soles of the feet to inhibit lower extremity extensor synergy postures. The resultant posture may include ankle plantar flexion and supination—a biomechanically unsafe position for weight bearing. This situation can be prevented with the use of plastic ankle–foot orthoses during standing and gait activities. Effective use of an ankle–foot orthosis requires sufficient support from footwear. A canvas deck shoe can support an ankle–foot orthosis when worn in the water. Because canvas material does not absorb a great deal of water, the shoe does not become heavy, impeding the swing phase of gait. The ankle–foot orthosis is used for proper foot positioning during the stance phase of the gait cycle rather than for ankle dorsiflexion assistance. Less neural input is required to create

BOX 7-1. Task Type Training Approach Activities Commonly Used to Improve Gait Dysfunction

Standing weight shift. Client stands and shifts weight from one leg to the other. Slight knee flexion should occur in the unweighted lower limb.

One leg up. Client stands facing the pool wall and lifts one leg repeatedly. Emphasis is placed on active hip flexion and passive knee flexion.

Marching. Client lifts and lowers one leg, followed immediately by the same on the other leg. Speed and coordination are emphasized.

Kick back. Client stands facing the pool wall and kicks one leg in a posterior direction repeatedly. Emphasis is placed on hip extension with knee extension.

Side kick. Client stands facing the pool wall and kicks one leg to the side repeatedly. Emphasis is placed on hip abduction and knee extension.

Straight leg kick. Client stands with side to the pool wall and swings one leg forward and back repeatedly. Emphasis is placed on hip flexion and extension, with knee extension on the swinging lower limb and hip and knee extension on the stance limb.

Walking with front support. Therapist stands in front of the client and provides bilateral support to the client's upper limbs.

Walking with side support. Therapist stands at the client's side and provides unilateral support to one of the client's upper limbs.

movement in the aquatic environment because of the effect of buoyancy. A reduction of neural input to the agonist reciprocally reduces antagonist muscle inhibition. Smoother, more reciprocal movement can result.

Community Aquatic Programs for Clients With Brain Injury

Wade and colleagues[40] demonstrated that even though physical impairments can be positively influenced with therapeutic exercise, function can decline beyond premorbid status when this activity ceases. Therefore, maintenance physical exercise programs are essential. Unfortunately,

architectural barriers and a lack of special population programs create difficulties for people with brain injuries to engage in fitness activities. Community aquatic exercise programs are ideal for brain-injured people. Studies and anecdotal reports indicate that community aquatic programs may even directly improve the participants' function.[41] However, when developing community aquatics programs, certain key decisions must be made:

Program objectives. The objectives should be clearly stated before implementation. Objectives include who the program will serve, participant characteristics that will be influenced, and to what degree the therapist will effect them. The most helpful program objectives are clearly stated, measurable, and goal oriented. These objectives can address both the physical and psychological needs of clients as well as those of their families (Box 7-2). When program objectives are clearly stated early in program development, decision making during the planning process will likely improve. In addition, specific goal-oriented program objectives provide outcome markers that help measure progress. The program can then be modified so that realistic, achievable goals are set.

Activity format. Programs can be customized to meet the specific client's needs, or all participants can participate in the same program. Because no two clients with brain injuries are identical, each client could be evaluated and provided with an exercise program that meets his or her specific needs. Although this approach should improve an individual client's outcome, such an approach is personnel intensive and therefore reduces the program's cost effectiveness. Also, an individualized program may provide less social interaction than a group exercise format. When participants exercise as a group, they are usually motivated and encouraged by others performing the same activities. The group exercise format is also cost effective because one staff member can simultaneously supervise a number of clients. Group customization seeks to meet the needs of the clients in the most individualized manner possible. Criteria for inclusion in a particular group attempt to ensure that the group is as homogeneous as possible. Several group formats

BOX 7-2. Stroke Aquatic Program

- The Spain Rehabilitation Center's Stroke Aquatic Program is scheduled every Tuesday and Thursday from 9:30 to 10:30 AM.
- Activities are conducted according to a group format, yet are designed with the special needs of stroke surivivors in mind.
- Entry into the 92°F pool water is ensured by use of a pool lift chair or walk-in ramp.
- All activities are supervised by a certified lifeguard.
- Cost of the program is $20.00/month.
- Participants must provide their own transportation and dressing assistance.

Philosophy

The Stroke Aquatic Program is designed to provide opportunities for improving general fitness, socialization, and health awareness to people who have experienced a stroke. In general, stroke survivors have common fitness, emotional, and educational needs. Because of the unique properties of water and its versatility in providing an effective exercise medium, the swimming pool is a logical choice for addressing these needs. We believe that the Stroke Aquatic Program should be designed to improve flexibility, endurance, and strength in a manner that is enjoyable. Additional benefits of such a group include providing an emotionally supportive environment for people who have experienced a stroke, their families, and friends.

Goals

1. Produce a positive influence on participants' overall endurance, strength, and flexibility (assessed by physical examination).
2. Provide a convenient, regularly scheduled opportuntiy for participants to exercise and socialize in a positive, fulfilling manner (assessed by participant survey).
3. Provide effective, worthwhile educational programs for participants, family members, and friends (assessed by participant survey).

Criteria for Participation

1. History of cerebrovascular accident.
2. Physician's written approval.
3. Signed consent form indicating that the participant is aware of risks involved and poor rules.
4. Before participating in exercises, the participant must undergo a screening evaluation by a physical therapist.
5. Participants must pay a monthly membership fee by the fifth day of each month. New participants may prorate the fee based on the starting date.

Activities

The exercise sessions will be conducted as follows:

A. Warm-up (5 Minutes)

Participants will perform low-level continuous activities to increase blood circulation gently. Examples:

1. Slow walking
2. Slow marching at wall
3. Slow cycling

(continued)

BOX 7-2 *(Continued)*

B. Stretching (10 Minutes)

Participants will perform slow, prolonged stretching activities. Each stretch will be held for 15 seconds, and active stretches are preferred to passive stretches. Examples:

1. Hip flexor
2. Hip adduction
3. Hamstring
4. Heel cord
5. Back extension
6. Shoulder flexion
7. Shoulder horizontal abduction

C. Movement Control (10 Minutes)

Participants will conduct activities aimed at improving control of muscular contractions to enhance smooth, effective joint movement. Activities will be conducted in standing positions whenever possible to challenge and improve postural stability. Clients are encouraged to move body parts at the quickest speed tolerated while ensuring correct, comfortable movement patterns. Examples:

1. Straight leg kick front
2. Side kick
3. Hamstring curl
4. Knee to chest
5. Back kick
6. Arm raise front
7. Arm raise side
8. Clap together
9. Arm circles—hemi-arm
10. Pendulum swing—hemi-arm
11. Marching
12. Hula
13. Knee bends
14. Leg circles
15. Toe-ups

D. Aerobic Activity (15 Minutes)

Participants will perform relatively vigorous, continuous activity designed to increase the participants' heart rates. The activities will be aimed to increase the clients' heart rates to 50% to 70% of maximum heart rate. Examples:

1. Water walking
2. Water running
3. Marching at the side of the pool
4. Cycling in the innertube
5. Cycling while held by a partner

E. Cool-down (5 Minutes)

Participants will conduct low-level, continuous activities to return the heart rate gently to a resting level. Examples:

1. Slow walking
2. Slow marching at the wall
3. Slow cycling

TABLE 7-1. Activities Included in the Spain Stroke Aquatic Program

Phase	Duration	Activity	Comment
Warm-up	5 min	Slow marching at pool wall	
Stretching	10 min	Hip flexor	Active stretched preferred to passive stretch
		Hip adductor	
		Hamstring	
		Heel cord	
Movement control	10 min	Straight leg kick front	Body parts moved at quickest speed possible, while ensuring correct, comfortable movement patterns
		Side kick	
		Hamstring curl	
		Arm circles—hemi-arm	
		Pendulum swing—hemi-arm	
Aerobic activity	15 min	Water walking	Activities aimed at increasing the client's heart rates to 50%–70% of maximum
		Marching at side of pool	
Cool-down	5 min	Slow walking	
		Slow marching at the wall	
Stretching	10 min	As before	

could be conducted at several times throughout the daily schedule (ie, beginner, intermediate, and advanced). Examples of program activities are provided in Table 7-1.

Criteria for participation. Because clients with brain injuries differ in their impairments and degrees of disability, program staff must decide if participants must demonstrate prerequisite skill before joining a group. Staffing decisions are critical here, because the greater the client's disability, the greater the staff needs (ie, number, skill, and credentials).

Staffing needs. As previously stated, criteria for participants influence a program's staff requirements. Because most community programs have limited potential for profitability, heavy use of skilled professionals (eg, OT, PT, ATC) may not be cost efficient. Aquatic rehabilitation attendants, volunteers, or family members can be used if program activities do not require specialized knowledge or skills. Most program activities should be supervised by a skilled professional. Nonprofessional staff require training to ensure client safety and program effectiveness.

Program location. Community user programs for brain-injured clients should be conducted at pools with appropriate characteristics with regard to accessibility, temperature, water depth, and safety. Accessibility considerations should include parking, dressing facilities, and entrances into the building and pool. The pool should have sufficient area at water depths compatible with program activities. If standing exercises and water walking are part of the exercise regime, a 3- to 4-foot water depth area, without a sloping surface, is best. Many recreational pools may be too cold for less active clients with brain injuries (ie, <86°F) and many therapeutic pools may be too warm (ie, >95°F) if endurance activities are performed. Pool temperatures between 88°F and 93°F allow a wide variety of populations and activities and are therefore ideal for community programs. Specific temperature selection will vary based on the pool's clientele. Appropriate safety equipment (eg, shepherd's crook, rescue tube, spine board) and lifeguard personnel must be present. Dressing facilities may pose a problem for clients who require assistance from their opposite-sex significant other. Solutions to this problem include putting up curtains in locker rooms or designating a third locker room as an assisted dressing area. Conveniently located reserved parking should be available for clients with special needs.

Liability. Issues of liability should be the concern of any community aquatic program staff. The participation of clients with brain injuries may increase the liability risks because of physical and cognitive impairment. This risk may be reduced if appropriate steps are taken. Signing a consent form may not protect the program staff in a court of law, but indicates that participants were educated regarding the rules, guidelines, and inherent risks of water exercise. Such a waiver should include (1) activity description and rationale, (2) potential risks involved with these activities, (3) contraindications to or precautions about participation in the program, (4) pool rules, (5) fee-for-service arrangements, and (6) a statement that all parts of the document had been read and understood. A similar form may also be sent to participants' physicians, and is particularly helpful when program staff do not have access to a reliable and comprehensive medical history. This document may contain information similar to that in the consent to participate (pool rules may not be necessary) and a statement that, to the best of the physician's knowledge, the client is appropriate for participation. The standard pool safety measures of posting rules and warning signs, providing lifeguards, purchasing safety equipment, and developing emergency plans and practicing them regularly, can also help reduce liability for the sponsoring people or agency.

Summary

Aquatic rehabilitation has been advocated as beneficial for clients with brain injury for many years.[5–12] Historically, aquatic rehabilitation activities for these clients have been designed to influence brain injury impairments (eg, hypertonicity, weakness, limited range of motion).[5–9] More recently, aquatic rehabilitation professionals have developed an expanded view of aquatic neurorehabilitation to include activities designed to influence brain injury disabilities directly (eg, gait training).[9–12] WATSU, the BRRM, the Halliwick method, and the task type training approach are examples of treatment approaches that are particularly helpful during aquatic neurorehabilitation.[12,21,25–28] In addition, aquatic community programs have been advocated as promoting life-long exercise that address the fitness needs of clients with brain injury.[41]

Although aquatic neurorehabilitation is believed to be beneficial for treating clients with brain injury, experimental evidence of its effectiveness is limited. Case study and single case design activities have been reported.[10,41] Continued clinical research and more elaborate experimental design activities are needed to improve the understanding and use of aquatic neurorehabilitation and to ensure future funding.

Acknowledgments
The author thanks Carol Leiper, PhD, PT, Rochelle Kober, MA, and Paula Owens for their assistance in editing and producing the manuscript.

REFERENCES

1. Gordon J. Assumptions underlying physical therapy intervention: theoretical and historical perspectives. In: Carr JH, Shepherd RB, Gordon J, et al, eds. *Movement Science: Foundations for Physical Therapy in Rehabilitation*. Rockville, Md: Aspen Publishers, Inc; 1987:1–30.
2. Horak FB. Assumptions underlying motor control for neurologic rehabilitation. In: Lister MJ, ed. *Contemporary Management of Motor Control Problems*. Alexandria, Va: Foundation for Physical Therapy; 1990: 11–27.
3. Duncan PW. Stroke: physical therapy assessment and treatment. In: Lister MJ, ed. *Contemporary Management of Motor Control Problems*. Alexandria, Va: Foundation for Physical Therapy; 1990:209–217.
4. Mills VM. Traumatic head injury. In: O'Sullivan SB, Schmitz TJ, eds. *Physical Rehabilitation: Assessment and Treatment*. 2nd ed. Philadelphia, Pa: FA Davis; 1988.
5. Duffield MH. *Exercise in Water*. London: Bailliere, Tindall, and Cassell. 1969:71–78.
6. Davis BC, Harrison RA. *Hydrotherapy in Practice*. New York, NY: Churchill-Livingston; 1988.
7. Campion MR. *Hydrotherapy in Pediatrics*. Oxford: Heinemann Medical Books, 1985.
8. Campion MR. *Adult Hydrotherapy: A Practical Approach*. Oxford: Heinemann Medical Books; 1990.
9. Hurley R, Lyons-Olski E, Sweetman NA, Yuenger JL. Neurology and aquatic therapy. *Clinical Management*. 1991;11(1):26–29.
10. Taylor EW, Morris DM, Shaddeau S, et al. The effects of water walking on hemiplegic gait. *Aquatic Physical Therapy Report*. 1992;1(2):10–13.
11. Morris DM. The use of pool therapy to improve the functional activities of adult hemiplegic patients. In: *Forum Proceedings on Issues Related to Strokes*. Alexandria, Va: Neurology Section, American Physical Therapy Association; 1992:45–48.
12. Morris DM. Aquatic rehabilitation for the treatment of neurological disorders. *Journal of Back and Musculoskeletal Rehabilitation*. 1994;4:297–308.
13. Schumacher K. Classification of stroke problems and the use of standard terminology in the care of persons with stroke. *Neurology Report*. 1991;15(15):4–8.
14. Shumway-Cook A, Woollacott M. *Motor Control: Theory and Practical Applications*. Baltimore, MD: Williams & Wilkins; 1995.
15. Schmidt RA. Motor learning principles for physical therapy. In: Lister MJ, ed. *Contemporary Management of Motor Control Problems*. Alexandria, Va: Foundation for Physical Therapy; 1990:49–61.

16. Winstein CJ. Designing practice for motor learning: clinical implications. In: Lister MJ, ed. *Contemporary Management of Motor Control Problems*. Alexandria, Va: Foundation for Physical Therapy; 1990:65–76.

17. Crutchfield CA, Barnes MR. *Motor Control and Motor Learning in Rehabilitation*. Atlanta, Ga: Stokesville Publishing Co; 1993.

18. Gentile AM. Skill acquisition: action, movement and neuromotor processes. In: Carr JH, Shepherd RB, Gordon J, et al, eds. *Movement Science: Foundations for Physical Therapy in Rehabilitation*. Rockville, Md: Aspen Publishers, Inc; 1987:93–154.

19. Higgins S. Motor skill acquisition. *Phys Ther*. 1991; 71:123–139.

20. Morris DM. Handle with care: providing patient security in the therapeutic pool. *Aquatic Physical Therapy Report*. 1994;2(3):6–9.

21. Dull H. *WATSU: Freeing the Body in Water*. Middletown, Calif: Harbin Springs Publishing; 1993.

22. Ballantyne B. Factors contributing to voluntary movement deficits and spasticity following cerebral vascular accidents. Neurology Report. 1991;15(1): 15–18.

23. Craik RL. Abnormalities of motor behavior. In: Lister MJ, ed. *Contemporary Management of Motor Control Problems*. Alexandria, Va: Foundation for Physical Therapy; 1990:155–164.

24. Giuliani CA. Disorders in motor synergies, initiation, and termination of movement. In: Montgomery PC, Connolly BH, eds. *Motor Control and Physical Therapy: Theoretical Framework and Practical Application*. Hixson, Tenn: Chattanooga Group, Inc; 1991; 110–120.

25. Boyle AM. The Bad Ragaz ring method. *Physiotherapy*. 1981;67:265–268.

26. Cunningham J. Applying the Bad Ragaz method to the orthopedic client. *Orthopedic Physical Therapy Clinics of North America*. 1994;3:251–260.

27. Levin A. The Halliwick method. *SYNAPSE*. 1995; 15(1):5–7.

28. Martin J. The Halliwick method. *Physiotherapy*. 1981; 67:288–291.

29. Nashner LM. Sensory, neuromuscular, and biomechanical contributions to human balance. In: Duncan PW, ed. *Balance: Proceedings of the APTA Forum*. Alexandria, Va: American Physical Therapy Association; 1990:5–12.

30. Sahrmann S, Norton BJ. The relationship of voluntary movement to spasticity in the upper motor neuron syndrome. *Ann Neurol*. 1977;2:460–464.

31. Hufschmidt A, Mauritz KH. Chronic transformation of muscle in spasticity: a peripheral contribution to increased tone. *J Neurol Neurosurg Psychiatry*. 1985; 48:676–685.

32. McComas AJ, Sica RE, Upton AR, Aguilera GC. Functional changes in motoneurons of hemiparetic patients. *J Neurol Neurosurg Psychiatry*. 1973;36: 183–193.

33. Horak FB, Shumway-Cook A. Clinical implications of postural control research. In Duncan PW, ed. *Balance: Proceedings of the APTA Forum*. Alexandria, Va: American Physical Therapy Association; 1990: 105–111.

34. Horak FB. Clinical measurement of postural control in adults. *Phys Ther*. 1987;67:181–185.

35. Schumway-Cook A, Horak FB. Assessing the influence of sensory interaction on balance: suggestion from the field. *Phys Ther*. 1986;66:1548–1550.

36. Esquenazi A, Hirai B. Gait analysis in stroke and head injury. In: Craik RL, Oatis CA, eds. *Gait Analysis: Theory and Application*. St. Louis, Mo: Mosby; 1994; 412–419.

37. Winter DA. Concerning the scientific basis for the diagnosis of pathological gait and for rehabilitation protocols. *Physiotherapy Canada* 1985;17:245.

38. Giuliani C. Adult hemiplegic gait. In: Smidt GL, ed. *Gait in Rehabilitation*. New York, NY: Churchill Livingstone; 1990:253–266.

39. Oatis CA. Perspectives on the evaluation and treatment of gait disorders. In: Montgomery PC, Connolly BH, eds. *Motor Control and Physical Therapy: Theoretical Framework and Practical Application*. Hixson, Tenn: Chattanooga Group, Inc; 1991;141–155.

40. Wade DT, Collen FM, Robb GF, et al. Physiotherapy intervention late after stroke. *Br Med J*. 1992;304: 609–613.

41. Morris DM, Buettner TL, White EW. Aquatic community-based exercise programs for stroke survivors. *SYNAPSE*. 1995;15(1):8–14.

8 Aquatic Rehabilitation of Clients With Spinal Cord Injury*

Christine Giesecke

"On the ground, gravity is a vise that presses on our joints, compresses the spine. But we levitate in the pool . . . "walking" in this water we have the illusion of power and freedom."[1]

SUZANNE BERGER

Sir Ludwig Guttmann, father of modern spinal cord injury (SCI) management, opined that "of the many forms of disability which can beset mankind, a severe injury or disease of the spinal cord undoubtedly constitutes one of the most devastating calamities in human life."[2] Up until World War II, it was not only devastating, it carried a virtually hopeless prognosis. Life expectancy was no more than 2 to 3 months. During the war, advances in medical care greatly improved the survival rate from SCI. As life expectancy improved, the concept of comprehensive treatment and rehabilitation began to develop. Radical changes in medical and psychological approaches to the problem of SCI were introduced, including early mobilization, prevention of previously fatal complications, and vocational training.

Today, mortality during the first few months after an SCI is perhaps as high as 20%, but those who survive the acute stage have a relatively low excess mortality compared with the non–spinal cord-injured population.[3] Health care professionals must focus on assisting the person with SCI achieve and maintain his or her maximum potential for health and function. As a result of metabolic changes from the injury and the drastic decrease in physical activity that often accompanies an SCI, this population is thought to be at a much greater risk for cardiovascular disease, obesity, diabetes mellitus, and osteoporosis.[4] Full-time wheelchair users must rely for their mobility on their upper extremities, which are notorious for their higher metabolic demand. R. M. Glaser states that " . . . arm exercise appears to be inherently inefficient and stressful to the cardiovascular and pulmonary systems."[5] Elevated physiologic demands may also be the result, in part, of lack of fitness.[5] Daily living activities are not intense enough to prevent deterioration of physical fitness.[4] Wheelchair users could find locomotion less stressful with a higher level of fitness.

To achieve a high level of fitness and maintain a healthy lifestyle, the person with SCI requires a comprehensive regimen of activity. Guttmann stated that, "swimming represents one of the most natural forms of remedial exercise and has proved invaluable in restoring the paraplegic's co-ordination, strength, speed, endurance and self-confidence . . . ."[2] The challenge of mastering the water and improving personal performance can help to overcome fatigue and inertia, two major enemies against which those with SCI battle. Aquatics therapy can be an integral part of a rehabilitation and fitness program for the achievement and maintenance of a healthy lifestyle.

This chapter assists the reader in understanding the problems associated with SCI and how an aquatics program of individual therapeutic

* Photos courtesy of Bryn Mawr Rehab, Malvern, Pennsylvania.

exercises, group exercises, recreational activities, and swimming strokes can assist these clients in reaching their maximum physical potential. What follows is a description of the neurologic and functional classifications of SCI, medical complications and common sequelae, therapeutic goals, precautions and contraindications, design of an aquatics program, methods of transfer, and aquatic techniques. At the completion of this chapter, the reader should be able to identify problems, set goals, and develop a comprehensive aquatics program for the client with SCI.

Neurologic and Functional Classification of Spinal Cord Injury

Spinal cord injury can have either a traumatic or nontraumatic origin. Using data collected between 1973 and 1985, the National Spinal Cord Injury Statistical Center published the following statistics concerning the SCI population in the United States.[3] Most traumatic injuries occur in teenagers and young adults. The most common etiologies of traumatic injuries are motor vehicle accidents, acts of violence, falls, and water sports. SCI occurs more frequently among men than women (with a ratio of about 4 : 1), and is slightly higher for African-Americans than whites.

Nontraumatic etiologies include, but are not limited to, neoplasm, bone disease, infection, arteriovenous malformation, stenosis, spondylosis, arachnoiditis, and congenital anomalies.

Classification of SCI† is based on the injury's neurologic level—that is, the most caudal segment of the spinal cord that exhibits normal motor and sensory function on both sides of the body. A complete injury is characterized by the absence of motor control and sensation below the neurologic level and in the lowest sacral segment. Tetraplegia results when interruption of spinal cord functioning occurs in the cervical segments. This affects sensation and motor control in all four extremities and the trunk. The greatest amount of cervical mobility occurs in the C5–C7 region, and this is the most common

area of injury in tetraplegia.[7] Injury to the thoracic, lumbar, and sacral segments and the cauda equina results in paraplegia. T12–L1 is the second most common area of injury.[3] Injuries below the thoracolumbar junction are relatively rare. The proportion of neurologically complete injuries declines below T12 as the spinal cord becomes more anatomically diffuse in the cauda equina (which begins anywhere from T12 to L3, depending on the individual).

A gross look at motor control at each segment reveals the following:

C2–C4: The person has no active movement in the upper extremities, but has some neck control. There is paralysis of the diaphragm resulting from loss of segmental innervation of the phrenic nerve at C1–C3. Injury above C4 requires ventilatory support.

C5: The person has use of the biceps, brachialis, rhomboids, and deltoids. This affords minimal scapular stability.

C6: The person has wrist extension, forearm pronation, and shoulder protraction by means of the serratus anterior.

C7: The person has weak triceps, pectoralis, and latissimus dorsi. This affords a stable scapula, allowing significantly greater functional potential.

C8: The person has full triceps, wrist flexion, and extrinsic hand muscles. The person presents with a clawed hand because of the loss of intrinsic hand muscles.

T1–T6: The person has full use of the hands. The lower the level of the injury, the better the person's respiratory status because of increasing function of the intercostals.

T6–T12: The person gains segments of abdominal muscles. At T12, there is complete trunk control.

L1–L3: The person has weak hip flexors and adductors, and knee extensors.

L4: The person has hip flexors and quadriceps, and tibialis anterior and posterior. The person presents with an equinovarus foot.

L5: The person has full extension and abduction of the hip and at least some knee flexion.

S1–S2: The person has full function of the lower extremity muscles.

Figures 8-1 through 8-3 give a complete description of segmental innervation for all muscles of the extremities and trunk.

Damage to the spinal cord occurs as a result of physical impingement, interruption of the

---

† American Spinal Injury Association (ASIA) definitions are used throughout. The term "tetraplegia" is the ASIA preferred term to "quadriplegia," and is used throughout the text.[6]

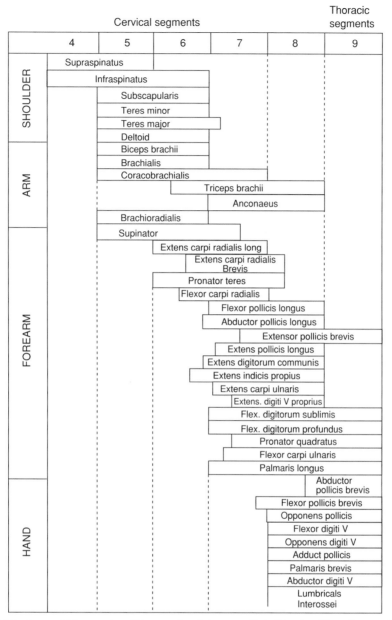

FIGURE 8-1. Segmental innervation of the muscles of the upper limb. (Reprinted from Guttman L. *Spinal Cord Injuries: Comprehensive Management and Research.* 2nd ed. Oxford: Blackwell Science, 1976.)

vascular supply, or, rarely, actual transection.[8] SCI is primarily a metabolic injury to neural tissue from edema and impaired circulation leading to ischemia and cell death. The ultimate extent of the damage is directly related to the severity of the initial insult, with cord necrosis occurring one to three segments above and below the actual area of injury.[8]

An incomplete SCI is defined as partial preser-vation of motor control or sensation below the neurologic level, including the lowest sacral segment. Incomplete lesions evolve from two different mechanisms of injury. The first involves pathologic processes affecting more or less all the neurons, both afferent and efferent, at a given level but without complete destruction. The second involves circumscribed processes affecting distinct parts of the cord. The most

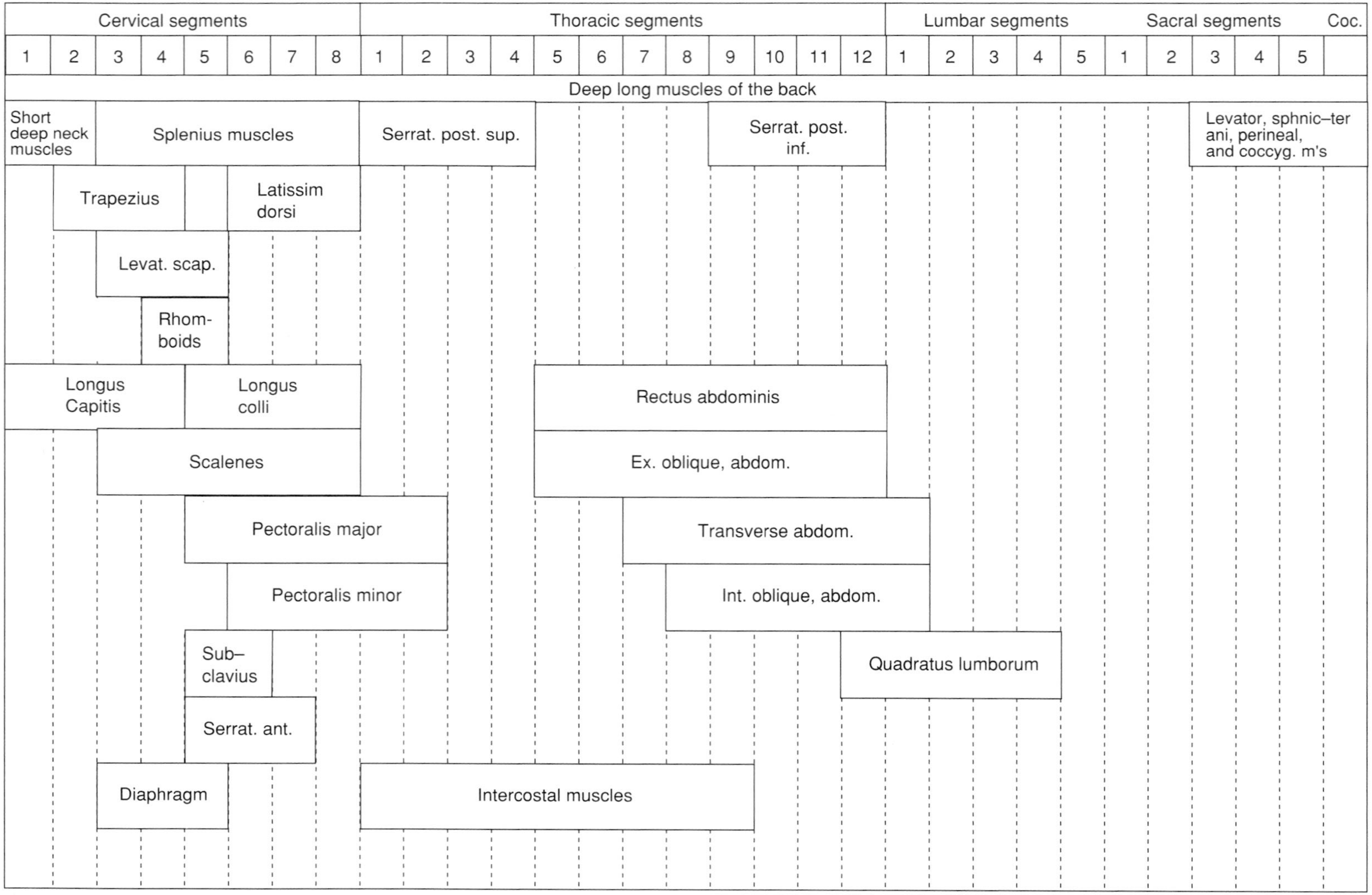

FIGURE 8-2. Segmental innervation of the trunk muscles. (Reprinted from Guttman L. *Spinal Cord Injuries: Comprehensive Management and Research.* 2nd ed. Oxford: Blackwell Science, 1976.)

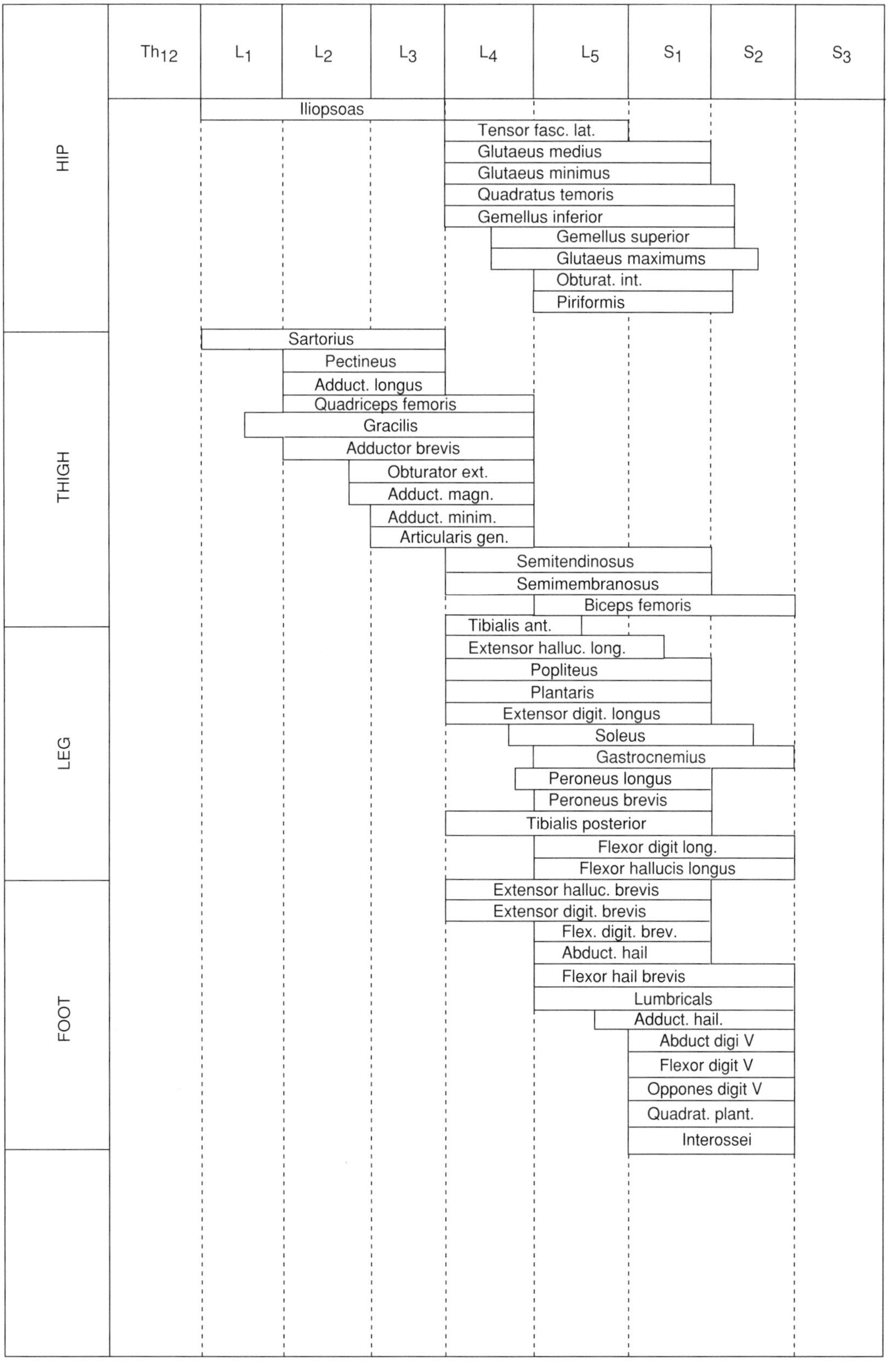

	Th$_{12}$	L$_1$	L$_2$	L$_3$	L$_4$	L$_5$	S$_1$	S$_2$	S$_3$

HIP
- Iliopsoas
- Tensor fasc. lat.
- Glutaeus medius
- Glutaeus minimus
- Quadratus temoris
- Gemellus inferior
- Gemellus superior
- Glutaeus maximums
- Obturat. int.
- Piriformis

THIGH
- Sartorius
- Pectineus
- Adduct. longus
- Quadriceps femoris
- Gracilis
- Adductor brevis
- Obturator ext.
- Adduct. magn.
- Adduct. minim.
- Articularis gen.

LEG
- Semitendinosus
- Semimembranosus
- Biceps femoris
- Tibialis ant.
- Extensor halluc. long.
- Popliteus
- Plantaris
- Extensor digit. longus
- Soleus
- Gastrocnemius
- Peroneus longus
- Peroneus brevis
- Tibialis posterior
- Flexor digit long.
- Flexor hallucis longus

FOOT
- Extensor halluc. brevis
- Extensor digit. brevis
- Flex. digit. brev.
- Abduct. hail
- Flexor hail brevis
- Lumbricals
- Adduct. hail.
- Abduct digi V
- Flexor digit V
- Oppones digit V
- Quadrat. plant.
- Interossei

FIGURE 8-3. Segmental innervation of muscles of the lower limb. (Reprinted from Guttman L. *Spinal Cord Injuries: Comprehensive Management and Research.* 2nd ed. Oxford: Blackwell Science, 1976.)

131

commonly seen incomplete SCI syndromes are Brown-Séquard, anterior cord, and central cord. Brown-Séquard syndrome results from damage to one side of the cord. These clients present with ipsilateral motor and proprioceptive loss and contralateral loss of pain and temperature two segments below the level of injury. Lower motor neuron signs, including areflexia and atrophy, occur at the level of injury. An anterior cord syndrome is characterized by loss of motor control below the injured segment, but only partial loss of sensation and intact proprioception. Central cord syndrome occurs almost exclusively in the cervical region, affecting only the central aspect of the cord. This results in greater paralysis and sensory loss in the upper extremities than in the lower. Careful evaluation is required to determine the exact nature of motor and sensory loss because each individual presents differently. The proportion of people with incomplete versus complete lesions has increased significantly over the years, presumably because of improved methods of emergency care.[3] An incomplete SCI often promises a better functional outcome.

Medical Complications and Common Sequelae

Spinal cord injury is a devastating form of trauma affecting many systems of the body, either directly or indirectly. A good understanding of the many complications is necessary to design a safe and comprehensive aquatics treatment program for these clients.

The most obvious direct result of a SCI is the loss of motor control. The trunk and limbs exhibit varying degrees of weakness, spasticity, or flaccidity. If muscle strength or spasticity is greater than that of its antagonist, there is abnormal posturing of the limb that can result in joint contractures. Weakness, loss of speed and timing in muscle reciprocity or cocontraction, and impaired sensation and proprioception lead to ineffectual movement and poor coordination in the affected limbs. When the trunk muscles are affected, there is a loss of balance in sitting and standing and a loss of the central stability on which the mobility of the extremities depends.

Loss or impairment of sensation and proprioception below the level of the injury can have serious consequences for those with SCI. Normal sensation provides feedback when there are noxious or potentially harmful stimuli or pro-

longed pressure in a specific area, and for the awareness of limbs in space. Without this system of feedback, the person is in danger of injury, contractures, and pressure sores. Constant vigilance is required to avoid these sequelae.

Impaired respiratory capacity is a serious threat to the person with tetraplegia or high paraplegia, in whom the muscles of respiration are compromised. Respiratory failure and infection is one of the major causes of death and morbidity.[3,9] Several respiratory muscles can be affected, depending on the level of injury. The diaphragm is mainly a muscle of inspiration, innervated by the phrenic nerve. The intercostals (innervated from the thoracic segments) and the accessory muscles (C1–C8) are also inspiratory muscles. The lower intercostals and accessories are usually active only in higher levels of ventilation.[7] The inspiratory capacity approaches normal as the level of the injury descends below the first few segments of the thoracic spinal cord. Those with tetraplegia below C4 have about 58% of normal vital capacity, whereas those with high thoracic paraplegia have about 73%.[9] The abdominals participate in a mostly expiratory capacity because they facilitate either a passive recoil of the diaphragm or forced expiration. Paralysis of the abdominals results in a poor respiratory reserve volume and consequently in reduced cough capability. A marked increase in the work of breathing can lead to early fatigue.

The neurogenic bowel and bladder, resulting in incontinence, is a chronic problem for almost all people with SCI. Sepsis due to infection was once a leading cause of death,[2] but better and more sterile techniques of management have reduced morbidity considerably. Normal function of the bowel and bladder depends on the interaction at several levels between components of the autonomic and voluntary nervous systems. The degree of impairment is not always predictable by the level of injury. Long-term management is usually accomplished by intermittent or indwelling catheterization, the use of external urine collection devices, timed voiding, and medication. Occasionally a suprapubic cystostomy is required.

Orthostatic hypotension is often found in the early stages in those with a higher level of injury. When coming to the upright position, the person experiences an increase in heart rate and a decrease in blood pressure secondary to venous pooling and deficient vasomotor reflexes. Both the systolic and diastolic pressures can drop as much as 30% to 50%,[7] causing the person to experience nausea, visual blurring, syncope, or even loss of consciousness. The cardiovascular system usually adjusts with time. This can be facilitated by slowly and incrementally adjusting the person to the upright position and by using an abdominal binder to reduce pooling in the visceroabdominal vasculature.

Autonomic dysreflexia (or autonomic crisis, autonomic hyperreflexia), usually seen with injuries above T6, is characterized by severe hypertension, bradycardia, diaphoresis, flushing, headache, miosis, nasal congestion, and sometimes chest pain and agitation. This is caused by massive sympathetic outflow in response to afferent stimulation below the level of the injury, most often from bladder or bowel distention, decubitus ulcers, or infection. It can also be triggered by cutaneous stimuli and muscle spasm. As many as 60% of those with tetraplegia and 20% of those with paraplegia are affected by this disorder.[9] The dangers of unchecked autonomic dysreflexia can be serious, including transient visual loss, seizures, subarachnoid hemorrhaging, and even death. Incidents can be managed by elevation of the torso to induce venous pooling in the legs, and immediate identification and removal of the trigger stimulus when possible. Immediate medical attention should be sought.

The body undergoes many cardiovascular and metabolic changes after SCI, many of them deleterious. Indeed, cardiovascular disorders have been implicated as the leading cause of death in those with SCI.[4,9] Deficits in muscular, respiratory, and cardiovascular response vary with the level of the injury. Alterations after injury include a lower resting blood pressure; decreased myocardial contractility; greater venous capacitance, which leads to peripheral venous pooling; decreased venous return, which lowers the cardiac output; and lessened cardiac reserve. Oxygen uptake, ventilation, and cardiopulmonary function diminish the higher the level of injury.[10] Reflex distribution of blood required for delivery of oxygen and fuels and the removal of waste by-products are partly mediated by sympathetic control. Injuries above T1 interrupt sympathetic outflow to the heart, which can limit cardiac output capability.[5] Prolonged immobility leads to decreased total hemoglobin and blood volume, increased body fat, and a significant decrease in high-density lipoprotein cholesterol levels, which is implicated in a higher risk for coronary artery disease.[4,11] Deep vein thrombosis can also occur, usually in the lower extremities, and is characterized by swelling, heat, and point tenderness. In this case, lower extremity activity is contraindicated for at least 72 hours after diagnosis to avoid dislodging the thrombus. Pulmonary emboli often arise from venous thrombi in the deep veins of the legs or pelvis. This is a serious condition, the symptoms of which are sometimes lacking or too subtle to detect in those with SCI, but may include transient episodes of shortness of breath, feelings of chest compression, tachycardia, tachypnea, unexplained fever or pyrexia, and a cough. If pulmonary embolus is suspected, treatment should be immediately discontinued and the physician notified, because this condition can be fatal.

Heterotopic ossification, a frequent occurrence in the spinal cord and traumatic brain injury populations, is a process of unknown etiology that causes inflammation of extra-articular soft tissue with subsequent deposition of cancellous bone. This can result in limitations of joint mobility and sometimes ankylosis. It develops below the neurologic level, most commonly in the hips, knees, elbows, and shoulders. Onset is most frequently observed between 1 and 4 months after trauma,[9] and can often precede clinical symptoms of local swelling, heat, erythema, pain, fever and radiologic changes. The process is usually self-limiting. There is still debate about the effects of exercise on the development of heterotopic ossification, but the literature implies that immobility facilitates the progression.[7] Other possible bony sequelae of SCI include osteoporosis, osteomyelitis, and spinal deformity.

Immobility itself has serious consequences for those with SCI. Decubitus ulcers are caused by prolonged pressure over bony prominences leading to oxygen starvation of the underlying tissues. By far the most common site for these ulcers is the sacrum, followed by the heels and ischium, respectively.[3] Other areas include the occiput, scapula, trochanter, malleolus, and the genital region. Contractures can occur if joints are not regularly mobilized and may be further facilitated by the presence of spasticity. Absence of movement also encourages fungal infections in warm, moist, poorly ventilated areas. Immobility leads to reduced endurance and excess fatigue.

There are a variety of pain syndromes associated with SCI. Pain arising from soft tissue damage or structural damage of the spine is the most obvious. People with SCI often undergo surgical management procedures, including fusion, open reduction, bone or skin grafting, halo traction, and tracheostomy, to name but a few. The client may experience neurologic or dysesthetic pain below the level of injury, pain from nerve root lesions, or hyperalgesia. Those with SCI are subject to strains, sprains, and myofascial pain syndromes secondary to overuse of residual muscle groups. People with tetraplegia often suffer shoulder pain. Traumatic SCI is often accompanied by a host of other injuries, including fractures, burns, internal injuries, and head trauma.

Consequent to all the problems previously discussed, the person with SCI suffers a severe loss of functional ability. The person is often restricted to a wheelchair or is severely limited in ambulation. Virtually all activities of daily living become more difficult or even impossible, depending on the level and extent of the injury. The person may not be able to return to previous employment, or has to change anticipated career plans. Previous forms of recreation may become impossible. The person's living environment may require expensive remodeling to be habitable. In addition, all of this places extra demands on the person's family or significant others. The emotional stress taxes coping skills severely. The person can suffer from depression, lack of initiative, loss of self-worth, and a poor body image, among other psychological dysfunctions. People with SCI go through many stages of mental, emotional, and physical adjustment over a period of years before finally coming to terms with their new lives.

Therapeutic Goals of Aquatic Exercise

The physical properties and comfort of warm water allow those with disabilities to move freely in ways that would be painful and difficult on land. Swimming pools are associated with enjoyable activities and do not hold the same connotations of hard work and pain that are often associated with "gym therapy." The person with SCI can work on balance with less fear of falling, can stretch and exercise limbs with less pain, and can achieve greater mobility with less effort in the pool. Therefore, many physical and functional goals can be facilitated in the pool.

Reduced Spasticity

The neutral warmth of the water combined with slow, rhythmic motions, rotation, and prolonged, gentle stretch can relax spastic muscles. The buoyancy of the water eases the constant resistance to gravity that aggravates spasticity. The warm temperature of the water is important because water that is too cool may worsen the spasticity.[12] Care must be taken as well with resisted exercise to uninvolved muscle groups because heavy effort can cause an increase in spasticity in affected muscles.

Strengthening

Good upper extremity strength is vital to the day-to-day functioning of those with SCI. People with incomplete SCI also need to strengthen residual muscles in the lower extremities to reach their maximum potential. Water is an effective tool in strengthening those muscles. Depending on the strength of the muscle, the buoyancy of the water can be used to assist, support, or resist the movement desired. Weaker muscles can be facilitated through the range of motion (ROM) by directing the plane of movement slowly across the surface of the water or from the bottom of the pool toward the surface. Stronger muscles can be resisted in several ways. Increasing the speed of movement creates turbulence and increases the effects of the water's viscosity against the limb. Buoyancy adds resistance when moving from the surface toward the bottom. Lengthening the lever arm and adding floats, weights, or paddles to the distal end also increases resistance to the movement. When exercising muscles that are affected by spasticity but have active movement, care should be taken to avoid positions or patterns that feed into the spasticity.

Increased or Maintained Range of Motion

Painful, restricted joints can seriously hinder the functional ability of those with SCI. These joints can be mobilized more easily and comfortably in the water. The warmth of the water reduces pain and relaxes spastic or guarded muscles to allow greater ROM. The hydrostatic pressure supports the limb uniformly, and buoyancy assists the desired motion.

Reduced Pain

It is not within the scope of this chapter to discuss the physiology of pain, but suffice to say that the warmth, sensory stimulation, relaxation, weight relief, and pleasure of being in water all help to reduce pain and its perception.

Improved Respiratory Status

Simple immersion with the head out of the water increases the respiratory rate and improves the ventilation–perfusion ratio of the lungs.[13,14] Studies indicate that ventilatory muscle strength and endurance can be improved with training,[4] which can help prevent respiratory failure. Mekarski and Pachalski[15] performed a 3-year study comparing the cardiorespiratory efficiency of 30 people with paraplegia performing a land-based training program, with 30 people with paraplegia performing a swim-training program. Using the Skibinski cardiorespiratory index, they found that there was a significantly greater increase in the vital capacity and decrease in pulse rate in those who were swim trained. The prone position facilitates better use of the diaphragm and lower chest muscles, and the humid air assists with clearance of mucus.[14]

Improved Peripheral Circulation

The hydrostatic pressure gradient during immersion to the neck causes a cephalad shift of peripheral venous blood, augmenting central blood volume[16] and decreasing systemic vascular resistance.[13] Peripheral circulation is improved with better blood supply to the muscles.[13,17] This can help to reduce the risk of deep vein thrombosis and venous stasis ulcers.

Improved Cardiovascular and Metabolic Status

Simple immersion in water increases cardiac output, stroke volume,[13,16] and the general metabolic rate.[17] When the body is in the horizontal position there is a reduction in the cardiovascular load.[18] Regular exercise in water has been shown to increase high-density lipoprotein cholesterol levels in those with paraplegia,[11] an important factor in reducing the risk of coronary artery disease.

Increased Aerobic Endurance

Haas and colleagues state that, "Although SCI subjects have impaired adaptation to exercise, an increase in an individual's activity is strictly correlated to the corresponding increase in physical fitness, suggesting that training effects can be obtained in these subjects."[10] Nilsson and coworkers[19] demonstrated in a study of seven people with long-standing paraplegia that strengthening and endurance training can improve aerobic power, maximal work capacity, and mechanical efficiency. Swimming is one of the activities that can fulfill the requirements for good aerobic training.[20] It is dynamic, high intensity, uses many muscle groups, and has a long performance time. It has been shown that in those with paraplegia, a work load of 50% to 60% of the target heart rate (as opposed to 60% to 70% in those without disability) contributes to the maintenance of cardiovascular fitness.[21] Because of the disruption of the sympathetic acceleratory effects of the heart, it may be impossible to reach the target heart rate during exercise.[22] Diminished sympathetic outflow can also result in a greater dependence on anaerobic energy, which would lead to early onset of fatigue and reduced thermoregulatory capacity.[5]

Improved Function

The ultimate goal of any kind of exercise training for those with SCI is not only good overall health, but efficient functioning in day-to-day life. Reduced fear of falling and lessened pain make the pool an excellent medium for restoring balance and coordination and practicing functional activities. Evenly distributed hydrostatic pressure around the trunk and the buoyant force of water supporting the trunk ease the work and allow the client more time to recover from loss of balance. Rolling, transfers, sit-to-stand, and gait can all be practiced and facilitated in the pool.

Psychological Benefits

Sir Ludwig Guttmann stated, "Every person who has suffered severe injury or illness develops certain adverse psychological reactions—he loses activity of mind, self-confidence, self-respect, and self-dignity. He resigns into his disability and becomes self-centered and anti-social. Nothing can prevent and counteract these adverse psychological reactions more than two measures: regular work and sport."[20] A person with SCI will often discover a new enthusiasm after pool activities. Researchers using the Profile of Mood Survey have discovered that the short-term effects after pool therapy include diminished tension, depression, anger, and confusion and improved vigor.[18] Aquatics can foster a growth of independence and self-expression and give people with disability opportunity to mix with the rest of society.

Contraindications and Precautions

Contraindications for bringing people with SCI into the pool include:

1. Fever
2. Infectious diseases
3. Skin rashes
4. Uncontrolled high or low blood pressure
5. Vital capacity of less than 1 L
6. Uncontrolled or very recent seizure activity
7. Tracheostomy
8. Uncontrolled bowel and bladder incontinence
9. Menstruation without internal protection

Several precautions and special problems should also be considered. Any open wounds must be small enough to be covered with a waterproof dressing. Ostomies (colostomy, ileostomy, urostomy), suprapubic appliances, and G-tubes (clamped) can be allowed in the pool with special handling. The trunk area around and including the stoma site should be wrapped with plastic wrap and then enclosed firmly in an abdominal binder. Indwelling and condom catheters should have bags attached to the leg and drain tubes clamped. Clients with severely limited endurance, cardiac involvement, respiratory compromise, orthostatic hypotension, or autonomic dysreflexia should all be monitored closely and start with short treatment sessions (eg, 15 minutes). Garvey[12] states that the client should be able to tolerate at least one-half hour of therapy in the gym before being considered for aquatics therapy. People with tetraplegia and high paraplegia cannot regulate temperature well and are therefore prone to both heat prostration and hypothermia.[2,9] Sweating and shivering are absent or greatly reduced below the level of injury. Consideration should be given to both the water and air temperature, and the client monitored closely. Physician approval should be obtained for anyone with orthopedic injuries in the acute stage. Clients with halo traction (if their heads are kept out of the pool), collars, and body jackets can be taken into the pool as long as replacements are available for those pieces that soak up water. Those with sensory loss should have their skin checked for abrasions before and after each session, especially if the client is ambulatory or if extremities are dragging on the bottom. Protective footwear and knee pads can be worn during activities where these body parts may be in contact with the bottom of the pool. The skin should be well dried after each session, especially between the toes, under the breasts, and in areas of skin folds, to prevent fungal or bacterial infections and chafing.

Designing a Therapeutic Aquatics Program

Because SCI presents uniquely in each case, there is no set protocol or "cookbook" therapeutic program to follow. There are, however, certain steps to follow to design an approach that will be effective in meeting the peculiar needs of the individual client with SCI.

1. Make a careful assessment of strength, muscle tone, sensation, ROM, pulmonary function, endurance, balance, functional ability, and medical complications.
2. Identify the problems that can be addressed with aquatics therapy.
3. Set goals. Be sure to consider and include the goals the individual has for himself or herself.
4. Using the properties of water (eg, buoyancy, hydrostatic pressure, viscosity), develop a program of activities that addresses those problems and meets those goals.
5. Reassess and modify the program regularly.

Several different approaches are discussed, including individual therapeutic exercises, swimming strokes, group activities, and recreation.

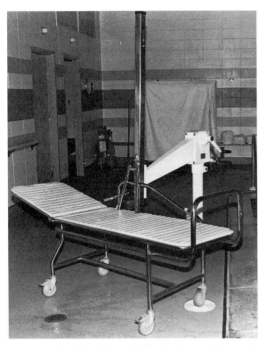

FIGURE 8-4. This hydraulic lift also has a chair attachment.

Methods of Transfer Into and Out of the Pool

Getting into and out of the pool may be the biggest challenge for those with SCI. Several options exist. A hydraulic stretcher (Fig. 8-4) or chair lift can easily, slowly, and safely ease the person in and out of the water with a minimum of assistance from others. The client can also be wheeled up and down a ramp in a shower chair (Fig. 8-5). If none of these options is available, a wheelchair-stool-floor transfer can be done with those with injuries at C7 and below. To perform this transfer, the client is parked facing the pool. A stool, approximately half the height of the floor to the wheelchair seat, is placed directly in front of the wheelchair and the client's legs are placed over the stool (Fig. 8-6). The client then eases himself or herself down onto the stool. The legs are then extended and the client eases himself or herself down onto the floor (Fig. 8-7). The client then sits at the edge of the pool with legs dangling and is assisted down into the pool from there (Fig. 8-8). This transfer may require anywhere from one to three people assisting at the shoulders and lower extremities, depending on the status of the lower extremities

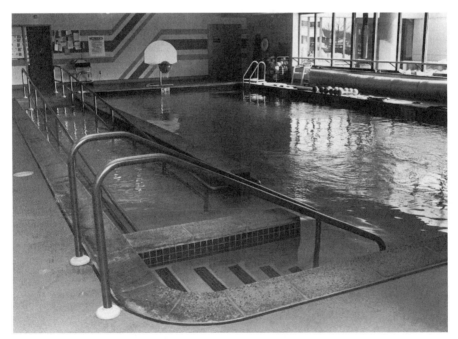

FIGURE 8-5. The client can be wheeled up and down a ramp in a shower chair. If the client is ambulatory, the stairs with railing can be used.

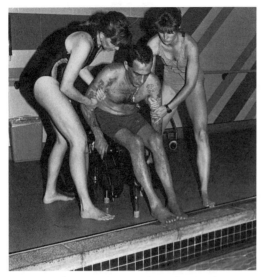

FIGURE 8-6. Wheelchair–stool transfer: initial setup.

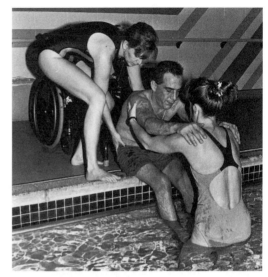

FIGURE 8-8. Wheelchair-stool transfer: client assisted into pool. Care should be taken not to scrape the legs across the rough edge of the pool.

and the strength and ROM of the upper extremities. If the client is ambulatory, steps with a railing or a pool ladder can be used (see Fig. 8-5).

Always give the person a few minutes to accommodate to the new environment when getting into the pool, especially the first time. Reassure the person of his or her safety and provide maximum physical and psychological support. Time to adjust to the water varies according to the level and extent of injury, age, physical condition, and premorbid comfort in the water and

swimming ability. Special consideration should be given to those whose SCI resulted from diving accidents and who may be experiencing fear of reentry into the water.

Therapeutic Exercises in the Pool

At this point, the therapist must transport the client from the edge to the area of the pool chosen for activity. If that person is not ambulatory, the therapist can float him or her over by cradling the head in the crook of the elbow and supporting the hips or the underside of the knees with the other arm. Activities can be performed sitting, kneeling, floating prone and supine, and standing.

What follows is by no means an exhaustive list of exercises and activities. All the various methods of assisting or resisting each movement in each position are not mentioned here in detail. The principles are discussed in the section on Strengthening, under "Therapeutic Goals," and should be individually applied as appropriate. The therapist should be stimulated to create and adapt techniques as the individuality of each client demands. The only limitation is the therapist's own imagination.

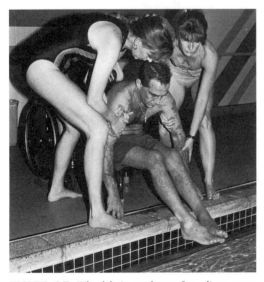

FIGURE 8-7. Wheelchair–stool transfer: client eases himself onto the edge of the pool.

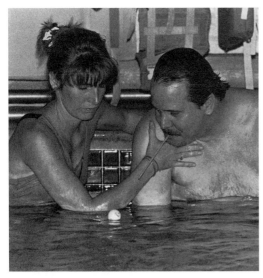

FIGURE 8-9. Client pushes ping-pong ball across pool with straw. The people pictured are sitting on a built-in bench in the 3-foot section.

Sitting on a Bench or Chair

1. *Action:* The client bends forward and puts the mouth and eventually the whole face in the water and blows bubbles. The client can also push a ping-pong ball across the surface by blowing through a straw (Fig. 8-9).
   Goal: The client learns breath control, and develops balance control (following the ball across the water).
2. *Action:* The client and the therapist bat a beach ball back and forth (Fig. 8-10).

Goal: The client learns balance, achieves upper extremity strength and coordination.

3. *Action:* The client sits unsupported while the therapist creates turbulence in various planes around that person.
   Goal: The client learns balance. Keep in mind that the client will be pulled toward the source of the turbulence.
4. *Action:* The client reaches for rings, displacing the shoulders out of the center of balance.
   Goal: The client learns trunk control and balance.
5. *Action:* Holding a polythene barbell, the client pushes it forward and back or rotates side to side (Fig. 8-11).
   Goal: The client achieves trunk and upper extremity ROM and strengthening, and active tone reduction of the trunk.
6. *Action:* The client performs active shoulder abduction–adduction, flexion–extension, and horizontal abduction–adduction to the surface of the water, and all elbow, wrist, and hand movements (also self-ROM).
   Goal: The client achieves strengthening and ROM of the upper extremities.
7. *Action:* The client with incomplete SCI performs active hip, knee, and ankle movements as sparing permits.
   Goal: The client achieves strengthening and ROM of the lower extremities.
8. *Action:* The therapist passively ranges all extremity joints.
   Goal: The client receives stretching to increase ROM.

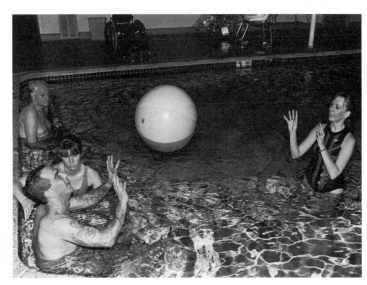

FIGURE 8-10. Client and therapist bat a beach ball back and forth. An extra person may be required to guard.

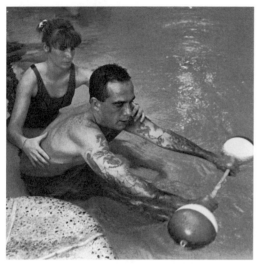

FIGURE 8-11. Client pushes polythene barbell forward and back, or rotates side to side.

9. *Action:* The client performs sitting push-ups and scoots from side to side (if on a bench).
   Goal: The client exercises the upper extremities, learns balance and trunk control, and practices for transfers.
10. *Action:* The client with incomplete SCI practices going from sit to stand with feet together, one foot in front of the other, and pausing half-way up and down. The therapist can assist from the front or the side (Fig. 8-12).

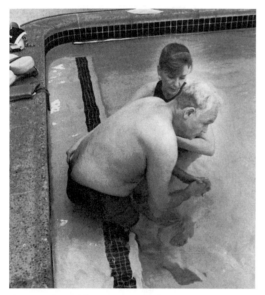

FIGURE 8-12. Therapist assists client to practice going from a sitting to a standing position.

Goal: The client strengthens the lower extremities and practices functional sit-stand. The buoyancy of the water assists part way to standing and eases down to sitting.

Kneeling

The client with incomplete SCI or low paraplegia can exercise in this position. The client may want to wear water shoes or socks and knee pads to protect the skin from abrasion (Fig. 8-13).

1. *Action:* The client performs active movements of the upper extremities unilaterally, bilaterally, and alternately, and chops and lifts with the hands clasped together (Fig. 8-14).
   Goal: The client achieves upper extremity ROM and strengthening, trunk and balance control.
2. *Action:* The client holds the barbell and rotates side to side, bats a beach ball with the therapist, reaches for rings, or resists turbulence created by the therapist (Fig. 8-15).
   Goal: The goals are the same as in sitting, with added challenge to additional hip and lower extremity muscles.
3. *Action:* The client squats and comes back up.
   Goal: The client strengthens hip and lower extremity muscles and develops balance control.
4. *Action:* The client works into and out of half-kneeling with each leg and balances in that position. Any of the above activities can be performed in this position as ability allows.
   Goal: The client develops balance control and works on skills necessary for ambulation and for coming to a stand from the floor.
5. *Action:* The client knee-walks with support from the therapist in the front, on the side, or in back or using a device (eg, barbells, ring, vest).
   Goal: The client strengthens trunk and lower extremity muscles and works on pregait skills.

Supine Float

Initially, in the back float the client may require three points of support—the head, the hips, and the lower extremities at either the knees or the ankles. The lower extremities may either float

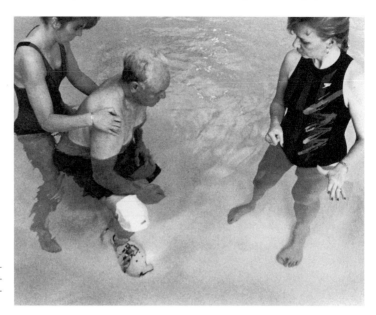

FIGURE 8-13. Knee pads and footwear worn for skin protection during kneeling and half-kneeling activities.

independently or sink. Support can be provided by the therapist, flotation devices, or a combination of the two, depending on the nature of the activity and the comfort level of the client. An excellent way to start for relaxation and security is for the client's head to be resting on the therapist's shoulder with the therapist's hands supporting under the lower trunk (Fig. 8-16). Unless that person is particularly dense, the lower extremities are kept afloat in this position as well without undue effort on the part of the therapist. As the client becomes more confidant, he or she may use flotation devices, which frees the therapist to move around the client to facilitate or resist different movements (Fig. 8-17). Eventually the client can learn to float independently, if possible (Fig. 8-18). WATSU cradling techniques are excellent for relaxation and easing of spasticity. Bad Ragaz techniques are excellent for strengthening as long as the resisted proprioceptive neuromuscular facilitation patterns used do not facilitate increased spasticity. Refer to the chapters on WATSU (Chap. 17) and Bad Ragaz (Chap. 15) for greater detail.

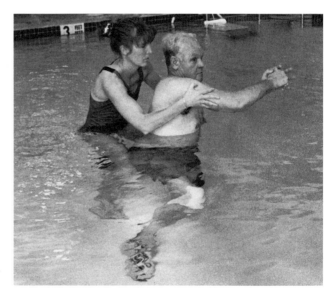

FIGURE 8-14. Client performs active movements of the upper extremities.

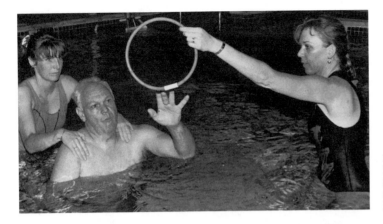

FIGURE 8-15. Client holds the barbell and rotates from side to side, bats a beach ball with the therapist, reaches for rings, or resists turbulence created by the therapist.

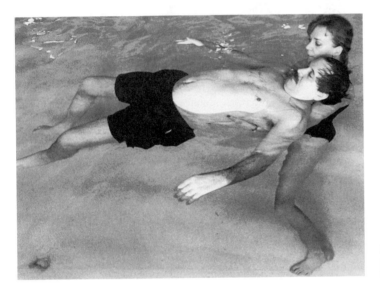

FIGURE 8-16. The therapist supports the head and trunk; the legs float independently.

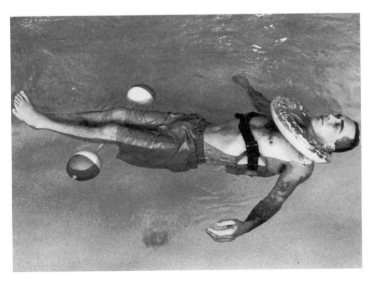

FIGURE 8-17. Client uses floatation devices so that therapist can move around. Many different combinations of devices can be used to accommodate support and activity.

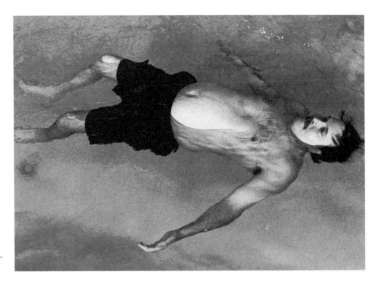

FIGURE 8-18. Client with tetraplegia floating independently.

1. *Action:* The client floats quietly or is moved slowly through the water by the therapist.
   Goal: The client achieves relaxation and reduction of spasticity and pain.
2. *Action:* The therapist, controlling at the shoulders, sways the client from side to side. This can be combined with deep inspiration at the point of maximum lateral stretch, followed by prolonged expiration through pursed lips (Fig. 8-19).
   Goals: The client achieves relaxation and spasticity reduction, and exercises muscles of respiration. The ability of the diaphragm to generate force is better in supine for those with tetraplegia. Using an abdominal binder

or resting a weight on the upper abdomen can also facilitate deeper inspiration.

3. *Action:* The therapist stabilizes the shoulders, while another person flexes the client's knees and hips and gently rotates from side to side (Fig. 8-20).
   Goal: The client achieves stretching for greater ROM and relaxation of spasticity.
   Caution: This may be contraindicated for those with open reduction and internal fixation or unstable fracture–dislocations of the spine. Medical clearance should be obtained first if there is any question.
4. *Action:* The therapist performs passive ROM to the four extremities.

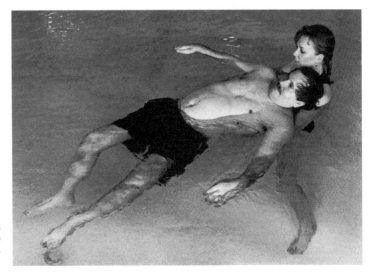

FIGURE 8-19. Therapist sways client from side to side to facilitate stretching, relaxation, and respiration.

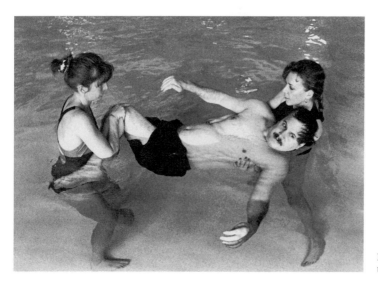

FIGURE 8-20. Passive trunk rotation.

Goal: The client receives stretching to increase ROM.

5. *Action:* The client performs upper and lower extremity motions within the water, bent knee bicycling, and straight leg kicking as neurologic sparing of muscles allows.

Goal: The client strengthens upper and lower extremities.

6. *Action:* The therapist stabilizes at the shoulders or the legs; the client swings himself or herself from side to side, curls up in a ball, or pulls knees toward one shoulder and the other (Fig. 8-21).

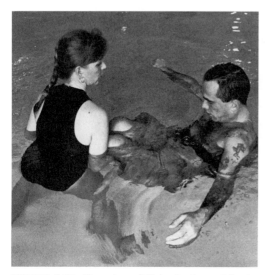

FIGURE 8-21. Therapist stabilizes the legs while the client performs trunk-strengthening exercises.

Goal: The client strengthens lateral trunk muscles, abdominals, and hip flexors.

7. *Action:* The therapist stabilizes at the shoulders while the client attempts to push his or her hips and legs down toward the bottom of the pool or isometrically into a float.

Goal: The client strengthens back and hip extensors.

8. *Action:* The therapist holds at the hips or shoulders and sways the client side to side while the client attempts to hold the trunk rigid.

Goal: The client strengthens trunk muscles isometrically.

The client can also hold onto the side of the pool or rail and perform many of these exercises there, with or without therapist assistance.

Prone Float

Because this position requires cervical hyperextension, it may be very difficult for those with tetraplegia who have restricted cervical ROM or weakness, or contraindicated for those with cervical collars, open reduction and internal fixation, or unstable fracture–dislocations. Medical clearance should be obtained first if there is any question. The client can be supported by holding onto a polythene barbell, kickboard, or the side of the pool, having a device under the axilla, and by support under the hips or legs by a device or the therapist. Any combination of these methods can be used. This position can be initially more stressful.

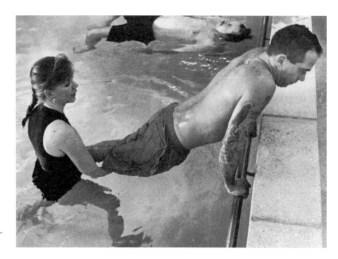

FIGURE 8-22. Client performs prone push-ups.

1. *Action:* The client holds the prone position.
   Goal: Just holding this position strengthens neck, back, and hip extensors and stretches the shoulders, abdominals, and hip flexors.
2. *Action:* The client performs lower extremity motions and kicking as neurologic sparing allows.
   Goal: The client strengthens the lower extremities.
3. *Action:* The client curls up into a ball, then extends straight out again, with the therapist assisting at the hips.
   Goals: The client strengthens abdominals, hip, and knee flexors then back, hip, and knee extensors.
4. *Action:* The client holds onto the bar or the side of the pool and with feet supported performs prone push-ups (Fig. 8-22).
   Goal: The client strengthens the upper extremities.
5. *Action:* The client places his or her mouth

and eventually the whole face into the water and blows bubbles (Fig. 8-23).
Goal: The client learns rhythmic breathing and improves respiratory status.

Standing

Standing activities and gait training may be possible for clients with incomplete SCI. They can be supported by the therapist, a ring, vest, or other flotation device, by holding on to the side of the pool, or within a set of submerged parallel bars.

1. *Action:* The client performs lower extremity exercises, including hip flexion–extension and abduction–adduction, leg and ankle circles, squats (bilateral and unilateral), up on toes, back on heels, and knee flexion–extension as neurologic sparing allows.

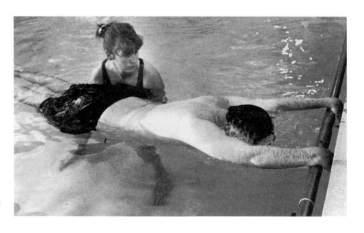

FIGURE 8-23. Client places his face in water and blows bubbles.

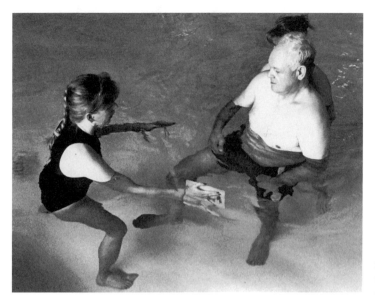

FIGURE 8-24. Client stands on one leg. Note paddles on therapist's hands to create turbulence.

Goal: The client strengthens the lower extremities.

2. *Action:* The client holds a polythene barbell out in front and twists from side to side.
   Goal: The client stretches and strengthens the trunk and shoulders.
3. *Action:* The client catches a beach ball, reaches for objects, or stands on one leg. The therapist creates turbulence around the client (Fig. 8-24).
   Goal: The client improves standing balance.
4. *Action:* Standing in neck-deep water, the client performs upper extremity motions.
   Goal: The client strengthens the upper extremities.
5. *Action:* Standing in neck-deep water, the client performs jumping jacks.
   Goal: The client works on total body strengthening, coordination, and endurance.
6. *Action:* Free floating upright in a flotation device, the client performs exercises with the lower extremities, including bicycling, scissors kicks, abduction–adduction, and hip and knee flexion–extension (Fig. 8-25).
   Goal: The client strengthens the lower extremities.

When gait training, the therapist must remember that the muscular dynamics of walking in a buoyancy-assisted, viscosity-resisted environment are different from those when walking in a gravity-resisted environment. Carry-over can occur, however, with such components of gait as weight shifting, heelstrike, sequencing, and step length. The depth of the water is important—too deep and the client tends to float; too shallow, and the effects of gravity negate the benefits of the water. Chest depth is about right for maximum support while keeping the feet on the bottom. Different devices can be used for support during gait, or the therapist can support from the front, back, or sides. The client can then walk across the pool at a consistent depth going forward or backward, sidestepping, or

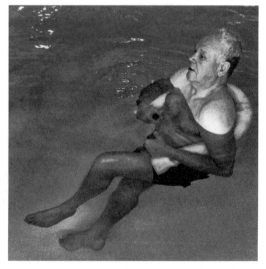

FIGURE 8-25. Client performs exercises for the lower extremities while free floating with the assistance of a floatation device.

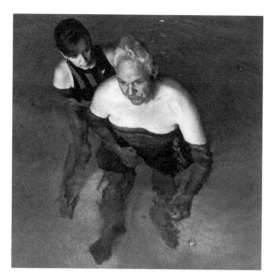

FIGURE 8-26. Client walks across pool.

braiding (Fig. 8-26). With increasing speed there is more resistance. If the therapist walks in front, the client gets pulled along in the wake. To progress in difficulty, the client can walk into shallower water. Ambulation in the pool is very encouraging to clients with incomplete SCI because they find it easier, less painful, and less fearful.

Recovery and Swimming Strokes

Swimming is one of America's most popular sports. Not only is it an enjoyable activity for those with SCI, it is a highly therapeutic one. Recreation, endurance, strengthening, ROM, co-

ordination, respiratory fitness, and reduction of spasticity are all benefits gained from a regular swimming program.

Before learning to swim after an SCI, the person needs to learn floating, recoveries, and rhythmic breathing (if performing prone strokes).

Recoveries for back float to stand, prone float to stand, prone to supine, and supine to prone are all performed as follows (information from seminar on "Aquatics for the Disabled," Rehabilitation Institute of Chicago, 1991):

Back Float to Stand

1. Tuck chin
2. Pull knees toward chest
3. Scoop hands forward
4. Thrust feet to bottom of pool

Prone Float to Stand

1. Pull knees toward chest
2. Press hands down
3. Thrust feet to bottom of pool and lift head

These skills are important for the ambulator.

Rolling Prone to Supine (Fig. 8-27)

1. Lower one shoulder
2. Turn head in opposite direction
3. Lead with elbow and look toward the direction of the roll

Rolling Supine to Prone (Fig. 8-28)

1. Lower one shoulder
2. Turn head in same direction
3. Bring opposite arm up and over chest

These skills are important for assuming the desired position for swimming and safely coming to a resting or stopping position.

Once the client has practiced rhythmic

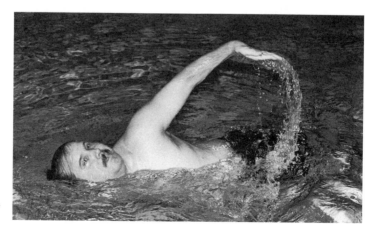

FIGURE 8-27. Rolling prone to supine.

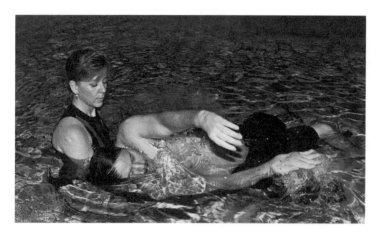

FIGURE 8-28. Rolling supine to prone.

breathing, as appropriate, floating, and recoveries, it is time to work on swimming strokes. One of the prime goals is eventual independence so that the person can continue swimming for lifelong maintenance of health and maximal functional ability.

For those with incomplete SCI, almost any stroke can be used, depending on muscle strength and ROM.

For clients with a complete SCI, the easiest way to begin is with the elementary back stroke (Fig. 8-29). It is performed on the back so that the face is out of the water and the symmetric stroke of the arms keeps the legs from rolling. Depending on client ability, this can be done with or without supportive floats.

People with paraplegia can perform almost any stroke with practice, including the back crawl, front crawl, and breast stroke. Indeed, those with paraplegia can reach a considerable degree of skill in the front crawl because even able-bodied swimmers use the legs minimally

in this stroke.[23] The breast stroke is excellent for shoulder ROM and strengthening back extensors. The front and back crawls promote rotation and trunk dissociation (Fig. 8-30). The main exception is the side stroke. The hips and legs tend to rotate and sink, and the lower extremities are required to perform this stroke effectively.[12]

People with tetraplegia can perform the elementary back stroke and the back crawl. Because the shoulders are often limited in flexion, abduction, and external rotation, the upper extremities may tend to swing out to the side and slap the water.[12] In later stages, the exceptional person with tetraplegia below C6–C7 can become proficient in the breast stroke and front crawl[20] if he or she is stable orthopedically and has sufficient cervical ROM and strength to turn the face out of the water to breathe.

Underwater swimming with snorkel and mask is appropriate for anyone with SCI and adds a new dimension to the sport. For more in-depth discussion, refer to Chapter 14.

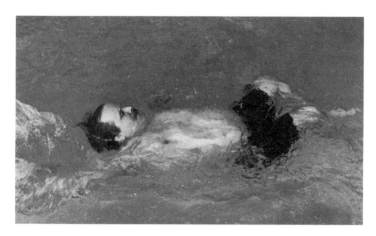

FIGURE 8-29. For client with a complete spinal cord injury, the easiest way to begin is with the elementary back stroke.

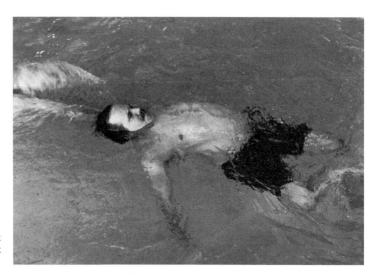

FIGURE 8-30. Front and back crawls promote rotation and trunk dissociation.

Group Exercises and Recreational Activities

People with incomplete SCI can benefit from group exercises. These could include many of the exercises already mentioned in standing, as well as aerobic water walking, jumping jacks, and running in place. The socialization makes the activity that much more enjoyable. Adding recreational activities like basketball, water polo, volleyball, and competitive swimming helps to achieve therapeutic goals with enjoyable activities (Fig. 8-31). A study done by Kennedy and Smith[24] using the Leisure Activities Blank compared the extent of involvement in 120 different activities in the past and in the expected future between those with SCI and the nondisabled. The study revealed that both men and women with SCI engaged in significantly more active leisure activities in the past than did the nondisabled, but had a significantly lower expectation for the same in the future. Kennedy and Smith also cited other studies that support their suggestion that greater attention on the part of health care professionals to encourage and assist people with SCI in active leisure activities "might help to reduce clinical depression, lessen re-hospitalisation, improve family interaction,

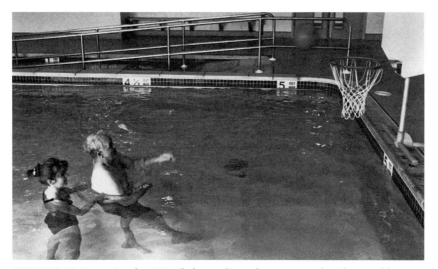

FIGURE 8-31. Recreational activities help to achieve therapeutic goals with enjoyable activities.

and prolong life expectancy among SCI patients."[24]

Summary

Aquatic activity is an excellent adjunct to land rehabilitation in meeting the psychological and physical needs of people with SCI. Sir Ludwig Guttman stated, "In the rehabilitation of paraplegics and tetraplegics, water therapy and training for water sport play a very essential part . . . ."[2] The client can achieve improvements in ROM, strength, coordination, and cardiovascular and respiratory fitness, as well as reduce pain and spasticity. These improvements can lead to better day-to-day function, a brighter psychological outlook, and a healthy adjustment to life.

REFERENCES

1. Berger S. Waterborne. *New York Times Magazine.* February 6 1994:14–15.
2. Guttmann L. *Spinal Cord Injuries: Comprehensive Management and Research.* Oxford, England: Blackwell Scientific Publications; 1973.
3. Kennedy EJ, ed. *Spinal Cord Injury: The Facts and Figures.* Birmingham, Ala: University of Alabama at Birmingham; 1986.
4. Hoffman MD. Cardiorespiratory fitness and training in quadriplegics and paraplegics. *Sports Med.* 1986; 3:312–330.
5. Glaser RM. Exercise and locomotion for the spinal cord injured. *Exerc Sport Sci Rev.* 1985;13:263–303.
6. American Spinal Injury Association. *Standards for Neurological and Functional Classification of Spinal Cord Injury.* American Spinal Injury Association; 1992.
7. Berczeller PH, Bezkor MF. *Medical Complications of Quadriplegia.* Chicago, Ill: Year Book Medical Publishers; 1986.
8. Somers M. *Spinal Cord Injury Functional Rehabilitation.* East Norwalk, Conn: Appleton & Lange; 1992.
9. Bloch RF, Basbaum M, eds. *Management of Spinal Cord Injuries.* Baltimore, Md: Williams & Wilkins; 1986.
10. Haas F, Axen K, Pineda H. Aerobic capacity in spinal cord injured people. *Central Nervous System Trauma.* 1986;3:77–91.
11. Sorg RJ. HDL-cholesterol: exercise formula. Results of long-term (6-years) strenuous swimming exercise in a middle aged male with paraplegia. *Journal of Orthopedic and Sports Physical Therapy.* 1993;17: 195–199.
12. Garvey L. Spinal cord injury and aquatics. *Clinical Management.* 1991;11:21–24.
13. Arborelius M Jr, Balldin UI, Liljaa B, et al. Hemodynamic changes in man with the head above water. *Aerospace Medicine.* 1972;43:592–598.
14. Skalnick B. Aquatic therapy. *Respiratory Therapy.* 1976;37–38, 47.
15. Pachalski A, Mekarski T. Effect of swimming on increasing cardiorespiratory capacity of paraplegics. *Paraplegia.* 1980;18:190–196.
16. Christie JL, Sheldahl LM, Tristani FE, et al. Cardiovascular regulation during head-out water immersion exercises. *J Appl Physiol.* 1990;69:657–664.
17. Haralson KM. Therapeutic pool programs. *Clinical Management.* 1985;5:10–12.
18. Weinstein LB. The benefits of aquatic activity. *Journal of Gerontological Nursing.* 1986;12:6–11.
19. Nilsson S, Staff PH, Pruett EDR. Physical work capacity and the effect of training on subjects with longstanding paraplegia. *Scand J Rehabil Med.* 1975;7: 51–56.
20. Jachheim K, Strohkendl H. The value of particular sports of the wheelchair disabled in maintaining health of the paraplegic. *Paraplegia.* 1973;2: 173–178.
21. Cowell LL, Squires WG, Raven PB. Benefits of aerobic exercise for the paraplegic: a brief review. *Med Sci Sports Exerc.* 1986;18:501–508.
22. Knutsson E, Lewenhaupt-Olsson E, Thorsen M. Physical work capacity and physical conditioning in paraplegic patients. *Paraplegia.* 1975;2:205–216.
23. Bleasdale N. Swimming and the paraplegic. *Paraplegia.* 1975;13:124–127.
24. Kennedy DW, Smith RW. A comparison of past and future leisure activity participation between spinal cord injured and non-disabled persons. *Paraplegia.* 1990;28:130–136.

ADDITIONAL READINGS

Bromley I. *Tetraplegia and Paraplegia: A Guide for Physiotherapists.* New York, NY: Churchill-Livingstone; 1981.
Lowman C, Roen S. *Therapeutic Use of Pools and Tanks.* Philadelphia, Pa: WB Saunders; 1952.
Mahoney M, McGraw-Non K, McNamara N, et al. Aquatic interventions for patients with spinal cord injuries. *Aquatic Physical Therapy Report.* 1993;1:10–20.
Skinner A, Thomson A. *Duffield's Exercise in Water.* 3rd ed. London: Balliere Tindall; 1983.

9 Aquatic Rehabilitation of the Pediatric Client

Jane L. Styer-Acevedo

Introduction

Use of Water in Pediatrics

Water has been enjoyed recreationally by children for many years, and the population of children with special needs is no exception. In fact, water is used both recreationally and as a therapy with children with amazing results. The best results occur when both areas merge into a single approach when working with children of all ages.

Current Use of Water Programs

There are a variety of water programs currently in use. The most common programs are those that teach adapted aquatic skills in school systems. This typically comes under the realm of physical education; however, some school systems employ physical therapists to work in the aquatic program. Alternatively, early intervention programs use therapists, volunteers, family members, teachers, and aides to assist in taking the children into the pool for exposure to water, water exploration, beginning safety skill development, play, and, when possible, to take advantage of the therapeutic effects of warm water.

Problem-Oriented Approach

It is not advisable to take the land-based program into the pool and duplicate its activities and exercises. This is rarely the best approach to use with water. A problem-oriented approach is possible when the properties of water are used to advantage (see Chap. 2). The problems, or areas of concern for the child, should be readily apparent from a land-based evaluation. It is then the therapist's responsibility to develop an aquatic program that addresses these problems using the water environment. This does not, however, preclude an assessment in the water. Therapists must always assess the child's response to the water, especially in the area of safety, every time the child is taken into the pool.

Land Versus Water Use in Pediatrics

A blend of land- and water-based therapy works well for most children. Working in water allows them to perform and learn movements that are too difficult to do on land. Returning to their land-based program on the same day or week provides them the opportunity to practice movements in which they have become more skilled in the water.[1] This also may be done immediately after the session if the child is not too fatigued. The author has replaced land sessions with water sessions when the child was making little or no progress with his land-based program, and was able to demonstrate progress in the water. This becomes increasingly important because many of the childhood illnesses tend to be chronic (eg, cerebral palsy, spina bifida, neuromuscular diseases). Aquatic therapy may be adjunctive (secondary) to land therapy for a portion of the year and then become the primary

151

therapy for a period of time. This decision should be made by the therapist in collaboration with the family and team, considering the child's best opportunity to become more functional and independent while maintaining high self-esteem.

This chapter includes (1) considerations specific to pediatrics regarding safety and behavior; (2) the evaluation procedures used to identify the child's strengths and problems; (3) problems typically encountered in pediatrics to set the basis for planning aquatic activities from a problem-oriented approach; (4) the clinical application of safety skills, emphasizing the need to teach the skills from two perspectives: safety in water, and goal-directed activities addressing the child's identified problem areas; (5) selected diagnoses, as examples only, for treatment activities; (6) specific treatment approaches and handling techniques that have proven useful with respect to specific problems; (7) a sample treatment plan with goals and activities to assist the therapist in setting up a child's therapy session; and (8) considerations for the future of aquatic therapy for the pediatric population.

General Safety Considerations

Oral–Motor Control

"Good breathing control is essential for all activity in water including swimming" (p 7).[2] It is imperative that children understand that they must blow out (exhale) when their mouth and nose go under water, *not* inhale. Inhaling is a frequent mistake that occurs when children are afraid or startled because their face has gone

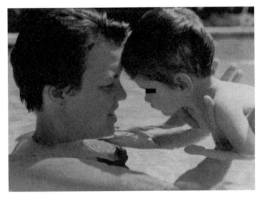

FIGURE 9-1. Demonstration and physical assistance for beginning bubble blowing.

under water or the water has splashed in their face. This results in choking and coughing and augments the child's fear of being in the water. To prevent this, explain and demonstrate to the child initially what to do in this event. If the child does not understand verbal instructions, rely on demonstration and physical assistance (Fig. 9-1). Humming or singing while the mouth is under water is a good way to teach exhalation. Blowing a ping-pong ball across the top of the water is an effective visual cue for blowing out through the mouth. The therapist should never submerge a child who is not water-safe (able reliably to close the mouth and exhale when submerged) or expecting the submersion. Therapeutic aspects of oral–motor control are addressed later in this chapter.

Chronic Ear Infections

Children who tend to get ear infections frequently can rinse their ears after the session with a solution of half alcohol and half white vinegar. The alcohol is a drying agent and the vinegar restores the correct pH balance. This is a common preventive measure against swimmer's ear.[3] There are no apparent dangers to children who have ear tubes in place[4]; however, it is advisable to keep their ears out of the water for most of the session.

Hyponatremia

According to *Stedman's Medical Dictionary*,[5] "hyponatremia" is an abnormally low concentration of sodium ions in the circulating blood. Hyponatremia occurs when a child swallows excessive amounts of water, reducing the serum sodium level. Symptoms can occur within minutes of water activity or hours later, and include restlessness, weakness, nausea, vomiting, polyuria or oliguria, muscle twitching, convulsions, and coma; death may occur.[6] Children younger than 9 months of age are especially vulnerable.[4] The author believes that any child with an atypical swallowing mechanism and poor oral–motor control is also at significant risk. Therefore, the therapist must determine the child's level of oral–motor control initially and monitor continually throughout subsequent sessions to prevent swallowing of excessive amounts of pool water.

Flotation Devices for Safety

Many children are fond of water wings, the inflatable upper arm flotation devices that provide for "independent" swimming and playing when the child is not yet "water safe." A note of caution with regard to use of this equipment: the shoulder girdle muscles must work continuously when the child is suspended in the water to keep her head above the water line. The shoulder muscles will eventually fatigue, and the child will encounter difficulty if she is in water that is too deep and cannot reach the side of the pool. Keep in mind that these flotation devices are *not* intended to save the child or keep her out of danger. Water wings have a definite place in therapeutic aquatics, and are addressed later in this chapter.

Behavioral Considerations

Age Guidelines

Pediatric aquatic therapy is used for all ages, from birth through adolescence and young adulthood. The emphasis in instruction to the pediatric population has been on younger and younger children since the early 1970s, and now includes preschool, toddler, and infant age groups.[2] With this shift in emphasis has also come the realization that water can be beneficial for children with special needs. Sweeney has used hydrotherapy techniques in the neonatal intensive care unit for therapeutic neuromusculoskeletal and behavioral benefits.[7] This chapter deals more with the infant/toddler through young adult age groups, and how to provide aquatic rehabilitation.

Some general guidelines to follow when dealing with the pediatric population include the following:

1. The infant/toddler and young child is not necessarily able to follow verbal instruction, and therefore therapists must rely on touch as well as handling skills to communicate with the child.
2. If the child is not yet toilet trained, he should wear a diaper in the pool to protect against the release of fecal matter.
3. Most young children are not safety conscious—the therapist must teach them the dangers and the rules of the pool.

4. Fear of the great expanse of water is common in the child and even in older children without prior exposure to this environment. Therefore, therapists should take great care to introduce the child to the pool slowly and to reassure the child that assistance will be provided if needed.[8]

Cognitive Status

The cognitive status of the child helps to guide the treatment. As mentioned earlier, when the child cannot follow verbal commands, the therapist must rely on other mechanisms. This condition may result from a variety of diagnoses, including mental retardation, developmental delay, or having sustained a head injury with subsequent neurologic damage. Therapy is more easily accomplished by game playing, imitation, or handling techniques.

Behavioral Concerns Related to Diagnosis

The person who has sustained a head injury goes through a recovery process that involves various levels of cooperation. It is advisable to consider the size of the child and her ability to cooperate when in the pool so that a dangerous situation is not created inadvertently. If the child is combative, defer aquatic therapy until she has passed through this stage and can work with the therapist.

Beginning Aquatic Therapy

Evaluation on Land

It is best to perform a "land evaluation" of the child before taking him into the water. This should include, at minimum, range of motion, strength, level of stiffness, balance, sensory awareness, functional status, and mobility according to the child's age. Subjectively noting previous exposure to water and skill level in water will help the therapist plan the treatment session. Therapists should also check for skin lesions and any contraindications to aquatic therapy.

In completing the subjective and objective evaluation, the assessment of the child should lead the therapist toward a list of strengths and a list of problems that need to be addressed. Prioritizing this list of problems helps guide the therapist in setting up a treatment protocol. The aquatic-based therapist must review evaluations and progress notes from the land-based therapist to incorporate the "land goals" into the aquatic activities as necessary.

Evaluation in Water

Having studied the results of the land evaluation, therapists are able to predict how the patient will float in the water as well as how she may manage her body in the water. For example, if the child has a right-sided hemiplegia, she will more likely float in supine with the right half of her body lower in the water because of the asymmetry in the density of the two sides. This causes rolling to the right and may indeed cause the face to become submerged. Therapists should always prepare the child verbally for what will happen in the water, even when they are not sure the child understands. The entry should be as independent as possible while maintaining the utmost safety. The water evaluation should begin by assessing the child's safety skills, especially the ability to exhale when the nose or mouth, or both, are under water, or at least the ability to close off the nasopharynx. This immediately indicates the child's comfort and skill levels should his face go under water. When the child is supported in a floating position, the following questions should be addressed: (1) how much control does the child have of each limb? (2) can he recover to vertical (getting his feet to the floor for a stable position from which to breathe comfortably)? and (3) what is the level of stiffness present and its distribution in the body: hypertonia, hypotonia, or fluctuating tone? The child's ability to roll from prone to supine, especially in the absence of functional lower extremities, demonstrates his ability to get air when necessary.

Carefully noting the child's safety skills, the therapist continues the assessment with active range of motion, strength, balance, sensory awareness, and mobility in the buoyant environment. How do the findings compare with the land evaluation? What movements are being assisted or resisted by the water? Answers to these questions help the therapist focus the aquatic activities as necessary to achieve the desired goals.

The aquatic rehabilitation or therapy goals may be completely separate from or directly related to the goals on land. For instance, ambulation with erect posture may be the desired outcome in both environments, and the depth of water and speed of ambulation determine how challenging the activity is in water. Or, the client may be working on a flutter kick in a supported supine position to strengthen the gluteus maximus in a buoyancy-resisted manner. This works toward the land goal of maintaining an erect trunk over pelvis during short-distance ambulation (such as in the classroom) while using both arms to carry a light object. Therefore, it is imperative to complete a patient problem list so that the aquatic activities are developed to address the appropriate areas of need.

Using Water to Address Problem Areas

In this section, aquatic activities are presented that use various properties of water to address specific problems. The problems are not presented in a diagnosis-specific context. When the therapist uses activities that directly affect the child's areas of need (problems), this approach will most certainly cross diagnostic groups.

Alteration in Stiffness

Stiffness is the length sensitivity of a muscle or the ratio of the change in force over the change in length.[9] Tone, the resistance felt to passive stretch, is frequently used to describe stiffness. In this chapter, a low level of stiffness is referred to as *hypotonia*, a high level of stiffness as *hypertonia*, and stiffness levels that vary over time as *fluctuating tone*.

Hypotonia

The hypotonic child may have an underreactive vestibular system whereby she does not process enough vestibular sensations and does not get the same "nourishment" as other children from body movement and play.[10] Ayres states, "If the vestibular system is disorganized, the muscles have low tone . . . " (p 72).[10] This child still has the same inner drive to explore and master gravity as other children, but typically does not have the same functional means of mobility; she also may be afraid of what might happen to him. These children may feel "lost in space" when there is a dysfunction somewhere in the vestibular system, and therefore fear movement such as jumping into the water because they are not quite sure how far they are from the water. Therapists should note that these children still love being moved about in the water. Lifting them quickly vertically out of the water with a splashing return, typically brings smiles and giggles. The return of the child into the water provides him with proprioceptive and tactile input that works closely with vestibular input. Some other children may appear afraid of movement because of the postural insecurity that is sometimes noted with hypotonia. It is up to the therapist to discern the child's response and individual needs. It is Burpee's opinion that "all of these systems impact on a basic level of arousal, attention, orientation, body awareness, coordination, etc." (J. Burpee, MEd, unpublished manuscript, 1994:11). The proprioceptive system helps the brain modulate the vestibular system, whereas muscle and joint sensations enable the brain to use vestibular input effectively.[10] The therapist can hop in the water while holding the small child so the two torsos are in close proximity to provide increased proprioceptive input while the head, trunk, and pelvis are held in proper alignment. If tall enough, the child can hop independently.

When working with the hypotonic child, therapists need to increase the child's level of stiffness. Swishing the child in a circular motion while prone or supine helps to accomplish this, enabling the child to activate the muscles more effectively. Changing the speed of the movement changes the tactile input the child receives by means of a change in the turbulence of the water, and produces a similar effect. Therapists must remember that the "vestibular system is a major afferent contributor to the facilitation and maintenance of muscle tone for (1) balance of excitation and inhibition and (2) muscle cocontraction for vertical postures, for smooth flexible movements" (J. Burpee, MEd, unpublished manuscript, 1994:159). The increase in muscle tone lasts for different amounts of time between sessions and during a single session for each child. The best approach to help a child gain active functional movement is to intersperse vestibular stimulation with active work/play in which the muscles are working immediately after receiving the facilitation. This repetition of vestibular stimulation may be required at any

given interval, or just at the beginning of the session. The child's response indicates whether there is a need to return to vestibular input. Caution is warranted any time vestibular stimulation is provided because it is powerful input, and may last for up to 6 to 8 hours. When the child is overstimulated, the therapist may see color changes, sweating, reddening of the ears, and other manifestations. To prevent discomfort, therapists should stop the input before these changes occur, or immediately on their observation.

Hypertonia

Neutral-warmth water, 92F to 96°F (33.5°C to 35.5°C),[11] assists in the reduction of stiffness. Rhythmic rocking or rotation of the trunk, most easily achieved in supine floating, decreases stiffness and is a good activity for immediate activation of the trunk musculature. Using an "adapted Bad Ragaz" approach (see Chap. 15 and section in this chapter) allows the therapist to switch the child from passive to active muscle work without a position change. The child may gain overall mobility in the water because the effect of buoyancy decreases the effort of movement.

Weakness

Strengthening can be achieved easily in the pool because of the large variety of positions possible that allow for buoyancy-assisted (movement performed toward the surface of the water), -supported (movement performed parallel to the surface of the water), or -resisted (movement performed toward the pool floor) exercise (see Chap. 2). Weakness is frequently seen in children with cerebral palsy and other neuromuscular disorders, traumatic brain injury, tumors, skeletal anomalies, failure to thrive, spina bifida, severe and profound mental retardation, and spinal cord injuries, and in children recovering from surgical intervention. When dealing with the pediatric population, greater success usually results when the child's focus is on play and not on exercise. Therefore, it behooves the therapist to know what position is necessary to gain the movement desired from the child and create an activity in that position. For example, buoyancy can assist a child in attaining a prone position by supporting the child's weight and arms when reaching (Fig. 9-2). Buoyancy-resisted gluteus maximus work can be achieved by kicking to-

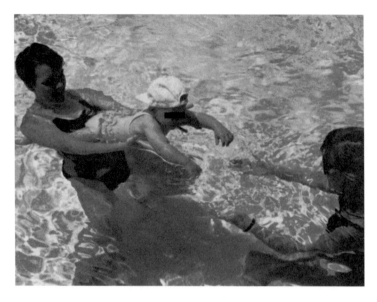

FIGURE 9-2. Reaching in supported prone position.

ward a colored tile on the pool floor while standing, or by doing a flutter kick in supine, as in performing the back crawl or when holding onto a kickboard with the upper extremities. The level of difficulty should be progressed through buoyancy assisted to buoyancy supported to buoyancy resisted as the child's strength indicates. The speed with which a movement is performed can be increased to increase the work required to complete the movement.

Range of Motion

Alteration in range of motion can manifest as either hypermobility (excessive range) or hypomobility. Range can be limited by weakness, increased stiffness, or contracture. When addressing hypermobility due to hypotonicity, the problem is best addressed initially by means of the vestibular system (see section on Hypotonia; Fig. 9-3), followed by coactivation around the specific joints. A vestibular activity that works well is the therapist jumping across the pool floor like a "bunny" with the child in his or her arms (Fig. 9-4). When the child's trunk needs to be assisted to remain in neutral, the therapist should hold the pelvis neutral with one leg flexed and the other extended (Fig. 9-5). This makes it easier for the child to maintain an erect, upright position. The child can push off the wall

of the pool with both feet in supported supine for coactivation through the lower extremities.

When range is limited, the therapist must identify the reason for the limitation and address

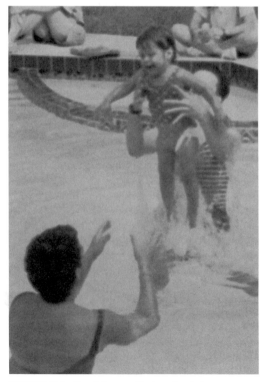

FIGURE 9-3. Providing vestibular stimulation.

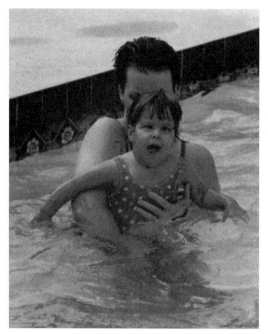

FIGURE 9-4. Secure position for "bunny hopping" across the pool.

it accordingly. When limited range is caused by weakness or hypertonia, as is typically seen in children with cerebral palsy, increased range can be achieved when buoyancy assists the movement, as in extending the hip for flutter kicking in a supported prone position for weak

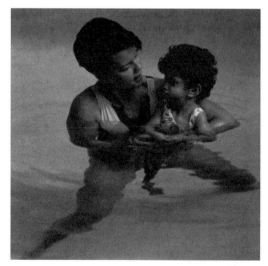

FIGURE 9-5. Fully dissociated lower extremities for a neutral pelvis position.

gluteals (Fig. 9-6). For limitation secondary to increased stiffness, the problem of the level of stiffness should be addressed first, followed by active movement in the newly acquired range. This "new" range must be actively used in the same session for expected carry-over outside of the pool (see Chap. 7). One example is the range limitation seen in lumbar spine flexion due to prolonged hyperextension. This posture is used by many children with cerebral palsy to stabilize the pelvis and spine using the quadratus lumborum. By lengthening the lumbar extensors in a rotated and horizontal position using the water for resistance, increased length can be acquired (Fig. 9-7). This can be followed by assisted supine recoveries to throw a basketball through a hoop, or a game in standing such as ring toss, to work on the balance of the trunk flexors and extensors. The depth of the water should be altered according to the amount of assistance the child requires to maintain muscle balance. When the child requires greater assistance, the water level should be higher on her trunk or chest. Use shallower water to progress the program and make the work harder for the child while she is engaged in play. Hip flexors can be lengthened in the horizontal position by the therapist turning herself and the child in the opposite direction from that shown in Fig. 9-7. Continue moving in a circular fashion and increase the speed to increase the stretch (Fig. 9-8).

Respiratory Problems

The problems most frequently encountered in the area of respiration are inability to control the oral–motor area for lip approximation to blow bubbles, inability to close the nasopharynx when submerging the face, intercostal muscle weakness, and limited vital capacity.

When the facial and oral–motor muscles are hypotonic, often noted as a slack jaw or an open-mouth posture, support can be given to the lower jaw before lowering the chin and lips into the water (Fig. 9-9). Imitation is frequently helpful to learn how to "blow" in the water (Fig. 9-10).[2] Singing a song under water requires exhalation and is an automatic response; therefore, there is less need for verbal cues. If there is increased stiffness in the oral–motor muscles, the warmth of the water assists in relaxation. Physical assist may be used, or the child can blow a ping-pong ball across the water with or

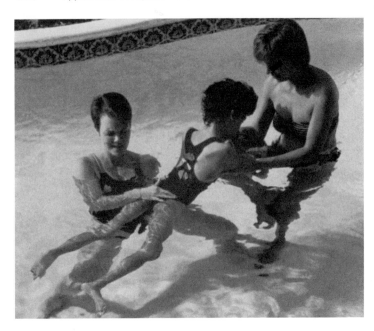

FIGURE 9-6. Buoyancy-assisted gluteus maximus work in supported prone position.

without a straw. This is helpful in gaining lip approximation and closure. It is an activity that directly assists the child who has difficulty, when feeding, in getting the upper lip down to clean off a spoon, or the child learning the bilabial sounds, "b," "p," and "m."

A person with a vital capacity of less than 1 L should be thoroughly assessed before entering the pool.[12] When hydrostatic pressure is too great to allow adequate rib cage expansion for inhalation, the child's activities should be conducted in supine, where the anterior chest wall is outside the water, or in vertical, where the level of water is at the lower rib cage or lower. Short work/play periods during which the rib cage is submerged act as resistive exercises for

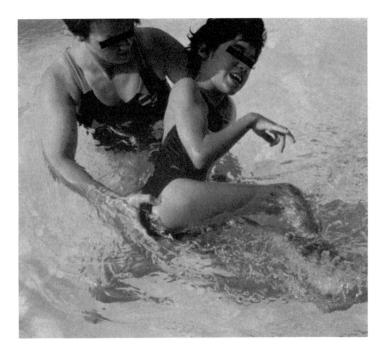

FIGURE 9-7. Lengthening the lumbar extensors in a rotated and horizontal position.

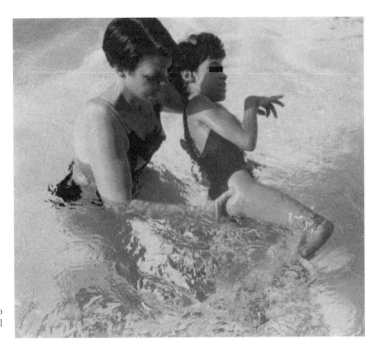

FIGURE 9-8. Lengthening the hip flexors in a rotated and horizontal position.

the intercostal muscles. *Monitor the child closely for comfort level and respiratory distress.*

When the problem is decreased cardiovascular endurance, as noted frequently in children with asthma and other chronic lung problems such as bronchopulmonary dysplasia, it is fun to work in a group for aerobic fitness. This can be done only with adequate staffing for children not yet independent in the water. The class can be structured in different ways depending on age and ability level, and may include such activities as aquarobics, step classes, deep-water jogging, and balancing, strengthening, and mobility activities in suspended vertical. Exercises using two kickboards or similar flotation devices for suspension should be done in deeper water so as not to allow unplanned rest periods by standing on the pool floor (Fig. 9-11).

Children with cystic fibrosis have compromised respiratory status because of thick mucous secretions that clog the airways. Airways are traditionally cleared of sputum with chest

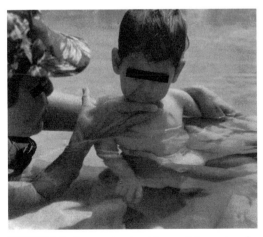

FIGURE 9-9. Support to shoulders and lower jaw for bubble blowing.

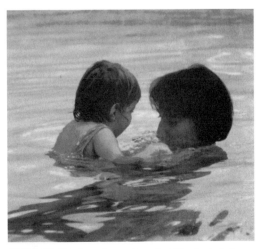

FIGURE 9-10. Learning to blow bubbles by imitation.

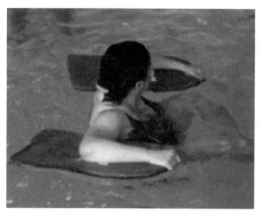

FIGURE 9-11. Exercises in suspended vertical position with two kickboards.

physical therapy, and the child is encouraged to cough during treatment. This procedure is time consuming for everyone involved and frequently leads to considerable tension by the time the child reaches adolescence. It has been found that aquatic physical therapy can increase the endurance of the respiratory muscles so children can better handle infections, and also facilitates airway clearance in some way.[13] Activities that might be appropriate are the same as those mentioned previously for cardiovascular endurance.

Arousal Problems

Movement through water can have stimulating effects on children who are difficult to arouse. This may typically be noted in children who had a traumatic brain injury or a severe neurologic insult. The movement should not be slow and rhythmic because this is relaxing and inhibitory. Instead, larger movements, vertical or horizontal, depending on the child's size, should be provided in an arrhythmic manner. Splashing of water also frequently arouses a child.

Sensory–Perceptual Difficulties

A limitation of active movement, from whatever cause, is likely to retard perceptual development, of which body image and spatial awareness are part.[2] The tactile and proprioceptive feedback afforded to the child while in the pool can help to improve the child's awareness of his body and spatial orientation. Emphasizing weight-bearing activities on the pool wall, floor, or floating objects such as a kickboard assists the child in feeling his extremities. Completing an obstacle course with tasks requiring up, down, around, over, under, and through helps the child learn the relations his body has with other people and objects around him.

The therapist can play games that require a change in speed of movement through the water to vary the tactile feedback the child receives, or play ball games to reinforce eye–hand coordination and bilateral upper extremity use. Burpee states, "rarely do we have isolated sensory system deficits which affect isolated developmental skills. More often there are numerous deficits, although they may be subtle and difficult to clearly discern or even differentiate sometimes" (J. Burpee, MEd, unpublished manuscript, 1994:22). Therefore, a multisensorial approach works best when treating a child with sensory–perceptual difficulties in the water.

Clinical Application of Safety Skills

Seven essential safety skills used in the treatment of children in the pool are rhythmic breathing (blowing bubbles), supine float and recovery, prone float and recovery, rolling, and changing directions. These skills are aimed at making the child as safe as possible in the aquatic environment and encouraging more independence for recreation and family outings. This section discusses ways in which these skills can be used therapeutically to achieve the goals set for and by the child.

Rhythmic Breathing

The necessity for controlled breathing and exhalation in water was discussed earlier in this chapter. Once the child has achieved the ability to control her breath, she knows that she can therefore control her body position in the water. By keeping her lungs filled with air, she floats higher in the water. When the lungs have less air in them, her body floats lower in the water. This knowledge and experience help to eliminate or decrease fear in the water. The techniques discussed earlier in the section addressing respiratory problems should be used to work on the safety skill of rhythmic breathing and bubble blowing. In this manner, the therapist addresses both the area of safety and the child's specific problems. It is the author's experience that many children with special needs have a difficult time learning how to control their breathing. Time should be spent in every session practicing these important skills, although progression through the other skills in the same session is strongly encouraged. Controlled breathing is not considered an absolute prerequisite for continuing to the other safety skills when the proper handling and assistance are provided.

Supine Float

The supine float should be taught before the supine recovery for the child to learn how to control the body in a horizontal position. The floating position depends on body composition and the level of stiffness and its distribution throughout the body. It is recommended that a flotation device not be used initially until the child and the therapist know how the child floats independently.[2] When there is asymmetry of stiffness and therefore alteration in floating, the stiffness problems should be addressed first, with a return to floating for an improved position. This may mean using the treatment techniques presented earlier in the Problem Areas section of this chapter; or, it may consist simply of changing postures so that the length of the arms is increased by extending the elbows and putting the arms up by the ears and head, and the length of the legs is decreased by flexing the knees. These actions themselves may be what the child needs to achieve improved function. For example, if a child has muscle tightness through the pectoral, teres major, and latissimus muscles, the therapist can encourage putting the arms by the ears in maximal shoulder flexion and abduction to bring the chest higher in the water. Such a position provides immediate feedback to the child and therefore reinforces that movement. Bending the knees while maintaining hip extension may shorten the heavier, longer lever arms and raise the lower half of the body higher in the water. This activity reinforces a pattern that is very difficult for many children with cerebral palsy. Doing this movement in the water helps to reduce synergy-dominated movement of the legs and may work toward improved gait on land.

Supine Recovery

Supine recovery is taught next, and is simply the return to vertical, placing the feet on the floor and achieving a stable position for safe breathing. In the event that the legs cannot be used (paraplegia, amputation, or overall height), the child can recover to the side of the pool and hold onto the railing or wall. Supine recovery "requires strong flexion of the cervical spine, trunk, hips and knees, with flexion of the shoulders in abduction followed by precise balancing of the head over the body to maintain the upright position" (p 27).[2] When verbal commands can be used with the child, saying "chin tuck, knees to chest, and feet to floor" in succession may help the child learn this skill. The therapist can use her hands on the child's abdominals from behind in an inward and upward motion, "telling" the child what is expected of him when verbal communication is not helpful (Fig. 9-12). In many children with cerebral palsy, relatively inactive obliques combined with an overactive rectus abdominis lead to a flaring rib cage (Fig. 9-13). By placing her hands on the bottom of the rib cage, the therapist can provide gentle pressure to bring the rib cage into alignment with the trunk. This assists the obliques in firing to help complete the supine recovery. This is a buoyancy-assisted activity for the abdominals and works well to balance the flexors and extensors of the trunk for function. When the child pushes his feet to the floor when in vertical, the motion is resisted by the buoyancy of water, providing resistance to the hip extensors. This is a good activity for children with cerebral palsy, especially because they typically have weak hip extensors and consequent poor trunk-over-pelvis posture in upright.

Prone Recovery

It is preferable to teach the prone recovery before the prone float because many children are either unsafe when putting their face in the water or are afraid to do so. The therapist can place the child's hands or forearms (according to the child's size) across the therapist's shoulders when facing the child, or allow him to hold onto the side of the pool. The therapist's hands

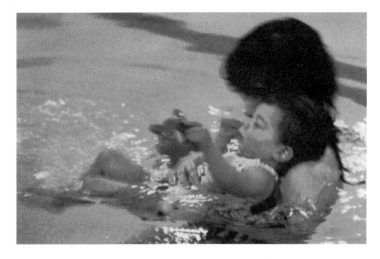

FIGURE 9-12. Using hand on abdominals for activation in supine recovery.

should reach to the abdominals to assist them to activate when the command is given to "bring your knees to your chest, head up, and feet to floor." The therapist's hands should be placed so as to activate the obliques without further assistance given to the rectus abdominis. As noted earlier, the therapist's hands may be the communication link to the child when verbal communication is not reliable or desired. Words should be used simultaneously in the event that the child might understand them, at that moment or in the future. Prone recovery is a buoyancy-resisted activity for the abdominals and should be used to strengthen them when the buoyancy-assisted position of supine recovery no longer provides adequate resistance to the movement. The hip extensors are resisted by the buoyancy of water, as in supine recovery, when the child pushes his feet toward the floor once he has achieved the vertical position.

Prone Float

When the child is ready (or safe from an oral–motor perspective), prone floating can be started. The child may keep her hands on a stable support surface such as the wall or the therapist (Fig. 9-14), and the therapist's hands can

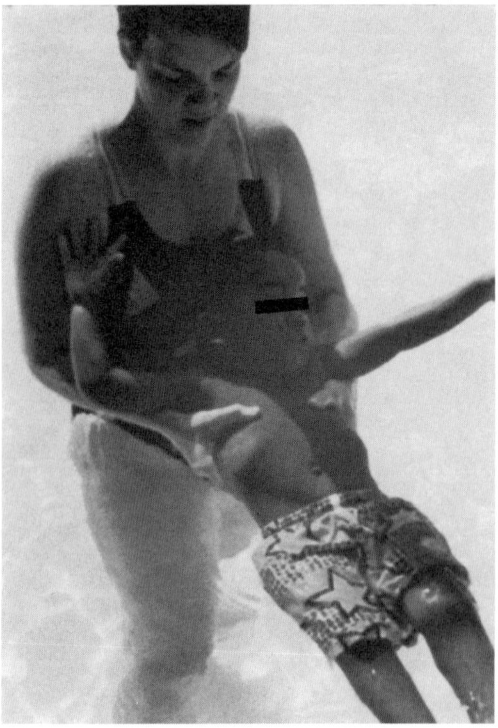

FIGURE 9-13. Flared ribcage in supported supine position.

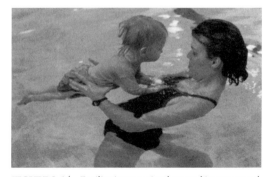

FIGURE 9-14. Facilitating proximal control in supported prone position with child's hands on therapist's chest.

facilitate proximal control through the obliques and hip extensors. This is a buoyancy-assisted position for hip extension.

Both recoveries are total-pattern body movements; that is to say, they begin with full extension, progress to full flexion, and end with full extension. For any child who already uses full flexion or full extension to initiate or perform movements, these skills should not be practiced repeatedly except with regard to the child's safety. They serve only to reinforce those patterns that make functioning more difficult for the child on land. Activities that promote flexion in one part of the body with extension elsewhere are indicated, as in the example given previously of supine floating with knees flexed while the hips remain extended.

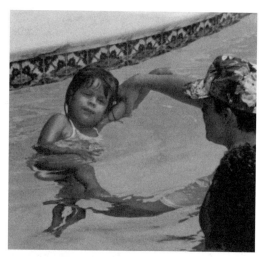

FIGURE 9-15. Assisted rolling with head supported out of the water.

Rolling

Rolling, or lateral rotation as it is referred to by Campion,[2] is used to get the face out of the water when the child is in prone and is unable to extend the cervical spine to get air. This is most commonly seen with extreme weakness of the neck extensors or a fusion of the cervical spine, as treatment for spinal fracture. When the head is turned to the side, the body follows and begins a roll. It is best that the child understand this so that during an activity, rolling does not occur unexpectedly. The child can initiate the roll from the head, the arms, or the legs. This is most easily taught from a supine position first, followed by the prone position. If the child is not safe when his face is in the water, his head may be supported out of the water (Fig. 9-15). Once the face is in the water, the therapist should never remove her eyes from the child's head during the learning phases. If the child signals that he is ready to receive assistance to return to supine and there is a short delay, mistrust develops immediately. Rolling or lateral rotation is useful to decrease stiffness in the trunk as well as to teach rolling for functional carry-over to land. To decrease stiffness, the child can be assisted at the shoulders or the upper trunk to complete part of the roll. He also can be assisted to initiate the roll at the pelvis or legs, thereby facilitating lower trunk rotation on the upper trunk. This should then progress immediately into active use of the trunk so the child can learn how it feels to use these muscles. Activities used might include rolling, supine recovery, elemen-

tary back stroke, back crawl, Bad Ragaz techniques, and the like.

Changing Directions

Changing directions becomes critical when the child is swimming in a crowded pool and needs to alter the direction in which she is going for safety reasons. It is often helpful to remember that for every action, there is an equal and opposite reaction (Newton's third law of motion). Therefore, if the child wants to turn to the right, she must pull with her right arm from the right side toward the left and back toward the feet. She may also compensate with her legs in the kicking pattern. This "pushes" her in the direction she would like to go. There may be alterations in the direction a child is swimming because of asymmetry in her body. This can be changed by remembering Newton's third law.

Special Considerations

"Smaller" Bodies

Having learned how to use the physical properties of water to the best advantage for the human body (see Chap. 2), the therapist now can apply such principles to a child-sized body. It is advisable for the therapist to learn how to use her own body in a variety of ways in place of typical equipment. For example, it could be difficult to

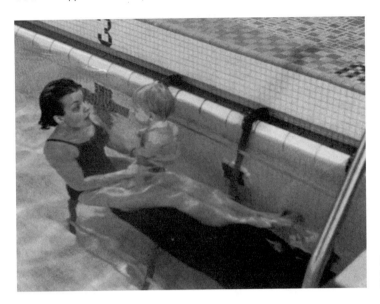

FIGURE 9-16. Supported standing using a submerged table to adjust for depth of water.

work on standing with a child in shoulder-deep water when the child is only 34 inches tall. To allow the child to stand on the pool floor, the water depth could not exceed 30 inches. Such a working depth would create uncomfortable working conditions for the therapist. Therapists can use a submerged table that can be adjusted to the appropriate height (Fig. 9-16), or work on a step (Fig. 9-17). In place of the table or step, it is often easier to stand the child on the therapist's thighs or abdomen (Fig. 9-18), with the therapist able to move to the appropriate depth for the child's activity. This can be done with a wide base of support, hip and knee flex-

ion, and posterior pelvic tilt so that the therapist is stable. This is of great help in cases of foot deformity such as equinovarus, because the deformity can be accommodated in weight bearing on the therapist's thigh with the toes pointed to the lateral sides of the thighs. A child can easily be seated on the therapist's one thigh for trunk and upper extremity activities when the therapist is standing on the opposite leg with her back supported against the pool wall. The child's pelvis can be assisted to remain in neutral by placing one of the child's legs in hip and knee flexion with hip external rotation (supported on the therapist's thigh), and the other leg in hip and

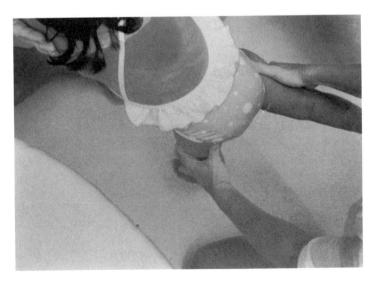

FIGURE 9-17. Adjusting to depth of water by working on a step.

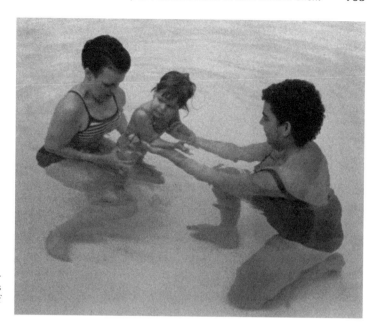

FIGURE 9-18. Working on standing with the child on the therapist's thighs to adjust to the depth of water.

knee extension (between the therapist's legs). With the pelvis stabilized, the therapist's hands are then free to assist the child's play or facilitate movement through the upper trunk and arms. The depth of water giving support to the child's trunk can be changed to increase or decrease the effort expended in remaining vertical or playing by the therapist simply moving to a different depth of water. Slowly tipping the child in any direction elicits a righting response, with buoyancy assisting the return to vertical (Fig. 9-19).

Fixed Deformity

As mentioned in the section on evaluation, it is imperative that the therapist know whether a change in structure is fixed. When working with the pediatric population, there is great potential for preventing deformity as the child grows. Therefore, the therapist must be sure that skeletal change noted is *definitely* fixed before deciding to compensate for that skeletal change. When fixed, the deformity must be accommodated during the treatment session (eg, foot deformity was mentioned previously in the context of upright weight bearing). Spinal deformity can be accommodated by handling the child so the head and face are held out of the water, as dictated by degree of oral–motor skill, or by using flotation devices to maintain the child's safety.

Thoracic kyphosis, for example, is more easily managed in a supine position, in which the head remains out of the water and buoyancy supports the spine. Using the arms for mobility is advisable because this may help to increase shoulder range for more independent function. Whenever possible, the child must be taught functional compensations for the fixed deformities.

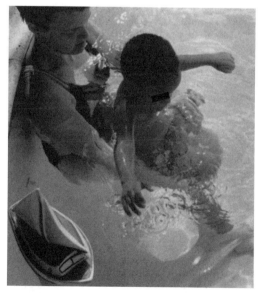

FIGURE 9-19. Eliciting anterior righting of head and trunk by tipping in the sitting position.

Parent/Guardian/Caregiver Instruction

The pediatric population differs from the adult population in that children require more intense supervision. It is unrealistic to assume that a young child can perform an exercise routine independently and reliably. It is therefore essential that someone other than the child be taught the child's program so that it may be carried out reliably and appropriately. It is recommended that the assisting adult enter the water with the child and therapist to learn the necessary skills, especially when the child is not independent in the water. A demonstration by the therapist followed by a return demonstration by the learner is the easiest way for the therapist to ascertain whether the adult is comfortable with the program. Poolside charts or waterproof pictures can be helpful to provide visual cues to the learner, as necessary.

Considerations for Specific Diagnoses

Spina Bifida

Spina bifida is defined as a limited defect in the spinal column, consisting of absence of the vertebral arches, through which the spinal membranes, with or without spinal cord tissue, may protrude.[5] The children with spina bifida most frequently seen in therapeutic programs are those with myelomeningocele, in which the spinal cord tissue protrudes and there is a lack of innervation to some part or all of the legs and accompanying sensory deficits. Typically, changes in the child's shape and density occur. Therefore, the therapist must plan in advance how best to support the child and facilitate movement. Campion lists the most common and frequent complications as (1) loss of density in the lower limbs leading to high floating of these limbs, (2) the ease with which vertical balance can be disturbed or lost, and (3) the rotational problems occurring because of asymmetric distribution of muscle power and deformity.[2] When developing a problem list for children with spina bifida, two major areas to be considered include the musculoskeletal changes, fixed or functional, and the need to increase upper body, trunk, and sometimes lower extremity strength for function. Activities suitable to address range deficits and strengthening programs in general were discussed previously. Specific to the child with spina bifida, an activity that works well is horizontal mobility in prone. The child is asked to hold onto a kickboard under each arm, in prone, with the face out of the water. A single kickboard is difficult to manage because of the small base of support. Tell or show the child how to move his hips up and down in the water. This can be called a "dolphin kick" because the legs follow wherever the hips are going. This activity requires buoyancy-assisted trunk extension followed by buoyancy-resisted trunk flexion while maintaining a stable base with bilateral use of the shoulder girdles. It works well as a strengthening activity for the trunk and shoulders, and provides mobility for the child who has not yet learned any swimming techniques.

Severe or Profound Mental Retardation

The issues most frequently encountered with children in this population include the fact that communication cannot be accomplished adequately by verbal means alone and that there often are multiple musculoskeletal changes to be considered. It is necessary to watch the child's facial expressions and feel the tenseness in the child's body when new or exciting things are introduced. Typically, there is a change in one or both of these measures to indicate positive or negative responses. Sounds, other than words, may be produced by the child. Changes in tone, pitch, and frequency of the vocalizations can provide clues to the child's response. Distinguishing between deformity versus stiffness and change in range of motion can assist the therapist in preparing the program accordingly. Knowledge regarding land goals for transfers and ambulation is helpful because upright weight bearing and movement are easier to perform in the water (Fig. 9-20). Therapists should also be aware of the psychological benefits of independent movement in water. For many children who are profoundly mentally retarded, this is the only opportunity they have to move on their own. A well positioned flotation device to provide safe positioning for the face and head may allow the child to propel herself around the pool without physical assistance. This may best be accomplished at the end of the session as "free play." Bailey has compiled a comprehen-

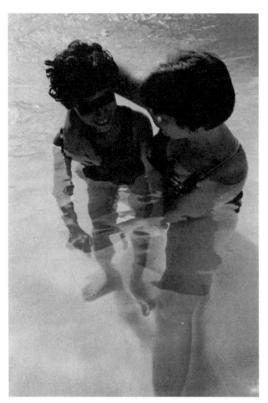

FIGURE 9-20. Maximally assisted ambulation in water to axillary level.

sive list of curriculum guidelines for teaching the student with severe or profound mental retardation.[14]

Postsurgical Issues

In pediatric practice, surgery often is performed to correct or maintain deformity or repair tissues that have sustained trauma. This is most commonly noted in children with cerebral palsy, spina bifida, and traumatic head injury. Most surgical cases result in pain, swelling, and inflammation at the site of surgery. The advantages of postoperative water therapy include pain reduction, quicker return to activity, and safer, more efficient workouts, according to Huey and Forster.[15] Water therapy can begin as soon as the wound is healed and there is no chance of infection. Because its buoyancy assists movement, children find playing in water much easier than on land once the casts or appliances are removed. Some physicians have strict guidelines about what movements may be done by the

child postsurgery and how much weight can be placed on the feet in an upright position. Table 9-1 presents general guidelines and suggested aquatic activities for the more common pediatric surgical procedures.

Treatment Techniques

"Adapted" Bad Ragaz

Chapter 15 addresses the Bad Ragaz method of aquatic therapy and should be read for a better understanding of how to use it. The original method requires that the patient respond to a verbal command by the therapist. In pediatric applications, it may be difficult to get the client to follow exact commands, and therefore the technique is modified when working with children. The therapist's hands become the vehicle of communication, and slight pressure or traction indicate to the child how she is supposed to move. The therapist may be able to hold the child without using flotation if she is small enough or buoyant enough (Fig. 9-21). This is preferable, because the technique can then be applied intermittently without having to don or doff flotation devices. An example of the use of this technique with children is to activate the lateral trunk and legs by beginning in supported supine, holding at the shoulders, elbows, or rib cage to provide stability. By quickly moving the upper trunk and shoulders side to side, the child can be helped to move her lower trunk and legs

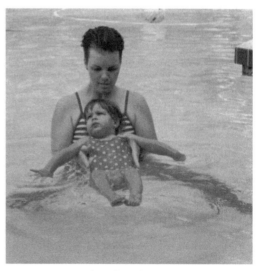

FIGURE 9-21. "Adapted" Bad Ragaz technique.

TABLE 9-1. Aquatic Activities for Children Who are Postsurgery

Identified Problems	Suggested Aquatic Activities
Varus Derotation Osteotomy	
Pain in hip Weakness of hip abductors Imbalance of hip abductor and adductor strength Decreased range Leg-length discrepancy (if unilateral procedure)	"Adapted" Bad Ragaz techniques to decrease pain, increase range, and progress to buoyancy-supported strengthening exercises for hips Prone flutter kicking, holding wall or kickboard Propel off wall in supine with two feet and continue with flutter kick Standing balance activities while playing various ball games Walk in lower, rib-cage deep water Suspended walking in deep water Swimming—front and back crawl Races—walking or swimming
Tendon lengthening such as hip flexors, adductors, hamstrings, triceps surae	
Weakness of muscle group where tendon was lengthened Imbalance of strength of the lengthened muscle to muscles on the opposite side of the joint Pain at incision site, at joint where surgery was performed, or throughout entire legs due to immobilization in cast Potential for increased stiffness into flexion with cast removal	"Adapted" Bad Ragaz techniques to decrease pain, increase range, and strengthen muscles Jumping across pool floor like a "bunny" Lower extremity exercises in suspended upright with kickboards under the arms Pushing off pool wall with both feet for flutter kicking in supine Water games: polo, basketball, volleyball, etc. Swimming strokes for lower extremity strengthening (using flutter and breast stroke kicks) Races: walking, running, swimming

to the sides. The water provides resistance to this movement. In this manner, the lateral sides of his trunk are lengthened and immediately activated. More success is noted when the rib cage is prevented from flaring and is held in line with the trunk for activation of the abdominals.

"Adapted" WATSU

Refer to Chapter 17 for details of this method of aquatic therapy. WATSU can be very useful with the severely or profoundly mentally retarded child and the child with increased stiffness. It is not indicated for children who are significantly hypotonic. It is a good method to intersperse with functional training skills in children who demonstrate significant stiffness and subsequent weakness. In these situations, WATSU can be used early in the session to "loosen up" the child in preparation for more active work.

Halliwick Method

Campion uses the Halliwick method extensively with the pediatric population with disabilities,[2] and goes into specific detail about how to use the method with children. The Halliwick method is designed for swimming instruction, but is effective for specific patient problems (see Chap. 16).

Individual Versus Group Treatment

Individual services provided to a child by the therapist usually allow for direct facilitation of movement in the buoyant environment for a functional goal. This is sometimes necessary because the child is too small to touch the floor of the pool, or is not water safe. Many programs use a one-to-one approach with the child, but can also involve families, teachers, aides, and volunteers to support the child in the water. Campion states that "the opportunity to work both individually and in groups provides the optimal situation for the child" (p 37).[2] These helpers are invaluable to the program and should be able to follow the therapist's directions once given. They should be trained in the water and must feel comfortable handling children in this environment. They are not, however, therapists, and should not be treated as such. When facilitation of specific muscle groups is indicated or programs require revision, the therapist should work with the child. Groups can be highly motivating for children; they enjoy playing games with other children such as Simon says, follow the leader, basketball, water polo, ring toss, volleyball, running obstacle courses, and so forth. Such activities may motivate the child to move more than she would typically, and do it in a fun-filled way. These games are a great way to work on cardiovascular fitness, especially when teams are set up for games such as water polo or basketball. This is useful for the older child with a diagnosis such as asthma or severe allergy who needs to work on her respiratory status. Care must be taken to ensure that all the children participating in the games are water safe or have an adult with them to give them the necessary assistance. Young children typically are not interested in or able to follow an exercise program with instructions given verbally or in a large group. They respond much better to a "fun" activity, either individually or as a group, and are therefore quite cooperative with such an approach.

Peer Group Activities

Many children and adolescents respond well to peer group activities. It is healthy for children with chronic disabilities to be able to join their peers for games and activities. This might consist of a group of children with similar disabilities, or might take place in the context of a local, community-based program such as at the YMCA or community center. The child may need assistance to join his peer group or to learn safety skills and activities that will allow him to be part of the group. The therapist plays an important role in getting the child to the point of joining the group safely and perhaps giving him the assistance he might need during group activities. Joining the peer group may be a primary goal during individual therapy because of the psychological benefit conferred on the child.

Competition

Competition can be healthy for children, especially when everyone ends up a winner in some way. Training children for participation in water and swimming activities can be rewarding, fun,

and therapeutic. The child may need to practice special skills in therapy to allow her to be safe in competing independently. This may in turn guide the therapy sessions to achieve the goal of independence. The psychological benefits of competition can be considerable for the child.

Family-Centered Activities

A goal of individual therapy should be to enable the child to participate as much as possible in family activities. This may mean teaching the family how to include the child and play with him safely and comfortably, and teaching the child how to play with the family. Most children need, at minimum, supervision, and at most, assistance to work and play in the water. When families can be included in this process, the therapeutic benefits are experienced throughout the week instead of only during the therapy session.

Community-Based Groups

A goal of individual therapy might be to include the child in community activities, typically at a YMCA or community center. This is especially helpful if the child's peers or siblings are involved in a program. It is more motivating to be able to join the others in activities, when possible. Again, the therapist's responsibilities are to ensure the child's safety skills and prepare the child in every way possible to be successful. The therapist should play an important role in assisting the child and family in choosing appropriate activities for fun and success, as well as prevention of deformity and dysfunction. If a child wants to learn swimming with the hopes of competition, but is prone to stiffness and flexion contractures of the lower extremities, the therapist should assist the child in choosing a swimming stroke that (1) does not increase her stiffness and flexion contractures, and (2) allows her to feel successful as she accomplishes her task. In such a case, the front crawl may be the stroke of choice because trunk rotation helps to keep the stiffness at a manageable level, whereas the flutter kick is a buoyancy-assisted hip extension exercise that works to decrease flexion contractures of the lower extremities. The breast stroke is not recommended because it is all straight-plane work of the trunk, and the lower extremities constantly return to the flexed position.

Box 9-1 provides a sample of goals with a possible treatment plan and activities.

Treatment Goal and Treatment Plan

As stressed earlier, it is imperative that the therapist know the child's strengths and problems. Equipped with this knowledge, the therapist can work with the child and family in deciding on the goal of aquatic therapy, which may be directly related to the land goal or completely separate, and thereby set up the treatment session.

Summary

Aquatic therapy is quickly becoming known as an effective, efficient method of physical therapy. For children in particular, it is fun, exciting, and different from traditional therapies. With increased cooperation on the part of some children, faster progress can be expected. It is expected that aquatic rehabilitation will grow in the field of pediatrics, as it is already doing in the

---

BOX 9-1. Treatment Goal and Treatment Plan

NAME: Mary
DIAGNOSIS: cerebral palsy, spastic diplegia with minimal severity

Strengths	Problems
1. Independent water safety skills	1. Minimal increase in lower extremity stiffness
2. G to N strength upper extremities	2. Imbalance of hip musculature: flexors and extensors; abductors and adductors, with flexors and adductors being stronger
3. Normal cognition	
4. Motivated to participate	
5. Enjoys swimming	3. Minimal decrease in proprioceptive awareness of lower extremities

Long-term goal (land) (6 weeks)
Mary will ambulate 25 feet independently while carrying her books to the library shelf with base of support at shoulder width and hip extension to neutral during stance phase of both lower extremities.

Long-term goal (water) (6 weeks)
Mary independently will use the back crawl to cross the pool for 15 feet with hip extension to neutral bilaterally while performing the flutter kick.

Pool session goal (1 hour)
Mary will demonstrate a handstand in lower rib-cage deep water (when upright) given moderate assistance and perform a symmetric lower extremity abducted split, and return to adduction once without losing the vertical position.

Aquatic Therapy Session Plan

1. Enter via jumping off deck from a sitting position near therapist
2. Turn around to place hands and feet on the wall, push off wall with feet, and continue with supine flutter kick
3. Supine recovery to do prone flutter kick back to the wall
4. Repeat steps 2 and 3 several times for trunk and lower extremity strengthening
5. Race across the pool using kickboards for upper extremity stability and flutter kick in either prone or supine
6. Perform an obstacle course with objects to retrieve from the pool floor using a surface dive, submerged vertical hula hoop to swim through, floating buoys to go around, submerged stool to ascend and descend when the water is between waist and chest depth, and a ring or ball toss station
7. Trunk and lower extremity exercises in suspended vertical with arms on two kickboards
8. Practice with simple hand stands
9. Handstands with controlled lower extremity movements into flexion/extension and abduction/adduction
10. Exit pool via staircase using two rails and assist as needed.

adult arena. There is still inadequate research to indicate whether a child will learn to ambulate faster, for instance, in the pool as opposed to on land, or whether the most efficacious method is to provide both land and water therapy. This question remains to be answered for all areas of functional skill in the pediatric population.

REFERENCES

1. Styer-Acevedo JL, Cirullo JA. Integrating land and aquatic approaches with a functional emphasis. *Orthopaedic Physical Therapy Clinics of North America*. 1994;3:165–178.
2. Campion MR. *Hydrotherapy in Paediatrics*. 2nd ed. Oxford: Butterworth-Heinemann; 1991.
3. Dull H. *WATSU: Freeing the Body in Water*. Harbin Springs, CA: Harbin Springs Publishing; 1993:15.
4. Burd B. Infant swimming classes immersed in controversy. *The Physician and Sports Medicine*. 1986;14: 239–244.
5. *Stedman's Medical Dictionary Illustrated*. 23rd ed. Baltimore, Md: Williams & Wilkins, 1976.
6. Kropp RM, Schwartz JF. Water intoxication from swimming. *J Pediatr*. 1982;947–948.
7. Sweeney JK. Neonatal hydrotherapy: an adjunct to developmental intervention in an intensive care nursery setting. *Physical and Occupational Therapy in Pediatrics*. 1983;3:39–52.
8. Fitness Column. Aquatic activities introducing your child to the water. *Exceptional Parent*. July/August 1990:54.
9. Walsh EG. Muscles, Masses and Motion: The Physiology of Normality, Hypotonicity, Spasticity and Rigidity. *Clinics in Developmental Medicine*. 1992;125.
10. Ayres AJ. *Sensory Integration and the Child*. Los Angeles, CA: Western Psychological Services; 1979.
11. Licht S, ed. *Physical Medicine Library*. Vol 7: *Medical Hydrology*. Baltimore, Md: Waverly Press, Inc; 1963: 242.
12. Skinner AT, Thomson AM. *Duffield's Exercise in Water*. 3rd ed. London: Bailliere Tindall; 1983:46.
13. Whitner T. Aquatic therapy in the management of cystic fibrosis. *Aquatic Physical Therapy Report*. 1994;2(2):6–7.
14. Bailey C. Curriculum guidelines for teaching profound and severely retarded students (IQ under 40) including those with physical handicaps. *The American Association for the Education of the Severely/Profoundly Handicapped Review*. 1975;1:1–17.
15. Huey L, Forster R. *The Complete Waterpower Workout Book*. New York, NY: Random House; 1993:304.

10 Aquatic Rehabilitation for the Obstetric and Gynecologic Client

Judy Cirullo

Throughout history, pregnant women have been encouraged to rest and refrain from strenuous activity. It was believed that active mothers had smaller babies and sedentary mothers had larger babies.[1,2] It was not until the middle of the 20th century that the benefits of exercise during pregnancy began to be appreciated. Although more is known about the physiologic, mechanical, and emotional changes of pregnancy, the effects of exercise on the pregnant woman and the fetus are not yet fully understood. The aquatic environment introduces its own set of questions in that regard:

- What effects does this environment have on the mother and fetus during vertical and horizontal exercise? Should all pregnant women exercise in the water?
- What is the recommended depth and water temperature?
- Is the water environment safe for high-risk obstetric clients?
- What conditions/restrictions should be considered for clients with osteoporosis?
- What is the difference between individual programs (one-on-one with a licensed health care practitioner) and group fitness classes for the pregnant woman?
- What legal issues arise either in rehabilitation or fitness programs?
- What are the guidelines for rehabilitative and fitness programming in a water environment?
- What are the advantages of recommending rehabilitative fitness programs for the pregnant woman in an aquatic environment versus conventional land programs?

Information does exist concerning program development and implementation of aquatic group exercises for low-risk pregnancy, but very little can be found about rehabilitation strategies. This chapter addresses some of these questions and suggests aquatic exercises for the more common musculoskeletal and medical problems of the obstetric client.

Maternal Anatomy and Kinesiology

Anatomically and physiologically, the pregnant woman undergoes massive changes. In the early months of pregnancy, the pelvis, sometimes called a basin, houses and protects the reproductive organs, including the uterus with its supportive ligaments. The pelvis, surrounded and supported by ligaments and muscles, is also affected by the changes of pregnancy. The two articulations of the pelvis are the sacroiliac joint and the symphysis pubis. The sacroiliac joint is synovial and the symphysis pubis has an interpubic disc of fibrocartilage. During pregnancy, this fibrocartilage becomes softened by the hormone relaxin and is at risk for separation with unsafe movements or exercise.[3,4] The ligaments supporting the uterus are the round ligaments, the broad ligaments, the uterosacral ligaments, and the transverse cervical or cardinal ligaments. The broad, round, and uterosacral ligaments are thought to maintain their positions within the pelvic cavity during pregnancy. If the increasing size of the uterus pulls on the round ligament, it can be a source of pain.[5]

The muscles of the pelvis include the perineum, as well as several that originate in the pelvis and insert in the lower extremity. Benson provides a complete review of the functional anatomy of the one and two joint muscles.[5] The pelvic diaphragm, or pelvic floor, has two parts, the upper and lower, which consist of muscle, ligaments, and fascia.[4] The muscle of the upper diaphragm is the levator ani and those of the lower diaphragm are the ischiocavernosus, bulbocavernosus, and transverse perineal muscles. The upper and lower diaphragms are interwoven for support and are perforated centrally by three openings, the urethra, the vagina, and the rectum, which enhance the sphincter-like action of the muscles. The function of the pelvic diaphragms is to support the internal organs.

As pregnancy progresses, greater demands are placed on the diaphragms. Without proper strength, the pelvic floor can sag, creating problems such as aching, heaviness, and urinary stress incontinence. Urinary stress incontinence differs from frequent urination in that it is the leakage of urine that may result from coughing, sneezing, lifting, or running. Dribbling can also result from a sudden increase in pelvic floor pressure on weak sphincters. The pelvic floor is a frequently forgotten structure in the prepartum and postpartum client. Benson[5] reports that at least 50% of women suffer from incontinence, and that 20% of all gynecologic surgeries are done to correct this problem. Recommendations for specific exercises are discussed in a later section.

The abdominal mechanism is also important during the prepartum and postpartum periods. This mechanism undergoes a tremendous challenge as the uterus grows and expands with the growing fetus. During and after pregnancy, this mechanism must be evaluated for its strengths and weaknesses and for the presence of a significant diastasis recti. A diastasis recti (a separation of the rectus abdominis muscle belly) occurs as the midline connective tissue attachment (linea alba) in the rectus abdominis stretches and separates. Hormonal changes combined with the growing fetus or increased abdominal pressure thin and widen the linea alba, leading to separation. Diastasis recti can progress to the point that the uterus is only partially covered by peritoneum, fascia, and skin.[6–9] Clinically, this situation can create potential problems with delivery, impair basic functions such as coughing, urination, defecation, and respiration, and affect trunk stability.[10] These effects on trunk stabilization, on support of the growing fetus, and on

delivery warrant consideration of the proper assessment of and recommended exercise for diastasis recti in the aquatic environment.

Of equal importance to the pelvic floor and abdominal mechanism is posture. The scapulothoracic region in the pregnant woman can be affected, causing a thoracic kyphosis and forward head posture.[10] This condition requires special attention to the middle and lower trapezius, thoracic spinal extensors, rhombi, pectoralis muscles, and cervical musculature. Evaluation for thoracic outlet syndrome may also be necessary. The feet and their many supporting ligaments can be affected by hormonal changes. Ligamentous laxity in the foot can be a primary source of pain and can also contribute to low back pain.

Increased lumbar lordosis is often associated with pregnancy. Low back pain that may be associated with increased lordosis is so common in pregnancy (48% to 56% of cases) that many practitioners consider it a normal symptom of being pregnant.[9,11] Onset of low back pain usually occurs in the fourth to sixth month.[9,11] These complaints are usually mechanical in origin. During pregnancy, the uterus expands, reaching the level of the umbilicus by the fifth month. Most of this mass is located anterior to the second sacral vertebra, potentially increasing lordosis. A variety of postural adjustments occur to compensate for the increasing curve and to maintain a postural balance.[12] Table 10-1 sum-

TABLE 10-1. Postural Changes in Pregnancy

Location	Change
Center of gravity	Nonpregnant: at S2 Pregnant: shifts anterior and superior
Feet	Increased pronation and stressed plantar arches
Hips	Increased flexion tends to increase
Knees	Increased extension tends to increase
Lumbar spine	Usually excessive lordosis
Thoracic spine	Kyphotic Rib cage tends to drop Breathing may change
Shoulders	Upper extremities (arms) may internally rotate Anterior chest tightens
Head	Can protrude forward
Gait	Increased base of support: waddling

marizes postural changes occurring during pregnancy at various anatomic locations. Studies have indicated that a correlation may not exist between low back pain and an increased lordosis.[13] Some pregnant women actually have a decreased lumbar lordosis. Other causes of back pain in pregnancy include intervertebral disc involvement, compression of lumbosacral nerve roots, vascular disorders, and transient osteoporosis.[14]

Effect of Physical Changes on Mechanical Loading

When establishing recommendations for appropriate exercise in an aquatic environment for the pregnant woman, the distribution of body mass and the overall loading effect on weight-bearing joints during functional activities must be considered. As the uterus reaches the umbilical level, at approximately 20 weeks' gestation, hip range of motion decreases. This reduction contributes to changes in lower extremity arthrokinematics. One study compared rising from a chair in pregnant versus nonpregnant women. In the pregnant woman, tibiofemoral force increases by 33%, tangential femoral force by 23%, and patellofemoral force by 83%. Quadriceps activity increases by 100%, and hamstring activity by 35%.[15] Using the upper extremities to assist in the sit-to-stand activity results in a reduction of tibiofemoral force by 20%, patellofemoral force by 57%, quadriceps activity by 57%, and hamstring activity by 40%. This illustrates the importance of strengthening both the upper and lower extremities and of educating the pregnant client on proper body mechanics. Examining postural adjustments further allows the therapist to focus on muscles that need strengthening and those that need stretching.

Physiology of Pregnancy and Fetal Development

Physiologically, the pregnant woman undergoes hormonal, cardiovascular, respiratory, nutritional, and thermoregulatory changes. The greatest hormonal effects on the musculoskeletal system are caused by the hormone relaxin. This hormone is present in the serum very early, peaks in the first trimester, and decreases before delivery. The effects of the relaxin, however,

take weeks to dissipate after delivery. As a result, the woman is more prone to injury during ballistic movements. In addition, there is an association between high relaxin levels and pelvic girdle pain, because the sacroiliac joint and symphysis pubis become hypermobile.[3,4,16,17]

Probably the most serious argument against sports and exercise during pregnancy concerns the intensity of the activity. As intensity increases there is an increase in body temperature. The heat produced by exercising muscles during vigorous exercise can rapidly elevate body temperature unless heat transfer to the outer environment occurs promptly. This could result in a rise of the core temperature above 39°C, which could be dangerous for the fetus.[18,19] Because the temperature of the fetus is 0.5°C higher than that of the mother, the fetus relies on the maternal circulatory system to dissipate heat.

Pregnant women can follow several specific guidelines to avoid hyperthermia:

1. Drink excess fluids (hyperhydration)
2. Monitor and maintain usual target heart rate
3. Improve breathing techniques
4. Monitor fetal movement after exercise
5. Avoid exercise when ill[20]

Perceived exertion has been gaining recognition as being easier to monitor and more clearly reflecting an accurate level of exercise intensity.[21] The use of perceived exertion can be helpful to a woman involved in aerobic conditioning in the water. Thermoregulatory cooling occurs at a faster rate in water than on land.[22] By the time the pulse is located, the exercise heart rate may have dropped. Thermoregulation during pregnancy relates to cardiovascular responses. The adequacy of blood flow to the fetoplacental unit is of great concern during aerobic conditioning and complicates understanding the implications of thermoregulation.

Cardiovascular changes occurring at rest in normal pregnancy include an increase of 15 to 20 beats/min in heart rate, at least a 40% increase in blood volume, and a 20% increase in oxygen consumption.[23] Vertical work increases oxygen consumption in direct proportion to the amount of weight that is gained. There are also changes in cardiac output with various positions in pregnancy that affect the treatment prescription and plan.[24]

Although exercise may be safe for low-risk, normal pregnancies, this may not necessarily be true for high-risk, problematic pregnancies.[25,26]

An obstetric client may be considered high risk if there is one or more of the following conditions:

- Premature rupture of the membranes
- Placenta previa or abruptio placentae
- Incompetent cervix
- Hypertension
- Diabetes mellitus
- Multiparity
- Premature labor

The American College of Obstetricians and Gynecologists lists risk factors of and contraindications to vigorous exercise and recommends that high-risk clients be excluded from exercise classes.[27] The scope of this chapter does not include the specialized area of care for high-risk antepartum clients. However, many high-risk, pregnant woman are not restricted to bed but are restricted from impact or high-intensity exercise, and may benefit from a specifically designed exercise program in an aquatic environment. Immersion may have important positive effects on volume disorders, from edema to preeclampsia.[28,29] No studies have established safe aquatic exercise guidelines specifically for high-risk antepartum clients. Indications for and contraindications to the aquatic environment should be established on an individual basis, with emphasis placed on the safety of both mother and fetus.

Physiologic and Anatomic Changes in the Postpartum Client

Dramatic physical changes occur within hours after delivery. Changing hormonal levels help the uterus, cervix, and birth canal to contract, and help establish lactation. Blood volume decreases and metabolic demands change. Specific exercises should begin within 24 hours of delivery and progress at a comfortable pace. Recommended exercises include deep breathing with abdominal wall tightening, pelvic tilting, bridging, modified curls, diagonal curl-ups, leg sliding, and foot and ankle exercises.[9]

A postpartum aquatic program becomes a viable exercise option. The land exercises performed before and after delivery can easily be incorporated into the aquatic environment at the appropriate time. Tears and episiotomies incurred during vaginal deliveries must be healed before initiation of the program. In addition, the

postdelivery discharge called lochia, which usually takes up to 4 weeks to cease, may be a limiting factor for entering the water.

Healing and returning to normal function takes longer after a cesarean section than with a vaginal delivery. A postcesarean section client should wait 6 to 8 weeks before beginning a vigorous exercise program. Initiation of land-based or aquatic exercise should be determined by the obstetrician. Before entering the water, all incision sites should be healed. Noble has outlined exercises for the woman after a cesarean section.[9] When appropriate, these exercises should progress to using the postpartum exercises recommended for a vaginal delivery. The main focus should be restoration of the abdominal wall, and this should be incorporated in all progressive exercises and postural retraining.

The Aquatic Environment and the Obstetric and Gynecologic Client

Hydrostatic pressure is probably the most influential property of water for the pregnant client immersed in the pool. Pascal's law states that fluid pressure is exerted equally at any level in a horizontal (lateral) directional. Based on Pascal's law, immersion exerts fluid pressure on all surfaces when at rest at a given depth.[30–32] This uniform pressure distribution pushes extravascular fluid into the vascular space, resulting in increased plasma volume.[33,34] The central volume increases and moves cephalad.[35] As intravascular volume increases, diuresis and natriuresis increase, with a positive effect on fluid retention problems. Katz and colleagues have shown that a loss of 300 to 400 mL of fluid can occur in a pregnant woman after 20 to 40 minutes of immersion.[36] Equally important with aquatic exercise and the pregnant woman are the assistive, resistive, and supportive properties of buoyancy.

The effect of hydrostatic pressure on the cardiovascular and pulmonary systems is an increase in venous return, increasing stroke volume by approximately 60%[37] and decreasing heart rate and blood pressure.[33,35] Studies of pregnancy, exercise, and immersion have provided initial guidelines for cardiovascular exercise and insight into the amount of weight bearing occurring during static and dynamic activities.[38,39] Studies comparing the effects of

BOX 10-1. General Health History/Information Form

Name _____   Age _____

Address _____   Phone # _____

Emergency Contact _____   Phone # _____

Physician _____   Phone # _____

Weeks Pregnant _____   Due Date _____

Delivery at (Circle one)   Home   Hospital   Birthing Center   Other

Are you exercising currently? If Yes, what type, frequency, duration, for how long?

Did you or have you ever been told you have any of the following:

High Blood Pressure _____   Arthritis   _____   Incompetent Cervix _____

Diabetes   _____   Heart Problems   _____   Varicose Veins   _____

Anemia   _____   Asthma   _____   Dizziness or Fainting _____

Shortness of Breath   _____   Vaginal Bleeding Episodes   _____

Lower Back or Other Joint Pain   _____   Separation of the Abdominal Muscles _____

Previous Pregnancies   _____   Number of Children   _____

Date of Last Pregnancy (Delivery) _____   Vaginal (V) or C-section (C)

Your Goals and Expectation from this Class   _____

Are You Concerned about Your Weight Gain: _____

Do You Currently   Smoke _____   Drink _____   Diet _____

Do you have any other concerns or questions about participating in an exercise class while pregnant?

I have answered the above completely and to the best of my knowledge and understand that all the data provided will be confidential.

Signature _____   Date _____

To Be Completed by the Physical Therapist

Diastasis Recti Present: Yes _____   No _____

Specific Precautions _____

Other Comments: _____

Physical Therapist _____   Date _____

© Integrative Aquatic Therapy™ 1989

BOX 10-2. Prenatal and Postnatal Exercise Referral Form

PRENATAL AND POSTNATAL EXERCISE REFERRAL

Patient Name _____   Date _____

Physician _____   EDD _____

Number of Weeks Pregnant as of Above Date _____

Precautions (Medical) _____

BOX 10-3. Sample Patient Waiver Form

WAIVER FORM

I understand that I am participating in this pre/post partum exercise class on my own, and have been medically released by my physician. I will not hold _____ or the class instructor responsible for any problems that may occur while participating in the class.

Signature   Date

water versus land aerobics demonstrate that the maternal heart rate, blood pressure, core temperature, heat storage, and recovery fetal heart rate are all lower during water exercise.[22,36,40] Urine volume, cardiac output, and end-diastolic volume are higher in water exercise.[28,40] These findings show that exercise while vertically immersed tends to put less strain on the uterine blood flow, reduces edema, and reduces weight bearing on the pelvis and lower extremities.

If an obstetric client requests participation in a community pool program without a referral or guidelines from a medical practitioner, the pool owner/manager or fitness instructor must decide how to guide the client in the aquatic fitness component. The client should have written approval or release from her physician, and should complete a general health screening form (Box 10-1). This form helps identify problems affecting safety and provides a means of communication with a physical therapist if a transition to or from a rehabilitation program is indicated. Two other standard forms (Boxes 10-2 and 10-3) may be needed to incorporate clients safely into an exercise program. This ensures the client understands that the program is not a substitute for the care received from her their medical doctor.

General Safety: Temperature and Equipment

Safety also plays an important role in aquatic rehabilitation and fitness training of the obstetric client. General facility safety concerns include pool and room temperature, humidity, pool chemicals used, and emergency rescue. General facility safety is discussed elsewhere in this book (see Chaps. 18 and 19), but pool temperature and the temperature humidity index are particu-

larly important for the obstetric client. Ventilation must allow for comfortable oxygen exchange.

Immersion in different water temperatures leads to various physiologic changes. Consequently, the goals of the exercise program determine the selection of water temperature. For the pregnant client, water temperatures below 25°C may be uncomfortable; temperatures over 34°C may cause excessive fatigue or nausea. For a more consistently moving exercise class, the ideal water temperature for the pregnant client is between 26°C to 30°C. For slower, therapeutic, one-on-one treatment, a temperature of 30°C to 32°C is more comfortable. Cool water dissipates body heat 25% faster than air. When immersed, a woman's core temperature does not rise as quickly in water as on land, depending on the water temperature, the air temperature, and the temperature–humidity index.

Katz and colleagues[41] found that immersed exercise for pregnant women in 30°C water for 20 minutes at 70% maximum oxygen consumption leads to significant physiologic effects on both the fetus and mother, compared with land exercises. These findings support the belief that there are potential hazards of maternal exercise to the fetus. These hazards include an increase in maternal temperature and a decrease in uterine blood flow due to decreased plasma volume and shunting of blood to exercising muscles. Katz and colleagues' study seems to support the need for close professional supervision to make the aquatic environment safe and beneficial for the pregnant woman.

There has been some question concerning the effects of various pool chemicals on the pregnant client. Because health regulations vary from state to state, the reader is advised to check with his or her local health department and request specific information on regulation of pool chemicals.

Safety for the obstetric client also involves using the appropriate aquatic equipment. Restrictive flotation equipment around the abdomen or chest should be avoided. Other flotation devices should be chosen with the idea in mind that the client can don or doff them easily and change positions in the water without excessive strain.

Physical Examination

Many of the evaluation procedures used for the nonpregnant woman are also applicable to the pregnant client. It is important to revisit and

BOX 10-4. Physical Therapy Musculoskeletal Examination

Patient Name _____   Date _____

Expected Date of Delivery/Date Delivered _____

Diagnosis or Reason for Referral _____

HISTORY: Include questions related to illness or disease of pregnancy
- Pre/postnatal complications
- Chronologic history or problem related to the current symptoms
- Questions regarding past pregnancies and deliveries
- Symptoms related to fever, urinary frequency, urgency, nausea and vomiting
- Prenatal problems: premature uterine contractions, episodic bleeding, incompetent cervix, urinary stress incontinence
- Postnatal: type of delivery, specific procedures or equipment used, episiotomy or C-section, and current stage of wound healing
- Current medications
- Current functional limitations or activities that are limited by problem

OBJECTIVE: Include areas of static and dynamic posture, active and passive mobility, tissue integrity and/or tenderness, muscle strength, and movements that provoke symptoms. Focus area for pregnancy (in addition to other objective tests that are normally done):

A. Upper Quadrant: presence of thoracic outlet syndrome
B. Lumbar Spine and Pelvis:
  1. Standing
    - Where is weight being carried?
    - Mobility of the ilium on the sacrum
    - Gait: are there signs of instability or muscle weakness?
  2. Sitting
    - Posture
  3. Supine
    - Testing periods in the second and third trimester should be broken up
    - Additional hip and sacroiliac joint provocation tests: fixation tests, Derbolowski test, ventral and dorsal gapping tests
  4. Prone: Normally not used after the first trimester
  5. Hands–Knees: A useful position for testing hip extensors and spinal flexion and extension in later stages of pregnancy

highlight areas that specifically affect how, when, and where the obstetric client is treated. Box 10-4 highlights focal points for a physical therapy examination of the obstetric client. The upper quadrant should be carefully examined using specific tests to screen for potential thoracic outlet syndrome.[42] This syndrome involves compromise of the brachial plexus, subclavian artery, and occasionally the subclavian vein. Frequently involved areas of this entrapment syndrome include the anterior and medial scalene muscles, the first rib, and the attachment area of the pectoralis minor muscle and the cora-

coid process. The forward head position, increased thoracic kyphosis, first rib elevation, and internal rotation of the humerus associated with pregnancy may lead to thoracic outlet syndrome. As pregnancy progresses, the increased weight of the breasts and abnormal costal patterns for respiration may also contribute to development of the syndrome.

In the pelvic girdle, mobility increases by two and one half times and the gap in the symphysis pubis at 9 months' gestation is approximately 9 mm. Too much softening of the symphysis pubis can lead to symptomatic rupture. When evaluating the gait of the pregnant client, it may be important to differentiate between normal pregnant gait and a significant problem with the symphysis pubis. A waddling or shuffling gait, a disorientation of the acetabulum resulting in external rotation of the lower extremities, a reduction of heel strike and swing phase, and pain at the symphysis pubis, sacroiliac joints, or adductor muscles are all clinical signs of rupture. Pain can also occur with contraction of the rectus abdominis muscle. Spasm can occur in the adductors and hamstrings, rendering the client unable to roll over.

Of interest in postpartum women is the continued effect of pregnancy on the internal organs and the pelvic floor. After delivery, women usually experience soreness resulting from stitches, bruising, and swelling. If care of the pelvic floor is not initiated and weakness is not resolved, prolapse, a dropping down or bulging of the uterus into the vagina, could result, affecting the bladder, urethra, uterus, and rectum. This increased pressure leads to either excessive laxity or pain in the muscles of the pelvic floor. The reader is directed to specialized texts for a more thorough knowledge base with regard to evaluation techniques.[42,43]

Testing and Recommendations for Diastasis Recti

A diastasis recti can be classified into three categories (Table 10-2). This classification allows the practitioner to determine how the abdominal wall is functioning and how it should be screened and tested periodically throughout the pregnancy. The therapist can easily teach the testing procedure to the pregnant woman. According to Noble's criteria, a measurement of two fingers or less is considered normal, and a measurement greater than two fingers is considered suggestive of a diastasis recti.[9] Although there is some disagreement as to the location of

testing along the linea alba, it is important to be consistent when reevaluating the client.[6,7,44] Testing procedures are as follows:

1. The client is supine with knees bent and arms stretched out at her side.
2. The client is instructed to raise her head and shoulders off the table until the spines of the scapulae leave the table.
3. Once in this position, the therapist measures for a diastasis by placing his or her fingers horizontally across the linea alba and determining how many fingers fit into the space between the borders of the two recti bellies.

The incidence of diastasis recti in postpartum women is high, and in many cases it does not resolve on its own. Noble describes specific exercises for this problem for both prepartum and postpartum clients.[9] Kendall and McCreary state that the use of supportive measures to reestablish and control normal alignments until the weakened muscles are strengthened is important when the weakness is associated with overstretching.[10] Both recommendations may need to be considered when creating an exercise or treatment program for the client in the water.

The Importance of Integrating Land and Aquatic Treatment

Before initiating an aquatic program, it is important to evaluate the client on land first, and orient her to the aquatic treatment program. Initiating specific exercise instructions on land allows for the stability needed to promote the initial stages of learning and to stimulate both proprioceptive and kinesiologic awareness. It also helps encourage carry-over for a home exercise program, where a pool may not be available. Unless the client cannot tolerate a land-based component, there should be continuous integration of land and aquatic treatment.

TABLE 10-2. Diastasis Recti: Classifying a Separation

Incomplete Separation	Incomplete, Complete Separation	Complete Separation
Fibers of the linea alba are attenuated or separated but not severed	Complete separation and division of linea alba from symphysis pubis to umbilicus. The fibers above the umbilicus are normal or only slightly separated	Complete separation of the linea alba from xyphoid cartilage to the symphysis pubis. The abdominal viscera are covered only by skin and peritoneum

Aquatic Applications

Therapeutic exercise for the prepartum and postpartum client can be performed in various positions, depending on the clinician's goals for treatment, medical precautions, stage of pregnancy, and the client's psychological responsiveness to the environment. In this section, activities and exercises that may be useful for various musculoskeletal problems are described by position, including suspended, supine reclined, supine, half-kneeling (cube), and standing-supported by the pool wall. With the problem identified and a thorough understanding of hydrodynamic effects on pregnant women, the clinician can then select a treatment program with both established goals and appropriate exercises and positions.

Suspended

In the suspended position, the client is non-weight bearing in a vertical orientation with the head out of the water. Flotation belts can be used early in the pregnancy or postpartum, if comfortable, although care should be taken not to push the client into trunk flexion. As the fetus grows, a more appropriate flotation location would be around the upper arms. The advantage to this placement is both safety and comfort, allowing increased freedom of movement to the trunk, pelvis, and lower extremities. The following are examples of suggested exercises in the suspended position.

Abdominal Mechanism

An exercise called the "chair sit abdominal" uses the assistive property of buoyancy. With flotation cuffs around the arms and a buoy in each hand, the client brings her lower extremities to 90 degrees of hip flexion and comfortable knee flexion to allow adequate balance (Fig. 10-1*A*). The client is instructed to contract the lower portion of the abdominal mechanism by pulling while exhaling and allowing the flexed lower extremities to pull up slightly. The release that occurs with inhalation is only a barely perceptible movement of the lower extremities downward (see Fig. 10-1*B*).

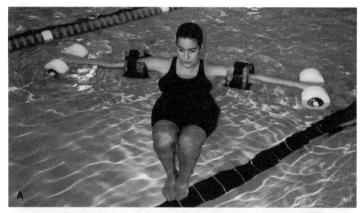

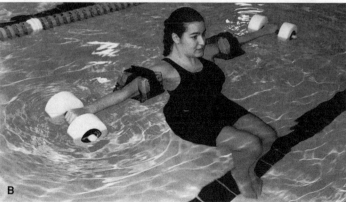

FIGURE 10-1. Chair sit abdominal; (*A*) front view; (*B*) side view.

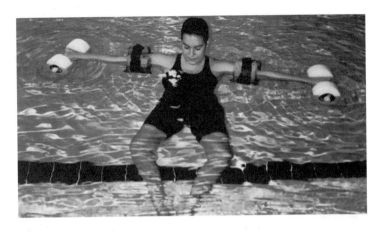

FIGURE 10-2. Pelvic floor exercise.

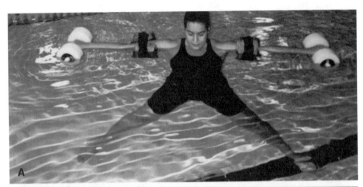

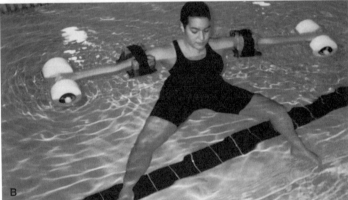

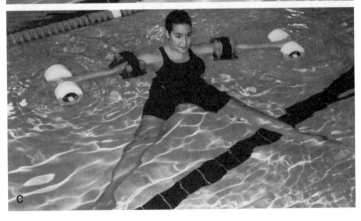

FIGURE 10-3. Adductor stretching: (*A*) hips neutral; (*B*) hips in flexion, stretching for one joint; (*C*) hips in flexion, stretching for two joints.

Pelvic Floor Exercises

In the same starting position as for the previous exercise, the client abducts and externally rotates the lower extremities, putting her feet together (Fig. 10-2). The pelvic floor exercises described by Noble can be performed in this position.[9] A slow contracting and holding of the pelvic floor for 5 (3) seconds is followed by a slow release. No more than five (three) repetitions are necessary at any one session to avoid fatigue of the pelvic floor.

Adductor Stretching

This stretch can be done for both the one- and two-joint hip adductor muscles. In the suspended position this can be done with hip flexion or hip extension. If done with the hips in neutral, hip adductors stretch across two joints and are buoyancy assisted (Fig. 10-3A). If done in hip flexion, adductor stretching is active and supported and can be done for both one-joint (see Fig. 10-3B) and two-joint (see Fig. 10-3C) adductor muscles. This also stretches the medial hamstring muscles, the semimembranosus, and the semitendinosus. The client should be instructed to keep the patellas and the feet perpendicular to the water surface, and the ankles dorsiflexed.

Suspended Cross-Country Stretch

This supported stretch offers simultaneous stretch to the quadriceps and hamstrings on the opposite lower extremities. While maintaining

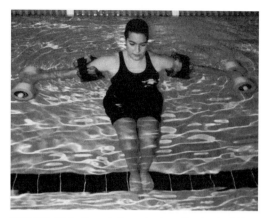

FIGURE 10-5. Scapulothoracic strengthening/stabilization.

the vertical position, one leg is brought forward (hip flexion) and the other brought back (hip extension). Slight flexion of the knees supports and encourages the stretch and assists in maintaining proper balance (Fig. 10-4). The trunk should be suspended vertically between the lower extremities. This position of the trunk should be maintained with abdominal mechanism contraction if the goal is to have the client focus on lower extremity strengthening using a reciprocal movement. This exercise can accomplish both strengthening and stretching.

Scapulothoracic Strengthening/ Stabilization

This postural and trunk stabilization exercise activates the scapular depressors and retractors. With the upper extremities at 90 degrees of shoulder abduction and neutral rotation (palms down), the client is instructed to push down about 1 inch into the water, activating the shoulder adductors and scapula depressors. The client is cued gently and simultaneously to squeeze the scapulae together to make the retractors active. A slow release back to the water surface also requires eccentric work by the muscles (Fig. 10-5). Holding buoys increases the resistance. This can also be done with the upper extremities in either external or internal rotation.

Lateral Trunk Flexor Stretch

The pendulum stretch is aimed primarily at stretching the lateral trunk flexors and the latissimus dorsi. This movement is initiated by pulling both lower extremities toward the ribs and then

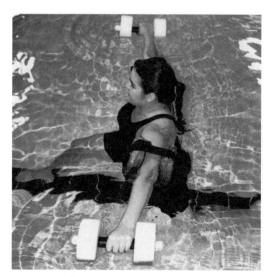

FIGURE 10-4. Suspended cross country stretch.

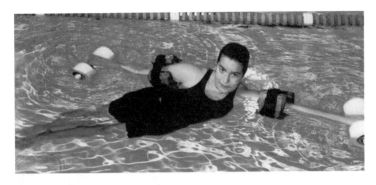

FIGURE 10-6. Lateral trunk flexor stretch.

pushing them simultaneously out to the side at approximately a 45-degree angle (Fig. 10-6).

Supine Reclined

This is a suspended position midway between vertical and horizontal. The midway point is determined by the client's comfort and the goals of the exercise chosen. If the true goal is the semireclined position, the head, upper extremities, and chest are at the surface edge and the trunk and lower extremities are deep. The equipment placement is similar to that with suspended vertical. The flotation devices should be around the upper body. Flotation pieces with less buoyancy can be used around the lower extremities of clients who tend to sink. This position affords a sense of relaxation and resistive work to the abdominal muscles.

Mini Crunch: Crossed Arm Protection

The abdominal mechanism can be activated against resistance in this position. This modification of the mini crunch requires splinting of the abdominal mechanism by crossing the upper extremities over the abdominals. This becomes necessary with a diastasis recti separation greater than two fingerwidths. To perform this exercise, flotation equipment may be needed under the knees and behind the head. A flotation board may also be needed under the pelvis for stability. The client should cross her hands over the abdominal area to support the two muscle bellies as contraction occurs with trunk flexion (Fig. 10-7). The client should exhale with abdominal contraction, and inhale on release.

Mini Crunch

If the client has been cleared to strengthen the abdominal muscles without arm protection, the beginning position is semireclined with hips and knees flexed (Figure 10-8A). The upper extremities are then extended toward the feet (see Fig. 10-8B). The cues to achieve the desired motion could be "push your waist down while your chest moves toward your thighs" (see Fig. 10-8C). This movement brings the trunk and extended arms longitudinally toward the feet. The release is back to the starting position (see Fig. 10-8A). Proper cueing not to flex or to extend the hips and knees toward the trunk, but to keep them stationary, is critical for exercise accuracy.

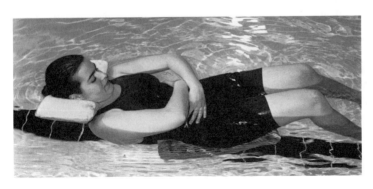

FIGURE 10-7. Mini crunch with crossed arm protection.

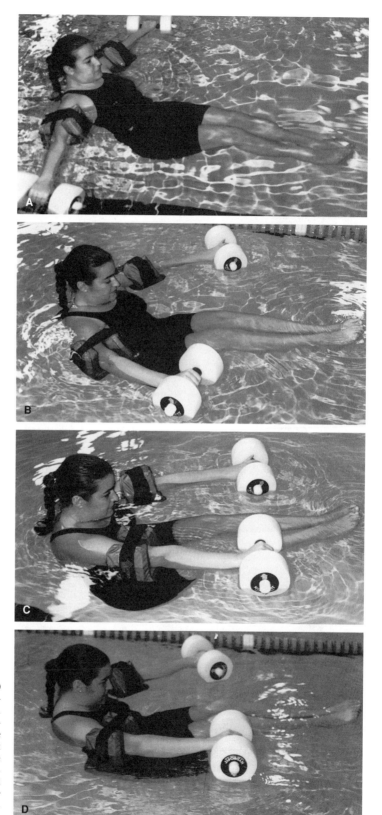

FIGURE 10-8. Mini crunch. (**A**) The beginning position is semireclined with hips and knees flexed. (**B**) The upper extremeties are extended toward the feet. (**C**) The client "pushes down" on her waist while moving her chest toward the thighs, bringing the trunk and extended arms longitudinally toward the feet. (**D**) A board placed under the pelvis before pushing downward creates additional resistance.

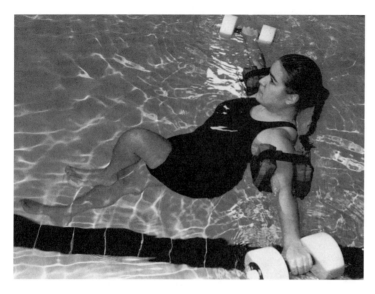

FIGURE 10-9. Alternate leg press.

Additional resistance can be added by placing a board under the pelvis before pushing downward (see Fig. 10-8*D*).

Alternate Leg Press

This exercise strengthens the thighs, hips, and abdominal mechanism. The upper body is supported comfortably with flotation equipment located at the arms and in the hands. In the semireclined position, both lower extremities should be flexed acutely at the hips. The movement involves alternatively extending and flexing the lower extremities with the heels below the water surface (Fig. 10-9). Buoyancy creates increased

resistance into extension and assistance into hip and knee flexion. Resistance can be provided by increasing the speed.

Bilateral Frog-Leg Press

The support position of the upper body is the same as in the alternate leg press. The starting position is knees flexed and hips flexed, abducted, and externally rotated with the feet together (Fig. 10-10*A*). As the dorsiflexed ankles push down through the surface of the water, the lower extremities adduct and extend (see Fig. 10-10*B*). The client should inhale and exhale with each cycle of movement.

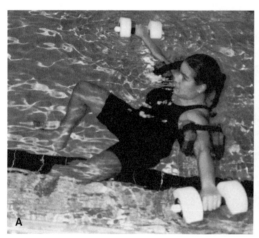
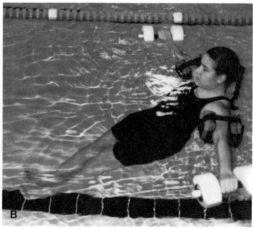

FIGURE 10-10. Bilateral frog-leg press. (*A*) The starting position is knees flexed and hips flexed, abducted, and externally rotated, with the feet held together. (*B*) The lower extremities adduct and extend as the dorsiflexed ankles push down.

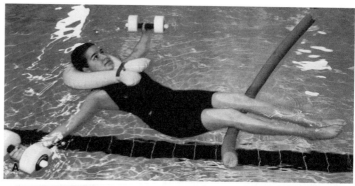

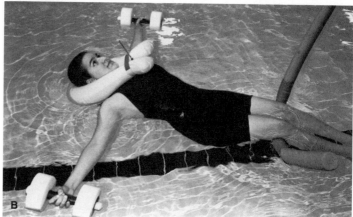

FIGURE 10-11. Scapular retraction. (*A*) The upper extremities are positioned at 90° of shoulder abduction. (*B*) The extended arms push down about 1 inch into the water followed by a slow release.

Supine

Supine, lying horizontally, is another non-weight-bearing supportive position. Most pregnant women float easily on their backs, but additional support may be needed around the neck, upper extremities, trunk, or lower extremities to maintain this position during the exercise.

Scapular Retraction

The supine position provides resistance to the scapular retractors and can also activate the thoracic spine extensors. The upper extremities are positioned at 90 degrees of shoulder abduction and in external or internal rotation, depending on the exercise goals (Fig. 10-11*A*). The extended arms are then pushed down about 1 inch into the water (see Fig. 10-11*B*). The release is slow and controlled. The longer the lever arm and the more distally the equipment is placed, the more resistance is produced.

Angel Wings

This exercise requires full range of glenohumeral joint motion. The feet can be hooked on a ladder or on the pool edge to prevent additional movement during exercise. The exercise begins with the upper extremities at the side, just below the water surface (Fig. 10-12*A*). The upper extremities are actively moved through full abduction range (see Fig. 10-12*B*), to the overhead position (see Fig. 10-12*C*), then adducted to return to the starting position. The upper extremities are to remain on the water's surface. This exercise should also incorporate breathing techniques, with inhalation during abduction and exhalation during adduction; this facilitates expansion of the chest wall.

Bridging

Bridging is used to strengthen the thighs, the buttocks, and the anterior and posterior trunk. The upper body should be comfortably supported with a neck collar. Equipment with mini-

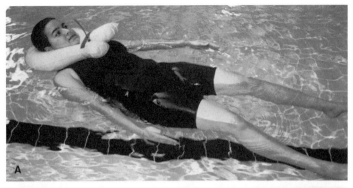

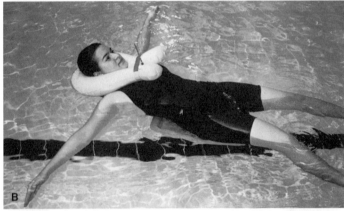

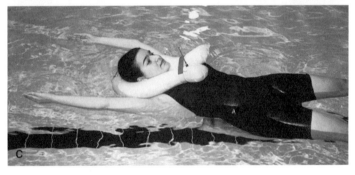

FIGURE 10-12. Angel wings. To begin, the upper extremities are held to the side, just below the water surface (*A*). The upper extremities are actively moved through full abduction range (*B*), to the overhead position (*C*).

mal flotation effects should be placed under the knees to provide additional sensory input and support during the exercise (Fig. 10-13*A*). The exercise begins with dorsiflexion of the ankles, contraction of the abdominal mechanism, and submergence of the feet about 1 inch below the water level (see Fig. 10-13*B*). This simultaneously activates the gluteus maximus, the erector spinae, the hamstrings, and the abdominal mechanism. For exercise accuracy, it is important to keep this motion small. The exercise should include coordinated breathing—exhalation with the contraction and inhalation with the retraction. After learning the proper technique,

pelvic floor exercises can be used in conjunction with this exercise.

Cube/Half-Kneel Standing

The cube position is a position of stability and can be used to accomplish several treatment goals. In a shallow pool, allowing submersion up to the level of C7, the therapist assumes a half-kneeling position. The client is positioned seated on the therapist's knee. Without assistance, the buoyant pregnant woman tends to float into vertical. The therapist can perform manual assistance and

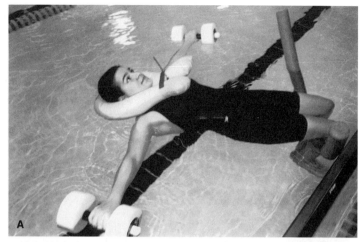

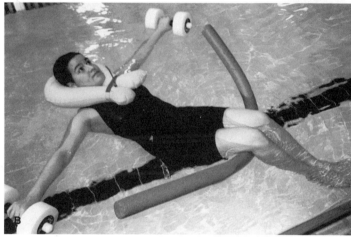

FIGURE 10-13. Bridging. (*A*) The upper body should be comfortably supported with a neck collar, and a minimal flotation device is placed under the knees for additional support and sensory input. (*B*) The ankles are dorsiflexed, the abdominal mechanism is contracted, and the feet gently push down about 1 inch into the water.

cueing through proper hand placement on the client's iliac crest (Fig. 10-14). This is an excellent position for activating and isolating the anterior and posterior chest/postural muscles. Depending on the treatment goals for the client, these exercises can also be done with the client in the half-kneeling position.

The Front/Back Chest Press

This exercise uses the upper extremities to challenge the postural muscles of the trunk. In the half-kneel position, the upper extremities are brought to 90 degrees of abduction with the elbows fully extended so that they are supported by the water. Anterior thoracic/chest musculature is activated as the upper extremities are pulled into horizontal adduction, performed with the shoulders externally rotated (Fig. 10-15*A*). The second phase involves internally

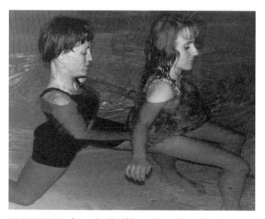

FIGURE 10-14. Cube/half kneel standing. The therapist assists through proper hand placement on the client's iliac crest.

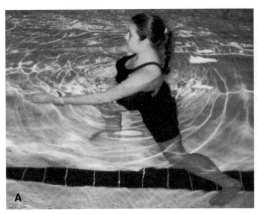
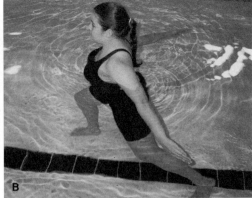

FIGURE 10-15. Front/back chest press. (*A*) In the half-kneel position, the upper extremities are brought to 90° of abduction with the elbows fully extended. The upper extremities are then pulled into horizontal adduction with the shoulders externally rotated. (*B*) The shoulders are internally rotated while moving into horizontal abduction.

rotating the shoulders while moving into horizontal abduction, emphasizing scapulothoracic musculature (see Fig. 10-15*B*). While performing this movement, simultaneous trunk stabilization occurs (see Fig. 10-15*A*). The speed and range of movement affect the degree of resistance, and equipment, such as a hand mitt or paddle, can provide additional resistance.

Bent Elbow Press-Back

This position is the same as in the previous exercise except that the elbows are brought into 90 degrees of flexion. As the elbows are pushed backward, the scapulae are retracted and the rib cage elevated (Fig. 10-16*A*). The pushing movement stretches the pectoralis and serratus anterior (see Fig. 10-16*B*). The release from this position occurs as the upper extremities move forward. The client should be encouraged to inhale as the upper extremities are pushed back and exhale as they come forward.

Shoulder Abduction–Adduction

The cube position can be used to activate the shoulder adductors and abductors. Begin with the shoulders abducted to 90 degrees, neutral to rotation, with elbows in full extension. The client pushes her arms down to her sides and back up. Buoyancy provides resistance to adduction and assistance to abduction. To increase

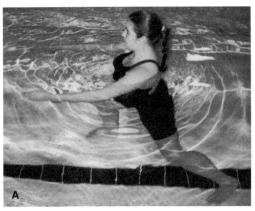
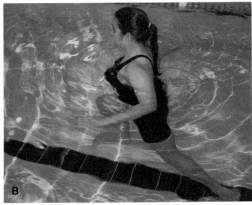

FIGURE 10-16. Bent elbow press-back. (*A*) This exercise is the same as the front/back chest press, except that the elbows are brought into 90° of flexion. (*B*) As the elbows are pushed backward, the scapulae are retracted and the rib cage elevated.

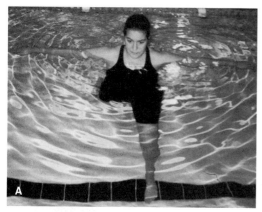
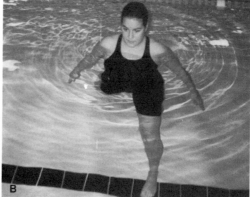

FIGURE 10-17. Shoulder abduction/adduction. (*A*) Beginning position is with shoulders abducted to 90°, neutral to rotation, with elbows in full extension. (*B*) The arms are pushed down to the sides of the thighs and controlled as they slowly return to the beginning position.

resistance to both muscle groups, increase the speed of movement (Fig. 10-17).

Protective Abdominal Contraction

This position can be used to teach the client how to splint (protect) the abdominals in a reversed curve position that initially provides more stability than the supine position. The hands are crossed over the abdomen. An eccentric contraction of the rectus abdominis is elicited as the client attempts to maintain trunk stability while moving into lumbar extension in the half-kneeling position (Fig. 10-18). The therapist usually needs to provide support for balance and stability at the iliac crests.

Standing by Pool Wall

Optimally, the client should be submerged to chest level. This position is effective for stretching the gastrocnemius–soleus and hamstring muscles, the hip adductors, and the ankles and feet.

Calf Stretch

This stretch can be done by facing the wall of the pool with both hands on the pool ledge. The leg to be stretched is placed forward with the ball of the foot on the wall and the heel on the floor. The knee should be straight but not hyperextended. The client is then cued to pull the

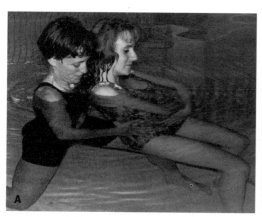
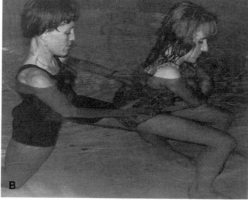

FIGURE 10-18. Protective abdominal contraction. (*A*) The client crosses her hands over the abdomen, with the therapist in half-kneeling, providing support at the iliac crest. (*B*) An eccentric contraction of the rectus abdominis is elicited as the client attempts to maintain trunk stability while moving into lumbar extension.

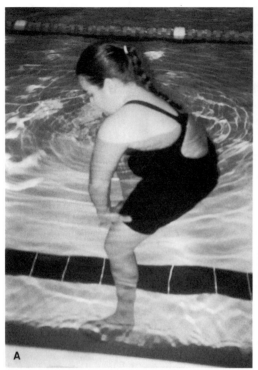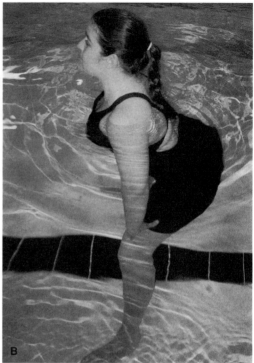

FIGURE 10-19. Standing pelvic rock. (*A*) The hands are placed on the thighs with the upper body perpendicular to the floor and the hips in slight flexion. The movement starts with a posterior pelvic tilt, then thoracic flexion, and finally cervical flexion. (*B*) The reverse motion consists of an anterior pelvic tilt, thoracic extension, and cervical extension.

body into the wall, keeping the pelvis facing the wall. This stretches the calf. The client may allow the back leg to float off the floor. With the knee flexed, this stretch isolates the soleus.

Resistive Squat

While holding onto the side of the pool, the client squats with legs abducted, maintaining a straight back. This exercise should be done slowly and rhythmically, incorporating proper breathing technique.

Bend, Lift, Straighten, and Drop

This exercise can be done first on two legs, then on one at a time, if desired. Facing the wall, the client performs the following sequence:

1. Bend both knees with feet flat
2. Lift heels off the floor
3. Straighten the knees
4. Lower heels to the floor

Standing Pelvic Rock

This closed-chain exercise allows the client to activate both the spinal and the abdominal musculature, and to mobilize the hips. The exercise begins in a standing position similar to the squat position. The hands are placed on the thighs with the upper body perpendicular to the floor and the hips positioned in slight flexion. The movement occurs sequentially, starting with a posterior pelvic tilt, then thoracic flexion, and finally cervical flexion (Fig. 10-19*A*). The reverse of this motion occurs with an anterior pelvic tilt, thoracic extension, and cervical spine extension (see Fig. 10-19*B*).

Swim Stroke Recommendations

Although swim stroke analysis is addressed in a separate chapter (see Chap. 14), it is important to address some aspects of stroke techniques relevant to the pregnant clients, whether therapeutic or recreational. A swimming program must fit the needs of the client and should follow these general guidelines[44]:

- Keep workouts moderate in intensity
- Keep water temperature between 80° and 83°F
- Never swim alone
- Make sure there is room to swim
- Monitor body response (how do you feel during and after the swim?)
- Swim only with a doctor's approval

With advancing pregnancy, the body's specific gravity changes and the woman becomes more buoyant, losing stability. Initially, movements should be slow and small to permit establishing and maintaining good body mechanics.

Crawl

Caution should be taken to avoid excessive kicking and splashing, which accelerate fatigue and increase rotation of the lower back. The recommended turn is the open turn and not the conventional flip turn.

Breast Stroke

This is an easy and relaxing stroke using a long glide, and is particularly recommended during the third trimester. The frog kick helps strengthen the adductor muscles. Emphasis can be directed to the upper body by increasing the parabolic arm motion. To compensate for the added buoyancy during pregnancy, the knees can be dropped down before extension to avoid breaking the water surface. Inhalation can take place during the arm pull as the shoulder widens, and exhalation as the face submerges and the upper extremities extend to the glide position.

Back Stroke

Many different arm motions can be used in the back stroke. The elementary back stroke and the inverted back stroke may be the easiest for the pregnant client. These variations call for simultaneous movement of both arms underwater. This stroke allows for easier breathing because the face remains above water. This stroke is also advantageous for correcting postural faults. If the single-arm stroke variation is used, hip swaying can be avoided by rotating the body toward the pulling arm. Rapid chest breathing (used in active labor) and transitional breathing can be incorporated with the arm movements.

Side Stroke

This stroke is excellent for all stages of pregnancy. It is of somewhat lower intensity and may be more comfortable than others in the later stages of pregnancy. This stroke position encourages practice of the cleansing breath used in labor. Exhalation begins while the lower extremities are tucked, and full exhalation takes place during the glide. A long glide after push-off enhances lateral trunk stretching.

Summary

The health care practitioner should think of rehabilitation for the obstetric client as taking place along a continuum from the initial stages of conception through postpartum. Exercise after delivery is just as important as exercise during pregnancy. Treatment in the aquatic environment can minimize some of the adverse effects of exercise associated with land programs.

In addition, health practitioners must recognize that the fitness community provide an important extension of care for the obstetric lient, continuing the emphasis on wellness and creating connections to community resources. The health care practitioner is challenged to establish a proactive approach in the evaluation and care of the obstetric client and integrate the aquatic environment into both rehabilitation and health maintenance in this population.

REFERENCES

1. Mittlemark RA, Gardin SK. Historical perspectives. In: Mittlemark RA, Wisewell RA, Drinkwater BL, eds. *Exercise in Pregnancy.* 2nd ed. Baltimore, Md: Williams & Wilkins; 1991:1–6.
2. Naeye RL, Peters EC. Working during pregnancy. *Pediatrics.* 1982;69;724–727.
3. Calguneri M, Bird HA, Wright V. Changes in joint laxity occurring during pregnancy. *Ann Rheum Dis.* 1982;41:126–128.
4. MacLennan AH, Nicols R, Green RC, et al. Serum relaxin and pelvic pain of pregnancy. *Lancet* 1986: 243–244.
5. Benson RC, ed. *Handbook of Obstetrics and Gynecology.* 8th ed. Los Altos, Calif: Lang Medical Publishers; 1983.
6. Boissonnault JS, Blaschak MJ. Incidence of diastasis recti abdominis during the childbearing year. *Phys Ther.* 1988;68:1082–1086.
7. Katorinos RK. Diastasis recti and review of the ab-

dominal wall. *Journal of Obstetric/Gynecologic Physical Therapy.* 1990;14(4):8–10.

8. Dunbar A. Restoration of the abdominal wall. *Journal of Obstetric/Gynecologic Physical Therapy.* 1990; 15(1):4–5.

9. Noble E, ed. *Essential Exercises for the Childbearing Year.* 3rd ed. Boston, Mass: Houghton Mifflin Co; 1988.

10. Kendall FP, McCreary EK (ed): *Muscles, testing & function,* 3rd ed. Baltimore MD: Williams & Wilkins, 1983.

11. Fast A, Shapiro D, Ducommun EJ, et al. Low back pain in pregnancy. *Spine.* 1987;12:368–371.

12. Berg G, Mammar M, Nielson JM, et al. Low back pain during pregnancy. *Obstet Gynecol.* 1988;71:71–75.

13. Magee DJ. *Orthopedic Physical Assessment.* 1st ed. Philadelphia, Pa: WB Saunders; 1987.

14. Bullock JE, Jull GA, Bullock MI. The relationship of LBP to postural changes during pregnancy. *Australian Journal of Physiotherapy.* 1987;33:10–17.

15. McNitt-Gray JL. Biomechanics related to exercise in pregnancy. In: Mittlemark RA, Wisewell RA, Drinkwater BL, eds. *Exercise in Pregnancy.* 2nd ed. Baltimore, Md: Williams & Wilkins; 1991:133–140.

16. Kubitz RL, Goodin RC. Symptomatic separation of the pubic symphysis. *South Med J.* 1986;79:578–580.

17. O'Connor L. The female pelvis. *Journal of Obstetric/Gynecologic Physical Therapy.* 1986;10:6–7.

18. Edwards MJ. Hyperthermia as a teratogen. *Teratog Carcinog Mutagen.* 1986;6:563–582.

19. Shiota K. Neural tube defects and maternal hyperthermia in early pregnancy: epidemiology in a human embryonic population. *Am J Med Genet.* 1982;12:281–288.

20. Drinkwater BL, Mittlemark RA. Heat, stress and pregnancy. In: Mittlemark RA, Wisewell RA, Drinkwater BL, eds. *Exercise in Pregnancy.* 2nd ed. Baltimore, Md: Williams & Wilkins; 1991:261–268.

21. White J. Exercising for two. *Physician and Sports Medicine* 1992;20:179–186.

22. Katz VL, McMurray R, Goodwin WE, et al. Non-weightbearing exercise during pregnancy on land and during immersion: a comparative study. *Am J Perinatol.* 1990;7:281–284.

23. Romem Y, Masaki DI, Mittlemark RA. Physiological and endocrine adjustments to pregnancy. In: Mittlemark RA, Wisewell RA, Drinkwater BL, eds. *Exercise in Pregnancy.* 2nd ed. Baltimore, Md: Williams & Wilkins; 1991:9–11.

24. Vorys N, Villery JC, Hamusek GE. The cardiac output changes in various postures in pregnancy. *Am J Obstet Gynecol.* 1961;82:1312–1321.

25. Campbell S, Griffin DR, Pearce JM, et al. New Doppler technique for assessing uteroplacental blood flow. *Lancet 2.* 1983:675–677.

26. Rauramo I, Forss M. Effect of exercise on placental blood flow in pregnancies complicated by hyperten-

sion, diabetes or intrahepatic cholestasis. *Acta Obstet Gynecol Scand.* 1986;67:15–20.

27. American College of Obstetricians and Gynecologists [ACOG]. *Exercise During Pregnancy and Postpartum Period.* ACOG Technical Bulletin No. 189. Washington, DC: ACOG; 1994.

28. Goodlin RC, Hoffman KL, Williams NE. Shoulder out of immersion in pregnant women. *J Perinat Med.* 1984;12:173–177.

29. Sibley L, Ruhling RO, Cameron-Foster J, et al. Swimming and physical fitness during pregnancy. *J Nurse Midwifery.* 1981;26:3.

30. Epstein M. Renal, endocrine and hemodynamic effects of water immersion in man. *Contrib Nephrol.* 1984;41:174–188.

31. Epstein M, Miller M, Schneider N. Depth of immersion as a determinant of the natriuresis of water immersion. *Proc Soc Exp Biol Med.* 1974;146:562–566.

32. Sheldahl LM, Wann LS, Clifford PS. Effect of central hypervolemia on cardiac performance during exercise. *Am J Physiol.* 1984;57:1662–1667.

33. Arborellius M, Balldin UI, Lilja B, Lindgren CEG. Hemodynamic changes in man during immersion with head above water. *Aerospace Medicine.* 1972;43: 592–598.

34. Behn C, Gauer OH, Kirsch, Eckert P. Effects of sustained intrathoracic vascular distention on body fluid distribution and renal excretion in man. *Pflugers Arch.* 1969;313:123–135.18

35. Greenleaf JE. Physiology of fluid and electrolyte responses during inactivity, water immersion and bed rest. *Med Sci Sports Exerc.* 1984;16:20–25.

36. Katz VL, McMurray RG, Berry MJ, et al. Fetal and uterine responses to immersion and exercise. *Obstet Gynecol.* 1988;72:225.

37. Westin CEM, O'Hare JP, Evans JM, et al. Hemodynamic changes in man during immersion in water at different temperatures. *Clin Sci.* 1987;73:613–616.

38. Harrison RA, Hillman M, Bulstrode S. Loading of the lower limb when walking partially immersed: implications for clinical practice. *Physiotherapy.* 1992;78: 164–167.

39. Harrison RA, Bulstrode S. Percentage weight bearing during partial immersion in the hydrotherapy pool. *Physiotherapy Practice.* 1987;3:60–63.

40. McMurray RG, Katz VL, Berry MJ, et al. Cardiovascular responses of pregnant women during aerobic exercise in water: longitudinal study. *Int J Sports Med.* 1988;9:443–447.

41. Katz VL, McMurray, Cefalo RC. Aquatic exercise during pregnancy. In: Mittlemark RA, Wisewell RA, Drinkwater BL, eds. *Exercise in Pregnancy.* 2nd ed. Baltimore, Md: Williams & Wilkins; 1991:271–277.

42. Wilder E, ed. *Obstetric and Gynecologic Physical Therapy.* New York, NY: Churchill-Livingstone; 1990.

43. O'Connor LJ, Gourley RJ. *Obstetric and Gynecologic Care in Physical Therapy.* Thorofare, NJ: Slack, Inc; 1990.

44. Katz J, ed. *Swimming Your Way Through Pregnancy.* New York, NY: Doubleday & Co., Inc; 1983.

11

Aquatic Rehabilitation of Clients With Rheumatic Disease

Roxane McNeal

The universality of rheumatic diseases, which affect all ages, has resulted in the formation of many foundations and support groups. These in turn have established many exercise programs, including aquatic programs, designed to provide physical, psychological, and social support for people suffering from these diseases. In general, these aquatic programs have provided needed incentives to millions of people who otherwise may never have become involved in any exercise program. The social benefits of such programs should not be underestimated.

Health care professionals, without denigrating the efficacy of the established programs, have devised variable procedures to accommodate individual needs. These programs and guidelines are designed to modify structured routines to the particular needs of the individual.

With a rigidly structured routine, it is assumed that all individuals will be served and that aquatic exercises are perfectly safe and injury free for all. This is not true. Participants may be told to hold a specific position regardless of the specific postural adaptations of each client, which could be injurious. A client without sufficient swimming skills, or an adequate fitness level, requires a personal program to perform in the water. Further, if the client experiences frustration and a lack of improvement, it can lead to discouragement and a lack of compliance. However, aquatic physical therapy can provide many additional benefits to the long- and short-term effects of regular, supervised, active exercise therapy. It combines the components and advantages of numerous treatment theories and exercise techniques, and has be-

come more widely accepted and used by medical professionals. The expansion and acceptance of this rehabilitation technique is largely a result of the positive client response and the high success rate of aquatic physical therapy. At times, it is the only medium that allows movement for clients with rheumatic disease.

The client's physician normally completes a physical examination before referral to the therapist for care. The therapist then evaluates the client to develop individual goals and a treatment plan before initiating an aquatic program. Based on the results of the evaluation, a program of exercise is designed that meets the individual's needs. Each session is monitored to determine fatigue and pain levels, client enthusiasm and motivation, and functional gains. Objective reevaluations should be scheduled on a timely basis to determine the client's progress using clinical methods and standards. This reevaluation, in conjunction with subjective measurements, is used to determine the attainment of current goals, the carry-over of client skills from water to land, and the establishment of new goals. The new program could include direction to more specific dysfunctions, emphasis on an isolated component of rehabilitation, or development of an independent program.

With the supervision of trained professionals, people in aquatic rehabilitation can be treated with positive results and can safely enjoy aquatic exercise. Also, because the client can perform exercises while standing in the water, holding the pool side, or using a flotation device, swimming skills are not a prerequisite.

Therapeutic routines may include any of the following:

- Isolated upper extremity, lower extremity, and trunk exercises for strengthening and range of motion
- Stretching exercises to increase flexibility
- Ambulatory drills for reeducation, proprioception, and initiation of weight bearing
- Positioning techniques used to decrease pain
- Lap work for general conditioning
- Complex movement patterns for coordination, balance, agility, and simulation of athletic or work skills[1]

Periodic reassessment is required to determine the need for treatment modification, and encourages regular compliance of clients.[2] To ensure continuation of the program, clients should be urged and assisted in participating in communal programs such as school facilities and the like. Instructors of water aerobic classes often allow people to participate and to complete specific exercises recommended by a physical therapist. This arrangement provides the continued psychological and social support of a group without forcing the client into an inappropriate exercise program. Abrupt discontinuation of the prescribed therapy can often lead to the ultimate loss of previous gains.

Aquatic rehabilitation can also be a form of mainstreaming. Clients are placed in an environment of social and recreational activity from which they may previously have been isolated. The camaraderie developed in this environment often flourishes into long-lasting relationships. In this manner, aquatic therapy also serves as a highly beneficial support mechanism.

Special Needs of This Client Population

Goals need to be established and the therapy directed toward meeting those goals agreed on by the health professional and client. The proposed program must consider all aspects of the activity, including the physical demands of the day. This includes the activity associated with getting to the facility, and changing clothes, showering, and walking to and from the parking lot. Clients need to be monitored closely for signs of overexertion, cardiovascular distress, fatigue and subsequent loss of exercise technique, and postural compensations. In addition, clients with rheumatic disease frequently have medical complications limiting their participation in aquatic rehabilitation. Fragile skin conditions often lead to open wounds with slow healing, as is common with use of steroid medications. Multiple fractures requiring bed rest interrupt regular visits. Depression of the immune system may make some clients more susceptible to infectious diseases, particularly the common cold.

Vascular disease or side effects of medication may cause changes in vision, requiring some compensation or adjustments in the treatment program. Negotiating elevations may be difficult because step height is difficult to assess under water. Contact guarding may be required for the safety of the client. Some clients have difficulty maintaining balance and equilibrium in water because their eyes cannot adjust to the constant movement of the water. Focusing on a fixed object such as the poolside wall may minimize this effect of changes in visual perception.

Aquatic and Land Physical Therapy

Aquatic therapy can be used as an adjunct to or as a substitution for traditional land physical therapy. However, a combination of both land and water exercises is preferred if it can be tolerated by the client. The ultimate goal is to progress the client to an independent exercise program designed to maintain/improve health and fitness at an appropriate level. Individuality is stressed, with modifications made as necessary through periodic reevaluations. With professional assistance, clients can learn to modify their exercise regimens and to follow instructions for maintenance-level programs after discharge from physical therapy. Some remain at highly controlled levels of exercise; other resume full activity/athletics.

Goals could also be short term and directed specifically to one joint complex (eg, one grade level increase in strength, a range of motion improvement, an increase in percentage of weight tolerance). Because aquatic exercises can be easily modified to accommodate the client's status, aquatic physical therapy can be used temporarily during transitional times in client rehabilitation. These transitional periods may include the following:

- Physical therapy not otherwise tolerated on land
  - Poor postural stabilization
  - Inability to stabilize surrounding joints to allow exercise

– Multijoint involvement requiring extensive exercise

– Poor tolerance of resistive types of exercise and antigravity movements

– Fragility of soft tissue precluding contact resistance forces

– Fragility of joint structures and bones precluding resistive gravitational forces

– Increased sensitivity to manual contact

- Before isokinetic or isotonic equipment is tolerated
- During nonweight-bearing or partial weight-bearing status
- In preparation for surgical procedures
- Before the return to other athletics/activities
- During remission for active exercise

Benefits of Aquatic Rehabilitation Specific to Clients With Rheumatic Disease

Common complaints are reported in a variety of rheumatic diseases. The similarities are especially noted with the musculoskeletal dysfunctions frequently treated with aquatic rehabilitation. Many clients with rheumatic diseases suffer from multiple complications of the disease, as well as side effects of the treatment (ie, medication and immobilization). These complications can be extensive, and include:

- Variable levels of pain and stiffness
- Symptoms related to muscle weakness
- Postural compensations
- Decreased cardiovascular endurance and increased fatigue
- Numerous joint complications
  – Multiple joint involvement
  – Joint laxity
  – Joint contractures and deformity
  – Alteration of biomechanical functioning
  – Extra-articular manifestations

Unfortunately, rheumatic disease is also associated with a strong tendency toward relapse and chronic inflammation.[3] Although the appropriate balance of rest and activity is necessary for reducing inflammatory disorders, immobilization of joints for more than 4 weeks may lead to increased joint stiffness and muscle atrophy.[3,4] Treatment, as always, should be focused on the specific needs of the client. Focusing on

the treatment goals may be a particular lenge with this client population because toms may fluctuate from day to day.

Pain and Stiffness

Frequently, subjective pain symptoms decrease while in the water. This may be attributed to any of the following:

- Increased sensory input from water turbulence, pressure, and temperature
- Decreased muscle activity and resultant relaxation gained from the water's buoyancy
- Decreased joint compression secondary to the buoyancy of the water
- Increased mental and social stimulation serving as a distraction from the pain

Buoyancy diminishes the effects of gravity. As a result, there is less compression on the joints and less muscle activity required while supported in the water. Water can be used for support, assistance, and resistance. With the body weight supported, central stability is achieved with less effort and postural control is increased. Distal limb movement is also assisted by buoyancy. The water can be used for resistance of movement as exercise becomes less inhibited by pain. Range of motion exercise is completed as tolerated and gradually increased. General mobility is increased, resulting in a decrease in the sensation of stiffness. Confidence in movement is restored with each completed exercise. Buoyancy allows for client relaxation, decreased pain, and easier movement.

Muscle Weakness

Aquatic exercise provides smooth engagement of resistance, full range of motion, and the opportunity to train at various speeds. These components make aquatic exercise an excellent method for increasing strength and power. The viscosity of water provides resistance to a body moving through it. Movement produces a resistance that is applied to the entire surface of a moving limb. This effect allows smooth resistance without an uneven pressure or a strong torque at the end of the limb. It is particularly beneficial when joint deformities limit other types of exercise using weights or other resistive devices. Clients with rheumatic disease may not tolerate pressure to fragile soft tissues from manual contact or even wrist and ankle weights. This pressure can be painful, disruptive to the skin, and, depending on the location and direction of the force, stressful to the joints.

Many aquatic exercises can alter the resistive forces without increasing the local stress to the joints and soft tissue. Turbulence is caused by irregular movement of fluids, and rapid, random movements create rotatory movements of the molecules, resulting in resistance to the direction of a moving body. Turbulence in a pool is inevitable and serves as increased resistance to the exercise, the movement pattern, and the proximal stabilization required.

A frequent change in direction of movement also increases resistance. Directional changes are slowed by the inertia of the water. A client is encouraged to change directions of an exercise quickly without stopping at any point in the range of motion. If less resistance is desired, stopping before reversing the direction of the exercise would be advisable. Assistive devices provide additional resistance. If hand paddles are used to increase resistance, the speed of the movement is reduced secondary to the increase in the mass of the water being moved.

Postural Compensations

The turbulence of the water demands central stabilization (cocontraction of abdominal and back muscles) before distal movement is allowed. Reeducating trunk muscles reinforces the importance of using the abdominal and back muscles for postural control on land.

Cardiovascular Endurance and Fatigue

Debilitation frequently occurs secondary to an overall decrease in physical activity. Aquatic rehabilitation can provide a safe method of increasing muscular and cardiovascular endurance (see Chap. 13) without the weight bearing, joint impact, and soft tissue trauma possible with other forms of exercise. The overall deconditioning experienced by many clients with rheumatic disease results in decreased tolerance to exercise.

Aquatic rehabilitation offers an environment that may be better tolerated than exercise on land. In general, the heart rate decreases be-

cause of the relative coolness of the water in a nontherapeutic pool, kept at 26°C to 28°C. This response is partly caused by peripheral shunting and increased venous return resulting in increased cardiac output. Horizontal positioning also increases the stroke volume and depresses the heart rate. Reports indicate a smaller oxygen uptake in the water as less muscle mass is demanded for stabilization, also accounting for lower heart rate.[5] Given these facts, a greater level of exercise may be tolerated in the water, while maintaining a lower heart rate, compared with other forms of exercise.[5,6]

Joint Complications

With most rheumatologic disorders, numerous complications occur in the joints. Specific joint lesions related to the disease process, or an orthopedic dysfunction secondary to abnormal stress on fragile structures, can result in trunk and upper and lower extremity dysfunction. These complications may be attributed to joint deformities and muscle weakness altering biomechanics of stance, gait, and active range of motion. Tendinitis, adhesive capsulitis, subluxation, and bursitis frequently occur. These conditions can be treated with an unlimited number of multidirectional exercises (open and closed chain) designed to increase strength and stabilization, range of motion, and to improve posture. The ability of a client to experience movement patterns that are not available against gravity on land can be both physically and psychologically rewarding. Correct posture can be maintained with the support of the water. This postural reeducation provides positive proprioceptive feedback to the client and allows proper positioning for extremity movements.

As controlled weight bearing becomes tolerated in various depths of water, normal gait patterns are more easily simulated. Dynamic stability and synergistic movements are developed early in the rehabilitation process. Functional reeducation involves multidirectional movement patterns rather than the training of individual muscle groups. The same physiologic principles of cocontraction and maximal resistance to mass movement patterns can be applied to exercise in water.[7,8] Water, which is 600 to 800 times more supportive than air, is an appropriate environment for education of proper body mechanics.[9] Aquatic rehabilitation offers a unique way of experimenting with movements and the simulation of athletic or work skills. Coordination of specific patterns can be practiced with the support and assie groups. The same physiologic principles of cocontraction and maximal resistance to mass movement patterns can be applied te groups. The same physiologic principles of cocontraction and maximal resistance to mass movement patterns can be applied to exercise in water.[7,8] Water, which is 600 to 800 times more supportive than air, is an appropriate environment for education of proper body mechanics.[9] Aquatic rehabilitation offers a unique way of experimenting with movements and the simulation of athletic or work skills. Coordination of specific patterns can be practiced with the support and assistance of the water to provide a means for designing a program for increased weight bearing. These effects can be monitored by gradually transferring the exercises to water of lesser depths and eventually to full weight bearing. The progression to increased resistance can then be accomplished without the fear of falling. The carry-over to land of aquatic rehabilitation may allow the performance of functional movements with increased confidence and an earlier return to work, activities of daily living (ADL), and athletics than might be expected with traditional land-based therapy alone.

Conditions

Numerous aquatic rehabilitation concepts are used to incorporate the appropriate treatment for each rheumatoid condition. The following examples show how clients with specific clinical diagnoses may benefit from aquatic rehabilitation.

Low Back Derangement

Incidences of low back derangement or dysfunction secondary to facet subluxations, disc prolapses, and postural compensations are commonly associated with rheumatic diseases.[3] The degenerative process leads to modifications in loading of the spine with subsequent remodeling of the bone and possible osteophyte formation.[10] These alterations contribute considerably to increased low back pain and a decline in functional ADL. Excessive loads are placed on the spine daily.[11] Aquatic rehabilitation minimizes the effects of gravity and provides active

exercise, resulting in less intense pain, an increase in trunk mobility, and an increase in strength with less potential for failure of the anulus fibrosus or endplates.[10]

Ankylosing Spondylitis

Clients with ankylosing spondylitis are subjected to the effects of gravity pulling the body into greater flexion. This posture is greatly lessened in the aquatic environment.[12] Extension exercises can be performed by people with greater ease in the water without compressive forces on the spine. The disease process is also associated with postural deviations, fibrosis, and ossification of joint capsules and periarticular soft tissue, which may also contribute to a decrease in lung capacity. Aquatic exercises to improve posture, coordinated with diaphragmatic breathing, may minimize these complications.[13]

Osteoporosis

Osteoporosis is a frequent occurrence in people with rheumatic disease, primarily because of low physical activity, immobilization, and the long-term use of prescribed medications (ie, corticosteroid therapy). For those suffering with symptoms of bone pain and multiple fractures, aquatic rehabilitation offers a method of exercise designed for pain relief, range of motion, and eventual strengthening. Because strong forces can be generated in the water with vigorous movements, exercises must be modified by incorporating gentle movements until the stress fracture sites are well healed. Clients with osteoporosis need to progress to a combination of partial weight-bearing and full weight-bearing exercises. The weight-bearing exercises provide the mechanical stress necessary to stimulate bone formation and to minimize the progression of the disease.

Fibromyalgia

Fibromyalgia, a condition included in clinical rheumatology, has been a professional challenge to many researchers and clinicians. The symptoms of fatigue, morning stiffness, sleep disturbances, widespread pain, and psychological abnormality are sometimes incapacitating. Few treatment modalities have been successful in managing the symptoms of fibromyalgia. Aerobic exercise and pain management techniques are supported as part of the team effort to treat clients suffering with these multiple clinical symptoms (Wolf F, unpublished observation, 1993). Aquatic rehabilitation does seem to offer strategies to assist in the treatment of clients diagnosed with fibromyalgia. The treatment would be directed toward general conditioning, pain relief, improving sleep patterns through physical exertion and relaxation, and postural improvement to correct long-term adaptations secondary to pain. Relaxation achieved from exercise and the support provided by the water can lead to significant improvements in subjective reports of pain and stiffness. A more positive mental outlook is often achieved with the accomplishment of exercise without pain. The camaraderie provided by the presence of other clients and the support of the therapist may also aid in the client's compliance. It is a primary goal of aquatic rehabilitation that the relief of symptoms produce a positive addiction to regular aquatic exercise and aid in maintaining long-term compliance. This may be one of the more important benefits in treating clients with fibromyalgia. The symptoms of the disease frequently require a long-term commitment to supervised treatment and independent participation in an exercise program.

Hemophilia

For people with hemophilia, aquatic rehabilitation can be used to increase range of motion and strength of limbs after an acute hemarthrosis. Isometric exercises are used after active bleeding stops, to prevent atrophy. Gentle range of motion is initiated as tolerated and progressed to resistive exercises. Aquatic exercise can be continued prophylactically without repetitive impact or high risk of trauma. Activities in the water also provide the opportunity for social interaction and participation in lifelong recreational sports.

Exercise Concepts Incorporated in Aquatic Therapy

Aquatic physical therapy can integrate many treatment techniques into a single form. Clients with rheumatic disease can be treated for a variety of dysfunctions, and the treatment can be focused on a particular joint complex or body area. However, functional movements are emphasized, using synergistic patterns, stabilization, postural corrections, and joint biomechanics. The flexibility of the program is limited only by the creativity of the therapist. This flexibility allows the incorporation of numerous types of exercise techniques used in combinations adapted to the individual client. Each technique contributes in some manner to the ultimate goal of normal synergistic movement patterns with appropriate joint stabilization. A brief discussion of selected exercise techniques is included to demonstrate the integration of land techniques with water techniques.

Passive Techniques

Passive range of motion may be indicated if active motion is not tolerated. Preservation of joint movement is critical in ensuring joint mechanics when active range is initiated. The comfort of the pool or whirlpool may encourage greater range, with the client assisted by the therapist. WATSU techniques may be helpful during this phase (see Chap. 17).

Active-Assisted, Active, and Resistive Techniques

The length of the lever arm has a significant effect in water exercises. The longer the lever arm, the greater the effect of both the assistance and resistance provided by water. For example, with the elbow extended when abducting the arm, the buoyancy of the water provides greater assistance, but also greater resistance when lifting the arm quickly through the same range of motion.

Adding or changing resistance permits progression of the therapy. Numerous techniques can be used to modify the resistance of each exercise:

1. Change the direction of the movement
2. Change the speed of movement
3. Increase the length of the lever arm
4. Increase the range of motion
5. Increase the displacement of the water

Various devices can be used to enhance the resistance already provided by the water, including, but not limited to, water wings, flippers, hand paddles, water barbells, and water mitts.

Isometrics

Isometric contractions are used extensively throughout the body with normal movement. They are useful in stabilizing the joint and in strengthening the muscle with minimal involvement of the joint complex. This type of contraction can easily be incorporated into any aquatic exercise protocol.

Istonics

Movement through the range of motion of a joint can be modified as needed for each client by varying the degrees of motion and the speed of the movement. This enables the client to adjust to his or her individual tolerance to resistance. If a client increases the speed of motion, a greater force is being applied. As the exercise is performed more vigorously, more resistance is felt.

Postural Stabilization or Concontractions

Postural improvement and control should be emphasized and addressed immediately. Proximal stabilization is essential before any advancement of range of motion and speed and variation of exercise patterns. Initially, stabilization must be acquired in a pain-free position, whether in flexion, extension, or neutral posture of the trunk. Because dysfunctional postures may result from compensations made to minimize a symptom of the disease, it may not be advisable to alter the adaptations to achieve a "perfect posture." This may risk an increase in symptoms. For example, with a client who has a flexed trunk, no lordotic curve in the lumbar spine, the thorax anterior to the pelvis, a posterior pelvic tilt, and a hamstring length of 70 degrees, compensations are frequently made to decrease weight bearing on painful facet joints. The goals for such a client should include:

1. Minimizing the progression of postural changes
2. Maintaining the range of motion or improving it to limits of symptom reproduction
3. Improving strength to control this posture

4. Addressing and challenging the person's balance and weight shift in various positions to increase safety when negotiating uneven surfaces and steps

Eccentric and Concentric Contractions

The transition from water to land requires a combination of concentric and eccentric movements. Because clients must be able to control their body weight against gravity, exercises should be designed that emphasize eccentric movements such as negotiating steps and ladders, transitional movements from sit to stand, and the like.

Closed- and Open-Chain Techniques

Open kinetic chain exercises are important when weight bearing through the distal extremity is not tolerated, and for range of motion, endurance, and strengthening. These exercises add to the functional aspect of treatment. Upper extremity closed-chain exercises can be added by holding onto a fixed object such as a pool ladder or leaning on a step or platform in the water. Lower extremity closed-chain exercises are completed in a weight-bearing position on the pool floor or platform with the client standing and stabilizing on one leg before moving to the other side. These exercises provide good joint cocontraction around lax joints, thereby reinforcing stabilization.

In the selection of a protocol, a mixture of exercise techniques should be incorporated throughout the session. The selection of exercises must be appropriate for individual goals and be tolerated by the client without increased symptoms. This variety may help to increase client compliance and decrease the time required for treatment. A balance of treatment techniques also helps to achieve multiple goals and to simulate functional movement patterns.

Pool Facility Requirements

Selecting a facility for aquatic rehabilitation requires a thorough understanding of the variables involved in treating specific clients and how easily client treatment can be managed in a public or private site (see Chap. 18). Although constructing a therapeutic pool is ideal, capital costs and operational expenses obviate this option for medical professionals. Because therapeutic pools can be very expensive and are unavailable to most people, public recreational pools may be a viable alternative. Facilities should be evaluated for location, ease of access, and staff support.

Area recreational pools (indoor or outdoor) can work well. Weather, time of day, and direct sunlight are factors that must be considered in scheduling treatment in outdoor pools. Water depth may vary but should include some areas of 1 to 1.5 m deep for walking and to increase the confidence of nonswimmers. Although water deeper than 2 m is unnecessary, it is helpful to provide an area for activities in nonweight-bearing positions (eg, water running and trunk stabilization with supportive devices). Wall space in standing depths of water is required to perform weight-bearing exercises. Although pool length is optional, the more advanced client progresses to various forms of lap work requiring a length of 25 m.

Aquatic rehabilitation programs directed toward active exercise can be managed in pool temperatures of 27°C to 30°C and air temperatures near 26°C. A client participating in the program for pain relief who is unable to exercise vigorously will become chilled in temperatures lower than 28°C.

Therapeutic pools frequently are heated to high temperatures, such as 33°C to 37°C. These pools are beneficial for people in considerable pain who can use heat for pain relief and gentle range of motion, but are inappropriate for active terrestrial-based exercise programs. The body temperature is normally controlled through convection, radiation, and the conduction and evaporation of perspiration. In heated water, these methods are compromised. Core body temperature may be increased because of heat gains from submersion in water of temperatures higher than the skin and from additional heat generated from metabolically active tissue.[14] In heated water, a general vasodilation of the capillaries may also cause a significant decrease in blood pressure.[15] In warmer water, exercising at an intensity level designed to increase strength may increase oxygen consumption and cardiac demands beyond a safe margin.[16] Heat is deemed an appropriate modality for client relaxation, and decreased anxiety may be achieved in warm, moving water.[17] It is, however, essential that the therapist consider the peculiarities and physical well-being of a person with rheumatic disease.

Client Selection for Aquatic Therapy

Indications

An exercise program as versatile as aquatic physical therapy can provide benefits to almost everyone motivated enough to participate. The following are some of the indications for aquatic physical therapy:

- High pain level
- Gait deviations
- Decreased mobility
- Weakness
- Coordination
- Limited weight bearing or poor weight shift
- Poor muscular endurance
- Decreased cardiovascular endurance
- Joint contractures
- Decreased flexibility
- Postural dysfunctions
- Poor proprioception
- Lack of knowledge of appropriate independent exercise program
- Need for motor skill simulation in a controlled environment
- Decreased client responsibility for management of health care
- Decreased recreational skills and social interaction[18-21]

Contraindications and Precautions

Possible contraindications to and precautions for aquatic therapy include:

- Fever
- Open wound
- Contagious skin rashes
- Infectious disease
- Severe cardiovascular disease
- History of uncontrolled seizures
- Incontinence of bowel or bladder
- Use of a colostomy bag or catheter
- Menstruation without internal protection
- Cognitive impairments that would prevent the client from safely entering the pool area or from transferring into the pool

- Tracheotomy, nasogastric, and gastrostomy tubes
- Decreased oral-facial control
- Acute orthopedic injury with resultant instability
- Pressure sores/decubitus ulcers
- Severe hypotension/hypertension
- Severely limited endurance[18-21]

Some limitations are also set depending on the following conditions:

- The type, location, and overall accessibility of the pool site
- The equipment available for transfers (Hoyer lift, mats, portable steps, platforms)
- The staff-to-client ratio
- The physical condition and level of independence of each client in the program

Initial Evaluation

The evaluation begins by obtaining a medical history. The following should be included: the onset of the disease, medical treatment, progress of disease, systemic involvement, length of repeated exacerbations and remissions, surgical intervention completed or recommended, previous physical therapy, current home exercise program, use of modalities at home, and compliance with current treatment. Past medical history should be noted and all current medications should be listed. It is important to note the schedule of the medications, which may influence the optimum time for active exercise.

During the evaluation, the therapist should direct the evaluation and assessment to the following suggested considerations:

1. Prioritize symptoms by importance to the client, and rate them on a scale of 1 to 10 (minimal to severe). Although pain may not be the most debilitating aspect of the client's condition, it may be a significant factor in compensatory postures.
2. Examine postural deviations and document corrections to be attempted in aquatic therapy sessions.
3. Assess possible causes of postural changes, including muscle weakness, muscle fatigue, joint malalignment, pain, soft tissue restrictions, or rigid bony adaptations.
4. Determine trunk and extremity range of motion and muscle strength of symptomatic areas.

5. Document joint deformities, crepitation, muscle atrophy, superficial heat and swelling, and observations of any dermatologic lesions and of the general condition of skin. Discuss the use of braces or supports, if appropriate.
6. Note the flexibility of all joints.
7. Assess overall mobility, balance, gait patterns, ease of weight shift, and appropriate use of assistive devices for ambulation and transfers.
8. Determine the capability of the client to transfer into and out of the pool without distress.
9. Determine functional status by evaluation or subjective report to establish long- and short-term goals. For each client, the specific needs of work and ADL need to be considered.
10. Record resting heart rate and blood pressure readings as a standard to compare with vital signs monitored at the pool site.
11. Document body weight, height, and chest expansion measurements.
12. Assess the respiratory capabilities of the client with exertion. Diaphragmatic breathing can be achieved even with little chest expansion and low vital capacities.

General endurance is a major consideration. The client must plan sufficient time for traveling to a facility, changing clothes, showering, and exercising, because these activities will place greater demands on his or her daily schedule. Exertion levels required to prepare for the treatment should not outweigh the treatment itself. The benefit of an aquatic active exercise program is directly influenced by the mental attitude, motivational level, psychological response to the disease, and the client's demonstrated adaptability to lifestyle changes and medical recommendations. The client needs to be aware that aquatic physical therapy requires a greater commitment than alternative therapy treatments. Poor self-esteem and depression are common for people undergoing major changes in everyday functioning, including displaced professional status and the inability to participate in previous recreational and social activities. Alterations in mental clarity and memory also affect client safety and ability to perform and remember appropriate techniques.

When a client is accepted into the aquatic therapy program, diaphragmatic breathing should be taught and practiced in sessions preceding the introduction to the pool. The client should be familiar with trunk stabilization techniques, including either a pelvic tilt or cocontraction of the abdominal and back muscles. These techniques should be demonstrated in various positions to ensure compliance in functional as well as resting positions.

General Guidelines for Aquatic Therapy

The following guidelines are given for initiating aquatic physical therapy. Modifications are always necessary because many clients are unable to tolerate even the most conservative exercises. Variations in exercises are needed to expand the program, to challenge the client, and to provide stimulation. The following guidelines are given as suggestions for initiating therapy.

Trunk Alignment and Stability

Trunk stability is encouraged throughout the exercise. Stability provides the base necessary for the extremity exercises to secure the pelvis, spine, and thoracic cage. Trunk control is obviously important to a client with low back disease. Variation from a perfect normal anteroposterior curve may be necessary at first for control of symptoms. Ideally, if not contraindicated, the client should progress to a point at which all positions of flexion and extension of the spine are tolerated and normal range of motion in all planes can be performed. A client without low back disease is instructed to maintain a posture with recommended anteroposterior curves in the cervical, thoracic, and lumbar spine.

Various exercises can be used to achieve trunk strengthening, range of motion, stability, postural correction, or symptom relief. The following are examples of various positioning techniques.

Flexion (Fig. 11-1)

- Wall slide/squats
- Posterior pelvic tilt with back to wall
- Hanging in corner, lower extremities flexed, back to wall
- Supine lap work, holding kickboard at chest
- Vertical stabilization with lower extremities flexed
- Walking backward, allowing flexion

Extension (Fig. 11-2)

- Facing wall, extension exercise
- Freestanding, holding extended posture
- Prone lap work
- Vertical stabilization with lower extremities extended
- Hanging in corner, lower extremities extended, facing wall
- Walking forward, allowing extension

Neutral (Fig. 11-3)

- Upright, neutral alignment, back to wall or freestanding
- Water running, pelvis under thorax, lower extremities under pelvis
- Freestanding, one leg in front of the other, shoulder width apart
- Walking, forward, backward, sidestepping, with neutral positioning
- Alternating lap work, prone and supine

Gait Training

Walking in the water offers many benefits. The client should be monitored carefully, however, to accomplish the goals of trunk strengthening, trunk rotation, a reciprocal gait pattern, and equal weight bearing. Normal weight shift to both extremities in a heel-to-toe gait should be encouraged in conjunction with bilateral and alternating arm swing, and trunk rotation. It is easy to lose the normal rhythm of upper and lower extremities in the water. Clients may have a tendency to push against the water by leaning, especially if change in speed is initiated. It is important to remind the client to maintain the desired trunk alignment (ie, thorax over pelvis), with appropriate anterior and posterior curves throughout the spine.

Body Positioning

A primary concern is to position the moving body part under water to benefit from the physical properties of water. For orthopedic reasons, depths should be changed to accommodate the desired joint weight relief. The stability of the body must also be considered. Greater buoyancy is achieved by increasing the volume of an object so that it displaces more water, such as by inhaling to expand the lungs and chest. Because muscle tissue is dense, less buoyancy is observed in a client with a muscular body type.

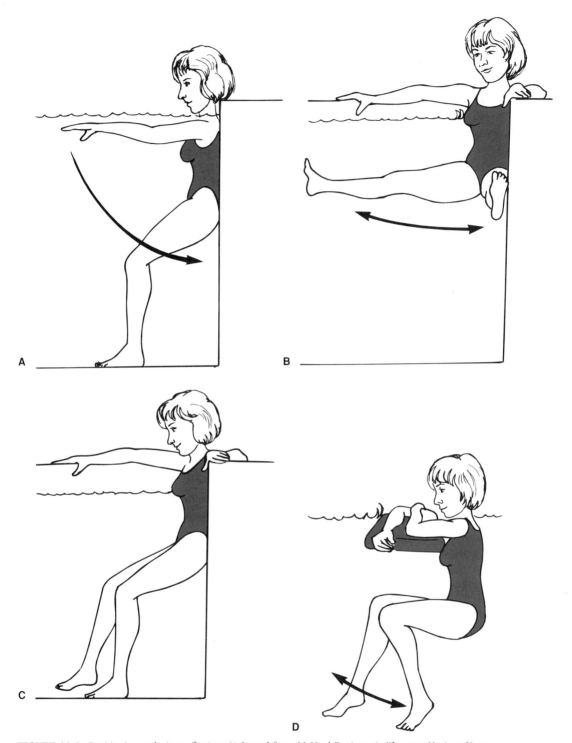

FIGURE 11-1. Positioning technique: flexion. (Adapted from McNeal R. *Aquatic Therapy: Various Uses and Techniques*. Abingdon, MD: Aquatic Therapy Services; 1988; with permission.)

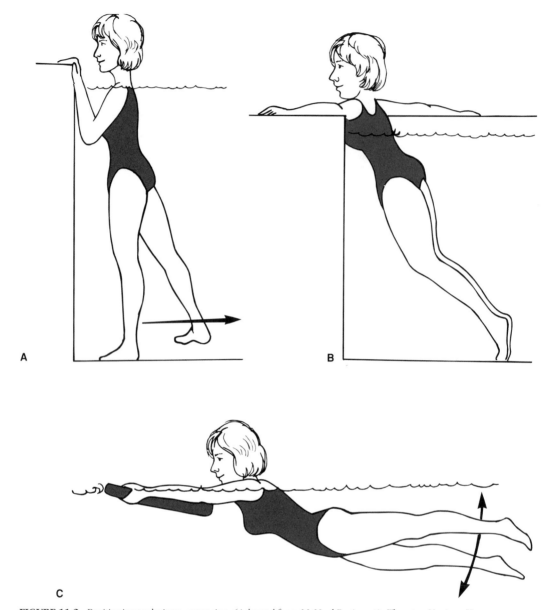

FIGURE 11-2. Positioning technique: extension. (Adapted from McNeal R. *Aquatic Therapy: Various Uses and Techniques*. Abingdon, MD: Aquatic Therapy Services; 1988; with permission.)

Overall stability is also decreased if standing in water above the level of T8–T11.[8] Therefore, individual initial capabilities may require modification of client positioning. Positioning for aquatic exercises may vary depending on the body type of the person and the difficulty demonstrated in attaining stability in the water. If the client experiences difficulty in maintaining the given position and "floats away," the therapist should recommend moving to less deep water.

Modifications may also be needed, if only temporarily, to acquire the posture or position desired or for pain relief.

Breathing Control

Diaphragmatic breathing should be incorporated throughout all exercises. The benefits of controlled breathing techniques include:

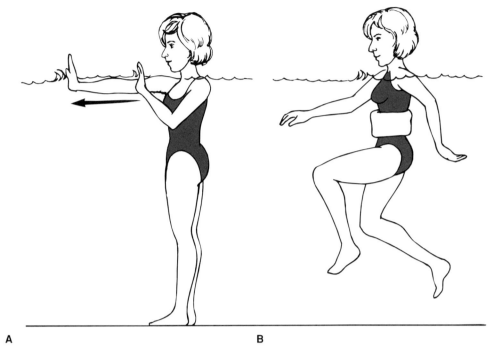

A   **B**

FIGURE 11-3. Positioning technique: neutral. (Adapted from McNeal R. *Aquatic Therapy: Various Uses and Techniques.* Abingdon, MD: Aquatic Therapy Services; 1988; with permission.)

- Prevention of temporary breath holding and the Valsalva maneuver
- More efficient inhalation and exhalation
- Greater gaseous exchange
- Awareness of the use of abdominal muscles

If appropriate, inhalation and exhalation should be coordinated with the movement pattern; otherwise, the breathing technique should be performed independent of the exercise.

Exercise Instruction

Exercises are performed in a rhythmic, fluid manner without stopping at any one point in the range. Stopping at one position results in a loss of resistance until the speed is reinitiated.

As a rule, the moving body part should be kept under water. The resistance is lost if the limbs break the surface of the water. However, if less resistance is desired, the body part should be only partially submerged.

The client's strength and ability to stabilize the body limit the speed at which the exercises are performed. Therefore, as the client becomes more efficient in performing exercises, the speed may be increased and consequently the resistance.

As noted, the difficulty or intensity of the exercise can also be changed by varying the range of motion of the pattern. With increased tolerance, there should be a gradual increase in the size of the movement for a greater level of exertion.

Further increase in resistance can be achieved with assistive devices such as water wings, water mitts, hand paddles, flippers, and water barbells. Water mitts are made with flexible fabrics or have fastenings that are more adaptable to clients with pain and deformities in the hands. Kickboards and flotation belts are used for various lap exercises, water running, and vertical stabilization (see Chap. 20). Later, swimming can be encouraged if techniques are monitored and modified as needed.

Client Education

Aquatic therapy sessions provide the time and environment for client education. People need to be aware of the long-term ramifications of the disease process and understand how treatment and care may be altered during various stages of exacerbation and remission. This education is critical in ensuring individual responsibility for the modifications needed in daily functioning and exercises when not supervised by a professional.

General Considerations

Depending on the current ability of the client, the program may last between 15 and 75 minutes. Compared with similar positions on land, less work is required to hold the body upright in the water, and is associated with a clinically documented decrease in heart rate.[5] Respiratory distress should be closely monitored because of the pressure against the chest wall during submersion and the increased physical demands of exercise. Aquatic exercise can also be deceiving. Initially it seems effortless compared with active exercise against gravity, but clients are often amazed at how fatigued and "heavy" they feel after treatment sessions in the pool. People with rheumatic disease may experience an exacerbation after extensive exercise, or extreme exhaustion and general malaise. For these people, energy conservation is advocated. They frequently overexert themselves with inefficient postures and movements related to weakness and poor biomechanics. An appropriate rest period balanced with appropriate exercise is key to managing the disease and progressing with set goals. It is always preferable to start slowly and progress gradually to allow time to adapt to an exercise regimen.

Exercises can usually be safely executed on a daily basis without difficulty. A minimum of three to four times a week is recommended. Strength gains have been documented with regular exercise sessions; however, improvements are not maintained if the regimen is discontinued.[2]

To a certain degree, muscle fatigue is desirable, as is gentle stretching. Pain, however, usually is an indication of a pathologic process, and should be acknowledged. The expression "no pain, no gain," should be especially discouraged with this client population. All exercises can be modified by changing the body position, range of motion, and intensity of the exercise. If the pain persists, the exercise in question should be deleted from the regimen. Improvements in strength, flexibility, and endurance may enable the person to perform the exercise at a later time.

❑ CASE STUDY 11-1

The subject of the case study is a well educated, 46-year-old woman, a registered nurse, diagnosed with vasculitis. Her progression from incapacitation to swimming laps and to scuba diving is inspiring. The case history follows the client through many years of the disease process and medical complications. The study briefly includes physical therapy, aquatic physical therapy, home exercise program, medical complications, and progression of ADL. Her return to a functional status and attainment of the established goals was satisfying to both client and therapist.

Symptoms of the disease initially appeared at an early age and over a period of years, and included anorexia, fatigue, low-grade fever, joint pain, and muscle pain. She did not attribute these problems to a disease process until she was diagnosed at age 40 years with vasculitis with involvement of the central nervous system. Although no conclusive diagnostic testing had been completed, in hindsight the facts become clearer and more understandable.

Vasculitis is a necrotizing inflammatory disease of the arteries, usually of unknown etiology. The disease frequently involves people of middle age with systemic features of fever, weight loss, malaise, and multiple organ involvement. Commonly seen are asymmetric polyarthritis, peripheral neuropathy, and kidney and central nervous system involvement.

Treatment includes the use of medications (corticosteroids and a cytotoxic agent to allow reduction of steroids after the disease is under control). Team management by medical and rehabilitation professionals is critical for these clients because of potential side effects of treatment and complications of the disease.

The client's complaints of weakness and joint pain progressed quickly from the age of 38. Her exacerbations were usually preceded by some gastrointestinal complication. She underwent extensive testing and prolonged hospitalizations for medication, intensive therapy, and bed rest. On discharge, she received home physical therapy and occupational therapy until she was able to receive treatment from an outpatient facility. From ages 41 through 44, she suffered frequent periods of increased symptoms, including hepatitis, osteoporosis with multiple fractures, cellulitis, ruptured diverticulum, colostomy, and seizures. This required extended time in hospitals and rehabilitation facilities.

After a 2-month period of intensive treatment, the client was discharged from a rehabilitation hospital at age 44. Functionally, she required a hospital bed, bedside commode, wheeled walker, stair glide, slider board, and shower bench. Home physical therapy and occupational therapy were frequently discontinued because of fractures. Thirteen months later, she was slowly regaining some strength and participated in outpatient therapy in a rehabilitation center. She then suffered an impacted fracture of the hip and was on bed rest for 3 months. Reversal of the colostomy 3 to 4 months later was mentally very uplifting for the client and seemed to be the turning point in her rehabilitation.

By age 45, this client returned to physical therapy at a private practice (2 years after her last visit for outpatient physical therapy). Functionally, she was still using two Lofstrand crutches, high-rest toilet seat, long-handled grabbers, and a wheelchair for long distances, and was unable to lift her leg to don pants. Her goal was to return to the pool! She loved being in the water for leisure enjoyment, and for the ease of movement. Her personal interests included scuba diving with her husband and with a dive club. Her ultimate goal was to travel to an island for scuba diving.

With medication, her pain level was 6 to 8/10 (1 minimal, 10 severe). For short distances without the crutches, gait deviations were numerous and based on pain and severe weakness. She demonstrated decreased weight bearing on the right side, increased lateral trunk shift, decreased trunk rotation, and poor swing phase. She was unable to sit erect without fatigue for more than 2 minutes or to lift her knee to chest in a hook-lying position.

After evaluation and client–therapist discussion, her goals for therapy were established:

Short Term
- Increase strength and endurance sufficiently to return to the pool (ie, walk from car, change clothes, manage five steps)
- Stand from toilet seat with minimal assistance from upper extremities
- Develop a home exercise program
- Increase tolerance for upright sitting to 5 minutes

Long Term
- Ambulate 500 yards without crutches
- Independent aquatic exercise, including swimming laps
- Normal ADL, including cooking and light housework
- Tolerance of travel by plane for vacation

Since returning to work was a desirable but unrealistic goal, she frequently looked for volunteer positions. She actively participated in the "Pet on Wheels" program for local nursing homes and initiated a local support group for clients with similar rheumatic diseases.

Initial physical therapy exercises were directed at increasing her central stabilization. A thorough mat program was initiated in hook lying, sitting, and side lying. Quadruped stance was not tolerated because of knee pain. Resistive exercises using manual contact, resistive tubing or band, or weights were used when available strength and positioning allowed. Standing postures were not incorporated because of the lack of trunk strength.

She was determined to begin aquatic rehabilitation. After approximately 1 month of land-based physical therapy, she started in the pool. Conserving energy, she used crutches, came dressed in her bathing suit, and avoided all stairs. Maximal assist with her upper extremities on the railing was required to enter the pool by the steps. Exercises were done initially with her back to the wall for stability and abdominal strengthening. She was positioned in chest-deep water. The buoyancy of the water at this depth minimized the effect of gravity, resulting in weight bearing of approximately 25% her body weight. Initially lower extremity movements were more demanding and were deferred until more pelvic stability was noted. Movements were done slowly through a small range of motion and gradually increased in intensity and range. Exercises were chosen using short lever arms, first in positions close to the body (ie, elbow flexion and extension, shoulder flexion and extension, shoulder abduction and adduction), and then to exercises away from the wall and with multidirectional movement patterns. Paddles were added to upper extremity exercises as long as trunk stability could be maintained. Walking was encouraged in between exercises to normalize gait and exercise the trunk muscles in a neutral position. Lower extremity exercises were added and completed in waist-deep water. The buoyancy of the water at this depth minimized the effect of gravity, resulting in weight bearing of approximately 50% her body weight.[22,23]

Lap work was initiated after 1 month of aquatic physical therapy. Freestyle was her personal choice for a swimming stroke, based on her goal of scuba diving and the similarities in the kicking pattern. A freestyle stroke demands considerable strength and requires smooth coordination of upper and lower extremities with the trunk. The client used a mask and snorkel to decrease the energy required to lift and turn her head with each stroke. The freestyle stroke requires out-of-the-water recovery of each arm. Initially this was too difficult, and some laps were done with kicking only to encourage a smooth reciprocating kick and to strengthen the lower extremities and the abdominal and back muscles. Compensation could easily occur with freestyle swimming because 80% to 90% of the propulsion is from the arm pull. Kicking the lower extremities is 80% body placement, with very little contribution to propulsion. She would also wear flippers while swimming, which aided in the body placement and the buoyancy of the legs without a steady kick. Because her lower extremities were always weaker than her upper extremities by at least a full grade, emphasis had to be placed on balancing the exercise regime to target her goals.

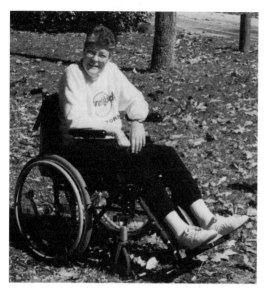

FIGURE 11-4. Client, 44 years of age, seen at home after discharge from the rehabilitation facility.

Four months after starting aquatic physical therapy, she was swimming 44 laps three times a week, walking on the treadmill at 1.5 km/hour, and using a cane only for stair climbing. She and her husband traveled to an island and went scuba diving with the sharks. For this client, returning to the pool meant resuming some normal phase of her life socially, physically, and emotionally. Swimming and aquatic exercise still provide her with

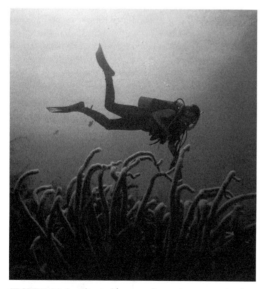

FIGURE 11-5. Client, 46 years of age, demonstrating her aquatic skills while on vacation.

that positive feeling of well-being and normality in a life that has been filled with strife and disappointment. Her personal will and determination are the factors that have driven her to be the successful women she is today (Figs. 11-4 and 11-5).

REFERENCES

1. McNeal RL. *Aquatic Therapy: Various Uses and Techniques.* Abingdon, Md: Aquatic Therapy Services; 1988.
2. Vignos PJ. Physiotherapy in rheumatoid arthritis. *J Rheumatol.* 1980;7:269–271.
3. Arthritis Foundation. *Primer on the Rheumatic Diseases.* 7th ed. Atlanta, GA: 1988.
4. Swezey R. Rehabilitation medicine and arthritis. In: McCarty D, ed. *Arthritis and Allied Conditions.* 11th ed. Philadelphia, Pa: Lea & Febiger; 1989:797.
5. Holmer I. Physiology of swimming man. *Acta Physiol Scand Suppl.* 1974;407:1.
6. Johnson B, Stromme S, Adamczyk J, et al. Comparison of oxygen uptake and heart rate during exercises on land and in water. Phys Ther. 1977;57:273.
7. Davis B. A technique of re-education in the treatment pool. *Physiotherapy.* 1967;53:57.
8. Boyle A. The Bad Ragaz ring method. *Physiotherapy.* 1981;67:265.
9. Martin J. The Halliwick method. *Physiotherapy.* 1981; 67:288.
10. Kurowski P, Kubo A. The relationship of degeneration of the intervertebral disc to mechanical loading conditions on lumbar vertebrae. *Spine.* 1986;11:726.
11. Nachemson A. The load on lumbar disks in different positions of the body. *Clin Orthop.* 1966;45:107.
12. Ball G. Ankylosing spondylitis. In: McCarty D, ed. *Arthritis and Allied Conditions.* 11th ed. Philadelphia, Pa: Lea & Febiger; 1989:934.
13. Harrison RA. Tolerance of pool therapy by ankylosing spondylitis patients with low vital capacities. *Physiotherapy.* 1981;67:296.
14. Atkinson GP, Harrison RA. Implications of the Health and Safety at Work Act in relation to hydrotherapy departments. *Physiotherapy.* 1981;67:263.
15. Golland A. Basic hydrotherapy. *Physiotherapy.* 1981; 67:258.
16. Kirby R, Kriellars D. Oxygen consumption during exercise in a heated pool. *Arch Phys Med Rehabil.* 1984; 65:21.
17. Levine B. Use of hydrotherapy in reduction of anxiety. *Psychol Rep.* 1984;55:526.
18. Duffield MH. *Exercise in Water.* London: Bailliere, Tindall and Cassell, Ltd.; 1969:1.
19. Fischer J, Jonkey B, Sharp D, et al. *Pool Therapy Seminar.* Presented at Glendale Adventist Medical Center; July, 1988; Glendale, Calif.
20. Haralson K. Therapeutic pool programs. *Clinical Management.* 1985;5:10.
21. Rodemers C, Gavin M. *Aquatic Symposium: European–American Philosophies.* Presented at the Aquatic Rehabilitation Center; December, 1988; Milford, Conn.
22. Whalen S, Berger M, Helm E, et al. *An Introduction to Aquatic Therapy.* Presented at the Bryn Mawr Rehabilitation Hospital; March, 1985; Malvern, Pa.
23. Huss D, Rud A. Pool weight bearing. Research in MCRH Therapeutic Pool, Memorial Hospital, Boulder, Colorado, 1986.

12 Aquatic Rehabilitation of the Athlete

Thomas Tierney

Modern athletes have a wide array of tools to assist in their quest to perfect their sport. High technology has infiltrated nearly every facet of training. An athlete can now experience every phase of a sporting event without stepping on the playing surface. Virtual reality technology or multiple-sense training is now a reality as a means of entertainment or as a rehabilitation tool.

Technology offers a great deal to a person striving for a physical or psychological edge. However, a naturally occurring medium exists that allows the replication of form and function, while negating the deleterious effects of a gravitational environment. The medium, water, is in daily use to cleanse and to replenish vital human systems. However, its immersive capacity and resistive qualities are frequently underused.

Many athletic organizations today realize the benefits of aquatic programming. Trends have shown the inclusion of aquatic facilities in professional team training centers and stadiums. However, few use it for more than a temporary rehabilitative medium. Considering the scarcity of literature about training or rehabilitation, this underuse may simply be the result of a lack of knowledge.

Historically, aquatic training for the athlete meant running in deep water. The buoyancy experienced in water unloaded the joints of the spine and lower extremities, negating the destructive vibration and compression forces experienced on land. The nature of today's athletic rehabilitation requires the clinician to be able to expand on this limited use through an in-depth understanding of aquatic rehabilitation. After the onset of injury, the athlete may be allowed a more rapid progression to full weight bearing than in the past. Any latency period may slow the athlete's return to unrestricted activity. Aquatic intervention can recreate the once-internalized functional movement patterns early in the rehabilitation process. In the early posttraumatic stages, the water environment may be more effective than land because of water's viscous qualities. Viscosity is the property of a fluid that makes it resistant to flow. Slow-motion movements negate undesirable compensatory activity.

The study of sport biomechanics has consistently produced research demonstrating the demands placed on the human body in sports. The literature provides substantial data correlating ground reaction forces with the number of athletic injuries.[1-4] The repetitive shock experienced in basketball, the shearing force of tennis, and the compression and distraction forces of football pose a potential threat to the athlete's continued participation. Studies of human motion have aided in understanding the mechanical and biologic mechanisms involved when the body is subjected to physical loads. The injurious effects of vibration and compression can be partially attributed to gravity, creating a dilemma for rehabilitation and training. This dilemma contributed to the introduction of cross-training. Cross-training, in turn, helped popularize the use of the aquatic medium as an alternative or an adjunct to traditional land formats. Today, the media provide intermittent segments on the many applications of aquatic intervention in athletic rehabilitation.

This chapter begins with a discussion of the benefits of aquatic programming relevant to the athlete. The following sections provide practical applications of aquatic physical therapy. The chapter concludes with guidelines for beginning aquatic programs.

Benefits of Aquatic Programming for the Athlete: The Principle of Unloading

The purpose of unloading the joints is to negate or lessen any forces that would interfere with a final goal. In rehabilitating an athlete, the structures to be unloaded are the articular cartilage and the cortical and cancellous bones. Special consideration may also be given the ligaments and muscle–tendon units to protect them from excessive torque or damaging vibrational forces. Premature loading or stressing of a damaged ligament, muscle, bone, tendon, or cartilage can cause a number of adverse chemical, metabolic, and vascular changes. The inflammatory process is nature's way of ridding the traumatized area of toxic substances. However, if prolonged, this process produces proteolytic enzymes that attack the joint tissues.[5] Clearly, the rehabilitation process progresses consistently when inflammation is kept to a minimum.

Unloading is critical to the athlete because the rehabilitation time may be minimized. Whether a high school, college, or professional athlete, time can mean the accomplishment of personal goals, a monetary scholarship, or a multimillion-dollar contract. The aquatic medium provides the athlete with opportunities for injury prevention and for immediate onset of safe and functional rehabilitation. This can minimize injury and reduce recovery time.

History of Injuries in Athletes and Prevalence of Injuries in Sports

The *National Collegiate Athletic Association Injury Surveillance System* has been publishing detailed information on injuries in 16 sports since 1982. Comparisons of biomechanics, age, gender, and body parts involved have been included. Some of the more detailed studies of gender include body composition, muscle fiber makeup, strength, and cardiovascular endurance capacity. The location of many injuries depends on the particular sport (Table 12-1). Garrick and Requa found that 90% of sport injuries occur to the lower extremities.[6] In a study of 1280 sports-related injuries, Whitman and Melvin found the knee to be the most common area of involvement and noted that 53.9% of those injuries were soft tissue in nature[7] (Table 12-2).

Most injuries to the upper extremities occur in sports that involve swinging, throwing, or swimming. Factors affecting shoulder injuries are the level of overhead activity, duration of activity, age, technique, conditioning level, and anatomic predisposition. In the upper extremity, the shoulder is the most common area of involvement, followed by the wrist. DeHaven and Litner found that 48.1% of baseball pitchers and 57% of world-class swimmers have experienced some form of shoulder dysfunction.[8]

Although sports injuries to the lumbar spine can be career threatening, few injuries to the low back occur during competition. Fairbank and colleagues found that students who avoided sports were more likely to have lower back pains.[9] A study performed by Fisk and associates compared people in sedentary positions and athletes performing heavy lifting for incidence of Scheuermann's disease.[10] Results showed that prolonged sitting was a key contributor to the disease. A review of all athletic injuries in various sports showed a significantly higher rate of injury in practice sessions than in various game competitions (Table 12-3). The only sports with lower incidence of injury in practice were men's ice hockey, baseball, and soccer.

The fitness boom, in combination with the enactment of Title IX, has encouraged female participation in sports. The anatomic and physiologic differences have resulted in differing incidence trends (see Table 12-3). The most alarming trend was the almost double incidence of knee injuries compared with men.[11] The higher incidence of stress fractures in women has been attributed to low bone density from menstrual dysfunction and poor nutrition.[12]

As athletes age, they encounter changes in the number and type of sports injuries incurred. Only 3% to 11% of all children in the United States participating in sports programs will be injured this year.[13] It is rare to find more than an isolated case of tendinitis in a young athlete. This finding has been attributed to the profound ability of the musculotendinous unit to absorb and transfer forces to the tendon apophysis. The

TABLE 12-1. Injury Rates per 1000 and Percentage in Practice and Games*

Sport	Women				Men			
	Injury Rate Per 1000	Total Injuries	Practice	Game	Injury Rate Per 1000	Total Injuries	Practice	Game
Gymnastics	8.59	1634	78%	22%	5.06	415	81%	18%
Lacrosse	4.25	871	68%	32%	6.05	2554	54%	46%
Basketball	5.13	281	61%	39%	5.61	3386	65%	35%
Soccer	7.90	2540	51%	49%	7.87	5194	47%	53%
Volleyball	4.79	2823	65%	35%	—	—	—	—
Field hockey	5.00	1526	59%	41%	—	—	—	—
Softball	3.90	1788	52%	48%	—	—	—	—
Spring football	—	—	—	—	9.59	2129	94%	6%
Wrestling	—	—	—	—	9.41	4992	66%	34%
Football	—	—	—	—	6.57	29217	58%	42%
Baseball	—	—	—	—	3.37	3837	44%	56%
Ice hockey	—	—	—	—	5.61	2908	32%	68%

* All data are shown as rate per 1000 athletic exposures in 1991 to 1992.
From the *NCAA Injury Surveillance System*. No. 9044. Overland Park, Kan: National Collegiate Athletic Association; November 1992.

TABLE 12-2. Injury Rates per 1000 as a Function of Body Part*

Sport (Sex)	Neck	Shoulder	Wrist	Hand	Lower Back	Hips/ Groin	Knee	Patella	Lower Leg	Ankle	Foot
Gymnastics (W)	0.22	0.41	0.30	0.05	0.96	0.35	1.48	0.03	0.49	1.91	0.71
Gymnastics (M)	0.00	0.50	1.00	0.10	0.50	0.60	0.10	0.00	0.40	1.00	0.20
Basketball (W)	0.02	0.21	0.05	0.09	0.33	0.21	0.92	0.10	0.24	1.38	0.27
Basketball (M)	0.07	0.14	0.07	0.06	0.40	0.35	0.78	0.14	0.19	1.83	0.30
Soccer (W)	0.32	0.25	0.07	0.01	0.27	0.37	1.27	0.08	0.71	1.76	0.41
Soccer (M)	0.40	0.19	0.11	0.03	0.25	0.46	1.39	0.09	0.54	1.75	0.46
Lacrosse (W)	0.00	0.03	0.03	0.03	0.21	0.45	0.63	0.06	0.66	0.84	0.27
Lacrosse (M)	0.08	0.56	0.07	0.06	0.23	0.38	0.90	0.04	0.28	0.99	0.10
Field hockey (W)	0.02	0.12	0.04	0.10	0.16	0.14	0.47	0.22	0.35	0.69	0.24
Volleyball (W)	0.02	0.40	0.01	0.07	0.38	0.12	0.52	0.15	0.15	1.17	0.11
Softball (W)	0.03	0.63	0.08	0.15	0.24	0.03	0.45	0.06	0.13	0.39	0.08
Spring football (M)	0.53	1.33	0.08	0.05	0.35	0.33	1.80	0.20	0.30	1.70	0.18
Wrestling (M)	0.60	1.18	0.09	0.10	0.38	0.12	1.66	0.11	0.17	0.75	0.06
Football (M)	0.28	0.83	0.06	0.10	0.29	0.34	1.26	0.08	0.21	0.97	0.16
Ice hockey (M)	0.07	0.82	0.13	0.06	0.20	0.42	0.89	0.04	0.13	0.26	0.13
Baseball (M)	0.02	0.80	0.09	0.08	0.07	0.10	0.29	0.04	0.11	0.32	0.05

* All data are shown as rate per 1000 athletic exposures from 1991 to 1992.
From the *NCAA Injury Surveillance System*. No. 9044. Overland Park, Kan: National Collegiate Athletic Association; November 1992.

TABLE 12-3. National Collegiate Athletic Association Injury Rate by Type of Injury

Sport (Sex)	Con-tusion	Tendin-itis	Ligament Sprain		Muscle–Tendon Strain		Frac-ture	Stress Frac-ture	Con-cussion	Heat Exhaust-ion	Inflam-mation
			In-complete Tear	Com-plete Tear	In-complete Tear	Com-plete Tear					
Gymnastics (W)	0.98	0.30	2.73	0.46	2.43	0.03	0.30	0.30	0.19	0.00	0.25
Gymnastics (M)	0.60	0.20	1.59	0.00	1.00	0.00	0.40	0.00	0.00	0.00	0.30
Basketball (W)	0.50	0.21	1.79	0.21	0.78	0.03	0.28	0.20	0.17	0.00	0.18
Basketball (M)	0.80	0.20	2.23	0.09	1.06	0.03	0.39	0.07	0.10	0.00	0.15
Soccer (W)	0.92	0.33	2.12	0.23	2.20	0.07	0.44	0.25	0.23	0.04	0.32
Soccer (M)	1.75	0.19	2.24	0.20	1.98	0.01	0.47	0.03	0.30	0.03	0.20
Lacrosse (W)	0.18	0.18	1.08	0.12	1.83	0.00	0.09	0.33	0.09	0.00	0.33
Lacrosse (M)	1.15	0.30	1.51	0.15	1.24	0.01	0.35	0.06	0.15	0.00	0.11
Field hockey (W)	0.84	0.33	0.88	0.12	1.10	0.02	0.33	0.10	0.08	0.08	0.18
Volleyball (W)	0.23	0.23	1.51	0.05	1.02	0.02	0.13	0.04	0.05	0.02	0.15
Softball (W)	0.51	0.30	0.55	0.11	0.86	0.03	0.34	0.01	0.10	0.00	0.06
Spring football (M)	1.25	0.18	3.23	0.25	1.98	0.03	0.55	0.03	0.20	0.00	0.13
Wrestling (M)	0.69	0.06	2.46	0.14	1.63	0.04	0.27	0.03	0.31	0.03	0.08
Football (M)	0.89	0.08	1.95	0.23	1.29	0.03	0.34	0.03	0.30	0.12	0.10
Ice hockey (M)	1.04	0.02	1.14	0.10	0.79	0.01	0.35	0.01	0.30	0.00	0.01
Baseball (M)	0.44	0.28	0.59	0.06	1.15	0.01	0.25	0.02	0.05	0.00	0.05

* All data are shown as rate per 1000 athletic exposures in 1991 to 1992.
From *NCAA Injury Surveillance System*. No. 9044. Overland Park, Kan: National Collegiate Athletic Association, November 1992.

young athlete tends to experience injuries in the form of sprains, strains, and contusions. In contrast, Grossman and Nicholas noted that knee injuries in the aged consist of chondromalacia patellae, ruptured patellar tendons, and degenerative arthritis.[14]

Therapeutic Intervention

Principles of Treatment

Although therapeutic management principles for treating athletic injuries are similar regardless of the specific injury, the implementation can vary a great deal (Box 12-1). The first and most important of these principles is complete diagnosis of the injury. A complete diagnosis includes the primary and any existing secondary anatomic and functional deficits. Knowing the mechanism of injury is necessary when evaluating an acute injury, whereas more in-depth questioning is necessary when evaluating a

chronic injury. An example of such a history could include multiple sprains of progressively increasing severity and any subsequent rehabilitation. In the choice between land or aquatic formats, an athlete's history is a significant factor in the plan and outcome of treatment. The second principle in injury management is early intervention. After trauma, an early objective is inflammation control. Methods of controlling inflammation have been conveniently summarized into the well known mnemonic, RICE'M—rest, ice, compression, elevation, and mobilization. Used in moderation, RICE'M can maintain the proper vascular flow vital to healing progression.[15] Genuario and Vegso found water to be advantageous for controlling swelling in injured athletes.[16] The hydrostatic pressure of water at the 4-foot depth more than doubles the pressure of the standard elastic bandage wrap.[16] The combination of a pressurized environment and buoyancy allows for early and safe therapeutic intervention, thus promoting a quick return to previous athletic function. A balance between immobilization for tissue healing and early mobilization for health of the tissue must be obtained. The deleterious effects of immobilization on soft tissue and bone are well documented (Table 12-4). Supportive devices such as neoprene sleeves, braces, or taping can be used on land and in the water to allow healing, and the aquatic medium can be used for controlled mobility.[17,18]

Maintaining or regaining an athlete's cardiovascular condition is also an important aspect of early intervention. Many studies have demonstrated the positive effects of continued exercise on healing tissues.[15,19–22] Some effects include increased blood flow and neurologic stimulation, with minimization of adjacent tissue weakness and adverse psychological effects. However, the athlete must understand and work within the constraints of his or her limitations.

The therapist or trainer implements either static or dynamic exercise techniques (Fig. 12-1), depending on the extent and stage of the injury. In the acute stage, and when indicated, it is customary to use static and isometric exercise. Dynamic activity may be contraindicated because of joint compression, vibration, and torsion forces that accompany these techniques. The athlete may be able to perform dynamic exercise earlier in the pool owing to minimization of some of these forces. Earlier intervention may result in a more rapid return to unlimited activity. The resistive component of dynamic exercise appears as isotonic or isokinetic resistance. Each of these resistance formats can have a concentric and eccentric capacity. A concentric contraction involves the generation of force as a muscle shortens; concentric contractions are commonly associated with accelerating movements in sports. Conversely, an eccentric contraction results when the external load exceeds the internal force, resulting in muscle

TABLE 12-4. Adverse Effects of Immobilization

Muscle	Ligament	Joint
Decrease in muscle fiber size	Significant decrease in linear stress, maximum stress, and stiffness	Reduction in water and GAG content, decreasing the extracellular matrix
Decrease in miliochondia size and number	Decrease in ligament libral cross-sectional area, resulting in a reduction in libral size and density	Reduction in extracellular matrix associated with decrease in lubrication between fiber cross-links
Decrease in total muscle weight		
Increase in muscle contraction time	Decrease in synthesis and depredation of collagen fibers	
Decrease in muscle tension produced	Haphazard arrangement of collagen fibers	Reduction in collagen mass
Decrease in resting length of glycogen and ATP	Reduction in load and energy-absorbing capabilities of the bone–ligament complex	Increase in collagen turnover, degradation rate, and synthesis rate
More rapid decrease in the ATP level with exercise		Increase in abnormal collagen fiber cross-links
Increase in lactate concentration with exercise	Decrease in the GAG level	Reduction in hyaluronic acid
Decrease in protein synthesis	Increase in osteoclastic activity at the bone–ligament junction, causing an increase in bone resorption in that area	

ATP, adenosine triphosphate; GAG, glycosaminoglycan.
Adapted from Andrews JR, Harrison GI. *Physical Rehabilitation of the Injured Athlete*. Philadelphia, Pa: WB Saunders; 1991.

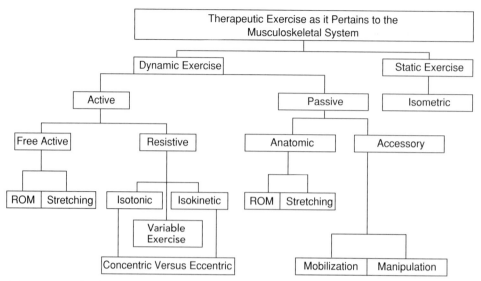

FIGURE 12-1. The characteristics of therapeutic exercise as it pertains to treatment of the musculoskeletal system. ROM, range of motion.

lengthening. These contractions are often found with decelerating movement patterns. Creating or regaining balance of the concentric and eccentric components of a movement pattern is an important component of athletic rehabilitation. As is discussed later, an aquatic program offers the opportunity to use these contractions early in the rehabilitation process.

The Proprioceptive Factor

Most sports consists of a series of movements assembled to create a skillful, coordinated activity. The success of many sports lies in the ability to repeat this skilled activity at high speeds. The high speeds in sports are also associated with compressive, distractive, and torsional forces of great magnitude. A finely tuned communication system integrates all the components of these high-speed activities. The lemniscal system, a component of the somatic afferent system, is responsible for the perception, transmission, and integration of messages to the central nervous system. These messages contain information about position and movement of joints, as well as muscle stretch and other vibratory and tactile stimuli. The mechanoreceptors perceiving the proprioceptive information are located in muscles, ligaments, tendons, and joint capsule. The threshold of excitation and the adaptation capabilities of these receptors vary and are critical to

the stabilization of a joint.[23] The onset of injury to a joint may cause an alteration or even disruption of mechanoreceptor activity, which may lead to changes in neuromuscular control. A variety of studies have shown significant alterations in the protective reflex arc, conscious detection of joint motion, or reproduction of joint position.[19–22] The human body has a tremendous capacity to compensate for such deficits and to accommodate to a multitude of situations. However, the extent of dynamic joint stability that can be regained through neuromuscular means is still unknown.

The process of retraining the athlete with proprioceptive deficits should center on the theme of awareness. The proprioceptive rehabilitation goal is to maximize sensory input with submaximal efforts. Through structured repetition, neuromuscular control can occur on the subconscious level. The joint must then experience the speed, amplitude, and extents in range necessary to recreate functional activity. Water can be an ideal medium to train for proprioception because of its viscosity. Viscosity provides a slow-motion, three-dimensional resistive environment that facilitates proprioceptive feedback through functional movement patterns. Viscosity allows acceleration and deceleration at protected submaximal levels that can be enhanced by increasing the speed of movement, increasing the surface area of resistance (resistive paddle), adding weight to the moving lever, or incorporating resistive tubing (Box 12-2). This proprioceptive activity enables the athlete safely to incorporate advanced levels of dynamic stabilization earlier in the rehabilitation schedule by decreasing both the demands of deceleration and the joint excursion.

Aquatic Approach to Vertebral Dysfunction in the Athlete

The prevalence of low back pain today has been well documented. Anderson noted that 50% to 80% of the general population will experience low back pain in their lifetimes.[24] The percentage of lumbar spine injuries is consistently lower than that of extremity injuries for specific extremity sports (see Table 12-2). However, the incidence of back injury increases significantly in sports such as gymnastics because of the mechanics involved. Keene and associates found that in collegiate sports, 80% of low back injuries occurred during practice; only 6% during competition; and 14% in the preseason.[25] Fifty-nine percent of these injuries were acute in nature, whereas overuse and pre-existing conditions accounted for 12% and 29%, respectively. The active child has a 4.4% incidence of spondylolytic injury, whereas the adult has a 6% incidence.[26] The young athlete is more prone to stress fracture, whereas the older athlete presents with injuries involving degenerative conditions. As such, an in-depth understanding of biomechanics for the involved joints and the sport is essential.

The three most basic mechanisms of injury to the spine consist of compression, distraction, and rotation. An axial compression load, commonly experienced in football and weightlifting, can fracture the endplate or the vertebral body. The intervertebral disc is commonly injured dur-

ing rotational forces, leading to tears in the anular fibers. Avulsion fractures within the spinous and transverse processes can also occur after twisting maneuvers. Secondary to the lordotic shape of the lumbar spine and the vector forces involved, the neutral arch is susceptible to stress fractures, or spondylolysis.

Correct diagnosis is essential to appropriate treatment. The evaluation should include in-depth subjective and objective examinations. The use of radiographs and scans can be helpful in the diagnosis of stress fracture, infections, or spondylolytic defects. One study noted a positive bone scan in 35% of young athletes treated for lower back pain.[27] Watkins and Dillin documented the presence of spondylolytic defects in 30% to 38% of routine radiographs.[28] Electromyographic and nerve conduction velocity studies would be introduced if peripheral nerve injury or entrapment was suspected. A well thought-out evaluation guides the mode of treatment as well as the initial speed of progression of activity.

As the various components of the injury are identified, specific treatment modalities can be implemented. During the acute phase, the use of the various ultrasound waves, high-voltage stimulators, and transcutaneous nerve stimulators has shown success in pain management, controlling inflammation and aiding the healing process, often in conjunction with oral or injected medications.[23,29,30] Aquatic therapy should also be considered at this time. The clinician needs a working knowledge of the physical properties and benefits of an aquatic medium, as well as an understanding of the timing of aquatic intervention, to attain the maximum benefit. It is important to remember that aquatic intervention is a treatment technique that can be used as an adjunct to a standard land protocol.

The cardinal rules for considering aquatic therapy for a client are as follows:

1. Aquatic treatment is only one component of the rehabilitation process. It is not an all-inclusive program.
2. Not every client is a candidate for aquatic treatment.
3. Functional transition from water to land must take place.
4. Fear of the water is an absolute contraindication.

The ultimate goals of an aquatic therapy program are the same as for any land program. Successful rehabilitation requires maintenance of a

TABLE 12-5. Outline of Four-Treatment–Progression Program for the Lower Back

Level I: Stabilization Phase
- Acclimation to the water environment
- Unload gravitational loads
- Progressive trunk stabilization

Level II: Mobility Phase
- Begin single-plane movement patterns
- Increase trunk stabilization endurance

Level III: Dynamic Phase
- Begin multiple-plane movement patterns
- Reciprocal upper/lower extremity

Level IV: Independent Phase
- Increase gravitational loads
- Increase speed and resistance
- Use sport-specific format

consistent, regimented protocol of objectives, as well as problem-solving skills. A goal-oriented rehabilitation format should be used, with specific attention to client outcomes. A home program must be implemented immediately, with a proposed exercise progression and time frame. This allows the athlete to visualize a continuum of events, and to take responsibility for attaining those goals. Because their athletic success before injury was attained by a regimented training program, athletes usually relish the opportunity to restore independence and take control of their program. The following is a four-level sample outlining various goals, techniques, and problem-solving situations typical of an athlete with a lower spine injury (Table 12-5).

Level I

The first level of aquatic intervention consists of pain control and mobility by unloading the vertebral segments and initiating vertical trunk stabilization. Because gravitational compression forces are minimized with immersion, the athlete's low back pain usually diminishes. The vertical position is used in this format because of its mechanical advantage and functional capacity. The mechanical advantage lies in a stabilization axis that is created at the midpoint between the center of buoyancy (T2–T4) and the center of gravity (L5–S2). The level of stabilization is progressed by decreasing the lateral assistance of the extremities (Fig. 12-2).

By using a vertical format, the athlete is able to decrease actions of the extremities while facilitating the trunk's ability to control the center of gravity. Further resistance can be provided by placing buoyancy cuffs on the lower extremities.

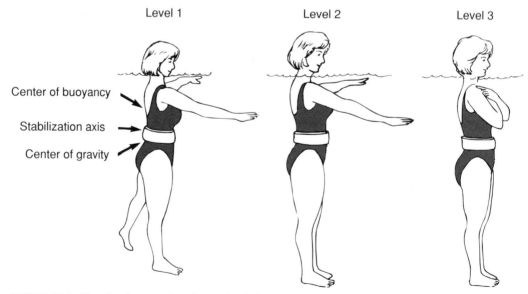

Level 1   Level 2   Level 3

Center of buoyancy

Stabilization axis

Center of gravity

FIGURE 12-2. Three-level progression of vertical stabilization.

Many functional positions, such as sitting, kneeling, and supine, can also be used to alter the length of tension relationships and add various levels of difficulty.

At this level, the client must be progressively challenged through functional movement patterns. The practitioner initially uses the client's body movements to facilitate these patterns, followed by use of equipment of many shapes and sizes. A variety of aquatic devices are effective in providing assistance or resistance as needed. In hopes of someday standardizing equipment design criteria, the following categories have been designated (Table 12-6). A surface-area–resistive device is a flat object, often made of rigid plastic, that creates resistance perpendicular to its surface when it is moved in water. These devices are made for the upper and lower extremities. The level of resistance is a function of the size of the device and the speed of movement. A gravity-reversed device is any product that floats in water. Most are made of various types of foam. The resistance from a gravity-reversed product depends on the energy expended to hold the product under water for a period of time. The devices with a round configuration provide only gravity-reversed resistance. However, some foam products are square or even triangular, and thus increase resistance by providing both gravity-reversed and surface-area qualities. All these devices can be effective in facilitating or inhibiting the desired muscle activity. A weighted glove, ankle or wrist cuffs, or resistive tubing also can add levels of resistance when implemented properly. In many cases, the therapist or trainer may wish to exploit the active-assistive qualities of buoyancy and not use weighted products. However, when dealing with an athlete, a weighted device can facilitate subtle, early, eccentric properties. Eccentric formats dominate the rehabilitation process in the later phases.

Level II

The goals at this level depend and build on the success of the previous level. An increasing level of integration is required as the athlete progresses from proximal to distal efforts. The program continues to emphasize kinesthetic awareness of the trunk region through altered positional alignments or use of resistive equipment. The level of aquatic intervention concentrates on patterns of mobility. The athlete is now introduced to a series of unidirectional extremity movement patterns to advance further the motor control learning process. These patterns are performed in waist-deep water to facilitate the movement and therefore lessen the stabilization demands on the trunk. A multidirectional format should be implemented, using assistive or resistive means to accomplish the desired effect. The speed and complexity of movement are kept to a minimum to maximize feedback and adaptation abilities. A variety of buoyancy ankle cuffs, resistive tubing bands, or resistive paddles can be applied to the upper or lower extremities. A qualitative approach must be maintained to discourage undesirable movement patterns. This level provides a measure of the clinician's problem-solving capabilities.

Level III

As the athlete continues to adapt to stabilization demands, more involved movement patterns are implemented. Altering the velocity of movement is now appropriate as a means of progression. An increased functional format is incorporated as upper and lower extremity movements are combined. The movement patterns are performed in an opposing fashion, to accommodate trunk stabilization. This includes the agonist and antagonist movements of the trunk, as well as functional reciprocal extremity movements. The active-assistive capacity (buoyancy) of water, combined with the force production capabilities of long lever arm movements, can create problems for the athlete at any level. For example, a repetitive straight leg movement pattern has the potential to increase nerve tension, leading to increased irritability. For this reason,

TABLE 12-6. Categories of Aquatic Resistance

Type of Resistance	Example
Surface area	Paddle, glove, boot (LE)
Gravity reversed	Foam dumbbell or cuff (LE)
Weighted	Weighted glove, ankle or wrist weights
Tubing	Resistive bands

LE, lower extremity.

a short lever arm approach for hip flexion–extension is more practical.

When the athlete gains the ability to stabilize the trunk during the reciprocal upper and lower extremity movement patterns, a variety of patterns can be formatted into a timed program. The timed programs should concentrate on speed specificity as well as functional cardiovascular training. A constant challenge can be provided by varying the intervals.

Level IV

The fourth and final level is the independent/resistive phase. The goals again relate to specificity of movement. However, unlike the unloading that characterized level I, the athlete must now progressively load the spine, to prepare for return to full unlimited activity. The athlete performs sport-specific activities in decreasing depths of water. A sport-specific effort is one that mimics a functional movement pattern, eventually recreating the type, force, and velocity of contraction.

Aquatic Approach to Lower Extremity Injuries in the Athlete

Much research exists on the subject of lower extremity injuries in athletics. The complex mechanical relationships that characterize the kinetic chain contribute to a high incidence of lower extremity injury. The biomechanical structure can further complicate the situation by predisposing the athlete to various lower extremity injuries. For clarity, the lower extremity is covered as a whole, and distinctions among the hip, knee, and ankle are provided as needed.

The athlete with a lower extremity injury immediately discovers the profound advantages of an aquatic environment. Similar to the experiences of the back client, the influence of buoyancy is instant and timely. The presence of hydrostatic pressure provides support to the lower extremity, and increased proprioceptive feedback. The pool environment allows better control of ground reaction forces, but significant shearing and compression forces can still be created. Therefore, proper footwear for shallow water workouts should be worn. Special consid-

erations for soft tissue healing may require the use of waterproof bracing as well.

Level I

The initial phase of aquatic intervention for lower extremity involvement is one of unloading and stabilization. Regardless of the area involved, the goals are to decrease overload and maintain proprioceptive input. The extent and type of injury determine the percentage of weight bearing allowed, as well as the timing of aquatic intervention. If an incision is involved, complete closure should be attained before entering the water. Surgical adhesives or biooclusive pads can hasten the latency period.

Initial concerns include range of motion, enhanced circulation, and decreased pain. Maintaining strength, endurance, and proprioceptive abilities are additional, secondary goals. Mobilization techniques, modality treatments, and various rehabilitative exercises are commonly used to accomplish these goals. However, the various constraints imposed by gravity and buoyant environments are the determinants for selecting an activity to be performed in one environment instead of the other. For example, in the early stages of a lower extremity injury, gait training is much more effective in chest-deep water than on land, whereas joint mobilization techniques are often more effective on land.

Initially, the athlete should work extensively on existing range of motion in gait deficits. The water can be used to facilitate muscle activity or inhibit compensatory movement patterns. The early application of progressive dynamic stabilization in a semiloaded lower or upper extremity is one of water's most valuable contributions. The therapist's or trainer's underwater analysis and feedback are imperative during this gait training progress.

The initial critical areas of stabilization are the pelvis and the hip. An athlete must first master sufficient proximal muscle control before attempting dynamic stabilization throughout the remaining kinetic chain. In the early stages, only unidirectional forces are applied, whether the format be open or closed chain. The varying effects of an open versus a closed kinetic chain format must be considered with respect to ligamentous injuries to the knee. Various methods of progression include altering the water depth, the speed or duration of the activity, and the lever arm length, or adding resistive devices.

Level II

This phase should incorporate a progressively dynamic format. The athlete continues to work on isolated exercises for range of motion, gait pattern (forward, backward, and side-to-side if indicated), balance, and cardiovascular conditioning. Functional exercises in a single plane may incorporate varieties of step-up, walking, running, or cross-country skiing patterns. Because endurance workouts are typically longer in duration, timed interval sessions can add more structure to the workout and are easier to communicate to the athlete and other treating clinicians. The athlete uses only minimal resistance in this level. A profound effort to achieve precision of movement is made before advancing to level III.

The therapeutic land program continues with mobilization of the involved joint tissues until full range of motion is achieved. Open and closed kinetic chain exercises can progress, correcting for any compensations. Various resistive devices or manually applied techniques should be implemented, pending the stability of the surrounding structures.

Level III

Training progressions with strong functional undertones dominate this level. Successful transition to full unrestricted activity requires the therapist or trainer to have a working knowledge of the phases and time frame of tissue healing. An unlimited variety of directional and resistance alterations are implemented to continuously facilitate or challenge the client. The athlete experiences a transition from deep to progressively shallower water. This transition can significantly increase the amount of joint loading and torque production. Protective footwear is likely needed to increase traction or to protect the feet from abrasive pool surfaces.

Cardiovascular training continues with emphasis on total-body conditioning. However, these activities can now be performed in increasing weight-bearing environments. As the athlete's stabilization capabilities continue to progress, the levels of torque, compression, and functional standing must increase concurrently. The functional training formats in water at this level could include static jumping, dynamic leaping, and multiple-plane trotting with frequent starts and stops. Emphasis should be placed on slower speeds to highlight quality of movement, as well as absorption of eccentric torque. The innovative use of aquatic equipment can further inhibit or facilitate such movement patterns.

Land training also takes on a more functional format. The movement patterns involved in the particular sport serve as a profile for the rehabilitation progression. However, the athlete should perform only isolated patterns at walking speeds, avoiding any jumping activities in full weight-bearing positions. The state of the injured tissue dictates the nature of any impactive activity starting at this stage.

Level IV

The rehabilitation program warrants structure and consistency throughout all phases. The transition back to gravity, speed, and multisurface training requires close supervision. The viscosity of water provides decreased eccentric overload, and therefore water is a good medium for functional capacity testing of the athlete. A high-speed, multidirectional format is recommended. An unlimited variety of sport-specific activities can be used, incorporating vertical or horizontal patterns of displacement.

The goals of aquatic programming mimic those on land. The physiologic aspects of training are the same and they provide a framework for the construction of a rehabilitation program. The principles of overload must be incorporated for segmental strength gains. However, athletic rehabilitation requires specific adaptation to imposed demands (SAID principle). The variables of frequency, duration, and mode of treatment are the tools available to fulfill those demands.

Aquatic Approach to Upper Extremity Injury in the Athlete

The rate of injury to the upper extremities is significantly lower than that to the lower extremity. Injuries to the shoulder account for 8% to 13% of all athletic injuries.[31] The anatomy of the shoulder complex allows extensive mobility at the cost of stability. An intricate balance between the two is necessary for the athlete to perform his or her skill. The most common mechanisms of shoulder injury include direct contact or repetitive microtrauma. The most common clinical presentations are glenohumeral instabilities, impingement syndromes, and eccentric tendon overload injuries.[32] The highest incidence of wrist injuries is found in gymnastics, whereas the elbow is the joint least injured because of its bony and ligamentous stability.

The concept of unloading the shoulder complex differs from the applications to the lower extremity and spine. The goal of decreasing gravity's compressive forces on bony articulations is no longer appropriate. Gravity applies a downward distractive force to the glenohumeral complex, which is counteracted by the upward pull of the soft tissues. Buoyancy can facilitate the deltoid for humeral head elevation and abduction. Therefore, buoyancy has the capacity to unload the downward pull of gravity on the shoulder complex. The contributions of buoyancy are most applicable when the client has trouble raising the upper extremity because of pain, tissue restriction, or nerve damage.

Before implementing any treatment to the athlete's shoulder, a number of considerations must be made, including the history, any previous injury, the mechanism of injury, and the findings of physical and radiographic examination.

Level I

The initial application of aquatic treatment for many shoulder injuries is to assist deficits of motion. The active-assistive qualities of water can facilitate upper extremity motion, preventing adhesion formation and increasing nutrition. This process can be further enhanced by the use of various foam dumbbells, barbells, or cuffs. When distraction is indicated, pool attachment devices such as the Aquatic Therapy Bar can facilitate progressive range of motion through appropriate distractive forces (Fig. 12-3).

The appropriateness of resistive exercise in water at this early stage depends on the constraints of the healing tissue, as well as the stage of the injury. A surface-area–resistance device (eg, paddle) can add progressive resistance. However, there is a strong tendency to overgrip this device, frequently causing excessive scapular elevation. This tendency can be overcome by using resistive gloves instead of paddles, thereby negating the influence of gripping. A gravity-reversed resistance device (eg, foam dumbbell) can be effective in resisting the agonist muscle group while providing assistance to

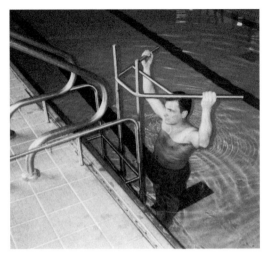

FIGURE 12-3. Pool attachment devices such as the Aquatic Therapy Bar can facilitate progressive range of motion through appropriate distractive forces.

the antagonist. Proper positioning of the body segment is critical to attain the desired effect. An air-filled ball held under the water at varied depths and positions can increase stabilization demands to the shoulder.

The therapeutic land program should continue to emphasize maintaining or regaining the full extensibility and strength of all involved tissues. A home program emphasizing static stretching as well as manual mobilization of surrounding soft tissue structures should be implemented.

Level II

The athlete should progress to an isotonic format in water in this phase. Both resistive formats (gravity reversed and surface area) can be used to isolate specific muscle groups. To increase the resistance, the athlete can either increase the surface area or increase the speed. The gravity-reversed product (eg, foam dumbbells) applies its resistance in an upward direction. To increase that resistance, the size of the foam material or the duration of the exercise should be increased. It becomes evident that the properties of buoyancy have multiple applications to the rehabilitation of the shoulder (Table 12-7). The same property that provided active-assistive qualities in level I now provides isotonic resistance and dynamic stabilization.

As the healing constraints of the tissue allow repetitive movements, the cardiovascular train-

TABLE 12-7. Applications of Buoyancy to the Upper Extremity

Type	Equipment Required	Desired Results
Assistive	Foam dumbbell Foam barbell Foam cuff	Increased range of motion Neuromuscular reeducation Decreased adhesion formation
Resistive	Small foam dumbbell Large foam dumbbell Triangular dumbbell Square dumbbell Air-filled ball	Scapulothoracic stabilization Glenohumeral stabilization

ing format should incorporate the upper extremities. The demands of using surface-area resistance over prolonged time periods make it unsuitable at this level. The gravity-reversed equipment is a better choice for initial endurance training.

Concurrently, the stabilization program should be progressed. The air-filled ball technique can promote progressive stabilization of both scapulothoracic and glenohumeral joints. Altering the position of the athlete with respect to the ball, introducing two balls, or varying the size of the balls adds difficulty. As the athlete masters increasing levels of stabilization, the duration of the workouts should increase accordingly. Closed kinetic chain techniques are commonly used to increase shoulder stability. These exercises require an apparatus for multiple gripping positions. A pool with a gutter system or installed grab bars can accommodate some of these requirements. Progression of exercises incorporating pushing and pulling maneuvers can recreate quick reversals from concentric to eccentric modes.

The goals of the land program at this level include full range of motion, proximal joint stability, and improved distal muscular strength and endurance. Precautions must be observed to protect the healing tissues. The quality of movement patterns must be closely supervised at all times. Isometric, isotonic, and isokinetic formats should be implemented as indicated.

Level III

The levels of resistance, duration, and functional content of the exercises should all be progressed in level III. As the athlete makes gains in strength, endurance, and the ability to stabilize

the proximal segments, functional capacity must be progressed. Whether the demands placed by the sport on the upper extremity are to throw, hit, or lift, the clinician must progressively recreate each phase of the pattern. The phases of sports activities routinely consist of acceleration (concentric emphasis), momentum, and deceleration (eccentric emphasis) components. Success in a sporting activity depends on the body's ability to control its pattern of displacement through rapid alterations in speed, direction, and resistance. The aquatic exercises continue to use increased levels of resistance and duration as progressing elements. However, more provocative functional positions are used. The closed kinetic chain techniques should be performed with increasing degrees of humeral abduction and rotation. Supervision must be maintained at this level to control the extent of torque and range of motion produced. Because the athlete is using his or her own body weight as resistance, the speed of the exercise is the method of progression.

The emphasis in land treatment should continue to be proximal stabilization of the scapulothoracic joint. Combinations of open and closed kinetic chain formats should be introduced and progressed according to the athlete's needs. Special considerations must be taken with closed chain techniques because of the joint compression demands. Advanced technology in biofeedback on land and in water provides worthwhile opportunities to increase specialized treatment as well as objective data.

Level IV

Level IV effects a transition from aquatic training to land training and finally to unrestricted activity by progressively increasing speed and functional content. The aquatic format up to this point has used patterns of movement below 90 degrees of elevation. Performing 180-degree movements of the upper extremity in water presents some problems. The difficulty of providing an air supply to a completely submerged vertical subject necessitates the use of alternative positions. To attain motion above the 90-degree plane, the athlete can use prone supine or side-lying positions. Performing aquatic activities for the upper extremity in supine negates efforts in the sagittal plane. Using a mask and snorkel in prone appears to be the most realistic alternative. Flotation belts are used to orient the trunk and lower extremities along with surface of the water. Progressions of single- to multiple-plane proprioceptive neuromuscular facilitation diagonal patterns should be used. Bilateral, reciprocal, upper and lower extremity patterns are used to help maintain trunk balance. Foam dumbbells are used to provide consistent resistance to the upper extremities. The athlete should progressively increase the speed and duration of the closed kinetic chain exercises. Increasing speed of the activity decreases the resultant reaction time. This prepares the dynamic stabilizers of the shoulder for the demands of athletic activity.

The athlete can experience further levels of progression by incorporating a format of sport-specific techniques. Many pieces of sporting equipment can either be used directly or adapted to the water (Fig. 12-4). The advantages

of using sports equipment in the water are two-fold. First, the surface area of the device promotes resistance throughout each component of the kinetic chain, enhancing strength and endurance gains. Second, the athlete experiences a superior level of neuromuscular re-education while working against the viscosity of the water. This is particularly beneficial for rehabilitating injuries to the elbow, wrist, or phalanx because of the fine motor movement patterns involved.

Land treatment at this level probably takes place on the athlete's field of play. The therapist or trainer is responsible for creating a regimented performance schedule. A strict time frame is enforced for this oriented program. The athlete must follow each level closely so that excessive forces are not applied prematurely.

Summary

The idea of using an aquatic medium to train an athlete has existed for many years, but the extent of its application was limited. The combination of increased biomechanical knowledge and access to an aquatic environment has opened the door to a wealth of opportunity for the health care provider. The acceptance of aquatic intervention as a tool for athletic training and rehabilitation has become widespread.

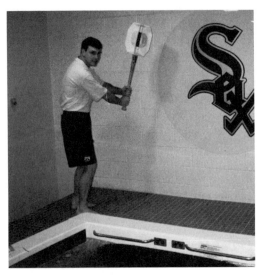

FIGURE 12-4. The athlete can experience further levels of progression by incorporating a format of sport-specific techniques.

REFERENCES

1. Overview. *Nike Sport Research Review.* July/August, 1988:1.
2. Valiant GA. Ground reaction forces developed on artificial turf. In: Reilly T, Lees A, Davids K, Murphy W, eds. *Science and Football.* London: E & F. N. Spon; 1988:406–415.
3. Nigg BM, Segesser B. The influence of playing surfaces on football and tennis injuries. *Sports Med.* 1988;5:375–385.
4. Korzick DH. Ground reaction forces in aerobic dancing. *Med Sci Sports Exerc.* 1987;19(Suppl 2):S90.
5. Knight K. The effects of hyperthermia on inflammation and swelling. *Athletic Training.* 1976;11(1):7.
6. Garrick JG, Requa RK. The epidemiology of foot and ankle injuries in sports. *Clin Sports Med.* 1988;7: 29–36.
7. Whitman PA, Melvin JA. Common problems seen in the metropolitan sports injury clinic. *Physical Sports.* 1981;9:105–110.
8. DeHaven KE, Litner DM. Athletic injuries: comparison by age, sport and gender. *Am J Sports Med.* 1986; 14:218–224.
9. Fairbank JC, Pynsent PB, Van Poortvliet JA, et al. Influence of anthropomorphic factors and joint laxity in the incidence of adolescent pain. *Spine.* 1984;9: 461–464.

10. Fisk JW, Baigent ML, Hill PD. Scheuermann's disease: clinical and radiological survey of 17 and 18 year olds. *Am J Sports Med.* 1984;63:18–30.
11. National Collegiate Athletic Association. *NCAA Injury Surveillance System.* Overland Park, Kan: National Collegiate Athletic Association; 1992–1993.
12. Protzman RR, Bodnari LM. Women athletes. *Am J Sports Med.* 1980;8:53–55.
13. Goldberg B. Injury patterns in youth sports. *Physical Sports Medicine.* 1980;17:175–184.
14. Grossman RB, Nicholas JA. Common disorders in the knee. *Orthop Clin North Am.* 1977;8:619–624.
15. Woo SL-Y, Buckwalter JA, eds. *Injury and Repair of the Musculoskeletal Soft Tissue.* Park Ridge, Ill: American Academy of Orthopaedic Surgeons; 1988.
16. Genuario SE, Vegso JJ. The use of a swimming pool in the rehabilitation and reconditioning of athletic injuries. *Contemporary Orthopaedics.* 1990;20: 381–387
17. Groppel JL, Nirschi RP. A mechanical and electromyographical analysis of the effects of various counter force braces on the tennis player. *Am J Sports Med.* 1986;14:195–200.
18. Ott J, Clancy WG. Functional knee braces: a review. *Orthopaedics.* 1993;16:171–176.
19. Roy S, Irvin R. *Sports Medicine: Prevention, Evaluation, Management and Rehabilitation.* Englewood Cliffs, NJ: Prentice-Hall; 1983.
20. Salter RB. *Continuous Passive Motion—CPM: A Biological Concept for Healing and Regeneration of Articular Cartilage, Ligaments, and Tendons, From Organization to Research to Clinical Applications.* Baltimore, Md: Williams & Wilkins; 1993.
21. Kibler WB, Chandler RJ, Stracener ES. Musculoskeletal adaptations and injury due to overtraining. *Exerc Sport Sci Rev.* 1992;20:99.
22. Frank CB, Hart DA. Cellular response to loading. In: Leadbetter WB, Buckwalkte JA, Gordon SL, eds. *Sports Induced Inflammation: Clinical and Basic Science Concepts.* Park Ridge, Ill: American Academy of Orthopaedic Surgeons; 1990:555.
23. Repachcoli MH, Benwell DA, eds. *Essentials of Medical Ultrasound.* Clifton, NJ: Humana Press; 1982.
24. Anderson G. Epidemiologic aspects on low back pain in industry, *Spine.* 1981;6:60.
25. Keene JS, Albert MJ, Springer SL, et al. Back injuries in college athletes. *J Spinal Disord.* 1986;2:190–195.
26. Watkins RG, Dillin WM. Lumbar spine injuries. *Sports Injuries.* 1994;50:878.
27. Watkins RG, Dillin WM. Lumbar spine injuries. *AJR Am J Roentgenol.* 1985;145:1039–1044.
28. Watkins RG, Dillin WM. Lumbar spine injuries. *Clin Sports Med.* 1985;4:85–93.
29. Bourguignon GJ, Bourguignon M, Bourguignon LWY. Effect of high voltage pulsed galvanic stimulation on human fibroblasts in cell culture: a model system for soft tissue healing [abstract]. *Research Section Newsletter.* APTA, Sept/Oct 1986.
30. Woolf C. Transcutaneous and implanted nerve stimulation. In: Wall PD, Melzack R eds. *Treatment of Pain.* New York, NY: Churchill-Livingstone; 1984:679–690.
31. Hill JA. Epidemiologic perspective on shoulder injuries. *Clin Sports Med.* 1983;2:240–246.
32. Bradley J, DiGiovine N, Tibone J. Shoulder biomechanics in the athlete. In: Pettrone FA, ed. *Athletic Injuries of the Shoulder.* NY, NY: McGraw Hill; 1995: 17–27.

13 Aquatic Rehabilitation of the Client With Cardiovascular Disease

Karen Congdon

In 1980, Eugene Braunwald wrote, "Today cardiovascular disease is the greatest scourge afflicting the population of the industrialized nations."[1] Current data confirm that this assessment is still valid.[2] In fact, 56 million Americans died from some form of cardiovascular disease, 0.5 million from cancer, and 0.3 million from acquired immunodeficiency syndrome. The American Heart Association has verified a significant reduction in death rate from sudden death, heart attack, and stroke of 47% since 1963,[3] and a 25% to 30% reduction over the 1980s.[2] Even with this significant reduction, the American Heart Association urges that more be done, especially in the area of disease prevention.

Statistically, the primary factors in the prevention and retardation of disease are the lowering of blood pressure (BP) and cholesterol and fat intake, the elimination of cigarette smoking, and an increase in regular exercise. The American College of Sports Medicine has made a concerted effort to emphasize the need for exercise. Still, 25% of Americans older than the age of 18 years report no leisure time activity. Independent of other risk factors, coronary heart disease is almost twice as likely to develop in physically inactive people than in active ones. In addition, a person who is less active or fit has a 30% to 50% higher risk for development of high BP.[2]

One of the major goals of cardiac rehabilitation[3–8] is the return of a person to a full and active lifestyle with an improved quality of life. Of equal importance to the economic benefits is the return of the cardiac-insulted person's sense of self-esteem and self-efficacy in the physical domain.[9,10] Aquatic rehabilitation programs provide a means to enhance this goal. They provide cardiovascular conditioning that can help limit coronary artery disease (CAD).[11]

This chapter explores the effects of aquatic cardiac rehabilitation treatment of CAD and myocardial infarction in the clinical setting.

Evolution of Cardiac Rehabilitation

In the early 1900s, cardiac rehabilitation was confined to passive treatment designed to reduce the workload on the heart. Autopsies of people who died after a myocardial infarction revealed a disruption of the myocardium, development of aneurysms, and congestive heart failure. Researchers advocated complete and protracted bed rest, often for several months.[3] It became known that survival is possible as long as less than 40% of the myocardium has been damaged. Greater damage results in complete pump failure. In the 1940s, "arm-chair treatment"[3] was advocated for coronary thrombosis on the assumption that the sitting position would decrease cardiac work by increasing venous pooling and decreasing preload. Controlled studies were not conducted regarding the efficacy of this treatment. It was assumed to be beneficial because there were no reported deleterious effects.

In 1968, a physiologic deconditioning study was performed on healthy male college students.[3] The participants were subjected to enforced bed rest. Results of the study included:

- A decrease of 25% in work capacity
- A drop in blood volume by 750 mL
- Orthostatic hypotension
- Reflex tachycardia
- Increased blood viscosity
- A decrease in muscle mass
- Negative nitrogen balance
- A 15% decrease in muscular contractile strength

This and other studies resulted in a redirection in the treatment and rehabilitation of clients with CAD. At the same time, dramatic changes in client care have contributed to a reduction in the actual size of necrotic tissue or have enabled intervention before any infarct occurs. Indeed, thrombolytic therapy has provided an opportunity to intervene in the infarction process as it happens, thus preserving myocardial tissue. The knowledge gained has increased the number of survivors[3] and has instilled a new awareness of populations now known to be at high risk for CAD. Some changes include the following areas:

Care

- Coronary intensive care units in the 1960s
- Pharmaceuticals in the 1970s and 1980s (Lasix [furosemide], β blockers, calcium channel blockers, angiotensin-converting enzyme inhibitors, and a new role for aspirin)

Aggressive Diagnostics

- Angiography
- Computer-enhanced imaging
- Exercise stress testing with radioisotopes

- Echocardiography
- Positron emission tomography
- Advanced electrophysiologic studies

Definitive Treatment

- Heart transplantation
- Coronary artery bypass graft surgery
- Coronary artery balloon angioplasty, laser intervention, pacemakers
- Automatic cardioverter–defibrillators

The American Association of Cardiovascular and Pulmonary Rehabilitation (AACVPR) defines cardiac rehabilitation as the process by which a person with CAD (including but not limited to clients with coronary heart disease) is restored to and maintained at an optimal physiologic, psychological, social, vocational, and emotional status.[12]

In the 1960s, cardiac rehabilitation programs admitted only noncomplicated survivors of myocardial infarction, and some clients with stabilized angina pectoris. The programs were confined to a gradual exercise regimen, with risk factor modification occupying a secondary position. Current programs accept a much broader range of clients (Table 13-1). Advances in technology have provided a wide range of aids to monitor body functions. These include on-site telemetry, transtelephonic equipment for home programs, and even waterproof telemetry for use in pool head-out water immersion (HOWI) activities (Fig. 13-1).

Pool activities can be initiated based on guidelines established by the AACVPR known as Cardiac Risk Stratification[3,4,13] (Table 13-2). These guidelines enable the clinician to determine the level of medical supervision and electrocardiographic (EKG) monitoring the client needs and

TABLE 13-1. Candidates for Cardiac Rehabilitation

Nonsurgical Candidates	Surgical Candidates
Postmyocardial infarction	Preoperative for any cardiac intervention
Stabilized angina	Coronary artery bypass
Survivors of sudden death	Rotoatherectomy ablation
Peripheral vascular disease	Heart transplantation
Congestive heart failure	Ventricular and aortic aneurysectomy
Myocardopathies, including end-stage renal failure	Ablation treatment for lethal arrhythmias
	Implanted automatic defibrillators
The elderly and medically complex	Pacemaker implantation
	Heart valve surgery (aortic and mitral)

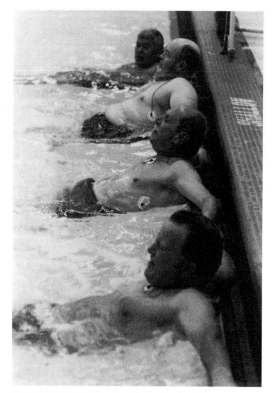

FIGURE 13-1. University of Rhode Island's Aquatic Cardiac Rehabilitation Program. Participants perform head-out water immersion exercises while on electrocardiographic telemetry.

the relative risk of sudden death.[3,10,14–18] Currently, cardiac rehabilitation programs have a holistic focus that fosters safe, appropriate, and independent exercise.[3,4,13,19,20]

Cardiac rehabilitation also seeks to change lifestyle parameters in an effort to ameliorate the effects of coronary disease. Many people are unable to make more than one or two major changes in their lives at a time. Aquatic programs facilitate several changes of lifestyle by extending the exposure of a client to the cardiac rehabilitation team. Over several months, the likelihood of behavioral changes occurring and becoming new habits is greatly increased. Pool aerobics (HOWI activities) should be part of a cardiac rehabilitation program. By their very nature, such activities imbue a much-needed element of fun and increasing independence into otherwise highly structured, medically supervised programs. Low- and moderate-risk people should be included. There is little research on aquatic rehabilitation for "high-risk" people. Typical candidates suitable for aquatic cardiac

rehabilitation would include those defined as low or intermediate risk (see Table 13-2) who have shown compliance with the exercise leader's instructions during terrestrial cardiac rehabilitation.[3,4]

Subjective Responses to Exercise in Water

One of the cornerstones of cardiac rehabilitation consists of reintroducing the "coronary-prone" person to his or her body's kinesthetic or conscious awareness of musculoskeletal movement. Another aspect of cardiac rehabilitation programs is to guide the person to an acceptable level of daily physical activity and fitness. Because the program can make use of physical measurements not available at home or work, it is necessary to provide a subjective means for determining an acceptable level of activity at home as well. Three such scales are available for this purpose:

Borg's Rate of Perceived Exertion (RPE) Scale[21]
The Fatigue and Dyspnea (FAD) Scale
The Pain Scale

These scales are presented in Table 13-3. All three subjective scales fall within the seven perceptual distinctions of Borg.*

People entering a rehabilitation program may be apprehensive or depressed. They begin with no knowledge of their activity limitations. The use of subjective scales should be introduced from the initial exercise stress test or certainly by the beginning of the rehabilitation program. This enables a cross-over of perception to the usual daily activities, increasing participants' control over both themselves and their disease.

The RPE and the FAD scales (see Table 13-3) should be used in conjunction with monitored exercises to provide a benchmark for the client to use. It is not uncommon for clients to experience anginal symptoms during home exercise, but not during rehabilitation classes. A careful recounting of the conditions before the appearance of symptoms usually reveals exercise levels beyond those assigned. Participants also fail to allow for the effects of environmental conditions

---

* Based on 40 years of psychophysiologic research, Borg concluded the human brain can make only seven perceptual distinctions. Although the RPE scale has 20 increments, there are only 7 descriptive levels.

TABLE 13-2. American Association of Cardiovascular and Pulmonary Rehabilitation (AACVPR) Guidelines for Risk Stratification

Risk Level	Characteristics
Low	Uncomplicated clinical course in hospital
	No evidence of myocardial ischemia
	Functional capacity ≥ 7 METs
	Normal left ventricular function; Ejection Fraction (EF) > 50%
	Absence of significant ventricular ectopy
Intermediate (moderate)	Segment depression (ST) ≥ 2 mm, flat or downsloping
	Reversible thallium defects
	Moderate to good left ventricular function; EF 35% to 49%
	Changing pattern or new development of angina pectoris
High	Prior myocardial infarction or infarct involving ≥ 35% of left ventricle
	Poor left ventricular function; EF < 35% at rest
	Fall in exercise systolic blood pressure or failure of systolic blood pressure to rise more than 10 mm Hg on exercise tolerance test
	Persistent or recurrent ischemic pain 24 h or more after hospital admission
	Functional capacity < 5 METs with hypotensive blood pressure response or ≥ 1 mm ST segment depression
	Congestive heart failure syndrome in hospital
	≥ 2-mm segment depression (ST) at peak heart rate ≤ 135 bpm
	High-grade ventricular ectopy

1 metabolic equivalent of task (MET) = 3.5 mL O_2 × kg^{-1} × min^{-1}.
From AACVPR. *Guidelines for Cardiac Rehabilitation Programs.* Champaign, Ill: Human Kinetics 1991. Copyright 1991 by American Association of Cardiovascular and Pulmonary Rehabilitation. Reprinted by permission.

TABLE 13-3. Subjective Test Scales

Rate of Perceived Exertion (RPE)		Fatigue and Dyspnea (FAD) Scale		Pain Scale	
Scale Factor	*Assessment*	*Scale Factor*	*Assessment*	*Scale Factor*	*Assessment*
7	Very, Very Easy	**1**	Mild, Noticeable	**1**	"Just Aware" Something Is Wrong, no Pain Yet
8		**2**	Mild, Some Difficulty	**2**	Definite Pain, Easily Distracted
9	Very Easy	**3**	Moderate, Can Continue	**3**	Definite Pain, not Distracted
10		**4**	Severe, Cannot Continue	**4**	Most Excrutiating, Agony Experienced
11	Fairly Easy				
12					
	Somewhat Hard				
13					
14					
	Hard				
15					
16					
17	Very Hard				
18					
19	Very, Very Hard				
20					

From Hall LK, ed. *Developing and Managing Cardiac Rehabilitation Programs.* 2nd ed. Champaign, Ill: Human Kinetics; 1995; and Wenger NK. Early ambulation after myocardial infarction: the in-patient exercise program. *Clin Sports Med.* 1984;3:333–348.

(temperature, pollution levels, wind, or precipitation). An added dimension of the problem is the marked tendency of coronary-prone people to suppress RPE below expected levels.

The subjective rating of the RPE correlates well with heart rate, oxygen uptake, $\dot{V}_E$ (expired volume), and power output. A subjective rating between 13 and 16 (Somewhat Hard to Hard +) shows correlation to the onset of blood lactate accumulation (70% $\dot{V}_{O_2}$ [oxygen consumption]).[4] Cardiac clients should be kept below this level.

Currently, more clients present for rehabilitation with congestive heart failure or silent ischemia whose only symptoms are fatigue or shortness of breath. The FAD scale (shortness of breath) provides a better monitor than heart rate response and a better measure than the other subjective scales. This technique also works well with concomitant or primary chronic obstructive pulmonary disease.[3,22–24] With these people, ST depression and severe ventricular arrhythmias could be occurring at low RPE levels. This makes correlation between RPE levels[†] and cardiac monitors most important during rehabilitation.

The third subjective scale, the Pain Scale (see Table 13-3), is used by the American College of Sports Medicine and the AACVPR. This scale is particularly useful in teaching pacing. Cardiac victims with stabilized angina and peripheral vascular disease tend to use denial as a major coping tool and ignore many symptomatic (somatic) messages. Pacing, using the Pain Scale, teaches these people that they can continue their activities, but at a slower pace. It provides them with the added benefit of regaining a modicum of control over their disease and symptoms.

Although all three scales apply to the aquatic setting, similar absolute workloads can result in lessened RPE responses in the water environment.[27–33] Fluctuations in air and water temperatures can provoke either angina or claudication from peripheral vascular disease. Some swimming strokes or HOWI walking exercises can also provoke symptoms. The FAD scale has proven more sensitive to a participant's homeostasis than EKG, lung sounds, or changes in vital signs.[25] FAD provides a better indication than the RPE because in the water environment

clients tend to focus more on breathlessness than they do on overall effort. Water exercise appears to mask a sense of effort and the signs and symptoms of ischemia.[27,28]

Blood Pressure

Monitoring BP (and rate-pressure products [RPP][‡]) in a pool environment is essential. A participant in a flume study showed variation in BP and heart rate at two different water temperatures, as shown in Table 13-4.[28]

The University of Rhode Island (URI) study group had an invariant 10% of subjects who had significantly elevated BP (systolic BP > 200, diastolic BP > 100) immediately after pool exercises. A poor cool-down immediately before exiting the pool could cause this phenomenon.[§] All were either recovering from or at risk for CAD, but not all had been diagnosed previously as hypertensive. Because the study occurred over a 7-year period, there were medication changes as well as some physiologic changes. After land exercise, several of the group experienced similar extreme BPs, but to a lesser extent. During water exercise, the temperature of the water was between 30°C to 32°C (86°F to 89°F). Of those being treated for CAD who were not known hypertensives, the terms "hot reactor" or "high cardiovascular reactivity" would apply.[35,36] Other potential contributors to a rise

TABLE 13-4. Effects of Water Temperature on Blood Pressure and Heart Rate

	25°C (77.0°F)	18°C (64.4°F)
Blood pressure (resting)	130/70 mm Hg	200/100 mm Hg
Maximum heart rate	115 bpm	105 bpm

[†] The somatic awareness effect works best in a cardiac population when attention is focused on the *words* of these three scales, and not the *numbers*.[4,5,25,26]

[‡] The RPP is the product of maximum systolic pressure times maximum heart rate at a given load, expressed in scientific notation (10^3).

[§] Because water is fun it is easy to disregard the hemodynamic effect a few extra arm strokes might have on the way to the stairs when class is over and the client is exiting the pool. Those with markedly high BP responses were advised to walk around the deck for a few minutes and always presented with repeat BPs that were adequately lowered.[34]

in BP are α stimulation and circadian (time of day) effects. Both cold water and exercise[10,37] are α stimulants, so some rise in BP is not surprising. Few of this population were being medicated with α-adrenergic inhibitors. Sessions were in the early morning, and many of the subjects had not eaten or taken their medications.

Temperature and Rhythm Disturbances

Aquatic rehabilitation programs must take into account the effects of temperature on energy costs.[38] Because of the vasodilation experienced from swimming in warm water of 35°C to 37°C (95°F to 98°F), subjects are likely to experience an increased heart rate. This is in contrast to the energy lost in water at 27°C to 31°C (80°F to 88°F), and the triggering of the mammalian diving reflex, which results in a lower heart rate. The effects of water temperature at 15°C to 20°C (59°F to 68°F) have also been examined. This environment provokes a higher ventricular irritability, regardless of apneic response (whether the person is diving or holding her breath).

Swimmers with a history of CAD experience serious rhythm disturbances even in more thermoneutral temperatures. Ten such people suffered fatal events while swimming.[39] Postulated causes are that the immersion forces and the horizontal body position in this population increase central volumes and pressures.[38] The same sequence could also be responsible for left ventricular overload with a subsequent decrease in the client's work capability.[38]

The large arm work component in swimming generates greater peripheral vascular resistance than does leg work at the same load on land.[38] At any given submaximal work load, arm exercise by a person with CAD in general results in a higher $\dot{V}o_2$, systolic BP, heart rate, and cardiac output. Peripheral vascular resistance is greater because there is relatively less vasodilation occurring because of the smaller vascular area in the pectoral and arm muscles. Simultaneously, relatively greater vasoconstriction occurs in the more extensive vascular beds of the nonexercising muscles (legs). This provokes a higher diastolic BP during arm activity than during leg exercise at matched submaximal work rates. A rapid rise in heart rate is partially the result of the difference in sympathetic response. Stroke volume augmentation is small because of the relatively small blood volume being pumped by the heart to and from the smaller muscle mass.[4]

In theory, the hydrostatic forces of water immersion should increase stroke volume and mitigate some of this effect. Studies indicate that the afferent branch of the reflex that produces bradycardia[||] in immersed humans appears to have multiple branches. These may include a specific facial receptor response actuated by cool stimuli, thoracic stretch receptors, and aortic or carotid sinus baroreceptors.[38] These immersion reflex changes are cardioinhibitory, leading to sinus bradycardia, sinus arrest (with junction or ventricular escapes), atrioventricular block, and atrioventricular nodal rhythms.[38]

Bradyarrhythmias can cause sudden death in clients with coronary heart disease. The ventricular fibrillation threshold is also lowered. Therefore, the diving reflex is potentially dangerous to people with CAD and to those at risk for sudden death.[38] All heart disease victims have a certain degree of risk for sudden death.[3,17] The risk is greater in those with left ventricular failure or malignant ventricular ectopic histories. These people should be excluded from activities in water cooler than 30°C (86°F) and prevented from diving or plunging their heads into cold water. Considerable caution should be exercised in allowing the untrained exerciser with a history of cardiac disease to swim the crawl.

Hot Tubs and Spas

Warmer water (>34°C [92°F]) causes peripheral vasodilation, which decreases diastolic coronary artery perfusion. This triggers earlier ischemia, similar to that seen in sauna settings.[40] Most jacuzzis and spas warn people with CAD not to exceed 15 minutes at 40°C (104°F). Studies of cardiac clients resting and exercising in 40°C water have identified physiologic changes and provided cautions and contraindications in the use of hot tubs:

Physiologic Changes

- Core temperature is increased 1°C (1.8°F) with exercise
- Lower peak heart rate and systolic BP during immersion than exercise on land
- A slight light-headedness on standing to leave the tub

[||] Heart rate < 60 beats/min.

- Rapid changes in sympathetic, vagal, and hormonal environments
- β Blockers (β_2 effects) inhibit heat tolerance[1,6]

Contraindications to Use of Hot Tub or Spa

- Use of β blockers
- Use of other hypertensive drugs such as diuretics and angiotensin-converting enzyme inhibitors because of massive interactions with the renin–angiotensin–vasopressin axis.
- Advanced age (particularly older than age 70 years) because of considerably lessened orthostatic responses and the extreme vasodilatory effect of hot tubs[41]
- Postural hypotension problems[42]

The conclusions of the studies were that people with stable CAD who are able to perform 8 METs (metabolic equivalents of task) should be able to tolerate 15 minutes in a hot tub at 40°C (104°F). They must sit quietly and be wary of transient hypotension on leaving the tub.

Swimming

Swimming has a place in cardiac rehabilitation, particularly as an adjunct to lifestyle improvement over a life span. The suggested selection criteria for inclusion in a swimming program are at least 2 months postinfarction, no residual ischemia or symptoms, and exercise tolerance of at least 100 watts (closer to 6 METs; Fig. 13-2) for 2 to 3 minutes (see Case Study 13-1). The suggested exclusion criteria are serious arrhythmias or latent cardiac failure, extensive myocardial infarction, and aneurysms.[38] Swimming is also helpful for those who are obese and those with lower limb impairments, muscular problems, pulmonary diseases, rheumatologic diseases, and hemophilia.

The subjective comfort and large muscle groups involved in swimming make it a good exercise. The high relative energy cost and failure to identify ischemic symptoms indicate caution in cardiac clients, especially if their swimming skills are poor.[28] This is corroborated by the 10-year data base at URI. The data also indicate the recommended temperature for cardiac rehabilitation activities to be 30°C to 33°C (86°F to 91°F). At these temperatures, peripheral vasodilation elicits a decrease in the normally high systemic vascular resistance present at least in the lower limbs. On entering the pool, there is a reduction in angina and peripheral vascular

disease symptoms. The participants perceive this as a comfortable temperature. During the first session, the use of water EKG telemetry and frequent BP measurements is strongly recommended. This can be accomplished safely at 4 months postcardiac event (6 months, preferably), which allows for complete cardiac remodeling.

The use of thromboembolytics and better perfusion imaging to identify the more asymptomatic CAD client enables improvement in early myocardial infarction treatment.[2,4,43] As a result, cardiac rehabilitation populations with good left ventricular function have increased significantly. This population particularly benefits from the greater variety and challenge of the pool environment. Those with congestive heart failure and poor left ventricular function (<35% ejection fraction or symptomatic at <3 METs) should be excluded from the rapidly changing hemodynamics brought on by the water environment. Also excluded should be those with serious arrhythmia, aneurysm, or myocardiopathies that have not been stabilized in a terrestrial cardiac rehabilitation environment.

Half the current cardiac population is older than 65 years of age. This population likely exhibits concomitant diseases such as hypertension, diabetes, chronic obstructive pulmonary disease, obesity, low back pain, and arthritis. The pool environment is probably one of the best media for their complete care. For those already well stabilized and healed after their cardiac insult, and well trained, controlled swimming is as good a cardiovascular training stimulus as running or biking.[28,44,45]

Water Exercise for a Cardiac-Based Population

The following guidelines should be considered in admitting and administering a water program for cardiac clients:

Contraindications

1. Unstable angina, symptomatic low ejection fraction (left ventricular failure), congestive heart failure
2. Frequent high-grade ectopy not medically corrected by medication, ablation, or AICD
3. Significant aortic or mitral valve problems
4. Cardiomyopathies

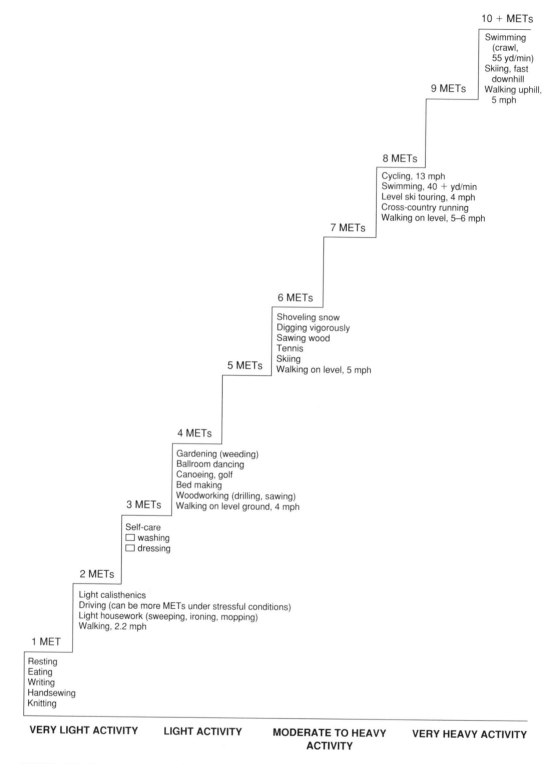

FIGURE 13-2. Energy cost, in metabolic equivalents of task (METs), of activities and exercises. (From Underhill SL, Woods SL, Sivarajan-Froelicher ES, Halpenny CJ. *Cardiac Nursing.* 2nd ed. Philadelphia, Pa: JB Lippincott; 1989.)

Before Entering the Water Program

1. Admit to the water program only after 4 months have elapsed since the cardiac event
2. Know the stabilized physiologic parameters through EKG-monitored, land-based cardiac rehabilitation before entering the water
3. Establish trust and rapport, if possible, before the water program to encourage the best possible communication between the participant and the staff
4. Admit to the program after training becomes comfortable at 5 METs (this should not be the maximum but the daily exercise capability)
5. Target heart rates should be 10 to 20 beats/min less than the land target heart rate (10 beats/min if client is taking β blockers, otherwise 20 beats/min; this ensures lower intensities and decreases the risk of a cardiac event[3])

After Entering the Water Program

1. Monitor via EKG telemetry and BP/RPP during the first exercise session and intermittently thereafter.¶ This is particularly important if the water temperature is greater than 35°C (95°F) or less than 30°C (86°F) when ventricular irritability is increased. It is critical to have the heart rate measured within 6 seconds of the BP measurement and at the last moment of exercise. This validates the RPP measurement,[46] and may require an aide to accomplish. It may be helpful to keep the RPP value 1×10^3 below the participant's normal arm ergometry RPP. A suggested program for a first session is given in the next section.
2. Remind the participants to speak up about symptoms of any sort, and that the most likely symptom will be shortness of breath.
3. Keep the pool between 30°C to 32°C (86°F to 89°F).
4. Use a gradual warm-up, beginning with shallow water walking and gradually increasing the depth and speed. Knowing the first-day data on maximum heart rate in water from RPP, RPE, and EKG measurements, as well as their known symptoms, each participant will be aware of his or her exercise limits. Initially, HOWI exercises should be 10 seconds in duration, with gradual increases and alternation between the upper and lower body. There should be frequent rest periods that can be used to measure heart rate.
5. Check heart rate frequently (at least every 5 to 10 minutes) depending on the needs of most of the class. Assign a second person to take the measurements of the slower members. Record the heart rate for comparisons between land and water readings.
6. Include some group activity with a ball (eg, inner tube basketball or water volleyball).[47–49]
7. Obtain a "resting" BP before entry and after exit from the pool, particularly for hypertensive clients.
8. Include a lap swim or extended walking time especially for a robust group.
9. Keep those who are short in stature in shallow water (hemodynamic effects are different above the waist-to-nipple line area).[41]
10. Discourage competition. Nothing is quite as potent as competition to provoke coronary-prone personalities.
11. Include a long cool-down period because malignant ectopy is most likely to occur at the end of exercise. This is the time of greatest catecholamine surge.[1]
12. Make it fun!

Initial Session Protocol

Obtain measurements on pre-exercise EKG, heart rate, and BP. During maximal exercise, obtain data on heart rate, BP, and RPE until either fatigue or symptoms are reached. Also obtain postexercise heart rate and BP. Observe and record the following responses:

1. Initial response to the water
2. A slow walk, short distance and long distance#
3. A fast walk, short distance and long distance
4. A fast walk in deep water (nipple high), using the arms
5. Easiest swimming stroke, short distance with head out of water (eg, back stroke, side stroke, dog paddle)

¶ This requires a little ingenuity. One method would be to tape a standard sphygmomanometer cuff to the arm and to follow the participant in shallow water with a staff member holding the bulb and its valve out of the water. For longer sessions, a plastic bag can be placed over the cuff in addition to taping it in place. The staff member can then inflate the cuff while the participant is exercising and take the reading as soon as the motion stops.

Short distance—width of the pool; long distance—length of the pool. URI data show the most common reason for discontinuing is shortness of breath and fatigue.

6. Easiest swimming stroke, long distance
7. Next easiest swimming stroke, short distance with head out of water
8. A slow crawl, short distance and long distance
9. A fast crawl, short distance and long distance
10. Stop when the participant:
    Exceeds his or her land exercise target heart rate
    Evinces symptoms
    Exhibits EKG changes

❏ CASE STUDY 13-1

Subject Definition and Medical History
- 62-year-old man, lifelong swimmer
- Preoperative complaint: air hunger while swimming leading to jaw pain and leg cramps
- Family history of hypertension and death by myocardial infarction (both parents)
- Employed as an executive (consultant during cardiac rehabilitation)
- Smoked since 20 years of age, and stopped before program entrance
- Triple-bypass surgery
- Medications: Cardizem (diltiazem), Persantine (dipyridamole), and Ventolin (albuterol) and Aerobid (flunisolide) inhalers

Postsurgery and Land Cardiac Rehabilitation History
- Records showed periodic occurrences of ventricular bigeminy
- Nocturnal asthmatic attack while in cardiac rehabilitation (emergency room visit); prescribed low dose of prednisone (1 to 2 weeks)
- Modest dietary changes; alcohol consumption lowered to once a day
- Sleep patterns good
- Work experience: job satisfaction high; house acceptable
- One month of standard land protocols, including resistance training
- At 5 METs and 50 watts at beginning of flume study
- Asymptomatic and without ischemia throughout cardiac rehabilitation

Flume Protocol
- Initiated at 1 mph and increased to 4 mph
- Water temperature between 27°C to 34°C (81°F to 94°F), mean of 32°C (90°F)
- Upright walking against current, adding arm movement in HOWI position
- Swimming: from head-out strokes to crawl against 4 mph current
- RPE between 9 to 11 (Very Easy to Fairly Easy)
- RPP at 13.9 × 10³ for land exercises and 15.5 × 10³ for water exercises

Flume Rehabilitation History
- At 7 METs and 70 watts on land at discharge
- Initial heart rate: 80 bpm; end of program: 100 bpm
- EKG showed 0 to 80 multifocal premature ventricular contractions during the exercise sessions
- One episode of unifocal ventricular couplet during land exercise, and frequent low-grade ectopy

The single anomaly occurred during the first flume session. By the fourth stroke of the crawl, there was sustained multifocal ventricular tachycardia separated by two regular beats. The episode ended when the participant stopped swimming and stood still. Subsequent sessions were kept at an RPP 3 × 10³ below the land level (13.9 × 10³). There followed a month of very gentle water exercise at a slow pace for 2 minutes, supplemented by home exercises, both land and water, without ectopy or signs of ischemia. After 3 months, he was able to do the crawl without ectopy at an RPP less than 2 × 10³ below the land level against a current of 4 mph. This was without being overwhelmed or fatigued, and he continued "feeling great."

Emergency Procedures for Cardiac Participants in Aquatic Programs

Clinicians should make therapeutic exercise programs as rewarding as possible without losing sight of serious safety concerns. Caution should be recommended to those with known coronary heart disease because of the increase in myocardial oxygen demand imposed by rigorous exercise. Statistics on the incidence of emergencies encountered in cardiac rehabilitation programs as a function of client hours are as follows:

Cardiac arrest: 1 per 100,000
Myocardial infarction: 1 per 200,000
Fatal incidence: 1 per 700,000

This translates to approximately 1 cardiac arrest every 4 years assuming 95 clients per year in a medically supervised program conducted 3 times per week.[14,50] People with coronary heart disease in an exercise program have a risk factor of seven times the rate for a healthy person.[16,17] This is the reason for medical supervision.

Land- and water-based cardiac rehabilitation programs demand thorough preparation. An aquatic program requires great emphasis on safety and prevention. Morbidity can be limited and mortality prevented by the following tools:

TABLE 13-5. Aquatic Cardiac Rehabilitation Emergency Plan

Procedure/Equipment Required	Remarks
Water rescue	Protect participant and personnel from electrocution during defibrillation[51]
Quick drying procedure	
On-site medical supervision (advanced life support)	Enables start of definitive medical treatment before tissue necrosis can occur
Advanced cardiac life support (American Heart Association)	
Emergency equipment	
EKG and BP monitoring	Initial entry, on request, or status change (eg, symptoms, medication change)
Slow warm-up, long cool-down	Particularly for those with stabilized angina
Education in warning signs	Participant knows when and how to recognize and report early warning signs
Establish rapport, trust, and communication with participant	
Adherence to target heart rates with frequent pulse checks	Every 5 to 10 min
Use Borg's RPE, FAD, and Pain Scales for PVD, CHF, chronic obstructive pulmonary disease, and angina	Stop exercise if: RPE scale exceeds 11 (fairly easy) FAD scale exceeds land norms or 3 (moderate but can continue)
Keep intensity low in high-risk clients	Obtain precise heart rate, rate-pressure product, and RPE parameters on first session
Minimize competition in games	Provokes catecholamine surge in coronary-prone personalities
Know individual patterns	To recognize symptoms obscured in water (eg, sweating)
Reduce intensity for those with CHF, PVD, and low ejection fraction	More likely to decompensate (lose pump function)
Prohibit hot showers at end of session for those with autonomic compromise or those on potent cardiac medications	Prevent rapid hemodynamic shifts
	Primary effect of many medications is blunting of portions of autonomic nervous system

RPE, Rate of Perceived Exertion; FAD, Fatigue and Dyspnea; PVD, peripheral vascular disease; CHF, congestive heart failure.

Risk stratification as defined in Table 13-2[3]

Borg's Scale of Perceived Exertion (see Table 13-3)[21]

Fatigue and Dyspnea and Pain Scales (see Table 13-3)[3,21]

Fully trained, alert staff

Emergency cart containing equipment and drugs, following American Heart Association advanced life support guidelines[51]

There is no reason that the resuscitation rate for land-based cardiac incidences (85%)[14] should be different for aquatic incidences. URI reports no life-threatening emergencies over its 10-year study of aquatic cardiac rehabilitation.

To reduce the incidence of cardiovascular complications, the AACVPR generated recommendations for cardiac rehabilitation in the water (Table 13-5). Table 13-6 provides a recommended list of standard cardiac rehabilitation equipment and plans that should be included in formalized procedures.

The first consideration in minimizing risk is the selection and instruction of candidates. It is advisable to remain conservative in the selection of participants (see Table 13-2), to use common sense and to consider each person individually. They should have completed phase II** (EKG-monitored) of a cardiac rehabilitation program, including a land program. This provides a good physiologic baseline for the beginning of the water-based program. The aquatic program provides:

• A change in modality while continuing the interface with the rehabilitation team

** Cardiac rehabilitation programs are usually conducted in three phases: I. immediate care, education, and training given while in the hospital; II. closely supervised, EKG-monitored physical training, education, and behavior modification, lasting 3 months; III. lifelong training and psychological support required to prevent another event, to ameliorate the current morbidity, and perhaps reverse some of the trends of the disease with continuing lifestyle modifications.

TABLE 13-6. Standard Cardiac Rehabilitation Equipment and Plans

Equipment/Plans	Remarks
Telephone and communication plan	Contact local emergency medical system and ALS for immediate transport
Standing orders following American Heart Association ALS guidelines	Signed by medical director
Portable defibrillator with backup batteries	Checked daily!
Chart recorder and cardioversion capability	

Portable oxygen unit with several modes of delivery:
  High-flow nonrebreather
  AmbuBag–valve–mask and tubing
  Mouth-to-mask unit
	With one-way valve for protection of rescuer

Intubation equipment Endotracheal tubes, airways, and laryngoscope Portable suction	Esophageal obturator no longer first-line device; acceptable as backup in prehospital environment
Intravenous equipment	Tubing, angiocatheter, and reservoirs of normal saline
Advanced life support (ALS drugs consonant with medical director, ALS provider, and state protocols for prehospital emergency care)	For example: sublingual nitroglycerin, epinephrine, lidocaine, atropine, glucose 25 G, dopamine, morphine, Valium, adenosine, Lasix, Narcan, and magnesium sulfate
Extra aneroid blood pressure cuff and stethoscope	
Standard first aid kit	Including ice packs
Absorbent blankets	
Secure cart/carrying case	Some ALS drugs are controlled substances requiring adherence to federal narcotics regulations
Document chart for emergency events	Added to session records Added to patient record Sent to receiving emergency facility

Documentation of
  Engineer checkout of equipment (every 6 mo)
  Routine daily checks	

ALS, advanced life support.

- Continuing behavioral modification and education
- Group support, permitting improvement in self-efficacy and self-esteem

In this known cardiac disease population, the possibility of sudden death is seven times greater than in a healthy exercising population. This mandates a knowledge of the incipient signs or symptoms and the appropriate actions or procedures to be taken if there is occurrence. Table 13-7 lists the danger signs for a cardiac incident.

Summary

Heart disease has been the leading cause of death in the 20th century. Much time, money, and effort have been expended in its diagnosis and treatment; this has covered all scientific areas, including pharmaceuticals, bioengineering, and surgical procedures (invasive and noninvasive). An added dimension is the area of prevention, which can decrease morbidity and mortality, and includes the consanguineous diseases of hypertension and diabetes. A powerful relationship exists between cardiovascular diseases and leisure-time activities.

Prevention includes ameliorating the conditions leading to the disease and rehabilitation of the afflicted after medical diagnosis and remedial action. Since the 1960s, the development and implementation of cardiac rehabilitation programs have kept pace with the science of cardiology.

These programs have progressed from cautious walking programs to resistive weight training with a full-body exercise component, and now include aquatics. A full array of services is designed and provided to redirect the cardiac client's attitude, beliefs, and behaviors.

TABLE 13-7. Signs and Symptoms of Potential Cardiac Events During Water Exercise

Condition/Observation	Action/Remarks
Anginal pattern change:	Discontinue water regimen
Type, duration, frequency, and response to medication	Notify physician
	Continue land-based exercises with electrocardiographic monitoring and physician's sanction
New onset of angina	Discontinue water regimen
	Notify physician
	Regular land-based exercises until stabilized, with physician's sanction
	Return to water program
Arrhythmia pattern change (dysrhythmia)	Temperatures > 34°C (92°F) provoke arrhythmia
Potential same for both land and water[30]	Temperature at 15°C (59°F) produces bradyarrhythmias
	Monitor rate-pressure product
	Measure blood pressure in the beginning and at the last minute of activity
New onset of arrhythmia (either atrial or ventricular)	Discontinue water regimen for that day
	Notify physician
	Doubt about stability—return to land-based exercise
Change in ST segment	Return to land-based exercise
Syncope in those >70 y of age	Change position slowly entering or exiting the pool
Transient ischemic attacks	If stable, see physician; if not abated, transport by ambulance
Increase or change in claudication pattern	Notify physician, monitor closely on land-based exercise
Change in Borg's Rate of Perceived Exertion Scale (work becomes harder)	Perceived effort for same MET level lessened in water—stop exercise, return to land-based exercise
	Use shortness of breath and FAD Scale (see Table 13-3)
Symptoms of congestive heart failure[3,12]	Chart appropriately—use group data sheet during session
Rales in lungs	Prepare and enter proper SOAP* note into permanent medical record
Increased complaints of fatigue and shortness of breath	
Change in sleep patterns	
Development of insomnia	

* SOAP and evaluation may be entered into permanent record later.
SOAP, subjective, objective assessment plan; FAD, Fatigue and Dyspnea

Control of water and air temperature is vital. Temperature extremes may have varying effects depending on the population under consideration. Table 13-7 lists some of the potential effects that must be considered when dealing with different populations in cardiac rehabilitation. Even in a thermoneutral environment, certain populations require special care (Table 13-8).

Swimming should be reserved to those who swam before experiencing cardiac dysfunction. It should be reinstated when no arrhythmia, ST changes, or symptoms occur, and RPP does not vary by more than 1×10^3 for the remaining session. The reinstatement should be gradual, starting for a few minutes as a substitute for upright walking. Few are able to swim because it is a very robust activity (8 to 10 METs). Non-swimmers would use too many accessory muscles, significantly increasing $\dot{V}>O_2$. The client should be monitored and EKG and BP (RPP) measured to preclude the effects of diving bradycardia (heart rate < 60 beats/min) and other arrhythmias. These measurements should be made while the person performs a gradual series of water exercises, culminating in the crawl with head immersed and the temperature thermoneutral.

Of special concern is the coronary-prone personality (type A behavior). By definition, these people are self-assertive, and care must be taken to ensure that they do not exceed instructions. The subjective scales (see Table 13-3) should be used to evaluate compliance. It is important that norms for the use of the subjective scales be

TABLE 13-8. Effects of Water/Air Temperature on Different Populations

Population*	Potential Effects
Temperature Extremes	
Stable CAD	Angina and arrhythmias
Diabetes	Negative effects from autonomic dysregulation
Peripheral or arterial limb obstructions and neuropathes	Negative effects, increased symptoms, decreased adherence, and discouragement
Key High Temperature	
Stable CAD	Syncope and arrhythmias
Thermoneutral	
Anemia	Blood shifts might increase shortness of breath, depriving myocardium of O_2 and leading to shortness of breath, angina, or heart attack
Chronic obstructive pulmonary disease and hiatal hernia	Lung impingement due to hydrostatic pressure around chest (restrain to shallow water)
Asthma	May benefit by humidified environment
Diabetes	Foot abrasions from walking on concrete bottom
	Hypoglycemic symptoms masked by water (eg, sweating)
Neuropathies	Hypotension and hypertension
	Fluctuations in heart rate

* All require long cool-down period.

established in the beginning during initial telemetry-monitored sessions. The client perceives his or her exertion in the water as much less than that achieved in land exercise.

Awareness of a client's medications is of utmost importance. With this knowledge, the staff can anticipate potential problems, for example, syncope due to the use of hypertensive medications.

Once the heart has healed from an attack or from surgery, cardiac-related diseases (eg, hypertension, diabetes) persist. An adjunctive aquatic program is an excellent way to continue a person's association with the cardiac rehabilitation team. This permits long-term behavioral modification. The attainment of an exercise habit requires more than the traditional 3 months prescribed for cardiac rehabilitation. Rising medical costs and limited resources could result in far less time to initiate the whole spectrum of lifestyle changes. An aquatic program can provide excellent variety to a seemingly dispiriting, drudge-like future of exercise.

Before any introduction of an aquatic program, procedures must be established and the means provided for dealing with emergencies.

A fully equipped "crash cart" should be available and should include advanced cardiac life support medications and a defibrillator. A means of drying and a safe area for treatment are essential. As with normal cardiac rehabilitation, special attention is necessary for "noncompliers," the very robust (>7 METs), and those with marked ST changes. Frequent practice sessions should be instituted and include not only the facility staff but the local emergency medical service staff and all its elements (fire, police, ambulance, and so forth).

Documentation is a necessity. It should follow the usual cardiac rehabilitation format and become part of the participant's legal medical record.

Cardiac rehabilitation can be safe and enjoyable in a water environment. For continuity, it can be provided by the same team in an overall land and water program. Precautions must be known and respected. Under these conditions, a cardiac aquatic program is a positive means for increasing client compliance with the difficult task of behavioral change, leading, ultimately, to a better, healthier life.

REFERENCES

1. Braunwald E. *Heart Disease: A Textbook Of Cardiovascular Medicine.* 2nd ed. Philadelphia, Pa: WB Saunders; 1984.
2. American Heart Association. *Heart And Stroke Facts: 1994 Statistical Supplement.* Dallas, Tex: American Heart Association; 1993.
3. Wenger NK. Early ambulation after myocardial infarction: the in-patient exercise program. *Clin Sports Med.* 1984;3:333–348.
4. Wenger NK, Hellersteiun HK. *Rehabilitation of the Coronary Patient.* 3rd ed. New York, NY: Churchill-Livingston; 1992.
5. American College of Sports Medicine (ACSM). *ACSM's Resource Manual for Guidelines for Exercise Training and Prescription.* 2nd ed. Philadelphia, Pa: Lea & Febiger; 1993.
6. Guzzetta CE, Dossey BM. *Cardiovascular Nursing: Holistic Practice.* St. Louis, Mo: Mosby Year Book; 1992.
7. Underhill SL, Woods SL, Sivarajan Froelicher ES, et al. *Cardiac Nursing.* 2nd ed. Philadelphia, Pa: JB Lippincott; 1989.
8. Wenger NK. Exercise testing and training of the elderly coronary patient. *Chest.* 1992;101(Suppl): 309S–311S.
9. Vidmar PM, Rubinson L. The relationship between self-efficacy and exercise compliance in a cardiac population. *Journal of Cardiopulmonary Rehabilitation.* 1994;14:246–254.
10. Steward KJ, Kelemen MH, Ewart CK. Relationships between self-efficacy and mood before and after exercise training. *Journal of Cardiopulmonary Rehabilitation.* 1994;14:35–42.
11. Powell KE, Blair SN. The public health burdens of sedentary living habits: theoretical but realistic estimates. *Med Sci Sports Exerc.* 1994;26:851–856.
12. American Association of Cardiovascular and Pulmonary Rehabilitation (AACVPR). *AACVPR Guidelines for Cardiac Rehabilitation Programs.* 2nd ed. Champaign, Ill: Human Kinetics; 1995.
13. Hall LK, ed. *Developing and Managing Cardiac Rehabilitation Programs.* Champaign, Ill: Human Kinetics; 1993.
14. Haskell WL. The efficacy and safety of exercise programs in cardiac rehabilitation. *Med Sci Sports Exerc.* 1994;26:815–823.
15. Thompson PD, Klocke FJ, Levine BD, et al. Task Force 5: Coronary Artery Disease. American College of Sports Conference: Recommendations for determining eligibility for competition in athletes with cardiovascular abnormalities. *Med Sci Sports Exerc.* 1994;26(Suppl):S271–S275.
16. Thompson PD. Cardiovascular hazards of physical activity. *Exerc Sport Sci Rev.* 1982;xx:000–000.
17. Thompson PD, Funk EF, Carleton RA, et al. Incidence of death during jogging in Rhode Island from 1975 through 1980. *JAMA.* 1981;247:2535–2538.
18. Morganroth J, Horowitz LN. *Sudden Cardiac Death.* New York, NY: Grune and Stratton; 1985.
19. Hartley LH. Exercise for the cardiac patient: long term maintenance phase. *Cardiology Clinics.* 1993;11: 277–284.
20. Verrill D, Bergey, McEleveen, et al. Recommended guidelines for cardiac maintenance (phase I) programs: a position paper by the North Carolina Cardiopulmonary Rehabilitation Association. *Journal of Cardiopulmonary Rehabilitation.* 1993;13:87–95.
21. American College of Sports Medicine (ACSM). *ACSM's Guidelines for Exercise Testing and Prescription.* 4th ed. Philadelphia, Pa: Lea & Febiger; 1991.
22. Mahler DA. The measurement of dyspnea during exercise in patients with lung disease. *Chest.* 1992; 101(Suppl):242S–247S.
23. Mahler DA, Horowitz MB. Perception of breathlessness during exercise in patients with respiratory disease. *Med Sci Sports Exerc.* 1994;26:1078–1081.
24. Rampulla C, Baiocchi S, Cacosto E, et al. Dyspnea on exercise: pathophysiologic mechanisms. *Chest.* 1992; 101(Suppl):248S–252S.
25. Friedman M, Rosenman RH. Association of specific overt behavior pattern with blood and cardiovascular findings. *JAMA.* 1959;169:1286.
26. Byrne DG, Rosenman RH. *Anxiety and the Heart.* New York, NY: Hemisphere Publishers; 1990.
27. Magser SA, Linnarson D, Gullstrand L. The effect of swimming on patients with ischemic heart disease. *Circulation.* 1981;63:979–985.
28. Magser SA. Swimming as an exercise for heart patients: caution advised. *Internal Medical News.* 1982; January:1–14, 24.
29. Campaigne BN, Lampman RM. *Exercise in the Clinical Management of Diabetes.* Champaign, Ill: Human Kinetics; 1994.
30. Fernhall B, Manfredi TG, Congdon K. Prescribing water-based exercise from treadmill and arm ergometry in cardiac patients. *Med Sci Sports Exerc.* 1992; 24:139–143.
31. Fernhall B, Manfredi TG, Congdon K. Prescribing water-based exercise from treadmill and arm ergometry in cardiac patients. *Journal of Cardiopulmonary Rehabilitation.* 1992;24:9, 10, 140.
32. Kurokawa T, Ueda T. Validity of ratings of perceived exertion as an index of exercise intensity in swimming training [abstract]. *Ann Physiol Anthropol.* 1992; 11:277–288.
33. Ueda T, Kurokawa T, Kikkawa K, et al. Contributions of differentiated ratings of perceived exertion to overall exertion in women while swimming [abstract]. *Eur J Appl Physiol.* 1993;66:196–201.
34. Myer JN. Perception of chest pain during exercise testing in patients with coronary artery disease. *Med Sci Sports Exerc.* 1994;26:1082–1086.
35. Okene IS, Okene JK, eds. *Prevention of Coronary Heart Disease.* Boston, Mass: Little, Brown and Co.; 1992.
36. Potema K. An overview of the role of cardiovascular reactivity to stressful challenges in the etiology of hypertension. *Journal of Cardiac Nursing* 1994;8(4): 27–38.
37. Guyton AC. *Textbook of Medical Physiology.* 7th ed. Philadelphia, Pa: WB Saunders; 1986.
38. De Meirleir K. Value of swimming in cardiac rehabilitation and internal medicine. In: Hollander AP, Huijing PA, de Groot G, eds. *Biomechanics and Medicine in Swimming.* International Symposium of Biomechanics in Swimming, 4th, Amsterdam, Netherlands. Champaign, Ill: Human Kinetics; 1982:17–27.
39. Samek L, Kirste D, Roskamm H, et al. Herzrhythmusstorungen nach Herzinfarkt: Beziehungen zur Bewegungstherapie, zu Funktionellen und Morphologischen Variablen. [Postmyocardial infarction arrhythmias in relation of exercise therapy, functional

and morphological variables]. *Herz/Kreislaus.* 1977; 9:641–649.

40. Parker JL, Oltman CL, Muller JM, et al. Effects of exercise training on regulation of tone in coronary arteries & arterioles. *Med Sci Sports Exerc.* 1994;26: 1252–1261.
41. Smith JJ. *Circulatory Response to the Upright Posture.* Boca Raton, Fla: CRC Press; 1990.
42. Allison TG, Miller TD, Squires RW, et al. Cardiovascular responses to immersion in a hot tub in comparison with exercise in male subjects with coronary artery disease. *Mayo Clin Proc.* 1993;68:19–25.
43. Kapoor AS, Singh BN. *Prognosis and Risk Assessment in Cardiovascular Disease.* New York, NY: Churchill-Livingston; 1993.
44. McMurray RG, Fiesilman CC, Avery KE, et al. Exercise hemodynamics in water and on land in patients with coronary artery disease. *Journal of Cardiopulmonary Rehabilitation.* 1988;8:69–75.
45. Fletcher GF, Cantell JD, Watt EW. Oxygen consumption and hemodynamic response of exercises used in training of patients with recent myocardial infarction. *Circulation.* 1979;60:140–144.
46. Gleim GW, Coplan NL, Scandura M, et al. Rate pressure product at equivalent oxygen consumption on four different exercise modalities. *Journal of Cardiopulmonary Rehabilitation.* 1988;8:270–275.
47. Sova R. *Aquatics: The Complete Reference Guide for Aquatic Fitness Professionals.* Boston, Mass: Jones and Bartlett; 1992.
48. Bolton E, Goodwin D. *An Introduction to Pool Exercises.* 2nd ed. Edinburgh, Scotland: ES Livingston; 1962.
49. McEvoy JE. *Fitness Swimming.* Princeton, NJ: Princeton Book Company; 1985.
50. American Association of Cardiovascular and Pulmonary Rehabilitation (AACVPR). *AACVPR Guidelines for Cardiac Rehabilitation Programs.* Champaign, Ill: Human Kinetics; 1991.
51. American Heart Association. *Textbook of Advanced Cardiac Life Support.* Dallas, Tex: American Heart Association; 1991.
52. Bleeson PB, McDermott W. *Cecil-Loeb Textbook of Medicine.* 13th ed. Philadelphia, Pa: WB Saunders; 1971.
53. Fernhall B, Congdon K, Manfredi T. ECG response to water and land based exercise in patients with cardiovascular disease. *Journal of Cardiac Rehabilitation.* 1990;10:5–11.
54. Manley L. Apnoiec heart rate response in humans. *Sports Med.* 1990:9:286–310.

14

Swim Stroke Training and Modification for Rehabilitation

Emily Dunlap

Swimming is an excellent form of exercise that offers minimal joint loading and permits great ease of movement. This may be why competitive and recreational swimming has been the most popular participation sport in the United States,[1-3] and over 2000 centers are using aquatic techniques for rehabilitative purposes.[1] However, many people do not realize that swimming is an advanced skill and, if done incorrectly or excessively, can place increased strain on the musculoskeletal system, delaying recovery or creating a new injury. Swimming-related injuries are being seen in ever-increasing numbers and are the result of inappropriate stroke mechanics, repetitive microtrauma (especially with competitive swimmers), and accidental impact loading.[1-6] Aquatic rehabilitation professionals can use swimming to achieve individual treatment goals if they understand the basics of swim training and modification. This chapter discusses a swim training progression that can be used for rehabilitating clients with a variety of injuries and disabilities.

General Issues

Why Would Swim Training Be Included in an Aquatic Therapy Treatment Plan?

Swimming has been used as a therapeutic technique for a variety of client populations.[7-20] There are many different reasons to include swim training in an aquatic therapy treatment program. Swimming offers an excellent means to work toward muscle conditioning and flexibility in a functional movement pattern. Open-chain trunk stabilization can be worked on through swimming. Motor control and body awareness are developed with this skill, which involves coordination of upper and lower extremity movement with floating balance and breathing control. Cardiovascular endurance can be accomplished with a consistent swim program. Pain management and relaxation can also be benefits of swimming. For clients who are not able to participate in a land exercise program such as walking, jogging, aerobics, or bicycling, their morale often improves when they work on swimming because they identify swimming with a more "normal" and athletic form of exercise. Clients may ask to have swimming be part of their treatment program, or they may start swimming on their own once they are in a pool. Often the client's swim stroke is not biomechanically efficient or safe for her disability or disease. It is important for the aquatic rehabilitation professional to be able to evaluate the client's swim stroke, assess which swim strokes are most appropriate for the person's rehabilitation, and be able to train the client in correct stroke mechanics, with any modifications dictated by the client's injury or disability.

Which Clients Are Not Suitable Candidates for Swim Training?

Some clients are not candidates for swim training as part of an aquatic therapy program. If a client does not have an interest in swimming, compliance is unlikely. When a client is fearful of the water or has no previous experience with swimming, the aquatic rehabilitation professional may not have adequate time to add this to the treatment program, and the time could be better spent on different areas of aquatic rehabilitation. A client who has difficulty with conventional exercise because of poor body awareness and poor coordination will have even greater difficulty with a complex task such as swimming. When the aquatic rehabilitation professional does not have adequate time to teach the basic water safety skills and swim strokes correctly, it is best not to include swimming in the treatment plan. To teach a client only partially about swimming could lead to accidents or injuries and greatly increase the therapist's or facility's liability.

Where Should the Aquatic Rehabilitation Professional Start With Swim Instruction and Modification?

An evaluation of the client's physical abilities along with information about his prior experience with swimming and his goals gives the aquatic rehabilitation professional an idea of at what level to begin the swim instruction. Even if the client says he is a good swimmer, a review of the basic water safety skills (discussed later in this chapter) is necessary before progressing to swim stroke instruction and modification. The aquatic rehabilitation professional should never start swim stroke instruction until she has observed the client properly perform all basic water safety skills. If the client is a good swimmer and has demonstrated good basic water safety skills, the therapist can start with any stroke and modify it as needed. If the client is a beginner or a new swimmer since an injury or disability, the following rules can help the therapist decide where to start: (1) supine strokes are easier for breath control because the access to air is constant; (2) motions that are closer to the midline are easier than motions farther away; (3) bilateral, symmetric motions are easier to accomplish than asymmetric motions; and (4) motions in which the limbs and trunk are submerged in the water at all times are easier than motions in which the limb lifts out of the water.

Which Swim Strokes Should Be Used for Rehabilitation?

The type of swim stroke selected depends on the muscle weakness, range of motion limitations, postural deviations, and motor control dysfunctions that are being targeted for rehabilitation. The aquatic rehabilitation professional should decide which swim strokes are most appropriate to help the client achieve his therapeutic goals. An example of this would be a client with rotator cuff injury who has restricted range of motion and strength in the right shoulder and pain with overhead activities, along with adaptive soft tissue restrictions on the right side of trunk causing an adaptive scoliosis. The side stroke with the right side down would allow the client to work on active-resisted overhead motion and lengthening of right trunk soft tissues while also working on cardiovascular endurance, without increasing pain symptoms.

When Should a Client's Swim Stroke Be Modified?

The decision to modify a swim stroke is made when the client cannot perform the traditional swim stroke because of deficits in range of motion, motor control, strength, or coordination, or when the correct stroke could cause increased pain or dysfunction. This decision should be based on the initial evaluation and response to conventional water exercise or swimming. An example of this would be a client with left hemiplegia due to cerebrovascular accident who does not have the range of motion or motor control in the left upper extremity to perform the elementary back stroke in the traditional manner. This client would need to learn how to compensate for the rotation caused by the hypertonic left side sinking by rotating the head away from hypertonic side or dropping the nonhemiparetic shoulder and pelvis to counterrotate the trunk. This client also has to compensate for the tendency to deviate to the left side with swimming due to insufficient power in the left upper extremity by laterally flexing the head away from the hemiparetic side, decreasing the arm pull of the nonhemiparetic side to match the weaker side, or kicking the legs with a directional force toward the hemiparetic side. Manual assistance or flotation devices may need to be used while the client is learning this compensatory technique. Another example would be a client with cervical facet irritation who cannot tolerate neck extension and complains of pain with the breast stroke. This client would need to be taught spine stabilization with this stroke to avoid extension of the neck with breathing. If the client is unable to maintain proper neutral spine position with breathing because of poor body awareness, poor swim coordination, or weakness, then a mask and snorkel should be used.

What to Expect From the Rest of This Chapter

The rest of this chapter describes a progression that should be used by the aquatic rehabilitation profession for basic water safety and swim stroke training and modification for the average client. The progression defined in this chapter is a combination of two forms of swim instruction, the American Red Cross method[21] and the Halliwick method.[22] Two swim strokes have been added that are not recognized by the American Red Cross—the basic stroke and the snorkel stroke. These strokes are useful for many client populations and are described later in the chapter. The butterfly stroke and diving are not mentioned in this chapter because these skills are more advanced and not frequently used in the rehabilitation of most injuries or disabilities. It is assumed that the reader is familiar with swim stroke mechanics as defined by the American Red Cross and is able to demonstrate each swim stroke in the traditional form. Typical swim stroke problems along with suggested corrections and modifications are given for each stroke and for specific client populations. The purpose of this chapter is to define swim training for rehabilitation, not athletic competition. Stroke modification is done primarily to reduce the strain on injured body parts or create a functional swim pattern for those with limited motor control. The modifications may or may not improve stroke efficiency.

Swim Training Progression

Table 14-1 indicates a logical progression for swim training. The first seven skills are areas of basic water safety that must be addressed before initiating swim stroke instruction. Each basic

---

TABLE 14-1. Swim Training Progression

1. Safe entry into and exit from pool
2. Mental and physical adjustment to the water
3. Breathing control
4. Recovery skills
5. Static floating control
6. Suspension skills
7. Changing directions
8. Swim strokes

---

water safety skill is described in more detail in the following sections, followed in turn by a discussion of the use of equipment with swim training. Next, each swim stroke is defined, and typical problems and modifications with each swim stroke are identified.

Safe Entry Into and Exit From the Pool

The client should be taught how to enter and exit the pool safely. This may include wheeling a wheelchair down or up a ramp safely, using a client lift, using stairs with or without a rail, or using a ladder. The client should demonstrate proper body mechanics while on pool deck and in the pool, and abide by all pool rules for safety (ie, no running on deck, no jumping or diving in pool).

Mental and Physical Adjustment to the Water

The client should demonstrate mental and physical adjustment to the water and effects of buoyancy. He or she should be comfortable moving around in the water and getting the hair, face, and ears wet. Activities to work on these areas include water walking, blowing bubbles, bobbing (an alternating rhythmic movement that involves exhaling while submerging under the water with inhaling when rising out of water), and submerging the face. Any signs of fear or apprehension with these basic activities indicate problems with continued swim instruction. If the client does not quickly adjust to the water with these activities, she may not be a good candidate for swim training.

Breathing Control

The client should demonstrate proper breathing control when the face is submerged. She should be able to submerge her face in all directions without having to hold her nose (face down in water, face sideways in water, and face up toward the surface, which is the most difficult position in which to control breath). The client should learn how to blow air out in a controlled manner when under the water so that it takes less time to breath in when the head comes out of the water. This skill is called rhythmic breathing and is essential for learning to swim in a prone position in which the head is under water for a portion of the stroke. If the client has difficulty with this, refer to the Chapter 16 on the Halliwick method for activities that work on breath control. Blowing bubbles and bobbing are good activities to encourage breath control under water.

Recovery Skills

Recovery skills are needed to make the transition from one position to another while in the water. More specifically, recovery skills allow a person to make the transition from standing to floating or from supine to prone while floating. Proper recovery skills are an essential part of the swim training progression. The client must master these skills before progress can be made to swim stroke instruction. The aquatic rehabilitation professional should demonstrate the proper recovery technique for the client and give verbal and manual assistance to the client as needed when learning these skills. The client should avoid using the wall when learning recovery skills because he can become dependent on it. The action of the head is the most important component, and should be emphasized when teaching these skills. If the client does not have previous swimming experience or is a new swimmer since a disability or injury, it may take a while to learn the recovery skills. Modifications for these techniques may be required for certain disabilities. Common modifications are listed after the descriptions of the recovery techniques. Refer to Chapter 16 on the Halliwick method for ideas on creative activities to work on recovery skills (Table 14-2; Figs. 14-1 through 14-6).

The most difficult transitions to teach are prone float to supine float and prone float to

TABLE 14-2. Recovery Skills

Transition	Mechanics
Vertical Transitions	
Stand to supine float (see Fig. 14–1)	Bend knees
	Pivot body vertically by bringing head back and legs up
	Let legs and head relax in floating position
Supine float to stand (see Fig. 14–2)	Arms abducted to side with palms down
	Bend knees up
	Pivot body by leaning head forward while letting hips sink down and pushing arms down then up in a semicircular fashion
	When in vertical position, straighten legs and stand up
Stand to prone float (see Fig. 14–3)	Bend knees
	Pivot body by leaning head forward, allowing hips to float up
Prone float to stand (see Fig. 14–4)	Arms flexed over head with palms facing down
	Bend knees
	Pivot body by lifting head and bringing knees forward while pushing arms down
	When in vertical position, straighten legs and stand up
Lateral Transitions	
Supine float to prone float (see Fig. 14–5)	Turn head in the desired direction, then lower the ipsilateral shoulder
	Facilitate the turn with an easy flutter kick of legs or sculling of arms when part way through the roll
Prone float to supine float (see Fig. 14–6)	Turn head in desired direction then lower the contralateral shoulder
	Facilitate the turn by easy flutter kick of legs or sculling of the arms when part way through the turn

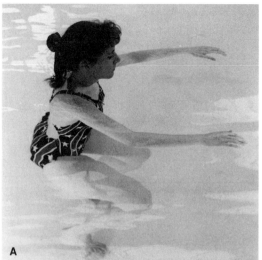
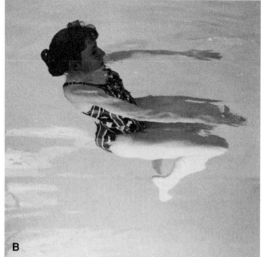
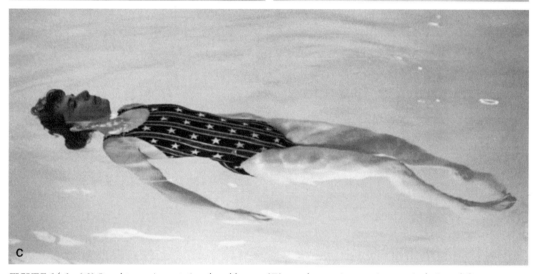

FIGURE 14-1. (***A***) Stand to supine rotation: bend knees; (***B***) stand to supine rotation: vertical pivot; (***C***) stand to supine rotation: supine floating.

stand, because the client is starting with his face in the water. These transitions may take longer to teach. With all transitions it is important to emphasize that the client should move slowly and allow the water to assist the transition rather than inhibiting it. Again, the action of the head is the most important component of each transition, and should be emphasized during training. These transitions should be completed with minimal physical exertion from the client. Recovery skills may require adaptation for certain clients; common modifications with recovery skills are listed in the following.

Recovery Skills Modifications

Modifications for Clients With Back or Neck Injuries

Clients who have back or neck injuries need to learn how to hold the trunk isometrically to maintain neutral spine stabilization throughout the vertical and lateral transitions. Hands-on assistance and verbal cues can be used by the aquatic rehabilitation professional to facilitate the desired motion. If needed, a cervical collar, lumbar support, or taping method (see section on Equipment for details) can be used to provide extra proprioceptive input for the client

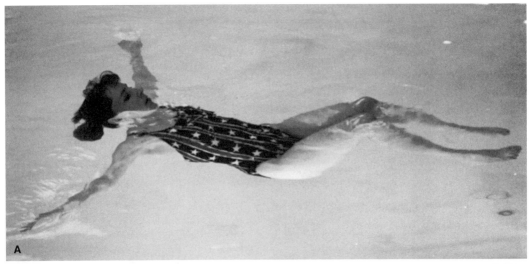

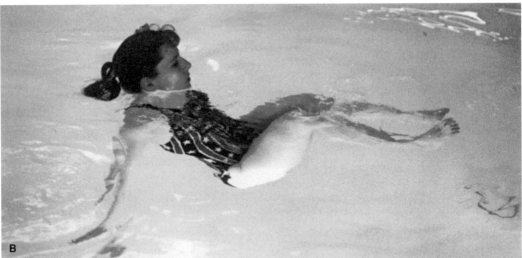

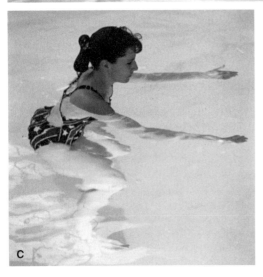

FIGURE 14-2. (***A***) Supine to stand rotation: bend knees; (***B***) supine to stand rotation: pivot body; (***C***) supine to stand rotation: vertical position.

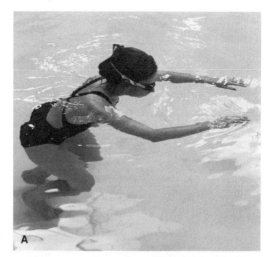

FIGURE 14-3. (***A***) Stand to prone rotation: bend knees and lean forward; (***B***) stand to prone rotation: prone floating.

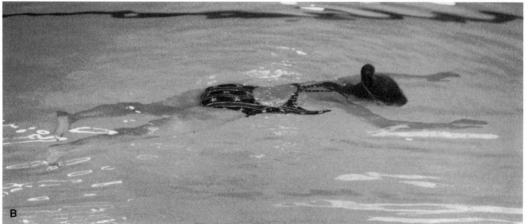

when learning how to maintain neutral spine position with these transitions.

Modifications for Clients With Imbalance of Motor Control

A client who has imbalance of motor control (eg, hemiplegia, amputation) needs to lean into the stronger side to prevent unwanted rolling with vertical transitions. It is easier to roll toward the impaired side with lateral rotations because the stronger arm can more easily facilitate the turn. With the supine float to prone float transition, the client should turn the head toward the impaired side and reach across the body with the stronger arm. The most difficult transition is prone to supine. In this transition, the client should turn the head toward the impaired side and reach across the body

then push with the stronger side across midline to help complete the turn.

Modifications for Clients With Spinal Cord Injuries

Spinal cord-injured clients need hands-on assistance and possibly the use of a personal flotation device or inflatable cervical collar while learning recovery skills. Even if these clients were good swimmers before their injury, they need time to adjust to the changes in their bodies that affect their ability to maneuver in the water.

Spinal cord-injured clients who do not have good trunk or lower extremity control and have very buoyant lower trunk and legs can complete vertical transitions and supine to prone float transitions by using the motion of the head to guide the motion. When making the transition

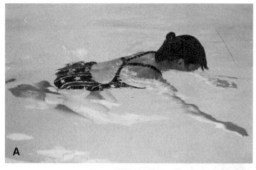

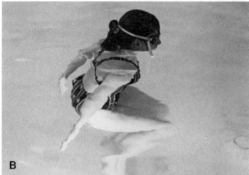

FIGURE 14-4. (*A*) Prone to stand rotation: bend knees and pivot; (*B*) prone to stand rotation: vertical position.

from supine float to a stand or vertical position, they need to move the head forward and lift the arms up and forward out of the water to allow the legs to sink. When transitioning from prone float position to a stand or vertical position, they need to bring the head back and scull their arms (fiqure-eight movement with arms used to maintain suspension of head above water) in front of them, and allow their legs to sink. Spinal cord-injured clients who do not have the ability to maintain a vertical position with the head out of the water can use the supine floating position as the position for safe breathing and relaxation between strokes. The prone to supine transition is the most difficult for spinal cord-injured clients. When prone, the client should turn the head in the desired direction, lower the contralateral shoulder, reach across the body with the contralateral arm, and push it across midline to help complete the turn.

Modifications for Clients Wearing a Flotation Belt

If a client is wearing a flotation belt for assistance with swimming, the head and arm motion need to be exaggerated to compensate for the upward force from the flotation device when changing from supine or prone float to stand.

Static Floating Control

The client should have good control in the floating position. The aquatic rehabilitation professional should learn how buoyant the client is and teach him how to position his body for maximum floating with minimal exertion. If he is a "sinker," the client can improve his supine float position by placing his arms overhead, lifting his hands out of the water, bending his knees, and taking a deep breath and holding it. If needed, the client can scull (figure-eight motion with arms) his arms or kick his legs just enough to stay afloat. Manual assistance under the thoracic area may initially be needed until the client relaxes enough to float alone. If the client's physical status does not allow floating without assistance, a flotation belt or cervical collar can be used. It is best to attempt to learn to float without flotation devices to avoid dependence on equipment. The client should be able to float comfortably before attempting to progress to swim stroke instruction.

Suspension Skills

Treading Water

Treading water is an important safety skill in a pool with a deep end. Treading water keeps the client upright in the deep water with the head out of the water. The client should learn to tread water in a relaxed manner with slow movements to conserve energy. Treading water is done by using the scissors kick or breast stroke kick (see section on Swim Strokes for definition of kicks) along with sculling movements (large figure-eight movements) of the arms and hands just enough to keep the head out of the water. Treading water may not be a necessary skill if the swimmer will swim only in the shallow water. If this is the case, the client should be instructed that it is not safe to swim in deeper pools or bodies of natural water that are over the head unless the client learns this skill. A client who cannot tread water because of physical limitations should be trained to float supine when she

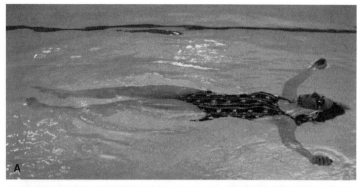

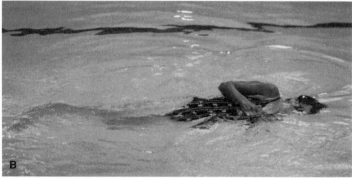

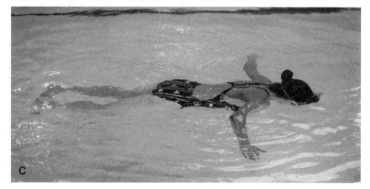

FIGURE 14-5. (***A***) Supine to prone rotation: supine floating; (***B***) supine to prone rotation: turning; (***C***) supine to prone rotation: prone floating.

needs to rest in the deep end, or use a flotation device when in the deep end.

Survival Float

The survival float is an important safely skill if the swimmer will be swimming in natural bodies of water over the head. The survival float is used if the client is away from the shoreline and in trouble (eg, exhausted, bad weather, cramping). To conserve energy, the client floats prone, lifts the head, and sculls the arms as needed to take a breath. This is done until the client has enough energy to swim to shore, or help arrives.

Changing Directions

Maneuvering

The client should be instructed in how to maneuver or adjust the path of direction with swimming. To maneuver during supine swim strokes, the client laterally flexes the head in the desired direction and strokes harder with the opposite arm. When maneuvering with prone swimming, the client reaches an arm in the desired direction, laterally flexes the head toward the new direction, and pulls slightly laterally with the opposite arm. The key is to use the head to facilitate the direction of movement.

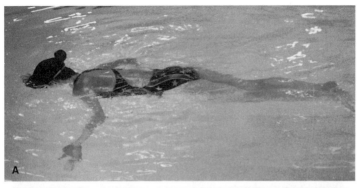

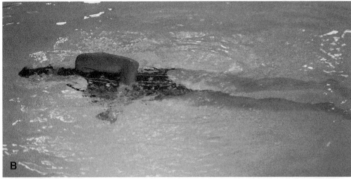

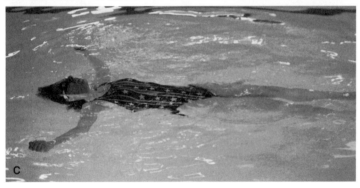

FIGURE 14-6. (***A***) Prone to supine rotation: prone floating; (***B***) prone to supine rotation: turning; (***C***) prone to supine rotation: supine floating.

Turns

The client should be instructed in open turns for lap swimming. Open turns involve stopping the stroke, making a vertical transition to stand, then pushing off the wall of the pool to change directions. Clients need to know how to complete the turn safely and efficiently. Flip turns are used only by more advanced swimmers such as athletes.

Basic Water Safety Skills

The seven previously mentioned basic water safety skills can be an excellent form of neuromuscular training. These preswim techniques are complex activities using many physiologic systems (vestibular, proprioceptive, neuromuscular), and they are therapeutic in and of themselves. The aquatic rehabilitation professional may chose to include basic water safely skill training in the treatment plan even if the client is not a candidate for swimming.

Swim Stroke Instruction

Once clients have learned the basic water safety skills, they are ready for swim stroke instruction. The aquatic rehabilitation professional should decide which swim strokes are appropriate for the client based on the treatment goals, and should modify the strokes as needed. The rest of this chapter provides information to assist the therapist with making these decisions. Swim skills are best taught by example, not words. The therapist should start with hands-on assistance if needed and progress to independent swimming as able, and avoid the use of equipment if possible. Once a client learns to swim with equipment, weaning can be difficult. In general, it is advised to teach the kick first, adding the arm portion of the stroke once the kick has been mastered. It is often helpful to teach the arm stroke while standing or when out of the pool. The stroke should be adapted to the client, not the client to the stroke.

Swim Training Equipment

When the decision has been made to use equipment with swimming, it is necessary to make sure the client (or client's attendant) can don and doff the equipment safely. The client should understand that it is not safe to swim without the equipment. Examples of equipment that are commonly used with swim training are given in the following sections, with the appropriate don–doff methods (Fig. 14-7). The reader can also refer to Chapter 20 on aquatic equipment for more ideas.

Flotation Belt

The flotation belt provides assistance with floating when the client is unable to float independently. The belt is easiest to don or doff when the client is standing in water at pelvis level or lower. The proper placement of the belt is around the pelvis/sacrum. Proper supine float to stand transitions need to be reviewed because they become more difficult with a flotation belt. If the client is not ambulatory, the belt can be placed around the pelvis/sacrum by the aquatic rehabilitation professional or attendant.

Mask and Snorkel

A mask and snorkel can be used with prone swimming to reduce the repetitive strain placed on joints with the breathing technique or to accommodate for poor motor control with the breathing technique. The mask must be adjusted for appropriate fit. To check the fit, the client presses the mask on the face and breathes in through the nose. If the mask forms a tight seal around the face, the fit is good. When using the mask and snorkel, the client needs to know how to defog the mask lens with saliva or soap solution. The client should be able to breath comfortably through the snorkel before placing the face in water. The aquatic rehabilitation professional may choose to have the client take the mask and snorkel home and practice breathing with the equipment in place to reduce the amount of time spent on this in the treatment session. The aquatic rehabilitation professional should teach the client how to blow out extra water in the snorkel and clear water out of the mask when under water. To clear extra water out of the snorkel, the client should blow forcefully through the snorkel, which removes most

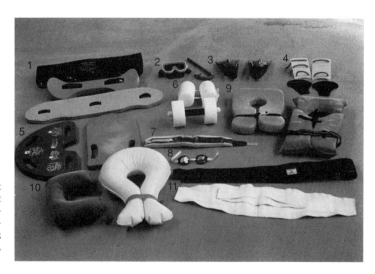

FIGURE 14-7. Equipment: 1, float belt; 2, mask and snorkel; 3, short fins; 4, gloves; 5, kickboard; 6, kickfloat; 7, soft cervical collar; 8, goggles; 9, personal flotation device; 10, inflatable cervical collar; 11, lumbar support.

of the water, then inhale slowly (so as not to inhale the remaining water in snorkel) and blow forcefully again to remove the remaining water. This can be repeated as often as needed to clear the snorkel. To clear water out of the mask when under water, the client should breath out through the nose while pressing the top of the mask into the forehead, allowing the mask to open under the nose. This will force the excess water out of the mask. A review should be given of proper stand to float transitions with mask and snorkel.

Short Fins

Fins are used with swimming to increase the surface area of the foot for lower extremity/ trunk strengthening, to increase kick power, or to facilitate proper leg motion with swimming. It is recommended that short fins be used because they provide enough increased surface area to accomplish the treatment goals while placing less strain on the body than full fins. The fins are easiest to don and doff if the client leans against the wall. The client should be able to stand and walk comfortably in the water with the fins. It is best to have the client start with small, slow kicks to assess his tolerance to the increased surface area at the end of the long lever. A review should be given of the proper stand to float transition, making sure the client dorsiflexes the foot with supine float to stand recovery to avoid catching the foot on the bottom of the pool.

Hand Paddles or Gloves

Hand paddles can be used to increase the surface area of the hand for increased upper extremity/trunk strengthening or increased power with stroke. Most gloves have webbed fingers and are held in place with a Velcro strap around the wrist. Most hand paddles are held in place on the palmar surface of the hand by rubber tubing that fits around the dorsum of the hand.

Kickboard

A kickboard can be used when teaching the kick portion of the swim stroke. When a client uses a kickboard, the therapist should be aware of the position stress on the body. For example, if a client with shoulder impingement holds the kickboard in front of him in the water, it may irritate his symptoms; it would be best to have this client hold the kickboard under his chest.

Kickfloat

A kickfloat is a float that can be placed between the legs to provide upward lift to the lower body when the swimmer wants to focus on the arm portion of the stroke or facilitate the trunk stabilizers with the stroke. To don the float, the client or assistant places it in between the client's lower legs when standing, and the client squeezes the float with the legs. The recovery skills need to be reviewed to avoid twisting with the narrow base of support. To doff the float, the client should release his or her hold on the float with the legs and allow it to float to the surface of the water.

Cervical Collar

A cervical collar can be used to provide proprioceptive feedback and support for neck position when training the client in recovery skills or swimming, and the emphasis is on neutral spine trunk stabilization. The client can don and doff the collar when standing.

Goggles

Goggles should be worn when swimming with face submerged to allow for better underwater vision and protection from pool chemicals. The goggles should be adjusted to allow for proper seal to prevent water from seeping in, without the strap being too tight. Most goggles can be adjusted with the strap between the eyepieces and the head strap.

Personal Flotation Device

A personal flotation device can be used when a client does not have enough motor control to float or swim independently. These clients are usually wheelchair dependent on land. The personal flotation device can provide a means of independent swimming rather than relying on manual assistance. It is best to don and doff the personal flotation device when out of the pool.

Inflatable Cervical Collar

An inflatable cervical collar can be used to give support to the neck with supine swim strokes. It is easiest to don and doff the cervical collar when standing with the head out of the water. The client should be instructed to hold the collar in place while making the transition from stand to supine float. The client should extend the neck and look at the ceiling when swimming to prevent the collar from slipping out behind.

Lumbar Support or Corset

A lumbar support can be used to provide proprioceptive feedback when log rolling with front or back crawl strokes. The client should stand at pelvis level or lower in the water to don and doff the lumbar support. It should fit snugly around the iliac crest, the base of the sacrum, and waist.

Taping

Lumbar taping (Fig. 14-8) can be used to provide proprioceptive feedback when log rolling with front or back crawl strokes.[1,3,6,18] The therapist should apply pretape compound to prevent skin irritation on removal of tape. The taping should be applied in crisscross strips, with the ends placed along the iliac crest and base of the sacrum, extending to the lower rib area.

The rest of this chapter describes the stroke

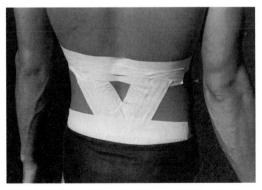

FIGURE 14-8. Example of lumbar taping.

mechanics, level of difficulty, and treatment goals that can be addressed with each stroke. Tables list typical problems seen with each swim stroke, as well as suggestions for corrections and modifications. The first set of tables (Tables 14-3 through 14-9) describes typical problems seen with all swimmers. The second set of tables (Tables 14-10 through 14-19) describes typical problems and modifications relevant to specific injuries or disabilities.

Swim Strokes

Each swim stroke is described in terms of stroke mechanics, including body motion; glide position (when appropriate); arm and leg motion, including power versus recovery phases of the stroke; breathing technique; and stroke coordination. The power phase of a stroke is that portion of the stroke responsible for propulsion. The recovery phase is that portion of the stroke that positions the limb for the next power phase. The level of difficulty is described for each stroke, as well as common treatment goals that can be attained. Typical problems and suggested corrections or modifications for each stroke are listed in the accompanying tables.

Basic Stroke (Fig. 14-9)

Stroke Mechanics

Body Motion. The basic stroke is a supine stroke with symmetric continuous movement of the arms and asymmetric continuous movement of the legs. There is no regular glide with the basic stroke; the arm and leg movement is continuous. If the swimmer needs to rest, he or she can glide in a streamlined position with arms in neutral at the side of the trunk with palms facing the thighs and the hips slightly adducted together, knees extended, and feet plantarflexed. The body is kept almost parallel to the surface with this stroke, except the hips and legs are slightly lower than the head and shoulders. The ears are submerged in the water with face out of the water.

Sculling: Arm Recovery and Power Phases. Shoulder and elbows are in neutral position along the side of the body, and the wrists are in mid-pronation/supination so that the palms are facing midline. The hands make the figure-

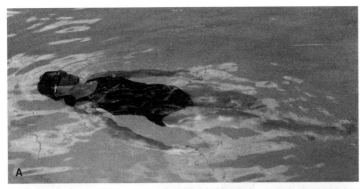

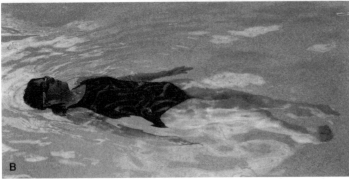

FIGURE 14-9. (*A*) Basic stroke power phase with arms pushing laterally; (*B*) basic stroke power phase with arms pushing medially.

eight motion by pronating and extending the wrist while abducting and internally rotating the arm, pushing the water laterally, and then supinating and flexing the wrist to neutral while adducting and externally rotating the arm toward neutral, pushing the water medially and caudally.

Flutter Kick: Leg Recovery Phase. The leg is extended down toward the bottom of the pool. The knee and ankle are relaxed

Flutter Kick: Leg Power Phase. The hip is flexed, allowing the knee to flex, then the knee is quickly extended with the ankle passively plantarflexed and inverted. The legs should be close together. The force of the kick is upward, as if flicking seaweed off the feet. Propulsion results from the pressure of the water against the dorsal surfaces of the feet and lower legs

Breathing. Because the client's head is out of the water with the entire stroke, he or she can breathe easily.

Stroke Coordination. The arms and legs move continuously throughout the stroke. Flutter kicking is a continuous, alternating movement that is initiated at the hip. The ankles should stay loose during the movement. As one leg is in the recovery phase, the other is in the power phase.

Level of Difficulty and Client Considerations

Very easy stroke, simple breathing pattern with face out of water, extremity motion is close to midline

Good for beginning swimmer and those with poor motor control and coordination

Good for pain management

Treatment Goals

Upper/lower extremity strengthening

Trunk stabilization

Endurance training

Relaxation training

Pain management

Table 14-3 lists the typical problems and corrections or modifications associated with the basic stroke.

Elementary Back Stroke (Fig. 14-10)

Stroke Mechanics

Body Motion. The elementary back stroke is a supine stroke with symmetric simultaneous movement of the arms and legs.

TABLE 14-3. Basic Stroke: Typical Problems and Corrections/Modifications

Typical Problems	Corrections/Modifications
Insufficient plantarflexion with kick causing poor propulsion	Instruct the client to keep foot loose and floppy and allow the foot to point when kicking
	Use short fins to facilitate proper kick and stretch into plantarflexion, but make sure client has sufficient lower extremity and trunk strength to counteract the rotational forces created by using fins
	If the client does not have the needed plantarflexion range of motion, he or she can compensate by increasing knee flexion with recovery phase to maximize the propulsion from the dorsal surface of the lower leg
Increased hip and knee flexion with kick and/or legs too stiff with kick causing poor propulsion	Tell client to keep legs "long but loose" and keep foot floppy with kick
Incorrect directional force with kick causing poor propulsion (ie, the force of the kick is posteriorly and cephalad, bringing the heels toward the buttocks)	Give cues that most of the force of the kick should be in the direction the person is facing: if the client is supine, the kick should be toward the ceiling
	Have client visualize pushing the water with the top of the foot when kicking, flicking seaweed off foot, or kicking a soccer ball
Improper head position causing sinking (ie, client flexing head and looking at feet)	Teach the client about the effect that head position has on the body when floating (ie, when lifting the head, the feet will sink)
	Instruct the client to relax neck and look at the ceiling rather than at the feet
Excessive muscle tension causing sinking	Review the basic water safety skills and make sure the client is comfortable with recovery techniques and floating. Excess muscle tension often is a sign that the client is not ready to progress
	Encourage client to relax with the stroke, give hands-on assistance under mid-thoracic spine or create drag in front of client to assist with floating until client learns to relax excess muscle tension. Drag can be created by positioning the therapist behind the client's head and walking backward while circling hands in a cephalad direction underneath the client's neck.
Client is a natural sinker, causing extension of spine	Aquatic rehabilitation professional can give hands-on assistance by standing behind the client's head, placing the palm of the hand to support the mid-thoracic spine, and walking backward to create drag, which assists with floating until the client learns to relax excess muscle tension and increase power of kick to improve lower body suspension
	Teach posterior pelvic tilt with increased kick power to reduce spinal extension
	Increase speed or efficiency of kick to help propel through water and reduce sinking
	Use flotation belt until the client is able to increase the power of the kick enough to propel through the water without sinking

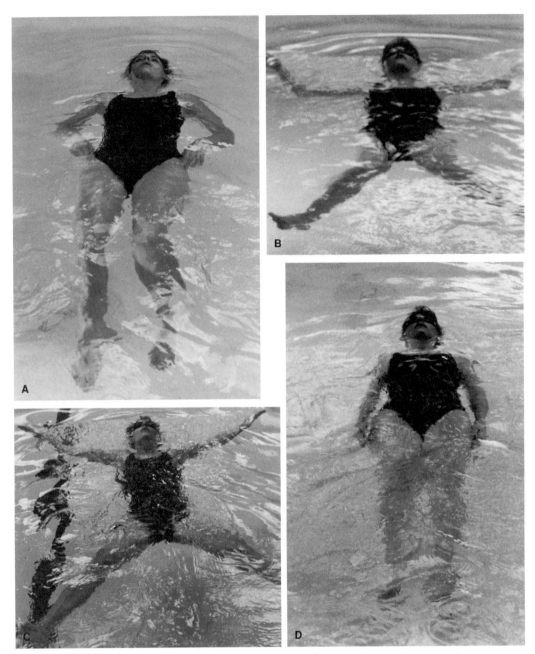

FIGURE 14-10. (*A*) Elementary back stroke mid recovery phase of arms and legs; (*B*) elementary back stroke end recovery phase—whip kick; (*C*) elementary back stroke end recovery phase—frog kick; (*D*) elementary back stroke glide after power phase of arms and legs.

Glide Position. The swimmer glides in a stream-lined position with arms in neutral by the side of the trunk with palms facing the thighs and the hips slightly adducted together, knees extended, and feet plantarflexed. The ears are submerged in the water with the face out of the water. The body is kept almost parallel to the surface, except that the hips and legs are slightly lower than the head and shoulders.

Arm Recovery Phase. From the glide position, the hand slides along the trunk up to the axilla, internally rotating and abducting the shoulder, while the elbow is flexing until the hand reaches the axilla. Then, the shoulder is externally rotated and the elbow extended so the hand reaches out to the side, abducting the shoulder to roughly 90 to 120 degrees,[21] with the elbow extended to almost full range.

Arm Power Phase. Both arms are pulled into adduction, keeping the elbow slightly flexed and the wrist in neutral flexion–extension and mid-pronation/supination so that the palms face midline.

Whip Kick: Leg Recovery Phase. The recovery begins with knee flexion and slight hip abduction. This motion brings the heels toward the buttocks while the knees are hip-width apart or slightly wider (depending on the swimmer's preference).[21] At the end of the recovery, the ankle dorsiflexes and everts. The ankles come underneath the water during the recovery and the knees may break the surface of the water slightly. The back and hips stay in about the same position as in the glide.

Whip Kick: Leg Power Phase. From the end of recovery, the whipping motion is initiated by internally rotating the hip so the feet finish lateral to the knees. Then, the plantar surface of the foot and the medial lower leg engage the water[21] while the knee extends and the hip rotates and adducts toward the glide position. The knee is almost fully extended when the feet are a few inches apart,[2] and the ankle finishes in plantarflexion. The ankle should describe a circular motion with this kick, and the legs should be under the surface of the water for the entire power phase.

The therapist may chose to modify the whip kick to the frog kick for most clients because it is easier to teach and places less stress on the knee, hip, and low back.

Frog Kick: Leg Recovery Phase. Recovery begins with knee flexion with hip external rotation and slight hip abduction. This motion brings the knees hip-width apart or wider (depending on the swimmer's preference) while the heels draw down together toward the buttocks. At the end of the recovery, the ankle dorsiflexes and everts. The ankles come underneath the water during the recovery and the knees may break the surface of the water. The back and hip stay in about the same position as in the glide.

Frog Kick: Leg Power Phase. From the end of the recovery, the hip internally rotates toward neutral rotation. Then, the plantar surface of the foot and the medial lower leg engage the water as the knee extends, the hip adducts, and the ankle plantarflexes and inverts, drawing the legs together. The legs finish in the glide position.

Breathing. Because the head is out of the water during the entire stroke, the swimmer can breath easily. Exhalation takes place during the power phase and inhalation during the recovery phase. Exhaling during the power phase keeps water from entering the nose during the forceful part of the stroke.

Stroke Coordination. The arms start their recovery just before the legs, but the arms and legs finish the power phase together.[21] The arms and legs pull up together slowly during the recovery phase and then quickly pull down in the power phase. There is no pause between recovery and power phases of the legs. The glide occurs when the body is in a streamlined position after the power phase and before the recovery phase. The client should glide until her momentum slows. The hips stay near the surface of the water during the entire stroke, and the arms stay in the water during the entire stroke.

Level of Difficulty and Client Considerations

Easy stroke, simple breathing pattern with face out of water, bilateral extremity motion, uses mass flexion and extension patterns

Good for beginner and those with poor motor control and coordination

Treatment Goals

Upper/lower extremity strengthening
Facilitate chest expansion
Trunk stabilization
Endurance training
Relaxation training
Pain management

Table 14-4 lists the typical problems and corrections or modifications associated with the elementary back stroke.

Snorkel Stroke (Fig. 14-11)

Stroke Mechanics

Body Motion. The snorkel stroke is a supine stroke using mask and snorkel with asymmetric legs and symmetric arms. The arm portion is

TABLE 14-4. Elementary Back Stroke: Typical Problems and Corrections/Modifications

Typical Problems	Corrections/Modifications
Poor coordination with kick or arms causing poor propulsion or fatigue	Instruct the swimmers that the arms and legs should work together: use cue "up-out-together-glide-2-3-4"
	Emphasize that the arms need to come *up* to the armpit before extending *out* to the side
Lifting arms too far overhead at the end of recovery or lifting arms out of the water, causing head to sink and poor propulsion	Teach proper arm placement at about 90–120 degrees abduction (not 180 degrees)
	Emphasize that the arms never come out of the water during the stroke
Improper head position causing legs to sink (ie, client lifts head and looks at the feet)	Teach the client about the effect that head position has on the body when floating (ie, when lifting the head, the feet will sink)
	Tell client to relax neck and look at the ceiling rather than at the feet
Excessive muscle tension causing sinking	Review the basic water safety skills and make sure the client is comfortable with recovery techniques and floating. Excess muscle tension often is a sign that the client is not ready to progress
	Encourage client to relax with the stroke, give hands-on assistance under mid-thoracic spine or create drag in front of client to assist with floating until the client learns to relax excess muscle tension. Drag can be created by positioning the therapist behind the client's head and walking backward while circling hands in a cephalad direction underneath the client's neck.
Client is a natural sinker, causing extension of spine	Aquatic rehabilitation professional can give hands-on assistance by standing behind the client's head, placing the palm of the hand to support the mid-thoracic spine, and walking backward to create drag, which assists with floating until the client learns to relax excess muscle tension or increase power of kick
	Teach posterior pelvic tilt with increased kick power to reduce spinal extension
	Increase speed or efficiency of kick to help propel through water and reduce sinking
	Use flotation belt until client is able to increase the power of the kick enough to propel through the water without sinking
Too much force created with recovery phase of stroke or too little glide time, inhibiting forward propulsion or causing early fatigue	Instruct client to bring arms and legs apart slowly, then together fast, then glide for rest. Explain that the powerful portion of the stroke is when the arms and legs are brought together

similar to the breast stroke arms, and the legs flutter kick in a way similar to the front crawl stroke. There is no regular glide with snorkel stroke; arm and leg movement is continuous. If the swimmer needs to rest, she can glide in prone streamlined position with hips and knees extended and ankles plantarflexed. The arms are flexed overhead and about 6 to 8 inches below the surface of the water, with the hands close together and wrists pronated so the palms are down. The head is positioned with the waterline near the hairline of the forehead. The trunk should be in a neutral position, nearly horizontal to arms and legs.

Arm Power Phase. From the overhead rest position, the shoulders internally rotate and the wrists pronate so the palms turn outward at a 45-degree angle to the surface of the water. With the elbow extended, the shoulder is adducted to press the palms lateral until the hands are spread wider than the shoulders. From this posi-

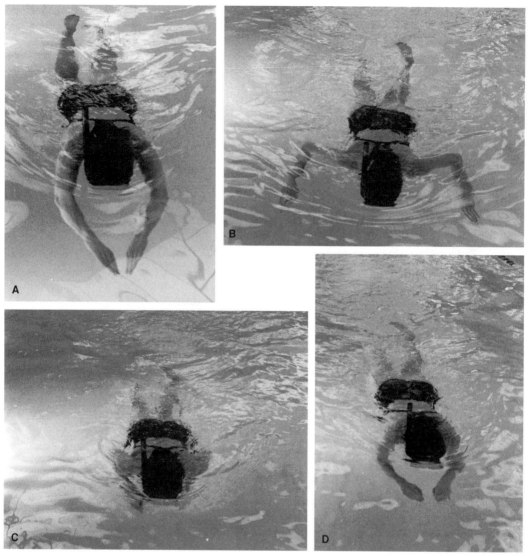

FIGURE 14-11. (**A**) Snorkel stroke—glide position; (**B**) snorkel stroke mid power phase of arms; (**C**) snorkel stroke end power phase of arms; (**D**) snorkel stroke—recovery phase of arms.

tion, the elbows are flexed and the hands pressed caudally and laterally until they pass near the elbows, with the forearms vertical. At this point, the wrists are supinated and the palms circumducted medially and cephalad until the palms are below the chin and facing each other, almost touching.

Arm Recovery Phase. Immediately after the power phase, the shoulders will horizontally adduct, squeezing the elbows together so the palms face each other. Then the arms reach overhead and the wrist pronate so the palms face down and end in the glide position.

Flutter Kick: Leg Recovery Phase. The leg is extended up toward surface of water until the heel just breaks the surface of the water. The knee and ankle are relaxed.

Flutter Kick: Leg Power Phase. The hip is flexed, allowing the knee to flex. Then, the knee is quickly extended with the ankle in passive plantarflexion and inversion. The legs should be close together. The force of the kick is toward the bottom of the pool, as if flicking seaweed off the feet. Propulsion results from the pressure of the water against the dorsal surfaces of the feet and lower legs.

Breathing. The client breathes continuously through the snorkel.

Stroke Coordination. The arms move slowly when in recovery phase and pull quickly in the power phase. Flutter kicking is a continuous, alternating movement that is initiated at the hip. The size of the flutter kick (distance the legs move up and down) ranges from between 12 to 15 inches, depending on the swimmer's height. The ankles should stay loose during the movement. As one leg is in the recovery phase, the other is in the power phase.

Level of Difficulty and Client Considerations

Easy stroke once the client masters the proper use of mask and snorkel

Good stroke for clients who cannot tolerate spinal extension/rotation and do not have adequate trunk stabilization strength to perform traditional prone strokes (breast and front crawl) in a neutral spine position

Good for clients who do not have sufficient motor control to perform the breathing technique with traditional prone strokes (breast and front crawl)

Treatment Goals

Upper/lower extremity strengthening
Trunk stabilization
Endurance training
Breathing control
Relaxation training
Pain management

Table 14-5 lists the typical problems and corrections or modifications associated with the snorkel stroke.

TABLE 14-5. Snorkel Stroke: Typical Problems and Corrections/Modifications

Typical Problems	Corrections/Modifications
Insufficient plantarflexion with kick causing poor propulsion	Tell client to keep foot loose and floppy
	Use short fins to facilitate proper kick, but make sure client has sufficient lower extremity and trunk strength to counteract the torque created by using fins
	If the client does not have the needed plantarflexion range of motion, he or she can compensate by increasing knee flexion with recovery to maximize propulsion from the dorsal surface of the lower leg
Increased hip and knee flexion with kick or legs too stiff with kick, causing poor propulsion	Tell client to keep legs "long but loose"
Incorrect directional force with kick causing poor propulsion (ie, client kicks posteriorly and cephalad bringing the heels toward the buttocks)	Give cues that the force of the kick should be in the direction the person is facing: if the client is prone, the kick should be toward the bottom of the pool; have client visualize pushing the water with the top of the foot when kicking
	Have client visualize flicking seaweed off foot or kicking soccer ball
Client is a natural sinker	Give manual assistance under abdomen or use flotation belt under hips until the client can create enough power with stroke to propel through water without sinking
Improper head position (ie, client looks in front, causing neck extension and sinking of legs)	Tell client to look at bottom of pool
Excessive muscle tension	Review the basic water safety skills and make sure the client is comfortable with recovery techniques and floating. Excess muscle tension often is a sign that the client is not ready to progress
	Encourage client to relax with the stroke, give hands-on assistance under abdomen or create drag in front of client to assist with floating until the client learns to relax excess muscle tension

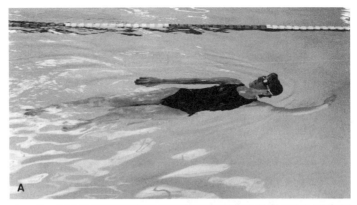

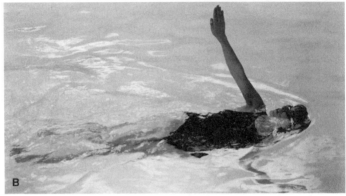

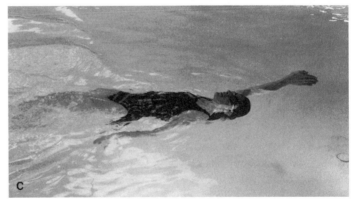

FIGURE 14-12. (*A*) Back crawl initial recovery of right arm; (*B*) back crawl mid recovery of right arm, power phase left arm; (*C*) back crawl end recovery of right arm—entry for power phase of right arm.

Back Crawl (Fig. 14-12)

Stroke Mechanics

Body Motion. The back crawl is a supine stroke with asymmetric movement of arms and legs. There is no glide in the back crawl. The waterline is at the top of the head, around the face to the chin line.[21] The ears are under water. The hips are slightly flexed so the feet can churn the surface of the water.[21] The body is supine in streamlined position, with the head and trunk aligned during the entire stroke.[21] The arms reach out of the water and the body rolls with trunk stabilization.[21]

Arm Recovery Phase. The arm is lifted out of the water by flexing the shoulder, and the wrist is positioned so the palm faces medially and the thumb and dorsal surface of the hand leave water first. The body rolls away from the recovery arm as the arm stays almost perpendicular to the surface of the water. During recovery, the wrist pronates and the shoulder internally rotates to allow the fifth finger to enter the water first. In the recovery phase, the arms and back muscles should be relaxed.[21]

Arm Power Phase. The arm enters in overhead flexion and internal rotation, with the fifth finger entering the water first. The body rolls toward the pulling arm at the same time the other arm starts its recovery.[21] The entry arm circumducts toward the bottom of the pool about 8 to 12 inches,[21] where the propulsion action starts. The hand sweeps downward and lateral while the elbow flexes and ends in roughly a 90-degree angle,[21] with the elbow pointing downward. Then the hand speeds up as it sweeps caudal while the elbow is extended and the shoulder is adducted, so the hand finishes below the buttock.

Flutter Kick: Leg Recovery Phase. The hip is extended down toward the bottom of the pool. The knee and ankle are relaxed.

Flutter Kick: Leg Power Phase. The hip is flexed, allowing the knee to flex; the ankle is relaxed. Then, the knee is quickly extended, whipping the foot upward into passive plantarflexion until the leg is completely extended and the toes reach the surface of the water. The legs should be close together. The force of the kick is upward, as if flicking seaweed off the feet.

Breathing. The head is out of the water for the entire stroke to allow for easy breathing. Inhalation takes place when one arm recovers, and exhalation when the other arm recovers.

Stroke Coordination. The arms are moving in constant opposition to each other. When one arms recovers, the other arm is pulling. This helps to counteract the rolling that occurs when one limb is lifted out of the water. Flutter kicking is a continuous, alternating movement that is initiated at the hip. When one leg is kicking upward, the other is kicking downward. At the end of the downward movement, the hip and knee flex and start the upward kick. The ankles are kept relaxed and the legs are close enough so that the first toes just miss each other. Most of the propulsive force comes from the upward kick as the dorsal surfaces of the foot and lower leg engage the water.[21] The kick also helps to stabilize the client by counteracting the motion of the arms and rolling of the body.

Level of Difficulty and Client Considerations

More difficult stroke, asymmetric extremity motion with arms moving out of water and away from midline

Client needs good body awareness and trunk stabilization strength, especially with rotation and extension forces

Client needs good shoulder range of motion to perform stroke correctly

May be stressful on shoulder injuries that do not tolerate repetitive resisted overhead motions

Client needs good body awareness to control swimming in straight line

Treatment Goals

Upper extremity range of motion/active stretching

Upper/lower extremity strengthening

Promote dissociation of the two sides of the body

Facilitate chest expansion

Advanced trunk stabilization

Endurance training

Table 14-6 lists the typical problems and corrections or modifications associated with the back crawl.

Side Stroke (Fig. 14-13)

Stroke Mechanics

Body Motion. The side stroke is a side-lying stroke with asymmetric arms and legs.

Glide Position. The glide position is side lying with the head just high enough to keep the mouth and nose out of the water. The bottom ears should be in the water, with the head, back, legs, and arms aligned. The body is nearly horizontal, except the legs are slightly lower in the water than the head.[21] The trunk is laterally flexed slightly, with the top portion of the body concave. The legs are extended with ankles plantarflexed. The bottom arm is flexed fully over the head so it is 6 to 8 inches below and parallel to the surface of the water, with the wrist pronated so the palm is down.[21] The top arm is extended by the side of the trunk with the wrist pronated so the palm is perpendicular to the thigh.

Arm Power and Recovery Phases. From the glide position the bottom arm starts its power phase and pulls down, with the shoulder moving into adduction and the elbow flexing to roughly 90 degrees,[21] so the hand sweeps cau-

TABLE 14-6. Back Crawl: Typical Problems and Corrections/Modifications

Typical Problems	Corrections/Modifications
Insufficient plantarflexion with kick causing poor propulsion	Instruct client to keep foot loose and floppy and allow the foot to point when kicking
	Have client visualize flicking seaweed off feet
	If the client does not have the needed plantarflexion range of motion he or she can compensate by increasing knee flexion with recovery phase to maximize propulsion from dorsal surface of the lower leg
Increased hip and knee flexion with kick or legs too stiff with kick, causing poor propulsion	Tell client to keep legs "long but loose"
Incorrect directional force with kick causing poor propulsion (ie, client kicks with a posterior and cephalad force, bringing the heels to the buttocks)	Give cues that the force of the kick should be in the direction the person is facing: if the client is supine, the kick should be toward the ceiling
	Have client visualize pushing the water with the top of the foot when kicking, as if kicking a ball
Improper head position (ie, client flexes neck and looks at feet, causing sinking of legs)	Teach the client about the effect that head position has on the body when floating (ie, when lifting the head, the feet will sink)
	Tell client to relax neck and look at the ceiling rather than at the feet
Excessive muscle tension causing sinking	Review the basic water safety skills and make sure the client is comfortable with recovery techniques and floating. Excess muscle tension often is a sign that the client is not ready to progress
	Encourage client to relax with the stroke, give hands-on assistance under mid-thoracic spine or create drag in front of client to assist with floating until the client learns to relax excess muscle tension. Drag can be created by positioning the therapist behind the client's head and walking backward while circling hands in a cephalad direction underneath the client's neck
Client is a natural sinker, causing extension of spine	Therapist can give hands-on assistance by standing behind the client's head, placing the palm of the hand to support the mid-thoracic spine, and walking backwards to create drag, which assists with floating until the client learns to relax excess muscle tension and increase power of kick
	Teach posterior pelvic tilt with increased kick power to reduce spinal extension
	Increase speed or efficiency of kick to help propel through water and reduce sinking
	Use flotation belt until the client is able to increase the power of the kick enough to propel through the water without sinking
Not knowing when to stop stroke	Instruct client on how to use landmarks on ceiling or side of pool to know when lane will end
Cannot control body roll with arm recovery	When arm is in recovery phase over the head, the other arm should be in power phase under water, which counteracts the rotational torque on the body. The client may need to be cued to push more with the underwater arm
	The therapist should teach proper trunk stabilization technique and log roll with the stroke. To accomplish this, the therapist may choose to place a kickfloat between the client's legs and have her practice log rolling while squeezing the float (this facilitates the trunk stabilizers). Cue the client to keep the shoulders and hips in line with rolling and to avoid twisting the midsection of the body. If client has difficulty with trunk stabilization, the therapist can use the Bad Ragaz ring method to teach and strengthen trunk stabilization while supine (see Chap. 15). The aquatic rehabilitation professional can have the client add the arm reach-back during the Bad Ragaz trunk stabilization exercise (the therapist's hand-hold is at the pelvis), and the therapist can assist with log roll at hips to simulate the back stroke pattern
Veering to one side with stroke	Check that client is log rolling in neutral position. Veering to one side can often be a result of lateral neck or trunk flexion with power phase of stroke
	If client has one side that is stronger than the other, have the client decrease the strength of pull on stronger side to match weaker side

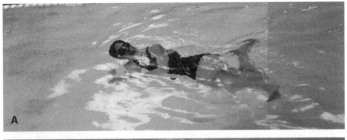

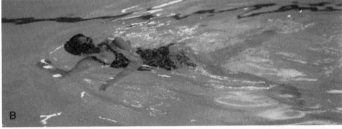

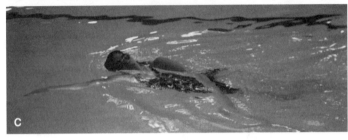

FIGURE 14-13. (**A**) Side stroke mid recovery phase for legs; (**B**) side stroke end recovery phase for legs; (**C**) side stroke glide after power phase of legs.

dal until the hand almost reaches the upper chest. During the power phase of the bottom arm, the top arm recovers by drawing up into shoulder/elbow flexion along the side of the body until the hand is nearly in front of the shoulder of the bottom arm.[21] The wrist stays pronated so the palm faces down. The two arms circle each other so the bottom arms ends up more medial than the top arm, and the bottom arm recovers by flexing overhead into the glide position. After the arms have circled and while the bottom arm is recovering, the top arm starts its power phase by sweeping caudal into the extended glide position.

Scissors Kick: Leg Recovery Phase. From the glide position, both legs recover by flexing the hips and knees so the heels draw up toward the buttocks. Then the legs prepare for the kick: the top leg dorsiflexes at the ankle and extends at the knee while the bottom leg plantarflexes at the ankle and extends at the hip and knee. The ending position before the power phase is with the top leg in hip flexion, the knee in extension, and the ankle near neutral or slight dorsiflexion,

while the bottom leg is in hip extension, partial knee flexion, and ankle plantarflexion.

Scissors Kick: Leg Power Phase. The top leg is pressed backward by extending at the hip and plantarflexing at the ankle while the bottom leg is pressed forward by flexing at the hip and extending at the knee. The water is pushed by the plantar surface of the top foot and the dorsal surface of the bottom foot. The legs end in the glide position.

Inverted Scissors Kick. This is the same as the scissors kick, except the top and bottom leg actions are reversed.

Breathing. The mouth is out of the water during the entire stroke, which makes breathing easy. The swimmer inhales through the mouth while recovering the top arm and exhales in the power phase of the top arm.

Stroke Coordination. From the glide position, the stroke is started with the sweep of the power phase of the bottom arm as the top arm and legs recover.[21] Then the legs and top arm push through the power phase as the bottom arm recovers into the glide position.[21] The swimmer glides until momentum slows, then starts the cycle again.

Level of Difficulty and Client Considerations

More difficult stroke, all four extremities have a different motion

The kick in this stroke may be difficult for clients who cannot tolerate spinal lateral flexion

Need good body awareness to maintain proper trunk position and coordinate arm and leg movements

Treatment Goals

Upper/lower extremity strengthening and active stretching

Promote dissociation of the two sides of the body

Elongation of trunk on underside

Endurance training

Table 14-7 lists the typical problems and corrections or modifications associated with the side stroke.

Breast Stroke (Fig. 14-14)

Stroke Mechanics

Body Motion. The breast stroke is a prone stroke with symmetric movement of the arms and symmetric movement of the legs.

Glide Position. The glide position is prone and streamlined with hips and knees extended and ankles plantarflexed. The arms are flexed overhead and about 6 to 8 inches below the surface of the water with the hands close together and wrists pronated so the palms are down.[21] The head is positioned with the waterline near the hairline of the forehead.[21] The trunk should be in a neutral position, nearly horizontal to arms and legs.

Arm Power Phase. From the glide position the shoulders internally rotate and the wrists pronate so the palms turn outward at a 45-degree angle to the surface of the water.[21] With the elbow extended, the shoulder is adducted to press the palms lateral until the hands are spread wider than the shoulders. From this position, the elbows flex and press the hands caudally and laterally until they pass near the elbows, with the forearms vertical. At this point, the wrists are supinated and the palms circumducted medially and cephalad until the palms are below the chin and facing each other, almost touching. Throughout the power phase, the elbows should point laterally and be higher than the hands and lower than the shoulders.[21]

Arm Recovery Phase. Immediately after the power phase, the shoulders horizontally adduct, squeezing the elbows together so the palms face each other. Then the arms reach overhead and the wrists pronate so the palms face down and end in the glide position.

TABLE 14-7. Side Stroke: Typical Problems and Corrections/Modifications

Typical Problems	Corrections/Modifications
Poor coordination with arms or legs	For arms, give cue "pick an apple and put it in the basket" For legs, give cue "up-out-together-glide-2-3-4"
Too much force created with recovery phase of stroke or too little glide time, inhibiting forward propulsion of stroke	Teach client to bring legs apart slowly, then together fast, then glide. Explain that the powerful portion of the stroke is when the legs are brought together and the top arm is pushing down
Insufficient plantarflexion or stiff feet with kick, causing poor propulsion	Have client keep feet floppy when bringing legs together If the client does not have the needed plantarflexion range of motion he or she compensate by increasing knee flexion of the bottom leg with kick to maximize propulsion off the anterior surface of lower leg
Incorrect head alignment (ie, client laterally flexes head so bottom ear is out of water)	Tell client to place ear on bottom shoulder Give cue to "rest your head on your arm like it's a pillow"
Inability to do side stroke on both sides with regular and inverted kick	It is best to teach regular and inverted kick on both sides for balancing of muscle training—usually clients are dominant one way, but this improves with practice

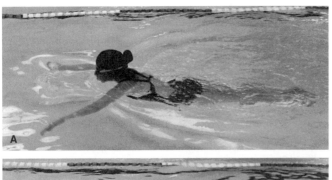
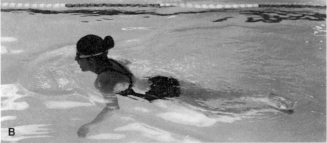
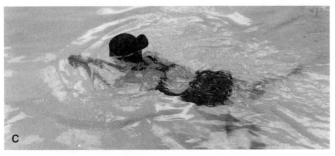
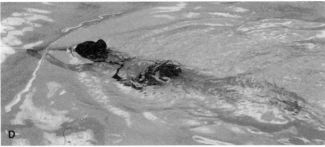

FIGURE 14-14. (**A**) Breast stroke early power phase for arms ("pull"); (**B**) breast stroke mid power phase for arms and recovery for legs ("breath"); (**C**) breast stroke recovery phase for arms and power phase for legs; (**D**) breast stroke glide after power phase for legs ("glide").

Whip Kick: Leg Recovery Phase. The recovery begins with hip and knee flexion with slight hip abduction. This motion brings the heel toward the buttocks while the knees are hip-width apart or slightly wider (depending on the swimmer's preference).[21] At the end of the recovery, the ankle dorsiflexes and everts. The ankles are just below the surface of the water at the end of the recovery and the hip is flexed to roughly 125 degrees.[2] The trunk remains in roughly the same position as in the glide.

Whip Kick: Leg Power Phase. From the end of recovery, the whipping motion is initiated by internally rotating the hip so the feet end up lateral to the knees. Then the plantar surface of the foot and the medial lower leg engage the water while the knee and hip extend, rotate, and adduct toward the glide position. The knee is almost fully extended when he feet are a few inches apart, and the ankle finishes in plantarflexion.[2] The ankle should form a circular motion with this kick, and the legs should be under the surface of the water for the entire power phase.

The therapist may choose to modify the whip kick to the frog kick for most clients because it is easier to teach and places less stress on the knee, hip, and low back.

Frog Kick: Leg Recovery Phase. The recovery begins with knee and hip flexion, with hip external rotation and slight abduction. This motion brings the knees hip-width apart or wider while the heels draw down together toward the buttocks. At the end of the recovery, the ankles dorsiflex and evert, ending just below the surface of the water with the hips flexed. The trunk remains in the same position as in the glide.

Frog Kick: Leg Power Phase. From the end of the recovery, the hip internally rotates toward neutral rotation, and then the plantar surface of the foot and the medial lower leg engage the water as the knee extends, the hip adducts, and the ankles plantarflex and invert, drawing the legs together. The legs finish in the glide position.

Breathing. The head is lifted to breath during the arm power phase. As the arms recover, the face lowers into the water and the swimmer should slowly exhale bubbles through the mouth. At the end of the arm recovery phase, the swimmer should explosively exhale the last of the breath and start lifting the head for the next breath.[21]

Stroke Coordination. The arm power phase starts from the glide position. At the end of the arm power phase, the swimmer lifts the head to breath and starts to recover the legs. Once the swimmer has taken a breath, she should immediately lower her face in the water and start to recover the arms while the legs are finishing the recovery.[21] When the arms reach about two thirds of their recovery, the legs should start the power phase.[21] The arms reach full overhead flexion just before the legs finish the kick.[21] The swimmer should glide briefly and start the next stroke before losing momentum.

Level of Difficulty and Client Considerations

- More difficult stroke, more difficult breathing pattern
- May be stressful on neck and back injuries that do not tolerate spinal extension (stroke

can be modified with use of mask and snorkel to reduce strain on back, neck, and shoulder with breathing technique)
- May be stressful on shoulder injuries that do not tolerate repetitive resisted motions
- Whip kick may be difficult on back or knee injuries (frog kick produces less torque on back and knees than whip kick)
- Need good coordination for this stroke—may be challenging for clients who do not have previous experience with this stroke
- Need good body awareness and trunk stabilization strength, especially with extension forces

Treatment Goals

- Upper/lower extremity strengthening and active stretching
- Trunk stabilization
- Endurance training
- Breathing control

Table 14-8 lists the typical problems and corrections or modifications associated with the breast stroke.

Crawl/Freestyle Stroke (Fig. 14-15)

Stroke Mechanics

Body Position. The crawl/freestyle stroke is a prone stroke with asymmetric movement of arms and legs. The trunk log rolls with this stroke and maintains a neutral spine position throughout the entire stroke. The log roll results from three movements: (1) the high recovery of one arm, (2) the downward sweep during the power phase of the other arm, and (3) the sideways force of the kicks as the legs roll with the rest of the body.[21] Log rolling is important to help relax the recovery arm and improve the propulsion with the power arm.[21] It helps to keep streamlined body position and assists with positioning for breathing. It also improves the overall rhythm of the stroke. The legs just break the surface of the water with the kick. The head and legs roll with the body to maintain a good streamline position.

Arm Power Phase. The arm enters the water with the shoulder flexed overhead and internally rotated, and the elbow flexed so point of entry is about three fourths as far as could be

TABLE 14-8. Breast Stroke: Typical Problems and Corrections/Modifications

Typical Problems	Corrections/Modifications
Poor coordination with arms or legs causing difficulty with breathing technique and poor forward propulsion	Give cue for arms "push down, around, then up and glide," and explain that arms will draw an upside-down heart
	Give cue for legs "up-out-together and glide"
	Give cues to start stroke with arms and finish with legs—"pull and breathe, kick and glide"
Too little glide time inhibiting forward propulsion of stroke and causing early fatigue	Stress the importance of gliding to prevent slowing down of forward momentum
Poor strength or propulsion with whip kick	Can work on motor planning and strengthening with the Bad Ragaz ring method lower extremity pattern (bilateral, symmetric hip flexion/abduction/internal rotation to reverse; see Chap. 15)

reached with full extension[21]; the wrist is pronated. The thumb and index finger enter the water first and the elbow enters the water last.[21] On entering the water, the arm extends fully at the elbow and sweeps caudally and laterally to just outside the shoulder with a flexed, pronated wrist. Then the elbow bends to a maximum of 90 degrees and the arm sweeps caudally and medially with a pronated wrist so it is directly below and perpendicular the chest.[21] From here, the arm finishes its sweep caudally and laterally with an extended, pronated wrist to end at the side of the thigh. The sweep forms an S-shaped pattern in the power phase with the left arm and a reverse S-shaped pattern with the right arm.

Arm Recovery Phase. The arm lifts out of the water elbow first, and then the hand exits the water little finger first.[21] The body roll is at a maximum at this point, which makes it easier to lift the arm in a relaxed manner. The shoulder lifts into extension and abduction out of water with the elbow high and relaxed forearm hanging down.[21] The hand then passes the shoulder and leads the rest of the arm to the entry point for the power phase.

Flutter Kick: Leg Power Phase. The hip is flexed, allowing the knee to flex. The knee is then quickly extended, with the ankle in passive plantarflexion and inversion. The legs should be close together. The force of the kick is toward the bottom of the pool, as if flicking seaweed off the feet. Propulsion results from the pressure of the water against the dorsal surfaces of the feet and lower leg.[21]

Flutter Kick: Leg Recovery Phase. The leg is extended up toward surface of water until the heel just breaks the surface of the water. The knee and ankle are relaxed.

Breathing. Breathing can take place each cycle (each time the right arm recovers) or every one-and-one-half cycles (the swimmer alternates the side on which he breathes). The breath occurs at the end of that arm's power phase, just as recovery starts.[21] The head turns with the trunk during the body roll, the opposite ear stays in the water, and the head laterally flexes slightly to that side to create an open pocket of air for the breath.[21] Once the swimmer has inhaled, he returns his face into the water and exhales bubbles slowly under water until the next breath.

Stroke Coordination. The arms move in constant opposition to each other. When one arm recovers, the other arm is pulling. Flutter kicking is a continuous, alternating movement that is initiated at the hip. The ankles should stay loose during the movement. As one leg is in the recovery phase, the other is in the power phase. The size of the flutter kick (distance the legs move up and down) ranges from about 12 to 15 inches, depending on the swimmer's height.[21] The arm recovery and power phases are not exactly opposite each other because the power phase takes longer than the recovery phase.[21]

Level of Difficulty and Client Considerations

More difficult stroke, difficult breathing pattern, asymmetric extremity motion with arms moving out of water and away from midline

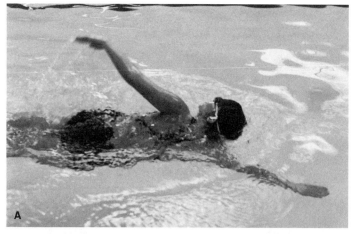

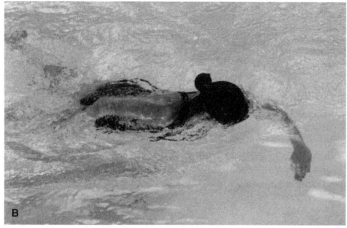

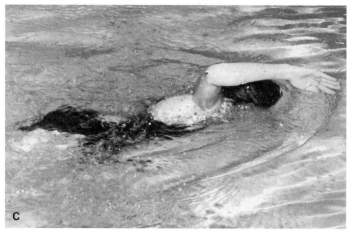

FIGURE   14-15. (**A**)   Crawl stroke—right arm beginning power phase, mid left arm recovery—breathing; (**B**) crawl stroke—right arm end power phase, initial left arm power phase; (**C**) crawl stroke—mid right arm recovery—no breathing.

TABLE 14-9. Crawl/Freestyle Stroke: Typical Problems and Corrections/Modifications

Typical Problems	Corrections/Modifications
Insufficient plantarflexion with kick causing poor propulsion	Instruct client to keep foot loose and floppy and allow the foot to point with kicking
	Have client visualize flicking seaweed off foot
	Use short fins to facilitate proper kick, but make sure client has sufficient lower extremity and trunk strength to counteract the torque created by using fins
Increased hip and knee flexion with kick or legs too stiff with kick, causing poor propulsion	Instruct client to keep legs "long but loose"
Incorrect directional force with kick causing poor propulsion (ie, client kicking with posterior and cephalad force, bringing heels toward buttocks)	Give cues that the force of the kick should be in the direction the person is facing: if the client is prone, the kick should be toward the bottom of the pool
	Have client visualize pushing the water with the top of the foot when kicking, just like kicking a ball
Improper head position (ie, client extends neck to take breath rather than log rolling, causing sinking of legs)	Have the client look at the bottom of the pool when face is under water and log roll, which positions head so client is looking at side of pool with face out of water to take a breath (do not lift head out of water to front, causing extension at neck)
	Have the client use the lane marker as an indicator of when to stop stroke—clients should not need to lift their head out of water to look in front of them when swimming
Excessive muscle tension	Encourage client to relax with the stroke, give hands-on assistance under mid-thoracic spine or create drag in front of client to assist with floating until he or she learns to relax excess muscle tension. Drag can be created by positioning the therapist behind the client's head and walking backward while circling hands in a cephalad direction underneath the client's neck
Client is a natural sinker	Therapist can give hands-on assistance by standing behind the client's head, placing the palm of the hand to support the mid-thoracic spine, and walking backward to create drag, which assists with floating until the client learns to relax excess muscle tension and increase power of kick
	Increase speed or efficiency of kick to help propel through water and reduce sinking
	Use flotation belt until client is able to increase the power of the kick enough to propel through the water without sinking
Difficulty with clearing face for breathing	Exaggerate log rolling—practice a complete roll from prone to supine to take breath with stroke
	Have client swim with kickfloat in between legs, using only arm portion of stroke with log rolling. As the client squeezes the kickfloat, he or she recruits the hip adductors, and the overflow facilitation will facilitate trunk stabilization with log rolling
	Emphasize arm reach toward the floor of the pool with power phase of stroke
Lateral flexion or rotation of trunk with breathing	This can be caused by poor breathing technique, with client lifting head up and to the side to breath. Instruct the client to look at bottom of pool when face is in the water, and log roll to side so the client faces the side of the pool to take a breath. The client never needs to lift the head out of water
	This can also be caused by the entry arm reaching past midline; instruct client not to reach past midline
	Teach proper log roll technique (see above)
	If the client does not have the range of motion to reach the arm into overhead flexion, it will difficult to maintain neutral position with this stroke. The client can compensate by allowing entry arm to enter water in some abduction or allow some lateral flexion with stroke, if this does not strain the spine

May be stressful on neck and neck injuries that do not tolerate spinal extension or rotation

May be stressful on shoulder injuries that do not tolerate repetitive overhead motions or do not have full extension–flexion or internal rotation

Can modify stroke with use of mask and snorkel to reduce strain on back, neck, and shoulder with breathing technique

Need good body awareness and trunk stabilization strength, especially with rotation and extension forces

Treatment Goals

Upper extremity range of motion and active stretching

Upper/lower extremity strengthening

Dissociation of the two sides of the body

Trunk stabilization
Breathing control
Endurance training

Table 14-9 lists the typical problems and corrections or modifications associated with the crawl/freestyle stroke.

Swim Stroke Progression: Typical Problems and Modifications Specific to Injury or Disability

Upper Extremity Amputation (Table 14-10)

Clients usually do not wear their upper extremity prosthesis in the water because they can learn to modify their stroke without the aide of a pros-

TABLE 14-10. Upper Extremity Amputation: Swim Stroke Problems and Modifications

Swim Stroke	Typical Problem	Modifications
Basic stroke	Uneven arm sculling causing deviation to the amputated side	Laterally flex head away from the amputated side
		Decrease arm pull on nonamputated side
		Kick legs with a directional force slightly toward the amputated side
		Place paddle on amputated limb if possible
	Trunk rotation with the amputated side up	Counterrotate low trunk with pelvis and legs
		Pull and recover with amputated upper extremity lower in the water if possible
Elementary back stroke	Uneven arm pull causing deviation to the amputated side	See basic stroke
		Decrease shoulder abduction and elbow extension of nonamputated arm
	Trunk rotation with the amputated side up	See basic stroke
Snorkel stroke	Uneven arm pull causing deviation to the amputated side	See basic stroke
		Pull nonamputated arm closer to midline and amputated arm slightly lateral
Back crawl	Uneven arm pull causing trunk rotation and deviation to amputated side	See basic stroke
Side stroke	Uneven arm pull strength causing difficulty maintaining side-lying position and poor propulsion	Swim with the nonamputated side down so the power phase of the bottom nonamputated arm helps to control rolling out of a side-lying position and assists with forward propulsion during lower extremity recovery
		Place paddle on amputated limb if possible
Breast stroke	Uneven arm pull causing deviation toward amputated side	Same as basic stroke
		Pull nonamputated arm closer to midline and increase intensity of pull
Crawl stroke	Uneven arm pull causing deviation to the amputated side	Laterally flex head away from the amputated side
		Pull the amputated arm slightly lateral of midline and nonamputated arm directly midline
		Place paddle on amputated limb
	Difficulty breathing toward nonamputated side	Increase log roll with nonamputated arm recovery overhead

thesis. In general, clients with upper extremity amputations need to compensate for asymmetric body position in the water and decreased force of arm pull on the amputated side by altering the motion of the nonamputated upper extremity when possible, and using the position of the head and the directional force of the lower extremity kick. The lower the amputation on the arm, the fewer modifications need to be made for swimming. Amputations that are higher on the arm require more modifications for swimming. If the amputation is very high on the upper arm, the client may have great difficulty mastering the breast stroke because the arm pull is essential to lift the upper body for breathing.

Lower Extremity Amputation (Table 14-11)

Clients with lower leg amputation may chose to wear a waterproof prosthesis when swimming, or they can learn to modify their stroke without the aide of a prosthesis. In general, clients with lower extremity amputations need to compensate for asymmetric body position in the water and decreased force of leg kick on the amputated side by altering the motion of the nonamputated lower extremity when possible, and using the position of the head and the directional force of the arm pull. The lower the amputation on the leg, the fewer modifications need

to be made for swimming. If the amputation is very high on the upper leg, swim strokes with flutter kicking (basic, snorkel, front and back crawls) are most appropriate; the client may not be able to progress to swim strokes that involve lateral movements of the legs away from midline (elementary back, side stroke, breast stroke).

Cerebrovascular Accident/ Hemiparesis (Table 14-12)

Clients with hemiparesis often require extensive practice learning recovery techniques. They need to use head movements to compensate for the rotation that tends to occur with recovery techniques and floating because of the lack of motor control and muscle tone changes on hemiparetic side. Clients with hemiparesis typically have difficulty maintaining a floating position because of the imbalance of muscle tone and range of motion. If the hemiparesis is not severe, the client can usually be trained in swimming with no flotation devices. If the hemiparesis is moderate or is severe in only one extremity, the client usually needs a flotation belt to assist with stability while floating, and strokes with easy access to breathing are most appropriate. If the client has both the upper extremity and lower extremity severely impaired, even modified swimming with flotation devices may not be attainable.

TABLE 14-11. Lower Extremity Amputation: Swim Stroke Problems and Modifications

Swim Stroke	Typical Problem	Modifications
Basic stroke	Uneven leg pull causing rotation in trunk with kick	Increase arm pull on amputated side
		Decrease intensity of kick and work on trunk stabilization with kick. The nonamputated leg should kick with a directional force toward midline
	Uneven leg pull causing deviation toward the amputated side	Laterally flex head toward amputated side
		Kick nonamputated leg with a directional force toward midline
		Increase arm pull on amputated side
Elementary back stroke	Uneven leg pull causing deviation toward the amputated side	Laterally flex head away from amputated side
		Increase arm pull on amputated side or decrease arm pull on nonamputated side
Snorkel stroke	Same as basic stroke	See basic stroke
Back crawl	Same as basic stroke	See basic stroke
Side stroke	Uneven pull of legs	Alternate scissors kick and inverted scissors kick
		Increase force of arm pull
Breast stroke	Same as elementary back stroke	See elementary back stroke
Crawl stroke	Same as basic stroke	See basic stroke

TABLE 14-12. Hemiparesis: Swim Stroke Problems and Modifications

Swim Stroke	Typical Problem	Modifications
Basic stroke	Rotation of trunk with hypertonic side down	Rotate head away from hypertonic side
		Drop "good" shoulder and pelvis to counterrotate trunk
		Use flotation belt or inflatable cervical pillow if needed
	Decreased hemiparetic arm sculling causing deviation toward hemiparetic side	Laterally flex head away from hemiparetic side
		Decrease arm pull of nonhemiparetic arm to match the force of the hemiparetic arm
		Kick legs with a directional force toward the hemiparetic side
	Poor motor control with flutter kick due to spasticity, causing sinking and poor propulsion	Emphasize small controlled movements versus rapid kicking
		Adjust position of kick to inhibit spasticity if possible (ie, increase knee flexion with kick to inhibit extensor tone)
		Give hands-on assistance or use flotation belt
	Difficulty maneuvering due to poor control of hemiparetic arm	Laterally flex head in desired direction and use "good" arm and legs for maneuvering; pulling arm towards the body (adduction) will turn the body in the opposite direction; pushing the arm away from the body (abduction) will turn the body in the same direction.
	Shortening of trunk on hemiparetic side, causing deviation towards hemiparetic side	Laterally flex head away from hemiparetic side
Elementary back stroke	Rotation of trunk with hypertonic side down	See basic stroke
	Decreased hemiparetic arm pull causing deviation toward hemiparetic side	See basic stroke
	Poor motor control with frog/whip kick due to spasticity, causing sinking and poor propulsion	Emphasize small controlled movements—decrease hip abduction and rotation with kick, and emphasize glide
		Emphasize relaxation with glide
		Adjust position of kick to inhibit spasticity if possible (ie, encourage glide with slight hip and knee flexion to avoid facilitating extensor tone)
		Give hands-on assistance or use flotation belt
	Difficulty maneuvering due to poor motor control of hemiparetic arm	See basic stroke
	Shortening of trunk on hemiparetic side causing deviation toward hemiparetic side	See basic stroke
Snorkel stroke	Rotation of trunk with hypertonic side down	See basic stroke
	Difficulty controlling breathing with mask and snorkel	If the client cannot comfortably and safely breath with mask and snorkel, this stroke is not appropriate for rehabilitation. See Equipment section earlier in this chapter for advice on how to train in use of mask and snorkel
	Decreased hemiparetic arm pull causing deviation toward hemiparetic side	See basic stroke
		Pull nonhemiparetic arm closer to midline
	Poor motor control with flutter kick due to spasticity	See basic stroke
	Difficulty maneuvering due to poor motor control of hemiparetic arm	See basic stroke
	Shortening of trunk on hemiparetic side causing deviation toward hemiparetic side	See basic stroke

(continued)

TABLE 14-12. *(Continued)*

Swim Stroke	Typical Problem	Modifications
Back crawl	Rotation of trunk with hypertonic side down	See basic stroke
	Decreased or painful shoulder motion for overhead recovery	If client does not have fairly good active shoulder motion, painful or subluxation, this stroke is not appropriate
Side stroke	Poor motor control or spasticity of hemiparetic arm	Swim with nonhemiparetic side down so the stronger arm is responsible for power phase of stroke when the legs are recovering and the hemiparetic arm does not have to reach into overhead flexion
	Poor motor control or spasticity of hemiparetic leg	Emphasize smaller controlled movements versus wide leg separation with rapid kick toward midline, which facilitates increased tone
		Emphasize relaxation with glide
		Adjust position of kick to inhibit spasticity if possible (ie, glide with hip and knee flexion to inhibit extensor tone)
Breast stroke	Difficulty with breathing control due to poor motor control or spasticity	Use a mask and snorkel with stroke
		Place flotation device (inner tube or belt) around thoracic area and underneath the axillae to prop the head out of the water for the entire stroke. This should only be done if the flotation device will not strain the shoulder joint
	Sinking because of decreased efficiency of frog/whip kick due to poor motor control or spasticity	Frog kick is easier to learn than the whip kick because there is less hip rotation, which tends to be a difficult motion for hemiparetic limbs
		Gives hands-on assistance until the client is efficient with the stroke, or use flotation belt
	Uneven arm pull due to poor motor control or spasticity	Same as snorkel stroke
Crawl stroke	Difficulty with breathing control due to poor motor control or spasticity	Exaggerate log rolling toward the breathing side; practice a complete prone to supine turn when taking breath
		Use a mask and snorkel with stroke
		Place flotation device (inner tube or belt) around thoracic area and underneath the axillae to prop the head out of the water for the entire stroke. This should only be done if the flotation device will not strain the shoulder joint
	Uneven pull of hemiparetic arm causing deviation toward hemiparetic side	See basic stroke
	Sinking because of decreased efficiency of flutter kick due to poor motor control or spasticity	See basic stroke

Spinal Cord Injury: Paraplegia (Table 14-13)

Clients with paraplegia need a lot of practice learning recovery techniques and floating control before advancing on to swim strokes. They need to use their neck, upper extremities, and trunk to compensate for loss of leg mobility with the swim progression. Manual assistance is needed while training, but if the client has good arm strength and trunk control, he should not need to use flotation devices or mask and snorkel once he has trained in swimming.

Spinal Cord Injury: Quadriplegia (Table 14-14)

Clients with quadriplegia need a lot of practice learning recovery techniques and floating skills before progressing to swim stroke training. They need to use their neck and any active upper extremity movement to compensate for loss of trunk and leg mobility with the swim progression. Typically, clients with quadriplegia need the use flotation devices or mask and snorkel for functional swimming and require supervision at all times for safety. When using mask and snor-

TABLE 14-13. Paraplegia: Swim Stroke Problems and Modifications

Swim Stroke	Typical Problem	Modifications
Basic stroke	Sinking legs due to spasticity	Lift chest, extend neck, and scull with arms abducted to counteract sinking legs
		Increase power of arm pull
Elementary back stroke	Sinking legs due to spasticity	Lift chest, inhale, and extend neck when arms are close to midline
Snorkel stroke	Sinking legs due to spasticity	Flex head toward bottom of pool and lift mid-back toward ceiling
		Increase power of arm pull
Back crawl	Unable to control rotation when performing arm reach over head	Increase force of underwater power arm to counteract the above-water recovery arm
		Laterally flex head in opposite direction to overhead recovery arm
Side stroke	Sinking	Keep head position as low in water as possible
		Increase power of arm pull
Breast stroke	Difficulty with raising body out of water for breath	Increase force of power phase to lift body out of water enough to take a breath with minimal neck extension
Crawl stroke	Difficulty with breath control	Breathe every few strokes if possible
		Increase force of power phase of stroke when preparing to take a breath
		Exaggerate log rolling toward the breathing side; practice a complete prone to supine turn when taking breath; use head, scapula, and arm motions to facilitate log rolling

kel, the client must be able to clear water from the snorkel (which may be difficult owing to low respiratory capacity) or learn to take the snorkel out of the mouth and roll supine for breath, if necessary.

Prognosis for Functional Swimming for Complete Spinal Lesions Causing Quadriplegia

C4 or C5: not functional

C6: can be functional with elementary back stroke and snorkel stroke

C7: can be functional with basic stroke, elementary back stroke, snorkel stroke, back crawl, crawl stroke

C8: can be functional with all strokes

Musculoskeletal Shoulder Injury (Table 14-15)

Swimming is an excellent way to strengthen the shoulder girdle. Cross-training with multiple strokes strengthens the musculature surrounding the girdle while displacing some of the repetitive strain of swimming. But cross-training alone is not enough, because all swim strokes have a much stronger internal than external rotation component. To compensate for this, the aquatic rehabilitation professional should complement the swim program with other therapeutic activities to strengthen the external rotators of the shoulder girdle. The aquatic rehabilitation professional should train all force-couples of the glenohumeral joint and the scapulothoracic joint to gain proper balance around the shoulder girdle. Clients with limited shoulder range of motion have more difficulty with back/front crawl and the side stroke, which call for greater range of movement. Clients with an unstable shoulder joint should not train with the back crawl and need to be careful with the front crawl (depending on level of instability) to avoid the risk of dislocation. Clients with impingement syndrome or rotator cuff tendinitis may have difficulty tolerating swim strokes that place the shoulder at the end range of forward flexion or abduction, as seen in the entry phase of the crawl/freestyle stroke.[4,5] Clients with shoulder injuries tend to compensate during the front and back crawl by allowing segmental rolling instead of log rolling. This type of compensation should be avoided because repetitive segmental rolling can strain and possibly injure the spine.[5] Hand paddles or gloves may be used to increase

(text continues on page 280)

TABLE 14-14. Quadriplegia: Swim Stroke Problems and Modifications

Swim Stroke	Typical Problem	Modifications
Basic stroke	Difficulty with sculling motion	If the client does not have fairly good shoulder rotation, pronation, supination, and wrist control, modify the figure-eight sculling motion for a simpler shoulder abduction/wrist extension to shoulder adduction/wrist flexion motion
	Sinking due to spasticity in LEs	Lift chest, extend neck, and scull with arms abducted as much as possible to counteract sinking legs
		Give manual assistance until client becomes more efficient with stroke, or use flotation belt
Elementary back stroke	Decreased arm pull due to lack of elbow extension	Increase shoulder internal rotation, which allows the water to extend the elbow passively when adducting shoulder during power phase
	Sinking due to spasticity in LEs	Lift chest and extend neck when arms are close to midline to counteract sinking legs
		Give manual assistance until client become more efficient with stroke, or use flotation belt
Snorkel stroke	Difficulty with breast stroke arms	Modify arm stroke to alternating reaching and pulling of arms under midline of body, like a long "doggy" paddle
	Sinking due to spasticity in LEs	Flex head toward bottom of pool
		Give manual assistance until client becomes more efficient with stroke, or use flotation belt
Back crawl	Difficulty with recovery due to lack of shoulder flexion with elbow extension	Allow client to have elbow flexed when reaching over head and lead with elbow into water, or modify overhead reach by using shoulder external rotation and abduction
	Sinking due to spasticity in LEs	Lift chest and extend neck to counteract sinking legs
		Give manual assistance until client becomes more efficient with stroke, or use flotation belt
Side stroke	Sinking due to spasticity in legs	Keep head position as low in water as possible
		Increase power of arm pull if possible to help propulsion; if not possible, this stroke is not appropriate for the client
Breast stroke	Poor arm pull due to lack of elbow extension	Increase shoulder flexion with recovery phase and abduction, internal rotation with power phase
	Difficulty with breath control due to poor neck extension strength and poor arm pull	Breathe every few strokes to conserve energy and increase force of arm power phase to lift upper body out of the water enough to take a breath with minimal neck extension
		Use mask and snorkel if necessary
		Use flotation belt around mid-thoracic area if necessary
Crawl stroke	Decreased force with power phase due to inability to extend arm out of water during recovery phase, also causing difficulty with breath control	Breathe every few strokes
		Exaggerate log rolling toward the breathing side; practice a complete prone to supine turn when taking breath; use head, scapula, and arm motions to facilitate log rolling
		Use mask and snorkel if necessary

LE, lower extremity.

TABLE 14-15. Musculoskeletal Shoulder Injury: Swim Stroke Problems and Modifications

Swim Stroke	Typical Problem	Modifications
Basic stroke	Usually no problem unless very sensitive to repetitive shoulder rotation motion	Take rests with arms as needed while continuing to kick legs
Elementary back stroke	Decreased abduction ROM in affected shoulder causing uneven arm pull	Have unaffected arm match the affected arm with pull—do not worry about overall power of stroke because the goal is to increase the affected shoulder's ROM and strength
		Make sure glide is complete before attempting to raise arms; this decreases the water resistance into abduction
	Insufficient external rotation to allow for arm extension from mid-recovery under axilla to late recovery with arm at 90-degree angle	Allow client to extend arm with internal rotation and decrease the angle of arm abduction for power phase of stroke
	Decreased strength in affected arm causing deviation to the affected side	Adjust pull of unaffected arm so both arms match
		If the goal is to increase shoulder girdle strength, do not have the client use legs to compensate for weak arm; rather, have the affected arm set the pace for the rest of the body
Snorkel stroke	Pain with breast stroke arm movement	Decrease reach of breast stroke to a comfortable range and have the unaffected arm match the reach for symmetry
		Modify arm stroke to an alternating long "doggie paddle"
Back crawl	Decreased shoulder flexion and internal rotation or pain with overhead recovery of effected side	If client does not have fairly good shoulder flexion and internal rotation ROM, this stroke may not be appropriate
		Increase log roll to decrease flexion range needed—have client bend elbow when reaching over head and lead with elbow into water (reduces flexion and internal rotation at the shoulder)
		Modify overhead reach—have client come into abduction for stroke, then modify the opposite arm reach to allow for symmetric overhead recovery to avoid directional deviation with stroke
	Decreased shoulder extension and external rotation ROM for underwater power phase of injured arm	If client does not have at least fairly good extension and external rotation ROM, this stroke may not be appropriate
		Log roll toward the affected arm during underwater power phase of stroke to decrease the external rotation and extension needed
	Unstable shoulder joint	Not appropriate stroke with clients who have history of frequent shoulder dislocations or joint instability
Side stroke	Decreased flexion ROM or pain causing poor reach with power phase for bottom arm	Modify reach to comfort level of client and have client increase reach as tolerated
		The client should alternate sides as needed to decrease the repetitive strain on affected shoulder
	Unstable shoulder joint	Bottom arm should recovery and pull anterior to the body (in flexion–abduction)
Breast stroke	Difficulty with arm movements due to pain or decreased ROM	Decrease reach of breast stroke to a comfortable range and have the unaffected arm match the reach for symmetry
	Difficulty with breathing due to insufficient arm strength to lift upper body out of water	Take a breath every few strokes to conserve energy
		Use mask and snorkel

(continued)

TABLE 14-15. *(Continued)*

Swim Stroke	Typical Problem	Modifications
Crawl stroke	Full overhead arm recovery in affected shoulder, but painful with repetition	Have client externally rotate arm occasionally with stroke (arm pushes through water leading with palm or dorsal surface of hand); this reduces the repetitive strain on arm
	Poor overhead reach due to pain or decreased ROM causing problems with breathing	Increase log roll with stroke to allow for less extension needed with arm recovery, lower arm during recovery, and allow hand to enter water farther away from midline
		Modify stroke to use mask and snorkel and keep arms under the water
	Pain in shoulder with power phase of stroke	Decrease force with power phase
		Adjust position of arm under body for more comnfortable stroke

ROM, range of motion.

resistance for upper extremity strengthening if all joints can handle the increased strain.

Musculoskeletal Elbow or Wrist Injury (Table 14-16)

A swimming program can assist with strengthening and stretching of the musculature around the elbow and wrist. The swim stroke intensity needs to be adjusted to the client's tolerance, and is especially an issue with chronic irritation syndromes such as carpal tunnel and chronic tendinitis. Clients with lateral epicondylitis are likely to have difficulty tolerating the excessive forearm pronation with an aggressive breast stroke.[2] Cross-training the strokes that require pronation in the power phase (breast stroke, basic stroke, top arm of the side stroke, snorkel stroke, back and front crawl strokes) with strokes that do not place as much repetitive strain on the pronators (elementary back stroke, and bottom arm of the side stroke) decreases the repetitive stress on the lateral elbow structures. Hand paddles or gloves may be used to increase resistance for upper extremity strengthening if all joints can handle the increased strain.

Musculoskeletal Hip, Knee, or Ankle Injury (Table 14-17)

Clients with hip and knee injuries typically have the fewest problems with the flutter kick and the most problems with the whip kick because of the torque created at the hip and knee with the power phase.[2] The whip kick should be avoided with these clients; the frog kick or flut-ter kick can be substituted. Clients with unstable ankle injuries may have difficulty with intense whip or frog kicks because of the ankle inversion during the power phase. Clients with ankle/foot extensor tendinitis may have difficulty with flutter kicking because of the repetitive passive stretch during the power phase.[2] Fins may be used to increase resistance for lower extremity strengthening if all joints can handle the increased strain.

Musculoskeletal Neck Injury (Table 14-18)

Clients with neck injuries need to be instructed in neutral spine stabilization during recovery techniques, changing directions, and swimming. Clients with poor tolerance for rotational activities should avoid or progress slowly with swim strokes that require rotational control, such as the back and front crawls. Clients with poor tolerance for cervical extension should avoid the breast stroke, which requires cervical extension during breathing, and should avoid or progress slowly with the front crawl stroke if they cannot maintain neutral stabilization with the breathing technique. Clients with neck injuries and limited or painful shoulder range of motion need to avoid or modify strokes that challenge shoulder flexibility and prevent them from maintaining a comfortable or neutral spine position. Cervical spine clients may require manual assistance or the use of flotation equipment until they learn the proper stroke mechanics to propel themselves through the water and prevent sinking, which causes spinal movement away from the neutral position.

TABLE 14-16. Musculoskeletal Elbow or Wrist Injury: Swim Stroke Problems and Modifications

Swim Stroke	Typical Problem	Modifications
Basic stroke	Inability fully to extend elbow or wrist during power phase of stroke due to contracture	Depending on severity of contracture, the client could compensate by abducting the shoulder and using internal and external rotation for sculling
	Pain with repetitive pronation/supination	Take rests with arms as needed while continuing to kick legs
	Uneven arm pull causing deviation to weaker side	Adjust pull on stronger arm to match weaker arm
	Weakness causing poor propulsion	Use hand paddle or glove to increase propulsion and provide increased resistance for strengthening
Elementary back stroke	Inability to extend fully elbow during power phase of stroke due to contracture	To compensate for this, the client can extend shoulder toward bottom of pool and pull with flexed elbow under water during power phase of stroke
	Uneven arm pull causing deviation to weaker side	See basic stroke
	Weakness causing poor propulsion	See basic stroke
Snorkel stroke, breast stroke	Inability to extend fully elbow or wrist during power phase of stroke due to contracture	Modify the arm stroke to the available range and have the opposite side match the pull for symmetry
	Uneven arm pull causing deviation to weaker side	See basic stroke
	Weakness causing poor propulsion	See basic stroke
Back crawl	Inability to extend fully elbow during stroke due to contracture, causing poor placement of upper extremity with power phase of stroke	Allow for lateral arm placement with elbow entering first
	Uneven arm pull causing deviation to weaker side	See basic stroke
	Weakness causing poor propulsion	See basic stroke
Side stroke	Inability to extend fully elbow during power phase of stroke due to contracture	Allow the client to modify his or her reach within available range
	Weakness causing poor propulsion	Use hand paddle or glove to increase propulsion and provide increased resistance for strengthening
	Pain due to repetitive strain	Switch sides so the affected arm has less repetitive strain, recognizing that the top arm will be pulling with more pronation
Crawl stroke	Inability to extend fully elbow during power phase of stroke due to contracture	Increase log rolling to allow for greater ease of entry with flexed elbow
	Uneven arm pull causing deviation to weaker side	See basic stroke
	Weakness causing poor propulsion	See basic stroke

TABLE 14-17. Musculoskeletal Hip, Knee, or Ankle Injury: Swim Stroke Problems and Modifications

Swim Stroke	Typical Problem	Modifications
Basic stroke, snorkel stroke, back crawl, crawl stroke	Pain with kicking	Slow speed of kicking and increase the arm pull, give manual assistance or use flotation device to improve propulsion to prevent legs from sinking
	Weak kick	To increase resistance for strengthening, use short fins if all joints can handle increased resistance
	Insufficient ankle plantarflexion causing poor propulsion with kick	Place short fins to increase ankle plantarflexion ROM if all joints can handle the resistance
Elementary back stroke, breast stroke	Poor tolerance for whip kick due to medial/lateral knee or ankle instability or poor tolerance for hip rotation	Use frog kick; if problems with frog kick, use flutter kick
	Difficulties with frog kick due to limited hip external rotation ROM	Avoid this stroke until sufficient hip ROM is achieved through other therapy methods
Side stroke	Pain with hip extension	Decrease hip extension with kick or decrease kick intensity
	Weak kick	See basic stroke
	Insufficient ankle plantarflexion causing poor propulsion with kick	See basic stroke
	Inability to do side stroke on both sides with regular and inverted kick, causing imbalance of muscle strengthening and stretching	It is best to teach regular and inverted kick on both sides as well as both legs—usually clients are dominant one way, but this improves with practice

ROM, range of motion.

Musculoskeletal Back Injury (Table 14-19)

Clients with back injuries need to be instructed in neutral spine stabilization during recovery techniques, changing directions, and swimming. Clients with poor tolerance for rotational activities should avoid or progress slowly with swim strokes that require stabilization control with rotational forces, such as the back and front crawls. Clients with poor tolerance for lumbar extension should avoid the breast stroke, which requires lumbar extension during breathing, and should avoid or progress slowly with the front crawl if they cannot maintain neutral stabilization with open-chain kicking and the breathing technique. Clients with back injuries and limited or painful hip range of motion need to avoid or modify strokes that challenge hip flexibility with kicking and prevent them from maintaining a comfortable or neutral spine position. Typically, clients with hip flexor tightness have difficulty with prone flutter kicking, and clients with hip rotation tightness have difficulty with the whip kick. Lumbar spine clients may require manual assistance or the use of flotation equipment until they learn the proper stroke mechanics to propel themselves through the water and prevent sinking, which causes spinal movement away from the neutral position.

When to Refer to a Community Swim Instructor

Not all clients need the expertise of a licensed aquatic rehabilitation professional for swim training. Clients who do not need specific swim stroke modification or do not have special precautions can be referred to a qualified swim instructor (eg, Red Cross, YMCA) for swim training. Another case in which a referral would be

TABLE 14-18. Musculoskeletal Neck Injury: Swim Stroke Problems and Modifications

Swim Stroke	Typical Problem	Modifications
Basic stroke	Poor neck positioning into flexion causing pain	Do not allow client to look at feet when swimming, tell client head should be submerged in water with ears and most of face wet
		Client may need manual support for head initially; if needed, provide support by use of inflatable pillow (but avoid use of equipment if possible)
		Instruct client in the use of landmarks on the ceiling or side of pool to avoid the need to turn head to find position in lane
Elementary back stroke	Poor neck positioning into flexion causing pain	See basic stroke
Snorkel stroke	Poor neck positioning into extension causing pain	Tell client to look at floor when swimming rather than looking in front
		Instruct client in the use of land markers on bottom of pool as indicators of when to change direction for lap swimming; this avoids the need to extend neck to look for end of lane
Back crawl	Poor neck positioning into flexion causing pain	See basic stroke
	Pain with cervical rotation during recovery	Teach client spine stabilization/log rolling in neutral position; have client hold a tennis ball under chin to avoid extension and rotation
Side stroke	Poor neck positioning into lateral flexion causing pain	Tell client to rest head on the bottom arm so bottom ear and face are under water; client should be looking in front and at the side of the pool to know his or her lane position
Breast stroke	Excessive or painful neck extension when taking breath	Instruct client in spine stabilization when lifting to breathe—"pretend to hold tennis ball under chin," "keep chin tucked in"
		Have client increase the downward push with power phase of arm stroke to lift body out of the water when taking a breath to minimize the need for neck extension
		Modify stroke with mask and snorkel
Crawl stroke	Poor trunk stabilization with breathing technique causing extension or rotation of neck	Instruct in proper spine stabilization or log rolling; see back crawl stroke for suggestions
		Teach client how to breathe on alternate sides every 3–5 strokes to avoid repetitive motions and promote even stretching and strengthening with stroke
		Modify stroke with mask and snorkel

appropriate is if the client is fearful of the water, has no previous experience with swimming, or has poor body awareness or poor coordination. In such a situation, a significant portion of the treatment time is taken up by swim instruction. If the aquatic rehabilitation professional does not think swim instruction is the best use of the time, but believes the client would benefit from swim training, he may chose to refer this client to a well respected community pool program that has an aquatics instructor who has experience with teaching swimming to the disabled and rehabilitation populations. When making a referral to a community pool, the aquatic reha-

bilitation professional should contact the swim instructor to discuss precautions and treatment goals for the client. The therapist should know the qualifications of the community pool instructor and be confident when making the referral that the instructor will teach and modify the swim stroke in a manner appropriate for the client. If such a program is not available in the therapist's area, she may want to develop one at her own facility. It is recommended that the therapist become familiar with the community programs in her area to be able to make such referrals when appropriate.

Swimming has always been a popular form

TABLE 14-19. Musculoskeletal Back Injury: Swim Stroke Problems and Modifications

Swim Stroke	Typical Problem	Modifications
Basic stroke	Poor trunk stabilization with flutter kick	Do not attempt swimming until the client has adequate stabilization strength with other open-chain activities
		Teach proper stabilization technique—pelvic tilt into neutral position with isometric hold; give cues for log rolling. Cue the client to keep the shoulders and the hips in line with rolling to avoid twisting the midsection of the body
		Use a lumbar corset or taping[1,3,6,18] of lumbar region for proprioceptive feedback for stabilization control. See Equipment section of this chapter for details on taping
		If client is a natural sinker, use flotation belt until the kick is strong enough to propel the client through the water in a streamlined neutral position
Elementary back stroke	Pain with whip kick	Use frog kick
		Emphasize proper trunk stabilization with kicking
Snorkel stroke	Poor trunk stabilization with flutter kick causing extension or flexion of spine	See basic stroke
		Modify the snorkel stroke kick to a bicycle motion
Back crawl	Poor trunk stabilization with flutter kick causing rotation of spine	See basic stroke. When teaching log rolling, the therapist may choose to place a float between the client's legs and have him or her practice log rolling while squeezing the float and using the arms (this facilitates the trunk stabilizers). The therapist may also use a lumbar corset or lumbar taping.[1,3,6,18] See Equipment section of this chapter for details on taping
Side stroke	Poor trunk stabilization causing lateral flexion or flexion–extension of spine	See basic stroke
	Poor tolerance for hip extension with kick	Decrease hip extension with kick or decrease kick intensity
	Shortening of trunk due to soft tissue tightness	Have shortened trunk in the down position to promote soft tissue lengthening if appropriate, have the shortened trunk in the top position if the client cannot tolerate lengthening
Breast stroke	Excessive lumbar extension with stroke	See basic stroke
		Check head position—keep chin tucked throughout stroke to minimize cervical/thoracic/lumbar extension
Crawl stroke	Poor trunk stabilization with flutter kick causing rotation or extension of spine	See back crawl

of exercise and recreation. The aquatic rehabilitation professional can use this fact to his or her advantage and include swimming as part of the client treatment plan. This chapter provides information for the aquatic rehabilitation professional so he or she may gain the skills necessary to evaluate and modify client swim programs for rehabilitation.

REFERENCES

1. Cole AJ, Moschetti ML, Eagleston RE. An aquatic sports medicine approach for lumbar spine rehabilitation. In: Tollison DC, ed. *The Handbook of Pain Management.* 2nd ed. Baltimore, Md: Williams & Wilkins; 1994:368–400.
2. Fowler PJ, Regan WD. Swimming injuries of the knee, foot and ankle, elbow and back. *Clin Sports Med.* 1986;1(5):139–148.
3. Cole AJ, Eagleston RE, Moschetti ML. Getting backs in the swim. *Rehabilitation Management.* 1992;August/September:62–71.
4. Ciullo JV. Swimmer's shoulder. *Clin Sports Med.* 1986; 1(5):115–137.
5. Cole AJ, Farrell FP, Stratton SA. Cervical spine athletic injuries: a pain in the neck. *Physical Medicine and Rehabilitation Clinics of North America.* 1994;5(1): 37–68
6. Cole AJ, Eagleston RE, Mochetti ML. Swimming. In: White, AH (Ed). Spine Care Diagnosis and Conservative Treatment. Vol. 1. St. Louis, MO: C.V. Mosby; 1995:727–745.

7. Harris SR. Neurodevelopmental treatment approach for teaching swimming to cerebral palsied children. *Phys Ther*. 1978;58:979–983.
8. Grace KJ. Hydrodynamics: rehabilitation of running injuries. *Topics in Acute Care and Trauma Rehabilitation*. 1986;1(a):79–86.
9. Genuario SE, Vegso JJ. The use of a swimming pool in the rehabilitation and reconditioning of athletic injuries. *Contemporary Orthopedics*. 1990;20: 381–387.
10. Garvey LA. Spinal cord injury and aquatics. *Clinical Management*. 1991;1(1):21–24.
11. Hurley R, Turner C. Neurology and aquatic therapy. *Clinical Management*. 1991;1(1):26–29.
12. Hughes D. Aquatic therapy in the management of low back dysfunction. *Sports Medicine Update*. 1992; xx:10–15.
13. Arrigo CA, Fuller CS, Wilk KE. Aquatic rehab following ACL-PTG reconstruction. *Sports Medicine Update*. 1992;xx:22–27.
14. Darden L, Fuller CS. Considerations for aquatic therapy with the Illizarov external fixators. *Sports Medicine Update*. 1992;xx:18–21.
15. Levin S. Aquatic therapy: a splashing success for arthritis and injury rehabilitation. *The Physician and Sportsmedicine*. 1991;19(10):119–126.
16. Thomas GJ. Swimming: an alternative form of therapy. *Clinical Management*. 1989;9(3):24–26.
17. Styer-Acevedo JL, Charness AL. *Considerations for Planning Adapted Swimming Instruction*. Course notes for Adapted Aquatic Workshop at Rehabilitation Institute of Chicago, Chicago, Illinois, Feb. 23–24, 1985.
18. Cole AJ, Martin L, Moschetti ML. *Aquatic Therapy: Stabilization Strategies for the Cervical And Lumbar Spine*. Course notes for Workshop at Timpany Center, San Jose, California, June 1, 1991.
19. Elkington HJ. The effective use of the pool. *Physiotherapy*. 1978;64:452–460.
20. Peganoff SA. The use of aquatics with cerebral palsied adolescents. *Am J Occup Ther*. 1984;38:469–473
21. American Red Cross. *Swimming and Diving*. St. Louis, Mo: Mosby-Year Book, 1992.
22. Martin J. The Halliwick method. *Physiotherapy*. 1981; 67:288–291.

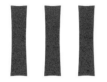

PHILOSOPHIES OF AQUATIC REHABILITATION

CHAPTER

15 | Bad Ragaz Ring Method

Gwen Garrett

The Bad Ragaz ring method is a collection of therapeutic techniques performed in the water that have been developed through the years in the thermal waters of Bad Ragaz, Switzerland. Still evolving, the method is used internationally for muscle re-education, strengthening, spinal traction/elongation, relaxation, and tone inhibition in the water. Water's unique properties of buoyancy, turbulence, hydrostatic pressure, surface tension, and thermal capacity are used to facilitate rehabilitation in a program of relaxation, stabilization, and progressive resistive exercises.

Since the 1930s, clients have used the spa waters of Bad Ragaz for active therapy. Clients with paralysis and limitation of movement in the joints were treated by performing range of motion exercises while supported on fixed treatment boards in the water. Straps were used to hold the client firmly in place, or rails were attached to the side of pool to provide a hand hold for clients exercising in the water.[1] In 1957, advances in techniques developed by Dr. Knupfer of Wilbad, Germany were introduced to Bad Ragaz by Nele Ipsen.[1]

Knupfer's exercises refined the method into a horizontal treatment technique in which the client was supported floating on his back by flotation rings around the neck and the pelvic region and under the knees and ankles.[1] The modified technique was used for stabilization or active resistive exercises. Knupfer incorporated the concepts of the neurophysiology of training, current at that time, and developed exercises that consisted of simple chains of movement passing from joint to joint, mainly in a single plane of motion. For example, while floating supine supported by rings, on command, the client would flex the knee and hip while the therapist held the client's foot. This active movement brought the client toward the therapist (the fixed point) in a single plane of continuous motion, in this case flexion. Here the role of the therapist as the stabilizing point in the water was established. Knupfer contended that active movements away from and back toward the fixed point of the therapist's hands facilitated stabilizing reactions adapted to the task circumstances, naturally occurring movement synergies, and isotonically resisted exercises of agonist and antagonist muscle groups. Furthermore, these patterns of movement provided the unique clinical opportunity to use closed kinetic chain exercise in a safe, supportive environment while enjoying the physiologic benefits of warm water. Before Knupfer, not all of the physical properties of water were used in pool exercises; after Knupfer, the use of buoyancy, turbulence, surface tension, and the thermal capacity of 92°F water to reduce pain, increase soft tissue compliance, reduce muscle tone, and promote relaxation were understood as unique clinical strategies that differentiated water from land exercise.

With the rapid growth and acceptance of proprioceptive neuromuscular facilitation (PNF), Dr. Zinn, medical director at Bad Ragaz and his medical team refined and modified Knupfer's exercises. Three-dimensional diagonal movements were developed and added to Knupfer's original exercise patterns. In 1967, physiotherapists Bridget Davis and Verena Laggatt incorporated Margaret Knott's PNF patterns, resulting in the technique known today as the Bad Ragaz ring method (BRRM).[2] The method continues to evolve, and is becoming increasingly popular in Switzerland, Germany, England, Australia,

289

South Africa, the United States, and elsewhere. For many years, BRRM training was difficult to obtain for therapists in the United States, and literature on BRRM was taught and published in German only. Some BRRM training is now offered in the United States by instructors who have been trained in the technique by European instructors.

Comparison of the Bad Ragaz Ring Method With Proprioceptive Neuromuscular Facilitation

Because many rehabilitation therapists are familiar with the concepts of PNF, a comparison of PNF with BRRM may improve the reader's understanding of the water exercise technique. The BRRM has incorporated many of the basic tenets of PNF, yet has modified them to suit the aquatic environment. The body, immersed in water, is no longer stabilized by gravity and moves freely unless stabilized by a therapist. With PNF, the client, who is lying on a plinth, is very stable. However, with BRRM, the client floats at the water surface supported by flotation devices. This can also be a stable position unless the client or the water moves. Any movement by the client's trunk or limbs from this stable position changes the floating client's metacenter (the balance of equilibrium between the client's center of gravity and center of buoyancy). Whereas PNF requires movement on the stability provided by gravity, BRRM requires movement on the stability provided by the therapist. The therapist's hands are the only points of fixation with BRRM. With PNF, resistance is applied manually; Movement through the water provides much of the resistance applied with BRRM. However, at times the therapist provides manual counter-resistance. A clinical constraint of BRRM compared with PNF is that although a terminal position of a joint can be achieved in water, a quick (passive) stretch cannot be exerted properly on lengthened muscles.[2] Such facilitory stretches are frequently used with PNF. The philosophy and techniques of PNF adapted by BRRM include the following:

1. Maximal resistance for isotonic and isometric exercise, throughout the range of motion, can be adapted to the client's capability.
2. Correct hand holds by the therapist serve to stimulate skin, muscles, and proprioceptors and likewise facilitate movement
3. Alternating "push" and "pull" patterns (approximation and traction, respectively) act on joint structures and sensory nerve endings to facilitate the muscle stretch reflex. Approximation facilitates cocontraction, whereas traction facilitates isotonic contractions.
4. Short, precise commands given by the therapist facilitate active movement.
5. Facilitation of strong muscles produces overflow/radiation to weak muscles, increasing activity of the weaker muscles in either the ipsilateral or contralateral limb.
6. Progression from proximal to distal holds increases the difficulty of performing the patterns, providing a natural gradation of exercise difficulty and, thus, strengthening.
7. By working dynamically with the client, the therapist is able to feel and assess the quality of client movement and make subtle alterations in resistance applied throughout the range of motion of any given pattern.
8. Muscles and joints are exercised in patterns of movement that are both natural and functional for the client.

Goals of Treatment

Because of its versatility, BRRM provides infinite possibilities for variation of exercise for the neurologic, orthopedic, and rheumatologic client. Aims of treatment include but are not limited to:

1. Tone reduction
2. Relaxation
3. Increasing range of motion
4. Muscle re-education
5. Strengthening
6. Spinal traction/elongation
7. Improving alignment and stability of the trunk
8. Preparation of the lower extremities for weight bearing
9. Restoration of normal patterns of upper and lower extremity movement
10. Improving general endurance
11. Training the functional capacity of the body as a whole

Technique

Stressing the need for the therapist to provide stability for the client and still be flexible with application, Margaret Campion[3] describes three ways in which the therapist acts in relation to the client:

1. *Isokinetically:* The therapist provides fixation while the client moves through the water either toward, away from, or around the therapist. The client determines the resistance encountered by setting the speed of movement through the water.
2. *Isotonically:* The therapist acts as a "movable" fixation point. For example, the client can be pushed or swung into the direction of his or her active movement. This action leads to an increase in resistance to that movement. Conversely, movement can be assisted by a therapist pushing in the direction opposite to the client's intended motion.
3. *Isometrically:* The client holds a fixed position while being pushed through the water by the therapist. This action promotes stabilizing contractions.

In addition, the therapist can move the client passively through the water for relaxation, tone inhibition, elongation of the trunk, and traction to the spine. In all four of these ways, the therapist acts as a fixed point throughout the activity.

Client Setup

Apparatus

The client wears a neck ring float and a large body ring or life jacket under the pelvis at the L5–S2 level. At times, several small ring floats are placed on the extremities. The neck ring float serves to keep the client's ears out of the water to hear the therapist's verbal commands. The small rings placed on the extremities prevent them from sinking, leading to improper spinal alignment. Care should be taken at all times to prevent hyperextension of the client's back, particularly in those with low back pain. The client is particularly vulnerable to hyperextension when moving from the vertical (standing) to the horizontal (supine) position. The therapist's hands should assist to support the client's low back when getting into and out of the flotation apparatus and when changing positions.

The Therapist

The Bad Ragaz technique is a one-on-one treatment situation, requiring the therapist to be in the pool with the client. The therapist stands in waist-deep water, not deeper than the T8–T10 or axillary level. Greater water depths destabilize the therapist, reducing his or her ability to serve as a fixation point. Wearing aqua shoes provides added traction and stability for the therapist. At times, wearing ankle weights may also increase the therapist's ability to stabilize. Therapists usually use a walk-stand position to provide a wide base of support (Fig. 15-1).

The therapist's feet should be shoulder distance apart, with the hips and knees slightly bent. One foot should be in front of the other to increase stability. The therapist should wear aqua tights or swim leotards that cover the legs

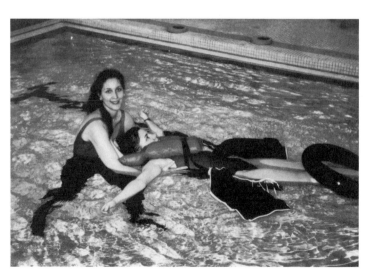

FIGURE 15-1. Walk-stand position.

to minimize skin-to-skin contact with the client and to provide a barrier to intimate contact with the client when the client is positioned between the therapist's legs.

Pool Size

A minimal pool area of 7 × 8 feet is required for BRRM activities. Davis recommends a pool not smaller than 170 square feet.[2] Water depth should be 3 to 4 feet, with a preferred water temperature between 92°F and 98°F.

Treatment Guidelines

Initial sessions of 5 to 15 minutes are recommended because the exercises often require maximal contractions and effort from the client and are fatiguing to client and therapist alike. As the client progresses, sessions are increased to a maximum of 30 minutes. Passive relaxation techniques to decrease hypertonicity may be integrated before active client exercise and whenever exertion elevates tone or muscle guarding in the session. Activity that increases spasticity in the neurologically involved client should be avoided. The physiologic effects of water immersion (ie, dehydration, dry skin) limit the period of time that a therapist should spend in the water. This author believes that the therapist should spend no more than 4 hours per day in the therapeutic pool.

Progression of Exercise

Davis states that resistance is provided by the movement of the client's body through the water.[2] When the body moves or is moved through the water, the resistance encountered is partly the result of the negative pressure produced behind the object. This negative drag results from eddy current production impeding forward movement. In addition, frictional forces are encountered in front of the movement object. Although not as effective in resisting movement, these forces do contribute to the turbulent drag encountered. The turbulent drag produced from movement is directly proportional to the client's speed of movement. Therefore, the faster the client moves, the more resistance he or she encounters. In this way, resistance to

movement is self-regulated by the client as opposed to applied by the therapist. If heavy resisted exercise is desired, clients should be instructed to move through the water at their fastest achievable speed.

Given these circumstances, resistance to movement can be progressively increased by:

1. Adding rings, floats, or equipment such as hand-held paddles
2. Using larger movements—for example, working from a fully flexed position to a fully extended position, or vice versa
3. Altering the shape of the limb or changing the lever arm
4. Moving from more proximal to distal hand holds on the client; this requires the client to exert more control over more body segments and therefore increases the difficulty of the activity
5. Increasing the speed of movement
6. Changing the direction of movement
7. Using quick reversals and reciprocal patterns, thereby working into and out of the negative drag effect produced, with cumulative increases in the overall turbulent drag
8. Decreasing the amount of flotation support

Indications and Contraindications

Indications

The BRRM is a versatile treatment method that lends itself to a wide variety of client problems and diagnoses. It is particularly indicated for:

1. Orthopedic and rheumatologic conditions, including presurgical and postsurgical conditioning for the trunk and the extremities, fractures, and soft tissue injuries. BRRM is valuable for all arthritic conditions, such as rheumatoid arthritis, osteoarthritis, fibromyalgia, and myositis.
2. Neurologic disorders including cerebrovascular accident, head injury, Parkinson's disease, paraplegia, and quadriplegia. Caution should be used with clients exhibiting hypertonicity. Rapid and fatiguing activities should be avoided because they increase spasticity.
3. Pain syndromes of the upper and lower extremities and back.
4. Reflex sympathetic dystrophy and similar problems in which sensory desensitization is indicated.

5. Mastectomy and cardiac surgery clients who benefit from performing bilateral upper quadrant stretching and strengthening.
6. Developmental delay symptoms like tactile defensiveness, because these clients benefit from the sensory bombardment and compression of the water.

Contraindications

Clients should be screened for all medical contraindications to aquatic rehabilitation activities.

1. Precaution should be taken to avoid excessive fatigue. Clients receive a great deal of vestibular stimulation as they are pulled, pushed, or turned in the water.
2. If a client is suspected of having vestibular problems, the therapist should move him or her slowly and continually monitor nystagmus. Some clients with poor tolerance to increased vestibular stimulation may be contraindicated from treatment altogether.
3. Special care must be taken with clients with acute conditions of the back, neck, and extremities. In many of the BRRM movements, clients move away from the therapist in a free movement that stops only when the limit of joint motion is reached. In the normal joint this is not a problem, but for the client with acute joint involvement, this could cause overstretching and subsequent joint damage. The technique can be modified by the operator stepping into the direction of the client's motion to stop the movement before reaching the end range of motion, by moving slower, and by using a shorter lever arm.

Sample Exercise Patterns

Bad Ragaz ring method exercises can be divided into patterns for the trunk, arms, and legs. They can also be categorized as unilateral or bilateral. Bilateral patterns are further defined as symmetric or asymmetric. Most patterns emphasize reciprocal movement patterns. Reciprocal movements are not always emphasized with certain client conditions and circumstances. For example, some neurologically involved clients are unable to perform reciprocal movements without facilitating hypertonicity (see Box 15-11 for an illustrative example). In general, the patterns are performed in supine floating, yet a few arm patterns are performed in prone and a few trunk patterns in side lying. The patterns described in Boxes 15-1 through 15-12 (on the following pages) are some of the most commonly used and versatile patterns, and have been adapted by the author to improve the reader's understanding. Because of the flexibility of the patterns and the adaptability of the technique, an almost infinite variety of exercises can be developed by the therapist to maximize client outcomes.

(text continues on page 304)

BOX 15-1. Trunk Pattern 1

A. Pattern: Trunk Stabilization in Neutral Alignment

Isometric

B. Starting Position

- Client in supine.
- Client aligns spine in midline, arms at the side.
- Rings: One ring or float at the L5–S1 level, a collar supporting the neck, and a ring around each of the client's ankles.
- Therapist: Positioned between the client's abducted legs (pelvic hand hold) or positioned at client's head (axillary hand hold).

C. Therapist Hold

- Pelvic hand hold: The therapist's hands are placed on the posterolateral aspect of the lower quadrant at the pelvis, knees, or ankles. Hand position can be moved proximal to distal (pelvis to knees to ankles) to require more effort from the client.
- Axillary hand hold: The therapist's hand hold can be moved to the posterolateral aspect of the upper trunk at the axilla. The hold can be progressed down the arm to the elbows bilaterally to increase client effort.
- The therapist turns the client in a circle through the water.

D. Verbal Commands

- "Hold your trunk in alignment."
- "Don't let me push you (out of alignment)."
- "Keep your body straight."

E. Finishing Position

- Client maintains alignment as therapist swings him or her in a circle to the right, to the left, or with quick reversals (ie, moving to the right then quickly to the left).

F. Progressions

The following adaptations can also be used to progress the activity:

- The client is required to maintain more control over body segments when the therapist's hand holds move distally, or from the pelvis to the axilla thus increasing the length of the lever arm.
- The client can hold the isometric contraption longer as the therapist swings him or her through the water.
- Repeated contraction techniques or repetition of the pattern.
- Rhythmic stablization techniques.
- Slow reversal techniques.
- Quick reversal techniques.

BOX 15-2. Trunk Pattern 2 (Fig. 15-2)

A. Pattern: Trunk Rotation

Isometric
Unilateral to the right or the left

B. Starting Position

- Client in supine.
- Client rotates trunk to left or right, bringing respective hip to the surface of the water.
- Rings: One at the level of L5–S1, a collar supporting the neck, and a ring around each of the client's ankles.
- Therapist: Positioned at the client's head.

C. Therapist Hold

- The therapist can use a pelvic or axillary hand hold (see Box 15-1) to start, and progress hold from proximal to distal to increase effort required from the client. The therapist turns the client in a circle through the water.

D. Verbal Commands

- "Turn your left (respective) hip up and hold."
- "Hold and keep holding."
- "Relax."

E. Finishing Position

- Client maintains trunk rotation until told to relax.
- Client returns to neutral trunk alignment (starting position) on command.

F. Progressions

The following adaptations can also be used to progress the activity:

- The therapist's hand holds can move to more distal locations.
- Clients can hold the isometric contraction longer as the therapist moves them through the water (sustained isometrics).
- The therapist moves the client more quickly, requiring stronger isometric holding.
- The client can be required to hold the isometric contraction longer as the therapist also moves him or her more quickly (sustained and stronger isometric holding).

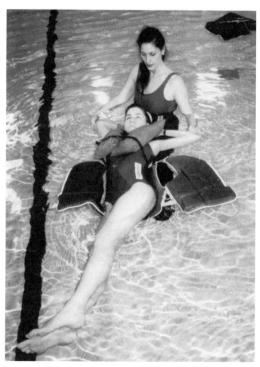

FIGURE 15-2. Trunk pattern: isometric rotation.

BOX 15-3. Trunk Pattern 3 (Fig. 15-3)

A. Pattern: Trunk Rotation With Flexion

Isotonic
Unilateral to right or left

B. Starting Position

- Client in supine.
- Client rotates trunk to the right or left while bringing the respective hip to the water's surface. On command, the client dorsiflexes the ankles and flexes the hips while maintaining knee extension.
- Rings: One ring at the L5–S1 level, a collar supporting the neck, and a ring around each of the client's ankles.
- Therapist: Positioned at the client's head.

C. Therapist Hold

- An axillary hand hold is used with a proximal to distal progression to increase client effort (ie, axillary hand hold to bilateral elbow hold).

D. Verbal Commands

- "Turn your right (or left) hip up and bend."
- "Bring your toes toward your left (or right) shoulder."

E. Finishing Position

- The client continues to hold trunk flexion and rotation until told to relax.
- The client returns to neutral trunk alignment and the starting position on command.

F. Progressions

The following adaptations can also be used to progress the activity:
- The therapist's hand holds move more distally.
- The client holds the contraction longer as the therapist swings him or her through the water.
- The therapist turns more quickly.

Precautions: Clients with spinal or upper extremity injuries may not tolerate this activity well.

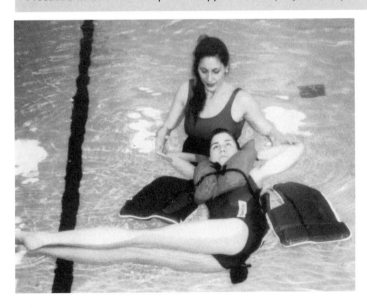

FIGURE 15-3. Trunk pattern: rotation/flexion.

BOX 15-4. Trunk Pattern 4 (Fig. 15-4)

A. Pattern: Trunk Rotation With Extension
Isotonic
Unilateral to right or left

B Starting Position
- Client in supine.
- Client rotates trunk to the right or the left, bringing the respective hip to the water's surface. On command, the client plantarflexes his or her ankles and extends the trunk and hip while maintaining knee extension.
- Rings: One ring at L5–S1 level, a collar supporting the neck, and a ring around the client's ankles.
- Therapist: Positioned at the client's head.

C. Therapist Hold
- An axillary hand hold is used, with progression from proximal to distal to increase client effort (ie, axillary to bilateral elbow hold).
- The therapist moves the client in a circle through the water.

D. Verbal Commands
- "Turn your right (or left) hip up and bend backwards."
- "Hold, hold, hold and relax."
- Clients may need to be cued to "point your toes and legs back."

E. Finishing Position
- Client continues to extend trunk, maintaining trunk rotation until told to relax.
- Client returns to neutral trunk alignment and the starting position on command.

F. Progressions
- Same as for Trunk Pattern 3.
Precautions: Clients who have been advised against back hyperextension should not try this pattern.

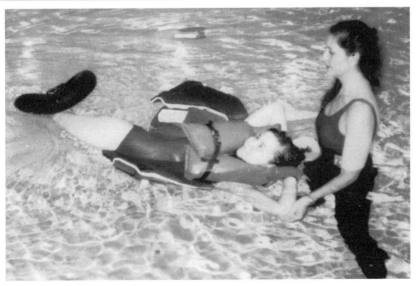

FIGURE 15-4. Trunk pattern: rotation/extension.

BOX 15-5. Trunk Pattern 5

A. Pattern: Lateral Trunk Flexion

Isokinetic

Bilateral symmetric

B. Starting Position

- Client in supine.
- Client aligns spine in the neutral position.
- Rings: One at the L5–S1 level, a collar supporting the neck, and a ring around each of the client's ankles.
- Therapist: Positioned between the client's abducted legs (pelvic hand hold) or at the client's head (axillary or bilateral elbow hand holds).

C. Therapist Hold

- A pelvic hand hold is used initially, with progression to an axillary hand hold and eventually to a bilateral elbow hold.
- The therapist stabilizes the client as he or she actively side bends laterally.

D. Verbal Commands

- "Bend to your right (or left) and then relax."
- "Bend and relax, bend and relax."

E. Finishing Position

- The client continues to laterally flex the trunk until told to relax.
- The therapist returns the client to the starting position.

E. Progressions

The following adaptations can also be used to progress the activity:

- Progress hand holds.
- Instruct the client to perform quick reversals to the right then left.
- This activity can be modified to make the exercise more resistive by swinging the client into the direction of his or her active motion, or less difficut by swinging the client in the direction opposite of his or her active motion.

BOX 15-6. Arm Pattern 1

A. Pattern: Shoulder Abduction, External Rotation, Wrist/Finger Extension Moving to Shoulder Adduction, Internal Rotation, Wrist/Finger Flexion

Isokinetic

Bilateral symmetric

B. Starting Position (Fig. 15-5)

- Client in supine.
- Shoulder in internal rotation and adduction, wrist and finger flexion.
- Rings: One ring at the L5–S1 level, a collar supporting the neck, and a ring around both ankles so that the legs are adducted.
- Therapist: Positioned in the walk-stand position at the client's head at an arm's length distance. The therapist positions deep in the water to submerge the client's hand while performing the pattern.

C. Therapist Hold

- The therapist hold is on the extensor surface of the client's hand for the proper sensory stimulus. The client moves away from the therapist.

D. Verbal Command

- "Push your fingers back, wrist back, and bring your arms over your head and relax."

E. Finishing Position (Fig. 15-6)

- Client's shoulder in full abduction, external rotation, wrist and finger extension.
- When the client relaxes, the therapist takes a step forward, returning the client's arm to the starting position.

E. Progression

- The speed of the client's active motion can be increased to progress the activity.

Precautions: Limitations in joint motion or spasticity require modifications in the activity. Clients with such conditions should perform a smaller active range of motion, and end range of motion momentum can be countered by the therapist's stepping forward into the direction of the client's active motion.

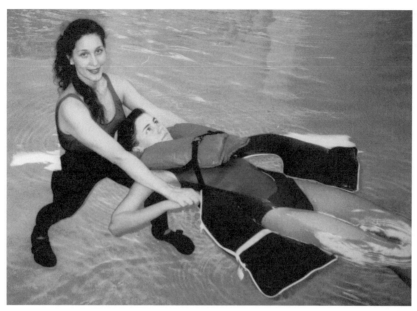

FIGURE 15-5. Arm pattern 1: start position.

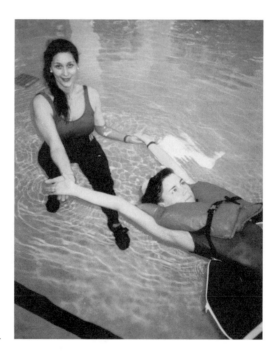

FIGURE 15-6. Arm pattern 1: finish position.

BOX 15-7. Arm Pattern 2

A. Pattern: Shoulder Flexion/Abduction, External Rotation, Wrist/Finger Extension and Abduction Moving to Shoulder Extension/Adduction, Internal Rotation, Wrist and Finger Flexion and Adduction (Elbow Moves From Extension to Flexion and Returns to Extension)

Isokinetic
Bilateral Symmetric

B. Starting Position

- Client in supine.
- Client's arms begin in shoulder external rotation, extension, forward flexion, and abduction.
- Rings: One ring at the L5–S1 level, a collar supporting the neck, and a ring around the ankles with the legs held together.
- Therapist: Positioned in the walk-stand position at the client's head at an arm's length distance. The therapist positions deep in the water to submerge the client's hand while performing the pattern.

C. Therapist Hold

- The client and therapist grip each other's hands. The therapist hold is on the client's palms to provide sensory input for the desired movement.

D. Verbal Command

- "Grip my hands, pull down and into your sides and relax."

E. Finishing Position

- Client's arms positioned in shoulder internal rotation, flexion, wrist/finger flexion and abduction.
- The therapist asks the client to relax. The therapist then takes a step back to return the client to the starting position.

F. Progression

- The client can increase the speed of his or her arm movement to progress the activity.
- Arm patterns 1 and 2 can be performed reciprocally.

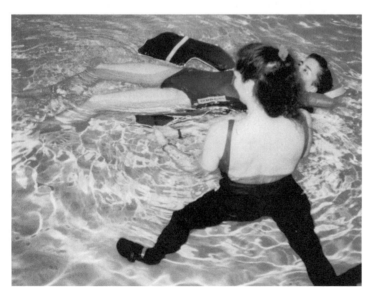

FIGURE 15-7. Arm pattern 3: start position.

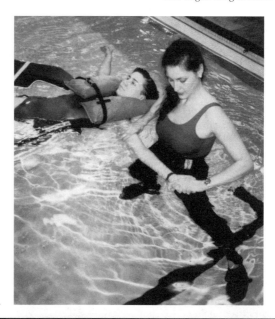

FIGURE 15-8. Arm pattern 3: finish position.

BOX 15-8. Arm Pattern 3

A. Pattern: Shoulder Extension and Adduction, Forearm Pronation, Wrist/Finger Flexion, Moving to Shoulder Flexion and Abduction, Forearm Supination, Wrist/Finger Extension

Isokinetic
Unilateral

B. Starting Position (Fig. 15-7)

- Client in supine.
- Client's arm begins in shoulder extension, forearm pronation, wrist and finger flexion with the arm positioned slightly behind the back.
- Rings: One ring at the S1–L5 level, a collar supporting the neck, and a ring around the ankles with the legs placed together.
- Therapist: Positioned in a firm stance with feet apart and one foot forward at the client's side. The client's active arm (ie, right arm) is placed over the therapist's opposite hip (ie, left hip).

C. Therapist Hold

- The therapist uses one hand to hold the client's axilla firmly. Therapist's other hand grips the client's hand over the extensor surface.

D. Verbal Command

- "Push your fingers back, wrist back, push and relax."

E. Finishing Position (Fig. 15-8)

- Client's arm moves to full shoulder flexion, abduction and forearm supination with wrist and finger extension.
- The therapist pivots forward, returning the client to the starting position.

F. Progression

- The client can increase the speed of his or her movements to progress the activity.

BOX 15-9. Arm Pattern 4

A. Pattern: Shoulder Flexion, Abduction, Forearm Supination, Wrist and Finger Extension Moving to Shoulder Extension, Adduction, Forearm Pronation, Wrist/Finger Flexion

Isokinetic
Unilateral

B. Starting Position

- Client in supine.
- Client's arm begins in full flexion, forearm supination, and wrist and finger extension.
- Rings: One at the L5–S1 Level, a collar supporting the neck, a ring around the ankles with the legs together.
- Therapist: Positioned in alignment with the client's body. The therapist's left leg is under client's right shoulder, or vice versa.

C. Therapist Hold

- The therapist stabilizes the anterior surface of the client's shoulder with one hand. The therapists other hand grips the client's hand on its palmar surface.

D. Verbal Commands

- "Grip my fingers hard."
- "Pull down hard."
- "Pull down and under your buttocks and relax."

E. Finishing Position

- The client's arm ends in shoulder extension, forearm pronation, and wrist/finger flexion.
- The therapist pivots backward returning the client to the starting position.

F. Progression

- The client can increase the speed of his or her movement to progress the activity.
- Arm patterns 3 and 4 can be performed reciprocally.

BOX 15-10. Leg Pattern 1

A. Pattern Moving Leg—Hip Adduction and Extension With Knee Extension Moving to Hip Abduction and Extension With Knee Extension

Holding Leg—Hip and Knee Held in a Neutral Position

Isokinetic
Unilateral

B. Starting Position

- Client in supine.
- Client's hip adducted with knee in extension.
- Rings: One ring at the L5–S1 level, a collar supporting the neck, and a ring float on the moving leg.
- Therapist: Positioned in the walk-stand position perpendicular to the holding leg.

C. Therapist Hold

- One hand on the medial surface of the holding leg at mid-thigh level and the other on the dorsolateral surface of the client's foot.

D. Verbal Command

- "Push your leg out (the working leg) and relax."

E. Finishing Position

- Client's hip abducted with the knee extended.
- The therapist steps forward with the holding leg, returning to the client the starting position.

F. Progressions

The following adaptations can also be used to progress the activity:

- The client can increase the speed of his or her movement.
- The pattern can be progressed to include internal and external rotation components in the following variations:

    Hip internal rotation and adduction with knee extension moving to hip external rotation abduction of the hip with the knees in extension

    or

    Hip external rotation and adduction with knee extension moving to hip internal rotation and abduction with knee extension

- Leg patterns 1 and 2 can be performed reciprocally.

BOX 15-11. Leg Pattern 2

A. Pattern: Hip Abduction and Extension With Knee Extension Moving to Hip Adduction and Extension With Knee Extension

Isokinetic
Unilateral

B. Starting Position

- Client in supine.
- Client's legs placed in hip abduction and extension with knee extension.
- Rings: One ring at the L5–S1 level, a collar supporting the neck, a ring float on the working leg.
- Therapist: Positioned in the walk-stand position perpendicular to the holding leg.

C. Therapist Hold

- One hand on the medial surface of the holding leg at mid-thigh level and the other on the dorsolateral surface of the client's foot.

D. Verbal Command

- "Pull your leg in and relax."

E. Finishing Position

- Client's leg is in hip adduction and extension with knee extension.

F. Progressions

The following adaptations can also be used to progress the activity:

- Client can increase the speed of his or her motion.
- The pattern can be progressed to incorporate internal and external rotation components (see Leg Pattern 1).
- Leg Patterns 1 and 2 can be performed reciprocally.

Contraindications: Clients with hip abductor hypertonicity are not candidates for this pattern.

BOX 15-12. Leg Pattern 3

A. Pattern: Knee/Hip Extension Moving to Knee/Hip Flexion

Isokinetic (working leg)
Isometric (holding leg)
Bilateral reciprocal/asymmetric

B. Starting Position

- Client in supine.
- Client's hips and knees are extended bilaterally.
- Rings: A ring float at the L5–S1 level and a collar to support the neck.
- Therapist: Positioned at the client's foot in the walk-stand position.

C. Therapist Hold

- One hand on the dorsal surface of the foot to provide appropriate sensory input.
- The other hand supporting under the plantar surface of the plantarflexed foot.

D. Verbal Command

- "Pull and relax."

E. Finishing Position

- Client's knee and hip are flexed on the working leg.
- The holding leg remains extended.
- The client's torso will have moved toward the therapist.
- The therapist takes a step back, returning the client to the starting position.

F. Progressions

The following adaptations can also be used to progress the activity:

- The client can increase the speed of his or her movement.
- Hand holds can be progressed more distally to a toe hold.
- Pattern can be modified to include diagonal movement by incorporating rotational components (ie, hip extension, adduction, internal rotation, with knee extension and ankle dorsiflexion moving to hip flexion, external rotation, abduction and plantarflexion).

Note: This pattern can incorporate a reciprocal "push" pattern to return to the starting position from the flexed finishing position. Alternating a "pull" and a "push" pattern promotes muscle balance.

Acknowledgment
Much of the information for this chapter is derived from the author's personal interviews, correspondence, and instruction from staff trained at Bad Ragaz, Baden-Baden, and Bath water physiotherapy departments over the past 14 years.

For more information regarding the Bad Ragaz ring method and instructional courses, inquiries may be addressed to: Gwen Garrett, 22 East Main Street, Smithfield, VA 23430.

REFERENCES

1. Zinn WM, Egger B. *The Role of Water in Rehabilitation Exercise in Water: A Revised Method Using Ring Floats.* Bad Ragaz, Switzerland: Bad Ragaz Department of Medicine; 1981.
2. Davis BC. A technique of re-education in the treatment pool. *Physiotherapy.* 1967;53(2):37–59.
3. Campion MR. *Adult Hydrotherapy: A Practical Approach.* Oxford: Heinemann Medical Books; 1991.

16

Halliwick Method

Jennifer Cunningham

The Halliwick method* is familiar to most aquatic rehabilitation professionals who have been involved in aquatics for any length of time. Those attempting to research the subject have realized that very little has been printed about this technique, and the written descriptions available are usually confusing. The late James McMillan, the man who developed and continued to refine this technique, offered courses throughout Europe on a regular basis, but actually presented only two papers describing his concepts. In an attempt to gather information concerning the Halliwick method and better understand the techniques involved, this author traveled to Bad Ragaz, Switzerland to attend the Basic Halliwick Course in 1992 and the Advanced Halliwick Method Course in 1993, taught by McMillan himself. Each course was a 5-day session with 8 hours each day being divided into lecture and laboratory time. The Basic Course fully explained the sketchy outline with which most American aquatic rehabilitation professionals are familiar. The course taught preswim skills through games in a group setting for pediatrics. The Advanced Course covered information not commonly available (if at all) in the United States. It focused more on one-on-one techniques to be used with adult client populations and for treating orthopedic and neurologic conditions.

McMillan, who was in his eighties at the time of this writing, readily admitted that he was an engineer and had no formal medical training. His concepts were developed using his knowledge of competitive swimming, his training as an engineer, his observations while working with the handicapped in the water, and many apparently lively discussions with the Bobaths and other members of the British and Swiss medical communities. He realized that the medical and therapeutic climates differ substantially in Europe and the United States. The treatment and documentation techniques described in this chapter are as he taught them in Switzerland. American aquatic therapists must adapt them so that they might be useful in treating their client populations. The Halliwick method uses the "general system theory" of teaching. This theory, which suggests that no information belongs exclusively to any one profession, is a multidisciplinary model that gathers information from many fields of study. McMillan's program for teaching the disabled to swim combines information from many fields, including fluid mechanics (engineering), neurophysiology (medicine), psychology, pedagogy (education), and group dynamics (sociology).

When approached about having his concepts possibly published in an American textbook, James McMillan, or "Mac," as he preferred to be called, seemed very pleased. His goal was to have Halliwick Clubs worldwide, with regular international swimming competitions. He explained that this author was the first American therapist to complete both the Basic Halliwick Course and the Advanced Halliwick Course under his direction. He was eager to spend extra time outside of the classroom to assist with this

---

* Editor's Note: This chapter contains excerpts from a speech given by James McMillan, creator of the Halliwick method, regarding the development of the technique. Since McMillan passed away during the time that this book was written, the editors were unable to consult with him regarding the excerpt contents. Therefore, the editors respectfully edited McMillan's speech to meet the needs of the manuscript.

chapter. He was interested in training additional American therapists and encouraged more to attend his courses. Unfortunately, James McMillan passed away before the completion of this book.

The following paper was presented by Mr. McMillan in São Paulo, Brazil in October 1993 at the I Congresso Internacional Degidroreabilitacao Terapias em Piscina E Natacao Terapeitica. The document is a brief overview of the beginnings and development of the Halliwick method. It also gives the reader a glimpse of the man himself. The remainder of this chapter is taken directly from the course notes and from conversations with "Mac." All quotes—unless otherwise noted—are his words. Illustrations are copies of his drawings on the chalkboard during the classes.

The Halliwick Concept
By James McMillan, MBE

This paper provides a brief introduction to the Halliwick Concept and its history. The Concept has two clearly defined elements: swimming and therapy.

First, an explanation is needed to describe the sequence of events that led to the development of the Concept. My training lies in the field of Engineering including the study of Fluid Mechanics. I have also followed the sport of swimming all of my life. In 1946, I had returned from a war and was older and not fit enough to swim competitively. So, I did what all of the older members of the club did—I taught the younger members.

My home and my swimming club is in North London. Located in this area is a home and school for physically handicapped girls—The Halliwick School for Crippled Girls. Many local organizations, including my swimming club, organized events to raise money for the support of the school.

What we were doing for the school was insignificant relative to the achievements of others. Furthermore, our efforts were passive. It was my opinion that we should take a more active and positive part in the improvement of the lives of these girls.

My statements to the club committee caused an uproar out of which came the question, "What should we do?" My answer—"teach them to swim" produced laughter among committee members. They said, "these girls are heavily handicapped spastics and no one, not even

medical professionals, will take them into the water."

I had seen only too recently, the tragedies of war. Comparing these events with the happiness of our young swimmers, I reflected on the situation of the Halliwick girls. I received the support of some members of the water polo team and we set out to teach the girls how to swim. The idea was to put them in the water with our young club swimmers—integration.

When I approached the Matron of the school with the idea, she said, "your idea is wonderful, but do you know what a spastic is?" I had no idea and said so. While she did not say no, she did defer to the Medical Officer responsible for the girls' health.

The project was started with the consent and good wishes of the Honorary Surgeon Oliver J. Vaughn-Jackson, FRCS (later Professor). Despite his blessing, considerable opposition to the project came from others. Perhaps this was understandable as we taught the girls to swim using no flotation aids. We believed that we should not merely replace adapted equipment used for movement on land with floatation devices. The water provides an environment where they can be free.

Then came the opposition from the medical professionals who believed that the "spastics" would become hypertonic in the cold water resulting in spasm. They never did. Then came the argument that I had no right to organize such a program. I was not medically qualified. My answer to these statements was simple, "one did not have to be medically qualified to teach swimming." Now attitudes are different, but I think in some places, I have never been forgiven!

The most important questions came from the Surgeon. "What was being done in the water that has improved their posture, head control, general movement, and above all their personal behavior?" In retrospect, he must have been surprised by my reply; "they are being taught balance in the water using principles of fluid mechanics, moments of inertia to control unwanted movement (especially around the midline), and body movement and shape by tactile stimulation." His reply was a classic one: "if you say that too loudly, you will be a large sized cat amongst the neurological pigeons." Readers must realize that this was in 1951, before man had gone into space and plasticity of the brain was discussed. Despite this, the encouragement of this great man was never diminished.

The opposition and difficulties we met were balanced by encouragement from parents and friends of the participants. The numbers coming to the Saturday afternoon sessions of the Halliwick Penguins Swimming Club were steadily increasing. It was obvious that we needed to expand to where we could use appropriate swimming facilities.

Working with the handicapped is a labor intensive operation and could become impossibly expensive if it were not for the principle of volunteer help. Would-be instructors came from parents and relations, Youth movements and other volunteers. Help with transportation and bathside organization came from the Lions and Rotary Clubs, the Round Tablers and their Ladies, the Red Cross, and St. Johns.

As the club system was established in 1952, a national teaching organization was formed to continue the development of the teaching method.

Four principles of instruction were established:

Mental Adaptation—Involves recognition of two forces acting on the body in water: gravity and upthrust. The combined effects of these forces lead to rotational movement.

Balance Restoration—Emphasizes the use of large patterns of movement, particularly with the arms, to restore and/or maintain balance. This use of moments of inertia coincides with the "primitive reflexes." Instruction involves the use of these wide ranging movements to move the body into different postures while maintaining balance control. The most important of these postures being the immediate response to movement around the midline axis.

Inhibition—The ability to create and hold a desired position or posture. When inhibition is developed, the swimmer is able to contain all unwanted movement.

Facilitation—The ability to create a mentally desired and physically controlled movement (eg, swimming) by any means without flotation aids.

These phases of learning are in an order by which the cerebral cortex learns all physical movement (eg, a developmental sequence) and are set out in a structure known as the Ten Point Programme. Unfortunately, teachers often remember the structure but not the importance of its sequence.

The most important step is learning to make a 360 degree rotation around the midline axis. This rotation is the most difficult to teach as it is in opposition to the body's natural reflex activity. The psychological change occurring with the student is most noticeable when perfecting this activity.

Instruction takes place in groups including no more than seven swimmers. Handicaps are mixed within each group yet principles of group dynamics are not overlooked. Each "swimmer" has an instructor who follows a program of games or water activity as directed by an experienced group leader.

Games and/or water activities contain teaching principles from the Ten Point Programme. By this means, essential movement and control is learned against a background of fun and games.

The Halliwick method has been criticized as being labor intensive. However, so is any activity used with the handicapped.

The Halliwick Method has two main purposes: (1) to teach the swimmers about themselves and their balance control in water; (2) to teach them to swim. The use of flotation devices such as rubber arm bands would negate these objectives. In some cases, their use could even be dangerous.

It has been our experience that helpers become competent when they understand handling principles and program activities. Many of our instructors have been working in their clubs for more than 30 years.

In 1959, a request came from an old, established organization caring for the handicapped: the Dr. Barnado's Homes. Their representatives stated, "We have the handicapped, we have the pool, but we don't know what to do. Even if we did, we don't have the staff needed."

We approached a local school, The Woodford High School for Girls. The Sports Teacher at the school pledged their support. The senior girls were taught the Halliwick Method and helped in the pool for the next few months on Saturday afternoons. The Barnado Dolphins S.C. was managed by Woodford High School for the next 30 years until reorganization closed the Home, the pool, and the club.

The concept of linking handicapped with nonhandicapped schools is called the Gemini (the twins) Scheme. This concept was encouraged as, apart from learning movement in water, it develops a social conscience and a sense of caring.

To stimulate the progress of the swimmers, and to encourage the growth of swimming clubs for the handicapped, competition was started among the clubs. The Halliwick Penguins had been competing within their club since 1951. Their experiences had already provided insights into the best approach to organized competition. The development of a competition system that could include all manner and degrees of handicapped participants so that each had an equal chance of winning was particularly challenging. Furthermore, competition organizers visualized an integrated competition with the able bodied for the future. This now takes place. For example, the Halliwick Association of Great Britain holds a national championship competition for all handicaps. The Australian Halliwick Association has started championship competitions including their able bodied champion swimmers. These activities are steps towards integration.

The ultimate in competition occurred in 1970, when a team of swimmers from our handicapped clubs in Great Britain were trained to swim the English Channel from France to England. It was a challenge to the handicapped to venture and test themselves.

This attempt was the first ever by a handicapped team. The team consisted of two amputees, two polios, one paraplegic and one hemiplegic with partial sight. The swim was particularly challenging as the sea temperature was 19 degrees celsius, the waves 1 to $1\frac{1}{2}$ metres high. Also, the swim was made at night.

The result was a successful crossing in 14 hours and 1 minute. This proved to be the fastest crossing of the year, so the team won the international trophy.

Clearly, the work that had been done in swimming revealed many advantages to those working in the field of hydrotherapy. Many attempts to interest therapists had met with little success. This apparent lack of interest led me to look for the bridges that could provide the answers.

Water as a medium of therapy has not had a very distinguished history. Claims for its healing powers that have been attributed to warm temperature, chemical structure, etc. were not based on sound theoretical evidence. The greatest weakness was the lack of understanding of the degree to which the human body adapts and changes its systems when immersed.

Water, when fully understood, can provide a very great contribution to the cause of therapy. However, water is a very challenging element in which to work, requiring great skill to get good results. The critical nature of water can be demonstrated when a person assumes a back lying position. If the swimmer needs to roll over, they merely need to laterally deviate their eyes to start the motion; even without motion of the head.

Because of its success, the principles of the Halliwick Method have created a firm foundation on which to build a more advanced idea of water. Support for its teachings came from recognition of the relationship of the metacentric principles of water and the rotational patterns observed with human physiology.

The therapeutic use of water lies in the art of carefully selecting to use the many physical properties of water in the most appropriate way to produce a sensible result. Misuse or careless application can mean that well intended therapy fades into merely tender loving care.

When lying on the back in water, there is no firm surface against which the muscles can react. Stretch reflex modulation is at a minimum if it exists at all. Further, the body is balanced around the midline, the most critical axis in water. Finally, after a period of some 15 minutes there is a reduction in muscle tone. This situation will cause the body to revert to an earlier system of learning and to be allowed to redevelop both movement and control. This can be shown in film and by demonstration.

The human body cannot be taught how to move. It knows how to move. Maturation or skill is achieved by being confronted with challenging movement situations. From its own experimental procedures, the body will find a resolution to the movement problem. Therefore, while in the water, the human body is in a learning situation that cannot be reproduced on land. However, it has been found that what has been learned in the water can be reproduced on land.

A logical approach to exercise must be followed in water. The first stage of this approach enumerates the treatment objectives. Those objectives in current use include to: (1) strengthen and/or improve weak muscle groups, (2) increase range of motion, (3) facilitate posture and balance reactions, (4) improve general physical condition, (5) improve mental adaptability, (6) reduce pain, and (7) reduce spasticity.

Treatment techniques which are specific to water are used to meet these objectives. The following techniques can be used individually or in conjunction with other techniques:

Upthrust/Gravity—Varying the water depth on the patient to either increase or decrease buoyant support. The critical depth appears to be the level of T11 on the patient.

Turbulence—Can be used to assist or disturb the control of balance in a very subtle way. It can also be used to move the patient through the water and may be helpful in swimming training.

Metacentre—Refers to the theory of balance for any floating object in water. It is a very powerful but gentle exercise technique.

Waves—Can be controlled to be large or small in size and/or wavelength and can create a smooth and strong working force.

In addition to the principles of fluid mechanics, other influencing factors include neurological reactions, some of which are impossible to apply to land treatment:

Skin Stimulation—Often used to obtain a very fine degree of posture control and/or movement.

Eye Deviation—Important in head control (eg, the client with athetosis).

Transference—A technique developed solely in water, and is the ability to create movement in one area of the body and transfer it to another area.

A plan of treatment must be developed including specific goals and activities to achieve an end result. A simple algorithmic technique can be used to evaluate the results.

It is firmly believed that the Halliwick Method represents a considerable evolution in swimming instruction and therapeutic practice. It has been developed on a general system theory approach. That is to say that knowledge from many disciplines have been brought together and synthesized around a specific objective.

The Basic Course

Underlying Concepts

As with most aquatic courses, the Basic Halliwick Course begins with an in-depth discussion of hydrodynamics. Mac addressed most of the topics explained in the traditional therapeutic aquatics courses taught in the United States (eg, relative density, Archimedes' principle, Pascal's law, viscosity, buoyancy, temperature of the water, turbulence, wave propagation, laminar flow, and the concept of metacenter). These topics are covered in Chapter 2 of this book. Mac's teachings correspond with most of the

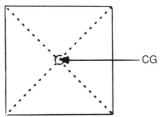

FIGURE 16-1. Center of gravity (CG) of a simple object.

chapter's contents. However, with his engineering background, Mac went into much more detail than what is given in most standard aquatic rehabilitation seminars, especially when discussing turbulence, wave propagation, and metacenter. This chapter discusses only those ideas that differ from or are not covered in Chapter 2.

One of Mac's early theories suggests that warm water temperatures are not entirely responsible for the decrease in muscle tone often observed with aquatic rehabilitation clients. This notion has been supported by aerospace research. Instead, tone is influenced by proprioceptive input stimulated by gravitational forces. In other words, tone is a function of weight. When a person is immersed in water above the T11 level, or lies horizontal in the water, the force of gravity is neutralized. Tactile sensory systems are then used to monitor body position and movement. After the effects of weight (gravitational force) have been neutralized by 15 minutes of immersion, a person's tone automatically decreases. This change in tone can also be noted for up to 1.5 hours after leaving the pool. Mac preferred to work in a cooler pool (below 29°C) and proposed that the first 15 minutes of any treatment should be devoted to allowing the body to adjust to the water environment. Any activity that involves movement through the water is an additional tactile stimulus contributing to the adjustment phase. With children, he usually pulled them slowly through the water in a zig-zag pattern to achieve this

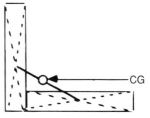

FIGURE 16-2. Center of gravity CG, of an irregular object.

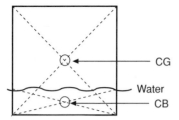

FIGURE 16-3. Center of gravity (CG) and center of buoyancy (CB) of an object in water.

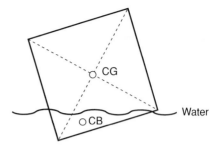

FIGURE 16-4. Center of gravity (CG) and center of buoyancy (CB) of tilted object in water.

goal. Adults may walk through the water, stand or sit and swing their extremities, or swim slowly to achieve the same results.

The concept of *metacenter* (meet-a-center), or human balance in water, is covered next in the Basic Halliwick Course. Metacenter is a naval architectural term and is defined as the intersection of two vertical lines, one through the center of buoyancy (CB) of a body in equilibrium, the other through the CB when the body is inclined slightly to one side. The distance between this intersection above the center of gravity (CG) is a measure of the initial stabilization of the body. Mac began with a description of the CB and the CG of differently shaped objects. The CG exists whether an object is submerged or is on dry land, and is determined by the shape of the object. It was defined by Bouguer in 1758 as the imaginary point around

which a pendulum swings. Metacenter can also be defined as the midpoint of an object at which it can be supported and be in perfect balance (Fig. 16-1). The CG of an irregularly shaped object may actually fall outside of the boundaries of the object (Fig. 16-2). The CG of a "normal" human body is at around the L2 level.

The CB can be considered only if an object is partially or wholly submerged. The CB is defined as the center of the displaced volume of water; it is always be under the surface of the water and inside the object that is displacing the water (Fig. 16-3). If the shape of the displaced volume of water is changed, the CB shifts to one side of the CG of the object. With the forces of gravity and buoyancy acting on the object, the object begins to rotate. The object rocks from side to side in an attempt to right itself and vertically align the CG and CB (Fig. 16-4).

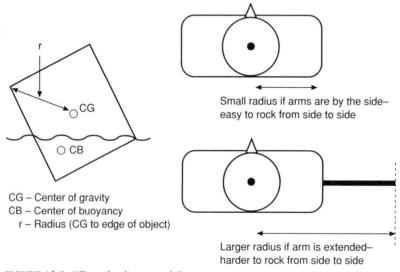

Small radius if arms are by the side—easy to rock from side to side

Larger radius if arm is extended—harder to rock from side to side

CG – Center of gravity
CB – Center of buoyancy
r – Radius (CG to edge of object)

FIGURE 16-5. Effect of radius on stability.

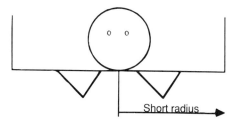

FIGURE 16-6. Arms extended with elbows flexed 90 degrees.

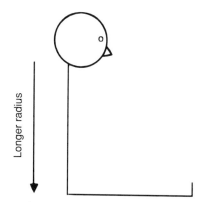

FIGURE 16-8. Body in sitting position.

Another important aspect of metacenter is the moment of inertia (MI) of an object. This is defined as the mass (m) of the object times its radius (r) squared (MI = m × r^2). The radius is measured from the CG outward to the edge of the object (Fig. 16-5). An object with a small radius is easy to move and to return to the upright position. Initiation of rotation is difficult with an object with a long radius, and the object is difficult to return to the upright position. Such objects tend to rock slowly from side to side.

Mac believed that the concept of metacenter is closely related to the influence of primitive reflexes on movement. In the water, the primitive reflexes are inertia patterns—they can be used to cause movement. On dry land, primitive reflexes are used to block movement—they are used to limit rotation. He explained that as the baby develops from the head down, he also develops around an ever-increasing radius. The baby has low tone and moves with small movements. Consider the symmetric tonic neck response (Fig. 16-6). As the child lies supine with his upper extremities positioned in 90 degrees of shoulder flexion and 90 degrees of elbow flexion, his movements are restricted by the boundaries of his arms. The movements are around a small radius. As the child develops, the asymmetric tonic neck reflex is noted (Fig. 16-7). This extends the radius about which the baby is able to move. He is then able to begin to roll. The next developmental step to consider

is when the child begins to sit (Fig. 16-8). The extended lever arm allows the child more freedom of movement. As he stands, the lever arm is at its maximum length, and the child can engage in multiple possible movements (Fig. 16-9).

The radius around which a baby moves is controlled by maturation of the muscles and the spine. One of Mac's most adamantly expressed opinions is that the primitive reflexes do *not* disappear, and he used them in his water treatment technique as inertia patterns to *achieve* motion. As a person lies in the water, there is no solid surface against which the muscles of the back can react. As a consequence, the person is like a baby in the water and is unable to use the higher levels of her cortex to monitor and control her movements. The person reverts to using her primitive reflexes. As a person lies supine in the water with her upper extremities stretched above her head in full flexion, the radius about which her body rotates is very small (Fig. 16-10). The person can gently lift first one hand slightly out of the water and then the other, and her feet will move about in an oval shape. The person can then lower her arms slightly to about 135 degrees abduction to lengthen the radius (Fig. 16-11). As she lifts first one hand slightly

FIGURE 16-7. Left arm extended with right elbow flexed 90 degrees.

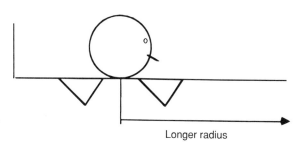

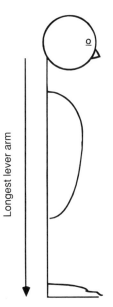

FIGURE 16-9. Body in standing position.

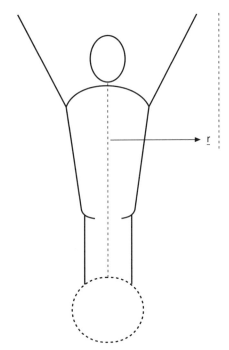

FIGURE 16-11. Radius with arms at 135 degrees.

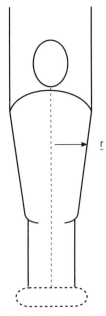

FIGURE 16-10. Radius with arms above head.

out of the water, then the other, the feet will move about in a more symmetric circular pattern. As the upper extremities are extended to 90 degrees of abduction, and the person lifts her hands alternately, the feet will move about in a large oval shape (Fig. 16-12). When the upper extremities are dropped to 45 degrees of abduction, the feet will move from side to side as the

hands are lifted alternately out of the water (Fig. 16-13). Once the person can control her movement around the smallest radius of the midline, she will be more comfortable with her active movements in the pool.

Mac often stated that "a person will not move unless they can first hold a position of stability." Therefore, balance reactions are needed more in the water than on dry land. If a person's symmetry is disturbed, then his balance is altered. Mac stated his four rules of metacenter:

1. If any part of the body is lifted out of the water, the body rotates to try to get that part back into the water (Fig. 16-14). If a person lies supine in the water and lifts the right upper extremity out of the water, then:
   a. he has changed the shape of the body and the CG moves up and out
   b. he has reduced the volume of the body under the water and the CB moves to the left
   c. the forces of gravity and buoyancy cause the body to rotate to the right in an attempt to submerge the right upper extremity. "Once a body moves beyond a certain angle of rotation it can't get back upright. That is what causes all fear."

2. If a weight is taken across the midline the

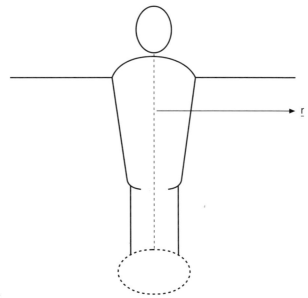

FIGURE 16-12. Radius with arms at 90 degrees.

body rolls with the weight (Fig. 16-15). As the right upper extremity is moved across the body, the CG moves to the left. The shape of the body under water is changed, causing the CB to move to the right. The forces of gravity and buoyancy rotate the body in an attempt to vertically align the CG and CB.

3. If the volume of the body is less on the right (as with an amputee), then the CB moves to the left, and the body rolls to the right (Fig. 16-16).

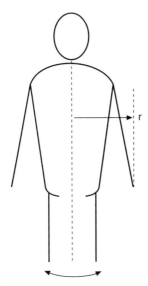

FIGURE 16-13. Radius with arms at 45 degrees.

4. The change of weight across the midline has a greater effect then the loss of buoyancy. Pelvic rotation has a greater effect than upper body rotation in the water.

The next topic of discussion in the Basic Halliwick Course is handling techniques, or how to hold a body in the water. Mac emphasized again that in the water the tactile systems and primitive reflexes are used by the client to monitor and control movement. Another of his most strongly voiced opinions is that "we have to stop holding and protecting patients, and let them use their survival reflexes to get these reflexes to work." He believed that therapists need to challenge their clients to allow the client to attempt to correct. All holds or supports should cover as small an area of the body as possible and avoid adding extra tactile stimulation. The support should be gradually taken away as the client becomes more independent with each skill. Consider the client in an upright position who requires a stabilizing hold in the area of the trunk. The CG for the "normal" body is S2 and the CG of the trunk area is T11. For handling a person in the upright position, the area between T11 and S2 is the ideal placement for the therapist's hands (Fig. 16-17). "If you are holding anywhere else, you will be adding unneeded pressure." As the client becomes stable, the therapist moves his or her hold progressively to a more distal location until the client is able independently to control the posture during activities. Examples of

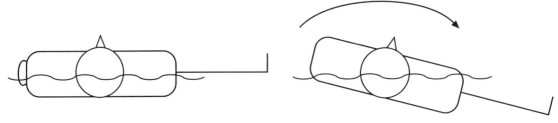

FIGURE 16-14. Rotation resulting from lifting right hand above surface.

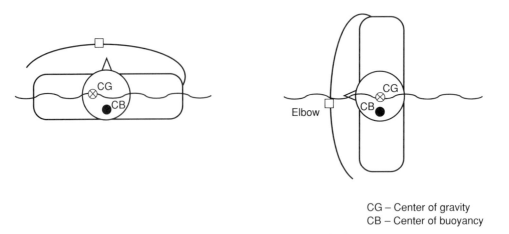

CG – Center of gravity
CB – Center of buoyancy

FIGURE 16-15. Rotation resulting from taking weight (elbow) across body.

more distal holds include forearm-on-forearm and moving the palm-on-palm support more distally before completely "disengaging" and allowing the client to perform the activity without support.

In treating a client in a supine position, the therapist's hands must be turned on edge with the thumb tucked into the palm so that only the lateral edge of the hand comes into contact with the client (Fig. 16-18). At times, the lateral portion of the forearm must be used. This hold, when used correctly, lends security to even the most frightened client, yet still provides minimal tactile stimulation. Before discussing the specific

hand placements for holding the client in a horizontal position, the actual desired starting position of the client must be described. The client should lie supine with the lower extremities in neutral extension and held together, the feet should be in dorsiflexion, the upper extremities should be held close to the sides, and the head should be in a slightly flexed position. Once this position has been assumed, the client's body responds automatically (without active movement) to the different placements of the therapist's hand in the following manner:

1. If the edge of the therapist's hand is placed midline above the client's T11 level, the

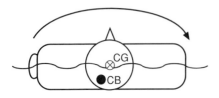

CG – Center of gravity
CB – Center of buoyancy

FIGURE 16-16. Rotation resulting from imbalance in body configuration.

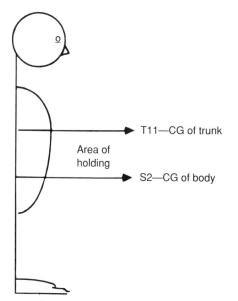

FIGURE 16-17. Center of gravity (CG) of body (S2) and trunk (T11).

client's lower extremities will drop to the vertical position.
2. If the support is moved to the T11 level, the client's lower extremities will drop to a 15-degree angle and stay there (Fig. 16-19).
3. Moving the support to the S2 (CG) level allows the client to float supine in a balanced position. Supporting slightly above the knee joints bilaterally facilitates activity in the hip flexors. Stronger hip flexion is invoked with support underneath both ankles. (Never hold on the lateral side of the ankles—this encourages hip abduction.)
4. If the client is very tall, these positions of support need to be adjusted slightly higher on the client.

5. Mac would often say, "Ears are not handles. Never hold the head!"
6. Do not hold the client's upper extremities either. This creates a closed kinetic chain and blocks the movement possibilities of the shoulders.

Mac noticed that all people respond in a similar way to tactile stimulation at certain points while lying supine in the water. These points of stimulation, "Voiter points," were charted by Mac. For example, If the cervical area is stimulated with a light touch, extension of the cervical spine is noted. Similarly, thoracic extension results from light stimulation in the area of the thoracic spine. Lumbar spine stimulation or light stroking along the dorsum of the metatarsal heads of the feet elicits hip extension. Hip extension can also result from tapping along the occiput of the skull and in the forehead area. Lightly stroking along the lateral surface of the smallest toe always is associated with lateral flexion of the trunk to the same side. If the body begins to roll, lateral flexion of the trunk occurs to stabilize the client. Tapping over the greater trochanter facilitates lateral rotation away from the stimulation. Touching directly under either eye causes the body to rotate. Experimentation with these "Voiter points" can be quite interesting.

When using the Halliwick method, the therapist's role is to direct the exercise, observe what happens, and correct what is undesirable. The client is the person performing most of the work.

The second day of class in the Basic Halliwick Course covers the *four aspects of rotation*. The human body moves in patterns of rotation. In water, there are two forces acting on the body, buoyancy and gravity. If the body is not in a straight line, then rotation occurs. The four aspects of rotation are (1) neurophysical, (2) de-

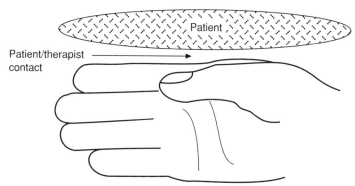

FIGURE 16-18. Minimal contact support of patient.

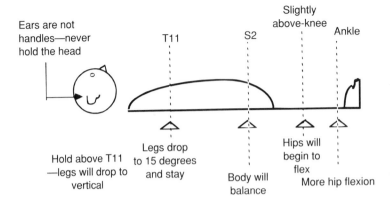

Ears are not handles—never hold the head

T11   S2   Slightly above-knee   Ankle

Hold above T11 —legs will drop to vertical

Legs drop to 15 degrees and stay

Body will balance

Hips will begin to flex

More hip flexion

FIGURE 16-19. Effects of support at various body locations.

velopmental, (3) basic imbalance—or the "handicapped effect," and (4) rotation/contrarotation—which is the metacentric effect that can bring an outside force to work for or against a person's movement.

The neurophysical aspect of the course involves a basic review of muscle and joint anatomy (muscles come across joints in patterns of rotation), muscle spindles, proprioception, and reciprocal innervation. Mac described the cortical brain as having seven layers, with three main areas relevant to the current discussion. He stated that stimuli are first received by the "earlier" or primitive brain. As the stimulus is repeated, the primitive brain processes it and refers the information to a higher level. Eventually the higher level learns to recognize the stimulus. This is the process of learning. This concept is very important because Mac believed that in the water, humans revert to using their primitive reflexes. The water is then a perfect place to begin

training or retraining the brain for movement. (This notion countered one of Bertha Bobath's main concerns about the Halliwick method. Bobath reportedly stated that "we are not little fishies, you know.") Likewise, if an incorrect movement is repeated over and over, it too will be registered in the higher levels of the brain. Therefore, therapists must teach correct movement patterns. The topic of how to teach is discussed in the section on the Ten Point Program later in this chapter.

To explain the concept of basic imbalance, Mac described three basic axes of rotation in the water: vertical, lateral, and combined. Vertical rotation occurs about the horizontal axis that runs across the hips (Fig. 16-20). This rotation is the easiest to control because it occurs about

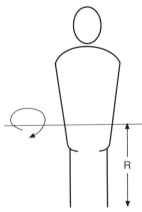

FIGURE 16-20. Vertical rotation about the horizontal axis. R, radius.

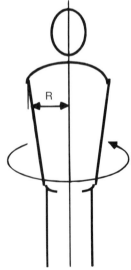

FIGURE 16-21. Lateral rotation about the vertical axis. R, radius.

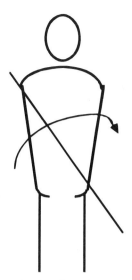

FIGURE 16-22. Combined rotation.

hemiplegia, amputations, and other asymmetric conditions are concerned. Combined rotation is movement about the previous two axes (Fig. 16-22). An example of this type of movement is when a person is sitting on the deck, falls forward into the pool (vertical rotation), and then rolls over onto his back into a supine float (lateral rotation). This axis of movement is used frequently by clients with severe scoliosis or spastic quadriplegia.

The rotation/contrarotation concept is the fourth aspect of rotation, and uses the metacentric effect that was discussed earlier in this chapter. When a client lies supine in the water and lifts the left hand out of the water, the body rotates to the left in an attempt to return that extremity to its original position under the water. The therapist can stop that rotation by supporting the client bilaterally under the legs or the ankles. But if the therapist supports this client only under the left heel, the client will laterally flex the trunk to the right to stop the rotation (Fig. 16-23). If the therapist supports the client only under the right ankle, the client can use contrarotation (rotate the opposite direction) to stop the rotation and hold the body in a stable supine float.

The Ten Point Program

After presenting this background, Mac discussed his "teaching structure," or what he has labeled his *Ten Point Program.* He divided his Ten Point

a long axis. Vertical rotation is most frequently used when treating clients with paraplegia, spina bifida, and mental disabilities. Lateral rotation occurs around the vertical axis that runs from the head to the coccyx (Fig. 16-21). This rotation is easy to initiate because it occurs around a short axis. However, if the body is floating supine and rotates over 18 degrees, it cannot bring itself back to supine. "Once a person learns to control lateral rotation he will no longer be fearful of moving in the water." This is the axis with which programs for clients with

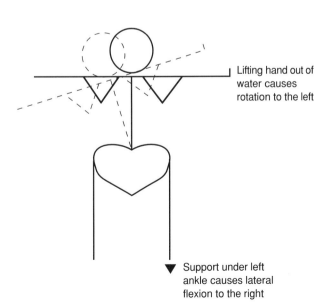

Lifting hand out of water causes rotation to the left

Support under left ankle causes lateral flexion to the right

FIGURE 16-23. Using contrarotation to stabilize body.

Program into four phases that reflect the order in which to teach. These four phases are:

1. Mental adjustment—or adaptation to being in the water
2. Balance restoration—which uses the primitive reflex activities discussed earlier
3. Inhibition—or posture control, as a client learns to hold his body still in the water
4. Facilitation—of mentally desired and physically controlled movement—not necessarily perfect movements, but movements within the client's ability

Mental Adjustment

One of the first things a person encounters on entering the water environment is difficulty in maintaining posture and balance. Therefore, the first point of this phase is called *mental adjustment.* As a person walks into shallow water, his or her posture is gravity controlled (Fig. 16-24). This upright posture is one that leans slightly forward, and the body adjusts the posture continuously according to the feedback it receives from the pressure on the feet and other joints. As the person proceeds into chest-deep water, the posture is affected equally by gravity and buoyancy (Fig. 16-25). As before, the person adjusts the posture as needed based on the feedback received from the feet and other weight-bearing joints. As buoyancy becomes more influential, the person begins to use more primitive processes to control posture and balance. Head positioning is also used to adjust posture. When the water level exceeds the body level of T11, the client is in a condition of flotation

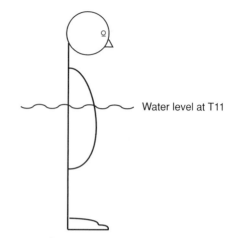

FIGURE 16-25. Gravity control on entering water.

dominance, and gravity no longer influences postural stability. The client uses the head to change direction and positions the hands forward. The deeper the client moves into the water, the more he needs to keep the arms out in front to maintain stability (Fig. 16-26).

As a person goes from the standing to a sitting posture in the water, the standard, comfortable sitting position is usually assumed (Fig. 16-27). Using the techniques of the Halliwick method requires that the client begin in the "working posture," or "cube position." This position is also a sitting one, but the knees and hips are specifically held in 90 degrees of flexion, the feet are placed flat on the bottom of the pool, with the feet and knees positioned together, the back is held upright, and the arms reach forward with the entire length of the arm slightly under

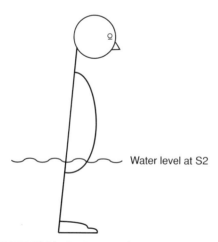

FIGURE 16-24. Gravity control on entering water.

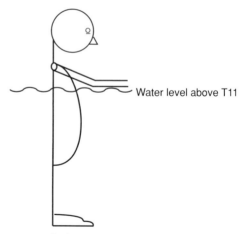

FIGURE 16-26. Maintaining posture in deep water.

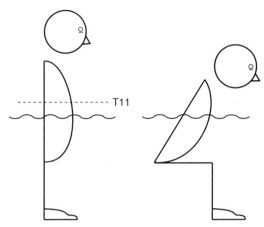

FIGURE 16-27. Transition from standing to standard sitting position.

the water (Fig. 16-28). The client will then be submerged in water above the T11 level, and will be controlled by buoyancy, facilitating the appearance of more primitive reflexes. Most people tend to fall backward when first placed in this position. However, if they are instructed to reach forward with their arms, they will be able to maintain their balance.

Another aspect of the mental adjustment phase is overcoming the often difficult time a person has with breathing while the chest is submerged. On dry land, atmospheric pressure only negligibly resists chest expansion. In the water, however, when the chest region is submerged, water pressure is added to the resistance against chest expansion during inhalation. The viscera are also pushed up into the diaphragm, adding resistance to the expansion of the diaphragm.

For some clients to be comfortable with breathing in the pool, negative-pressure breathing must be taught. The client is instructed to push the breath out in an exaggerated fashion. This exhalation is followed by a large inhalation. Negative-pressure breathing is one way to strengthen the musculature for breathing.

The third point of the mental adjustment phase is the concept of disengagement. "Engagement" refers to when a client is supported by the therapist; "disengagement," then, is the gradual removal of the support that the therapist gives the client. The goal is the client's complete independence. Mac emphasized that disengagement refers not only to physical support but to mental support. He said that most clients, and the mentally disabled in particular, prefer to face the therapist for most activities. Part of the mental disengagement process is to have the clients perform activities with the therapist's support behind them, or devise activities in which the client moves behind the therapist. When treating the client in a vertical position, physical disengagement begins with the therapist holding the client high on the thorax, about the level of T11. As the client gains control of movements, the therapist slowly moves the hand holds toward the S2 level of the trunk (Fig. 16-29). As more control is achieved, the therapist moves the hands more distally, beginning with arm-on-arm support (Fig. 16-30). The therapist progresses to forearm-on-forearm and finally to palm-on-palm holds before removing physical support completely. When supporting the client, the therapist's hands should rest gently on the client.

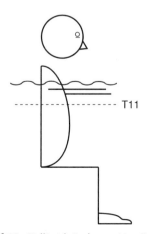

FIGURE 16-28. Halliwick "cube position."

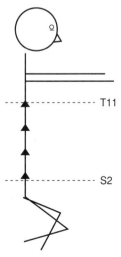

FIGURE 16-29. Holds on trunk for disengagement.

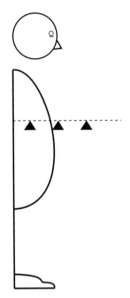

FIGURE 16-30. Arm-on-arm support.

Tightly gripping holds should be avoided (Fig. 16-31). As each new principle is taught, the client should be fully engaged, so that he is allowed to learn each activity with maximum support, and disengagement proceeds as the client achieves more and more control of each activity.

Balance Restoration

The second phase of the Ten Point Program is *balance restoration*. Balance is achieved as the client gains control of rotation about the three

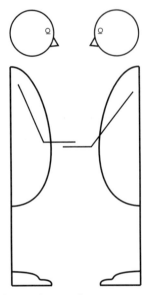

FIGURE 16-31. Palm-on-palm support.

axes discussed earlier. Learning to control these rotations ensures that the client will always be able to achieve a comfortable breathing posture. *Vertical rotation control* occurs about the horizontal axis, which is also a land axis. Control of this rotation is the most easily mastered because it moves about a long axis. Vertical rotation occurs when a client moves from the vertical, standing position into the supine position, and to the standing position again. The client must first be able to hold the upright position steady with his arms in a forward position. When proceeding to the supine position, a person cannot simply lie back in the water. First, the radius about which he is rotating must be reduced by flexing into the sitting position, and reduced even more by pulling the knees up toward the chin. As the person extends the head to lie back slowly, the arms will extend out to the side to help slow the rotation. Once the client's knees have reached the surface, he may gently extend the lower extremities. The process is reversed to return to the upright standing position. A client who is unable to flex the lower extremities can simply place the arms at his sides and lift the hands out of the water. Because of the metacentric effect, the client's hips will sink until they come to an upright vertical position. Because the mouth tends to submerge slightly in the process, this activity should be taught only after the client has developed head and breathing control in the upright posture. Mac noted that movement in vertical rotation mimics the Moro reflex with regard to the head and upper extremity movements.

Lateral rotation control is the fourth step in the Ten Point Program, and is "the most important maneuver you will ever teach anyone!" This rotation occurs about a "water axis." Lateral rotation occurs around a small radius and is difficult to learn to control. Mac emphasized that when a person lies supine in the water, there is no solid support in contact with the dorsal area of the body, and therefore no stretch reflex activity occurs along the muscles of the back. The body and mind return to more primitive controls. Mac believed that all primitive reflexes actually develop to assist the infant to learn control of rotations. The reflexes reappear when the client is in the water medium. When first learning to roll in the water, head rotation should lead. The reflex action associated with turning the head is the arm extending out sideways to the same side (eg, asymmetric tonic neck response posture). Performed in the water, however, extension of the lever arm blocks the rotation. Therefore, to accomplish rolling to the left, the client must consciously place the left arm behind the body while turning to look to the left. The client may also throw the right arm across the body, but the elbow (CG of the upper extremity) must cross the midline of the body or the body will roll to the right (using the principle of metacenter). If the right arm is thrown across the body higher than shoulder level, the body actually laterally flexes and also blocks the rotation. Similarly, the client can use the pelvis to rotate the spine by crossing the lower extremity in the same direction of the upper extremity. If the legs are allowed to abduct at any point during the rotation, they will increase the lever arm and stop the rotation. This concept can also be used to stop unwanted lateral rotation.

Combined rotation control occurs about a "water axis" and is often used to "roll out of trouble." Consider the client who is learning to come to standing from a supine float. If the client overrotates, she will fall forward as she attempts to get her feet on the bottom of the pool. The client can be taught to continue to fall forward (vertical rotation) and turn the head so that she rolls over to where her face is up (lateral rotation). She will then be in a supine float and a safe breathing position (Fig. 16-32).

Mental inversion is the last point in the balance restoration phase. Mac said that if the first five points have been taught correctly, this step will be easily accomplished. Mental inversion is the process of learning that the force of buoyancy is an upward thrust that brings objects, including the client, to the surface of the water. One method of teaching this concept is to have the client push a small ball under the water and then release it and watch it pop to the surface. The same maneuver can be repeated with larger and larger balls. Next, an adult can curl into a ball and allow the client to push him under the water and watch as the adult floats back to the surface. The final aspect of this point is to have the client submerge and learn that he, too, floats to the surface, where he can use one of the rotations to come to a comfortable breathing position.

Inhibition

"Balance is stillness" represents the only point in the third phase—*inhibition.* This phase teaches clients to hold a posture when events in the pool, such as currents, might be trying to move

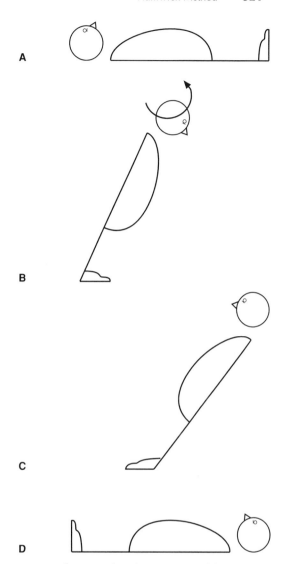

FIGURE 16-32. Combined rotation control (***A*** to ***D***).

their bodies about. Activities used in this phase challenge a client's balanced position to encourage him gently to correct himself. An example of such an activity is when the client is able to stand upright in the water at the T11 level with the arms forward. The therapist can then challenge the client's balance by causing gentle turbulence behind the client. This pulls the client backward, facilitating an attempt to correct the posture by stretching the head and arms forward (Fig. 16-33). Turbulence can be applied from any direction to challenge the client to hold a steady posture in any position (standing, cube position, kneeling, and supine). Once a client

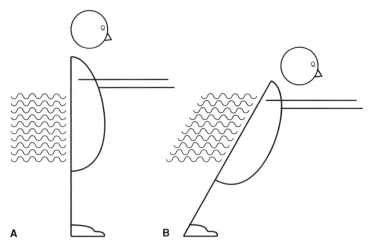

FIGURE 16-33. Restoration of balance in presence of turbulence in standing position.

is able to hold the posture without giving in to a disturbance, the client has mastered this point.

Facilitation

Turbulent gliding is point number eight, and is in the fourth phase, called *facilitation*. The phase of facilitation is concerned with controlled movement through the water. Turbulent gliding teaches the client to hold a balanced position while being passively moved through the water. This is accomplished by having the client lie in a supine float with the therapist standing at the client's head. The therapist produces turbulence under the client's shoulders. The client begins to move toward the therapist (Fig. 16-34). As the therapist steps backwards and continues

producing turbulence, the client must work to maintain a balanced supine float position while being pulled along. If the client is unable to achieve a supine float initially, this technique can be made easier by placing the client in a diagonal position with the feet on the bottom of the pool. As the client is pulled along, the feet will eventually float to the surface (Fig. 16-35).

Simple progression is the ninth step of the Ten Point Program. As the client learns to maintain a balanced posture while being moved passively through the water, she can begin to attempt gentle active movements to propel herself through the water. In a supine float position, the client can gently begin a sculling action, moving the arms gently in and out. Mac warned that in

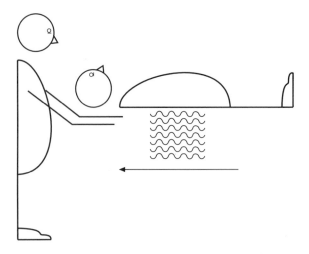

FIGURE 16-34. Restoration of balance in presence of turbulence in supine position.

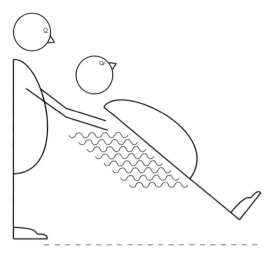

FIGURE 16-35. Turbulent gliding from oblique position.

this stage the movements of the client's hands should be restricted to the area bordered by T11 and S2, and later expanded to a larger range of motion (Fig. 16-36).

Once a client can control the balanced posture and progress through the water with this sculling-type movement, the client is ready to progress to the tenth and final point—*basic movement.* In this step, the client is taught actual swim strokes, beginning with a double-arm backstroke. All movement must be controlled as the posture is held in a balanced position.

Mac urged the therapist to "take time" in teaching these ten points. "It is very important to teach in this order and not leave anything out." One step must not necessarily be mastered before moving on to the next step. Steps may

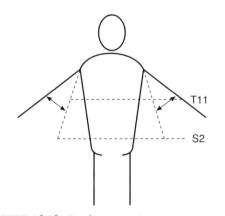

FIGURE 16-36. Simple progression—arm movements restricted to the area of T11–S2.

overlap, yet Mac suggested that therapists work on no more than three steps at any time.

The Halliwick method uses this Ten Point Program to teach people to swim using a group format. Mac devised many games to teach each of the ten points. He encouraged each of the therapists in his classes to devise other games on their own that would be pertinent to their client populations. As he stated, "We learn so much when we play games. All over the world children play games. Games are all devised around our bodies and how we move. The pool is a handicapped person's playground. It is the only place they can learn to move. They cannot be taught how to move and balance but can be encouraged to do activities where they have a chance to feel and learn movement and balance. They must practice and learn correctly. Then give them situations to use what they have learned mentally and physically." He often treated adults in the same manner because "when we put people in the water they become children again." When devising games to teach the Ten Point Program, four aspects should be considered for each game:

1. The game should have a name.
2. A checking system should be in place.
   a. Begin with the therapist helping the client
   b. Progress to where the client is able to do the activity independently
   c. Give the client a situation in which the objective is not known—can the client do the activity alone?
   d. If the client cannot, then go back through the entire process
3. The game should involve music and rhythm.
4. Know who your clients are and use appropriate activities.

Within the group, each client is paired with a trained instructor. Instructors may be therapists, swim instructors, volunteers, parents, spouses, and so forth. The ideal group size is five pairs. Each group has a leader. The leader gives instructions in short commands and the instructors work with their specific clients. Each client may accomplish the activity in a slightly different manner. This arrangement allows for individual attention in the group instruction. Each game lasts no longer than 3 minutes. Therefore, games should be planned ahead of time and instructors should be well trained in this technique. Campion details many games that can be used for teaching the Halliwick method.[1]

At the Halliwick School, these group activities

occur once a week for 30-minute sessions. Groupings are usually revised every 7 weeks. A variety of diagnoses can be grouped together, as long as they are developmentally at about the same point of the Ten Point Program. As clients progress beyond the tenth point of basic movement and learn actual swim strokes, competitions can be arranged. Regular swim meets are scheduled in many European countries. Mac ultimately envisioned all countries being involved in international multihandicapped Halliwick swim meets.

After the week-long Basic Halliwick Course, the participants are encouraged to practice the techniques for at least a year before enrolling in the Advanced Halliwick Course.

The Advanced Course

The Advanced Halliwick Course begins with a review of the Basic Halliwick Course's principle of human balance in water and the Ten Point Program. Water-specific exercises were devised using the principles of fluid mechanics as the working forces on the human body rather than the use of any form of manual manipulation. "This technique precludes the use of any flotation equipment."

Eye Deviation

The Advanced Halliwick Course elaborates on the concept of *eye deviation*. When a client looks straight ahead and focuses on an object,

both eyes are an equal distance from the object and focus easily under normal instances. If the object is moved such that one eye is further from the object, the eyes focus differently on the same object. This situation is uncomfortable for the client and leads to head rotation toward the object to bring the eyes again into equal focus. After head rotation, the entire body then turns toward the object (Fig. 16-37). The concept of eye deviation illustrates that rotation begins with the eyes, moves to the head, and continues with the shoulders and on to the spine. Therefore, the class is encouraged to instruct the clients to avoid looking at the therapist and instead look straight ahead, if the object of the treatment is to have them stay in midline when in the water. Mac added that the eyes are closely related to the vestibular system: another exteroceptor. Movement of the eyes has an effect on the otolith organ of the vestibular system. Therefore, if the therapist is treating a client who is displaying excessive movement, the first thing that must be accomplished involves fixing the client's eyes on a stable object. The client then gains control of the head movement and consequently of the shoulder and arm movements.

Mac described true trunk rotation as occurring down to the level of T12 only. Rotation is different in the lumbar spine. Likewise, the pelvis is a fixed structure that also limits rotation. Mac explained that the pelvis, together with the lower extremities and the floor, comprise a four-bar chain, and a four-bar chain is a power structure. In the water, the upper body is used for

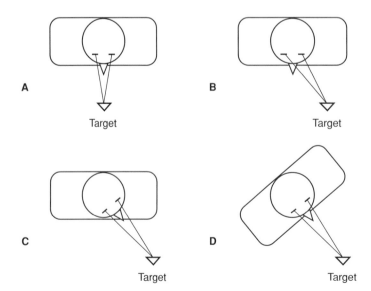

FIGURE 16-37. Eye deviation. (**A**) Target straight ahead, eyes in equal focus; (**B**) target moved, eyes in unequal focus; (**C**) head rotates, eyes in equal focus; (**D**) body rotates.

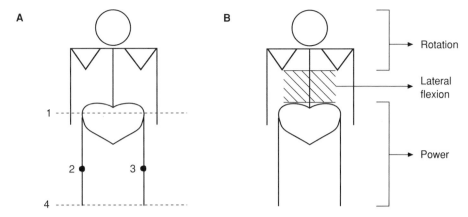

FIGURE 16-38. (**A**) Power structure. The pelvis (1), lower extremities (2 and 3), and floor (4) comprise a four-bar chain. (**B**) Lateral flexion occurs between the upper and lower body.

rotation, the lower body is used for power, and in between the two, lateral flexion occurs (Fig. 16-38). Lateral flexion is made up of rotation in the upper spine and flexion–extension in the lower spine. Mac said that this lateral flexion is not seen on dry land. Consider a person lying supine in the water with the left upper extremity abducted and the left hand out of the water. According to rule number one, the body will rotate to the left, attempting to submerge the elevated left hand. To maintain a stable supine float, the body will rotate to its right or laterally flex to the right to bring the center of buoyancy

under the left upper extremity (Figs. 16-39 and 16-40).

The Logical Approach to Exercise in Water

After this review, a new concept is introduced: *the logical approach to exercise in water.* Mac began this discussion by saying, "If you can do it on land, don't do it in the water!" Treatments in the water should be an extension of or complement to land treatment. Clients must be able

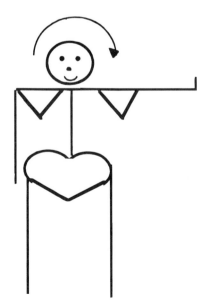

FIGURE 16-39. The body rotates to the left, attempting to submerge elevated left hand.

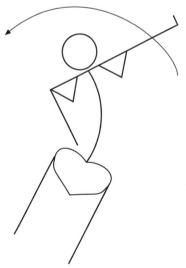

FIGURE 16-40. The body rotates to its right or laterally flexes to the right to bring the center of buoyancy under the left upper extremity.

to meet the movement requirements of numbers one through six of the Ten Point Program of the Halliwick method before the logical approach to exercise is used.

When faced with planning a treatment in the water, the therapist must first identify treatment objectives to be accomplished. Mac identified six basic *treatment objectives* usually addressed using the Halliwick method:

1. Strengthen weak muscle groups (+WMG)
2. Increase range of motion (+RM)
3. Facilitate posture and balance reactions (FPBR)
4. Improve general physical condition (+GPC)
5. Reduce pain (−P)
6. Reduce spasticity (−Sp)

Using these abbreviations, Mac would describe the preoperative treatment objectives of a client undergoing hip replacement as including: (1) decrease pain (−P); (2) strengthen weak muscle groups (+WMG); and (3) increase range of motion (+RM). After surgery, the same client would be listed for these treatment objectives: (1) +WMG, (2) +RM, (3) FPBR.

The second aspect of the logical approach to exercise in water involves identifying the *rotational planes* about which the client will work during the treatment—vertical rotation control (VR), lateral rotation control (LR), or combined rotation control (CR). To do this, the therapist simply pictures how the diagnosis has affected the client's body symmetry. A hemiplegic usu-

ally is effected on one complete side. Therefore, this client should begin work in LR in an attempt to teach the affected side to move like the uninvolved side. A paraplegic is effected only in the lower half of the body. Therefore, this client should begin work in VR. A client with diagnoses such as athetoid cerebral palsy or scoliosis usually exhibits an altered symmetry affecting more of the body, and should begin with CR activities (Fig. 16-41).

The *five starting postures* are identified as the third aspect of the logical approach to exercise in water:

1. Standing
   a. N + is used to document a client standing in the water above the level of T11. At this level there is little weight on the feet, and the client must use his or her head and outstretched upper extremities to maintain balance.
   b. N − is used to document a client standing in the water below the level of T11. This depth allows more weight bearing and proprioceptive input.
   c. N + is the neutral point and is used to denote a client standing in the water at the T11 level.
2. Sitting/kneeling: The sitting position, or the cube position, is described as placing the hips and knees in 90 degrees of flexion, holding the back upright, placing the feet flat on the bottom of the pool, bringing the feet and

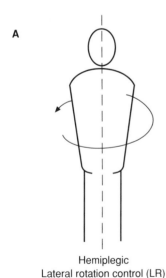

A

Hemiplegic
Lateral rotation control (LR)

B

Paraplegic
Vertical rotation control (VR)

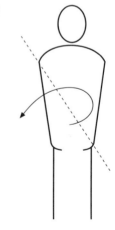

C

Cerebral palsy – scoliosis
Combined rotation control (CR)

FIGURE 16-41. Rotation control.

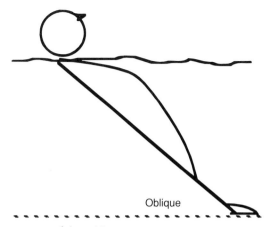

Oblique

FIGURE 16-42. Oblique position.

knees together, and stretching the upper extremities out in front with the entire length of the upper extremities and shoulders just below the surface of the water. In kneeling, the client's upper extremities are also outstretched in front with the entire length of the upper extremities and shoulders just below the surface of the water, the back is upright, and the hips are in a neutral position while the client rests on the knees.

3. Supine: This position places the lumbar spine in a slightly flexed position. The client should place her hands at her sides, the head in neutral or slightly flexed, the hips in neutral extension, the lower extremities together, and the feet in dorsiflexion.
4. Prone: This position places the lumbar spine in an extended position. It is seldom used.
5. Oblique: This position has the client supine with the body in neutral extension but with the feet on the bottom of the pool, and the body angling diagonally with the face floating above the surface of the water (Fig. 16-42).

There are *four exercise patterns* to be considered as the fourth aspect of the logical approach to exercise in water (Fig. 16-43).

1. Symmetric: Both sides of the body are performing the same activity
2. Asymmetric: Only one extremity is performing an activity
3. Cross-lateral (or heterolateral): The upper right and the left lower extremity perform the activity, or the left upper extremity and right lower extremity

4. Bilateral: Both upper extremities or both lower extremities perform the same activities

Now the client is in position for his treatment. The therapist must decide which technique to use as the treatment. These techniques constitute the fifth aspect of the logical approach to exercise in water. *Seven techniques* are listed:

1. Gravity dominant: When the client is placed in the water level below T11, and weight bearing is desired
2. Upthrust dominant: When the client is placed in water level above T11, and weight bearing is not desired
3. Turbulence assisted: Accomplished when the therapist applies manual turbulence to the client to help him to complete an activity; the client is drawn toward the turbulence
4. Turbulence resisted: Uses turbulence manually created by the therapist to challenge the movements or posture the client is attempting to maintain
5. Metacentric (MC): When a body part is lifted slightly out of the water and the body rotates to try to place that part of the body under the water; the client must resist that rotation to hold a position of balance (or stillness)
6. Wave of transmission: Used for stabilization; for example, as the client takes one step forward and stops, the incoming wave will push him from behind, and he must hold his posture stable until the resistance has passed
7. Neurologic techniques
   a. Eye deviation—Movement is facilitated with eye movement. Looking to the side with the eyes causes the body to begin to rotate. Having the client "look up" causes the body to extend, and looking down causes the trunk to flex.
   b. Kinetic chains (primitive reflexes)—A four-bar chain is established with the client's extremities and the therapist or the side or bottom of the pool. This technique reduces unwanted movement (Fig. 16-44)
   c. Specific skin stimulation (Voiter points)—Skin receptors adapt rapidly. Therefore, Mac suggested that therapists use only a few light strokes, tapping, or changing areas frequently (Fig. 16-45).
   d. Transference—This is when the client performs an activity with the extremity that is unaffected by his diagnoses. This movement is followed by an attempt to perform the same activity with the involved extremity.

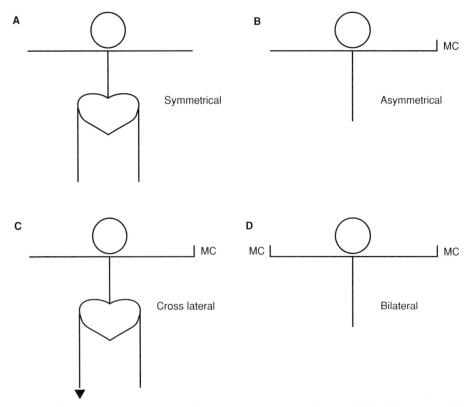

FIGURE 16-43. Four exercise patterns. (The arrowhead in part **C** indicates a holding force supplied by the physical therapist supporting the client under the right heel. MC, metacenter [fingers out of water])

When all five aspects of the logical approach to exercise in water are considered, over 30,000 possible activities are available for use during a therapy session. The final step in the logical approach to exercise in water would include *swimming instruction*, or swim correction if a

client needs to alter his usual stroke to adhere to therapeutic principles for his diagnosis.

Based on the information just presented, the therapist can plan a treatment for a many types of clients. Several examples follow.

Client A is a woman who has undergone a

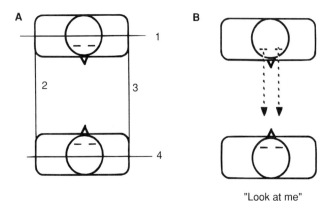

"Look at me"
"Put your hands on my shoulder"   **FIGURE 16-44.** Kinematic chains.

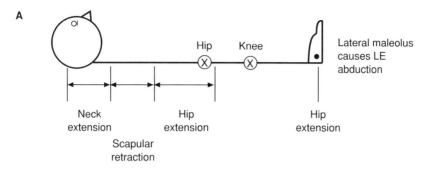

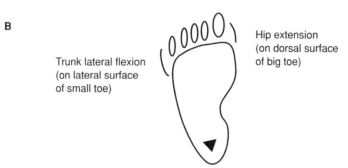

FIGURE 16-45. Voiter points. (**A**) If the therapist taps the greater trochanter, the body will roll away from the stimulation (trunk rotation). (**B**) Approximation for lower extremity stretch toward heel.

total hip replacement. The following is a reasonable treatment program for this woman:

Treatment objective (TO): −P, +RM, FPBR, and +WMG
Rotational plane (RP): VR
Starting position (SP): standing
Depth of water (WD): N + progressing to N − (begin in water above level of T11 and progress to water level below T11 to increase weight bearing as the client progresses)
Exercise pattern (XP): symmetric
Treatment technique (TT): wave of transmission

This client is placed in the water at a level above T11 in a standing position. She is then instructed to take one hop forward, regain her standing posture, and hold it until the wave of transmission has passed. She can repeat this activity across the pool. This activity encourages hip flexion while jumping, followed by full hip extension in standing. In addition, the activity challenges the hip musculature to hold her position against the resistance of the wave of transmission.

This treatment program could also be used for the same client:

TO: −P, +RM, +WMG
RP: VR
SP: standing
WD: N +
XP: symmetric
TT: Halliwick method point three (vertical rotation control)

Again, the client begins in the standing position in water above the T11 level. She is instructed to flex into the sitting (cube) position, lean her head back, and move her arms out to the sides as she rotates into the supine float position. As her knees reach the surface of the water, she is told to extend her knees and hips so that she would be in a completely extended and stable supine float. The therapist could support the client as needed with the edge of his hand at the S2 level. The client is then instructed to reverse the movement—to flex her body, pull her arms forward and slightly out of the water, and flex her head forward until her body is rotated to an upright standing position. She then can extend her hips and knees into a vertical upright position. This activity encourages full hip range of motion and strengthening of the hip musculature.

Client B is a man with a diagnosis of athetoid cerebral palsy. An appropriate treatment program for this client might include:

TO: −SP, FPBR
RP: VR
SP: standing, progressing to oblique
WD: N + progressing to N±
XP: symmetric
TT: neurologic (kinetic chain)

This client begins his treatment with 15 minutes of gentle movements through the water—the therapist can pull him through the water in a supine position—to allow muscle tone time to reduce. He is then placed in a standing position with the water level above T11 and told to look at the therapist in front of him to fix his eyes. He is then instructed to put his hands on the therapist's shoulders to form a four-bar chain. His arms must be completely under the water so that viscosity can be used to dampen his arm movements. Once the unwanted movements have been reduced, he is instructed to flex into the cube position and to let go of the therapist's shoulders and swing his arms slowly out to the sides as he extends his head. His body extends, but his feet remain on the bottom of the pool, so that he is in an oblique position. He is then instructed to flex his head forward, bend his hips and knees, and return his hands to the therapist's shoulders. He looks directly at the therapist and returns to an upright and balanced standing posture. This routine is repeated over and over until the client can control the movements.

As Client B progresses, his program can be adjusted like this:

TO: FPBR
RP: LR
SP: standing
WD: N± progressing to N −
XP: asymmetric
TT: wave of transmission

As Client B learns to control his posture in standing, he can begin to work on ambulation activities. He is instructed to take one step forward and hold his posture until the wave of transmission has passed. As the client begins to work in this activity, he may need to be sup-ported by placing his hands on the therapist's shoulders. As he progresses in this activity, the therapist can move to support the client by holding him from behind between the T11 and S2 levels, and finally completely disengage. Once the client has mastered that activity, he can begin to take two steps, then stop to hold his posture until the wave has passed. This activity is repeated until he is able to walk across the pool with controlled movements and posture. He can then move into more and more shallow water so that he can learn to control similar movements with more weight bearing until he is able to walk on dry land.

Client C is a woman with a diagnosis of chronic low back pain. The following is a possible treatment plan for her:

TO: −P, +WMG, FPBR
RP: VR
SP: sitting (cube position)
WD: N +
XP: symmetric
TT: MC

After the initial 15 minutes of slow movement through the water—perhaps just slowly walking back and forth—this client is placed in the cube position with the water level above T11. She is instructed to lift both hands slightly out of the water and attempt to maintain the cube position. As the hands are lifted, her body attempts to rotate forward to put the hands back into the water. The client must use her back extensors to resist that forward rotation and maintain the stable cube position. When her hands are returned below the surface of the water, her trunk musculature must readjust to continue to maintain her position. Once she is able to control this activity, she is instructed to lift both hands out of the water and turn her palms forward. This causes her body to be pulled forward, and she has to use her back extensors to resist this movement and maintain her posture. She is then told to turn her palms toward her face. Her body will be pushed back. She has to use her abdominals to resist this movement and maintain the cube position. Alternating the palm forward and palm toward her face movements challenges her trunk musculature to work in synchrony.

Client D is a man with a diagnosis of right-sided cerebrovascular accident causing left-sided hemiparesis. This is one of the many treatments that can be planned for him:

TO: $-$ Sp, $+$ RM, FPBR
RC: LR
SP: supine
WD: N $+$
XP: asymmetric
TT: MC

After the initial 15 minutes in standing to adjust to the reduced weight-bearing condition, Client D is placed in a supine position. The therapist supports the client first at the T11 level and slowly moves her support down the client's body to the S2 level. Support would then be moved to slightly superior to the knees and then to the ankles as the client learns to maintain a balanced supine float position. The therapist would then move her supporting hand to under the client's left heel only. This handling technique results in the client extending the left lower extremity and contrarotating to the right in an attempt to maintain a balanced supine float position.

The treatment technique of transference can also be used. While the therapist supports the client at the S2 level, the client is instructed to turn his head to the right and abduct his right arm with as much effort as possible, and to concentrate on how that position feels. He is then told to turn his head to the left and try to get the same feeling of abduction with his left arm. The left arm is thereby facilitated to perform abduction.

Summary

This chapter must be understood as a brief summary of the 2 weeks of classes on the Halliwick method; it is not possible to include all of the material presented in those classes in a single chapter of a textbook. Before Mac's death, it was strongly recommended that those therapists truly interested in his ever-evolving technique travel to Switzerland while he still taught, or train under someone who had received such instruction. For information concerning the seminars offered in Switzerland or by this author, the reader can contact the Aquatic Physical Therapy Section of the American Physical Therapy Association.

REFERENCE

1. Campion MR. *Hydrotherapy in Pediatrics.* Oxford: Heinemann Medical Books; 1985.

SUGGESTED READINGS

Campion MR. *Adult Hydrotherapy: A Practical Approach.* Oxford: Heinemann Medical Books; 1990.
Campion MR. Water activity based on the Halliwick method. In: Skinner A, Thompson A, eds. *Duffield's Exercise in Water.* 3rd ed. London: Bailliere Tindall; 1983:180–196.
Martin J. The Halliwick method. *Physiotherapy.* 1981;67: 288–291.

CHAPTER

17

WATSU*

Harold Dull

WATSU, or Water Shiatsu, was created in 1980 when the author began floating people in a warm pool, applying the stretches and moves of the Zen Shiatsu he had studied on land in Japan, and had come to Harbin Hot Springs to teach. Zen Shiatsu is more eclectic and creative than traditional kinds of Shiatsu, which focus strictly on points. In Zen Shiatsu, Shizuto Masunaga has integrated several Eastern body–mind practices. Passive stretches, joint mobilization, and hara-work are used as well as pressure on tsubos (acupoints) to balance flows of energy through the meridians (pathways of energy). Centering and connecting with the breath are essential. The emphasis is on *being* with someone rather than *doing* something to them, on their whole body being with the practitioner's whole body, and on spontaneity and creativity. Each session is a meditation.

Zen Shiatsu and WATSU use many terms and concepts alien to Western medicine. Also, Eastern philosophy embraces a mind–body relationship that is not always accepted in traditional aquatic rehabilitation. Terms such as "unconditional acceptance," "meridians," and "yin and yang" are used in WATSU schooling but not developed in this chapter. While reading this chapter, it would behoove the reader to remain open minded and consider the mechanical techniques independent of a belief system. The reader is encouraged to examine other books and writings about Zen Shiatsu for definition and use of specific terms.

WATSU was created as a massage or wellness technique that was not necessarily designed for "patients" as they are classically defined. However, aquatic rehabilitation therapists have applied the approach to clients with a variety of neuromuscular and musculoskeletal disorders and report empiric success.

One of the most beneficial results of WATSU is effective stretching. Through stretching, the meridians are believed to come closer to the body's surface, where the energy they carry can be released. These effects are embellished by rotational movements that release blocked energy. The client remains completely passive and often experiences a profound relaxation from the water's support and the continual, rhythmic movement of the various flows. Usually, the therapist stabilizes or moves one segment of the body through the water, resulting in a stretch of another segment due to the drag effect. A WATSU comprises a specifically prescribed transition and sequence of movements. Once the transitions are learned, the therapist can creatively adapt to most restrictions or specific limitations encountered. According to Morris,[1] "WATSU can be best described as a muscle reeducation approach because specific impairments (usually tight muscles and joints) are targeted for treatment with little regard to the models of motor control."

In addition to the immediately apparent effects of the stretches and mobilizations in warm water, many of the principles of Zen Shiatsu have also found a place in WATSU. In particular, "connecting" with the breathing takes on new dimensions in water. On land, the breathing is coordinated with the practitioner leaning into

*WATSU is a registered trademark. All photographs in this chapter from Dull H. *WATSU: Freeing the Body in Water*. Middletown, Calif: Harbin Springs Publishing; 1993.

points on the client's body. In water, the most basic move is the Water Breath Dance, in which the client floats in the therapist's arms and, as both exhale, they sink a little and then let the water return them upward as they inhale simultaneously. Repeated over and over at the beginning of a WATSU, this creates a connection that can be carried into all of the stretches and movements that follow. This Water Breath Dance and its stillness is returned to, or "come home to" throughout the session.

Although each person is unique, every time they sink and rise with the breaths, and surrender to the water together with the therapist, a nurturing and empowering connection is often formed that is not related to any doctor–patient, parent–child, lover or partner role. WATSU is bodywork, and in 1993 the Worldwide Aquatic Bodywork Association was formed to make the benefits of both giving and receiving aquatic bodywork available to as many people as possible.

The Flows of WATSU

The sequences, or flows, of WATSU, and the ways in which they are taught, have been developed and fine tuned in countless classes in the United States and in Europe. This chapter presents the Transition Flow and a subset of it, the Simple Flow. The Simple Flow incorporates the moves that can be performed with people who are not flexible enough for WATSU's more complex positions. Also, the Expanded Flow, which expands the three sections of the Transition Flow with additional stretches and pointwork, is discussed. Additional expansions and variations are included in the author's book, *WATSU: Freeing the Body in Water.* Besides these three flows, advanced techniques include Free Flow. WATSU has always interwoven stillness and movement, the yin and the yang. In Free Flow, the stillness that has been returned to over and over continues into the movement. Free Flow is stillness moving.

The Transition Flow

In WATSU the transitions, or means of moving from one position to another, are as important as the positions themselves and the specific movements performed in each. The transitions create the sense of continuity, of flow, that builds trust and helps the client relax. This chap-

ter explains how to maintain and adapt that flow to each person through all of WATSU's major positions. In the Transition Flow there is an Opening, a set of basic moves, three sections, and a Completion. The basic moves, which begin with the Water Breath Dance previously described, establish a powerful connection with the breath that continues throughout the session. These basic moves, and their stillness, are returned to after each section.

There are two kinds of positions in WATSU, simple and complex. The simple moves include the basic moves and Free Float. Other simple positions are named for the body part that is supported by the therapist's shoulder or upper arm, and they include Upper Head, Under Shoulder, Under Hip, and Under Leg. The complex positions are called cradles. In a cradle, the therapist captures or cradles the client between his body and one arm, thereby freeing the other hand to work the rest of the client's body. Each of the three sections begins with a cradle and ends with simple positions. The sections are sequenced in such a way that each cradle is somewhat more difficult than the previous one and introduces a slightly higher level of nonsexual intimacy. In a session, by the time the opening and the basic moves are completed, it is determined whether the client has enough flexibility to be put into the first cradle, and so on through each section. Thus, a WATSU Transition Flow consists of an Opening, basic moves, three sections (Head Cradle; Under Far Leg, Shoulder and Hip; and Near Leg Cradle) and a Completion, described in the following sections.

In the full Transition Flow there is typically one move, rock, or stretch that is done on arriving in each cradle, and another that initiates the flow into the next position. In the Expanded Flow, for which the Transition Flow becomes the framework, more detailed pointwork and stretches are introduced in each position.

In the text that follows, Section I begins and Section II begins and ends with instructions on how to simplify the appropriate part of the Transition Flow with clients who cannot be put into the upcoming cradle. In first learning the Transition Flow, these simpler versions should be mastered first. Like the Transition Flow, this Simple Flow is made up of the Opening, the basic moves, the simple positions of each section, and the Completion. A simple cradle, which requires less flexibility and is not as size-graded as the other three cradles, can be included in the Simple Flow. Thus, the ability of WATSU to be adapted to each individual client is inherent in its program.

Before Starting

Before initiating WATSU treatment, the client should be evaluated for any conditions in which pressure or stretching are contraindicated. It must also be determined if the client is comfortable floating supine with the neck in extension, or if the neck will need continual support (which should be given in any case).

Opening

As described, a WATSU session begins with an opening (Fig. 17-1). If there is a pool wall that can be leaned against, the opening consists of the Wall Beginning, described in the next paragraph. If the pool does not have a suitable wall, the client can sit on the steps or the shore. Otherwise, begin standing in the middle of the pool. Another way to begin is to float the client off a shallow ledge. In whatever case, start the WATSU from the place that the client will be returned to at the end.

Beginning at the Wall. WATSU is best performed in water close to skin temperature, 34°C to 35°C (94°F to 96°F) and at a depth midway between the practitioner's navel and chest. When beginning a WATSU, the therapist gives the following instruction to the client:

Find the most comfortable position you can to lean back flat against the wall. Keep your legs spread to give yourself a wide base. Focus on the straightness in your back. Feel how good the support of the wall feels. Notice whatever feeling of rising there might be in your spine when you feel its straightness. Later, when you feel the wall at your back again, you will know the WATSU is complete. Focus again on this straightness and the rising. Now, you're about to enter into a different world where you will feel a totally different kind of support than that of the water. Keep yours eyes open and step away from the wall.

Surrendering to the Water. The therapist stands in front of the client, just far enough away that his arms, floating out in front, do not touch those of the client. The legs are spread while standing in one place, letting the body sink and rise with the breath. The therapist then says, "Watch me. Each time you breathe out, sink into the water like I do. Sink up to your chin. As you breathe in, let the water lift you without effort. Don't push your body up any higher than the water lifts you. Feel how the water accepts you back in as you breathe out. You don't have to do anything. Surrender to the water. Let it do everything". When it appears as if the client has surrendered to the water as much as possible, the next verbal commend is "Close your eyes and keep letting the water breathe you up." The therapist then steps forward to face the client's right side, placing his left arm over the client's right arm, allowing it to float out behind the therapist's back. The therapist's dorsal right forearm is placed under the client's coccyx to elevate the body toward the surface as the client inhales. This is the first position and it is the first time physical contact is made. The therapist can begin the WATSU from the right or left depending on hand dominance. In this description, the positions are performed on the right first and then altered to the left.

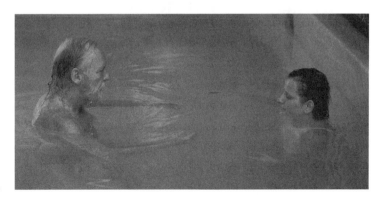

FIGURE 17-1. Opening.

Basic Moves

Water Breath Dance

The therapist maintains both forearms in a relaxed pronation position with the left arm under the client's head, and the right forearm under the coccyx (not under the lumbar spine, which could cause increased extension; Fig. 17-2). The therapist keeps low in the water with a wide, stationary stance, continuing sinking and rising with the client to the same breath rhythm as before. On exhalation, caution should be taken so that the client's head is not submerged enough to allow water into the eyes or mouth, and the legs should not completely sink.

During simultaneous rising with inhalation, the client's head should not come up so far that the ears come out of the water, and the rest of the body should rise to just under the surface. When working with someone so buoyant the body will not sink, the therapist can apply his forearm across the abdomen to help the client sink with each exhalation. If the legs are stiffened, placement of the right arm under the client's knees encourages the client to flex and relax, and arm support can be returned to the position under the coccyx. With a client who is very dense, before the therapist fatigues the next basic move, the Accordion, can begin.

Accordion

This basic move allows easier balancing of the client's weight. After completing the breath dance (or when the right arm is about to tire), the therapist slowly opens his arm as both participants inhale. The left forearm, pressing

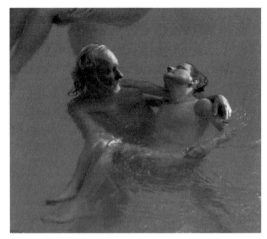

FIGURE 17-3. Accordion.

against the occiput, pulls the client away from the right forearm, which is then placed under the knees (Fig. 17-3). During exhalation, the client's trunk sinks a little. The process is repeated with opening the arms on inhalation, and closing on exhalation, allowing the client's hip to sink a little deeper. The client's knees should gradually come closer to the chest without effort. However, if tightness or holding in the knees or hips restricts the folding inward, the knees can be bounced gently, and the torso can be maneuvered into a more vertical alignment with each exhalation, encouraging the hips to flex by shifting the weight forward. If there is still holding, the therapist can try rotating the near leg for a moment to encourage relaxation (bouncing and moving it if it is still tight) before returning to the Accordion. As the knees are brought closer to the chest, with exhalation, the

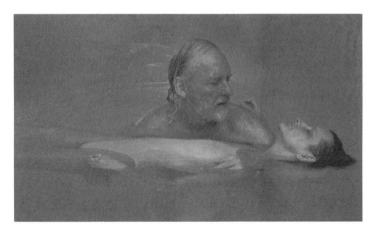

FIGURE 17-2. Water breath dance.

therapist increases the length of time that his arms are together, staying longer at the bottom of the breath. Similarly, his arms open wider with each inhalation. Any extraneous movements that could cause distraction from the breathing patterns should be avoided.

Rotating Accordion

Once the client's knees have come as close to the chest as possible, the opening and closing of the "Accordion" is continued to the breath. After each opening of the arms, the therapist stands higher and leans forward, sweeping the right arm out over the client's left side as they exhale, allowing the hips to swing toward the therapist's body. After each closing, the therapist rocks back and opens his arms as he inhales, the hips swinging away (Fig. 17-4).

Near Leg Rotation

Following out of the Rotating Accordion, as the therapist starts to rock back to open the arms, the client's far leg is allowed to slip off his arm (Fig. 17-5*A*). Without breaking the rhythm, the therapist leans forward to rotate the near leg up toward the left shoulder, concomitant with exhalation (see Fig. 17-5*B*). The rocking motions should become progressively larger, sinking back into the water with inhalation. While the right leg is rotated in this way, supported by the therapist's right elbow, a stretch is applied to the far (left) leg through the resistance of the water as the therapist moves the client around in a clockwise direction. If the client's knee does not come close enough to the chest to perform the next cradle, continue with the Simple Flow instead of the full.

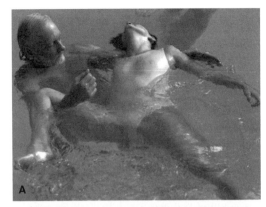

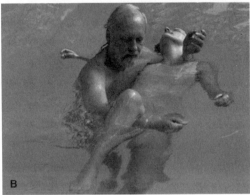

FIGURE 17-5. Near leg rotation. (*A*) The client's far leg slips off the therapist's arm. (*B*) The therapist rotates the client's near leg up toward the left shoulder.

When first learning these moves, the next step is the Completion, described later in this chapter. Each section of the Transition Flow should be mastered along with the Completion before returning to the pool to learn to combine it with the subsequent section.

Section I: The Head Cradle

Simple Flow. While rotating the near leg, and abducting it as much as possible, the therapist slips his arm out from under the client's knee and places his hand, palm up, under the "float point"—that point under the upper back where the client can be floated and balanced on one hand (the support of the forearm under the lower back can be added for those who sink). The left arm is removed from under the client's neck, and the therapist uses his left hand to slip the client's right arm out from behind his back. Once the arm is free and positioned between the two participants, the therapist supports the

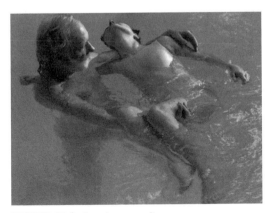

FIGURE 17-4. Rotating accordion.

client's head in the left hand and the sacrum in the right. The WATSU can than progress to those moves described later in the subsections on Stillness, Free Movement, and Hip Rock.

Full Flow. When holding a client in a cradle such as the Head Cradle (see the following three subsections), it is important to stay as low in the water as possible, with the client's chin partially submerged. Once again, it is important to keep the client's nose out of the water, and the participants should never stay in any of these cradles any longer than is comfortable. If any sensation of straining is noted, the transition to the next position should be made. In the Simple Flow, Stillness, Free Movement, and Hip Rock are done from both sides; in the Full Flow they are done just once.

Capture

After the Opening and basic moves, when the near leg is at the widest part of its rotation, the therapist keeps his left arm extended to allow the client's neck to slip out from the forearm so that the head can be supported by the hand (Fig. 17-6). The back of the right knee is held with the heel of the right hand between the hamstring tendons; grasping causes greater arm fatigue. The knees are flexed toward the chest as the client is turned toward the right side until the right arm slips free from behind the therapist's back. (If it does not float out by itself, the therapist assists by straightening the right leg and floating the client with the right hand under the "float point" in the upper back. The head is released and, with the left hand, the arm is pulled from behind the therapist's back.) When the

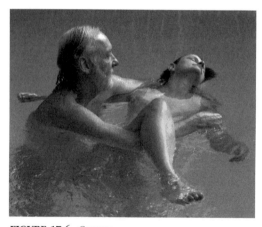

FIGURE 17-6. Capture.

client's right arm hangs free in front of the therapist's, and the head is supported in the left hand, the therapist remains low in the after and slips his right shoulder under the head, with the back of the client's neck placed snugly against the therapist's neck and shoulder. Both participant's heads are positioned to the same side that is still holding the knee. With the client's right arm still positioned under the therapist's, this capture motion should continue as an uninterrupted flow into the following moves.

Arm Leg Rock

As soon as the head is cradled (Fig. 17-7A), the therapist reaches over the upper left arm to grip it with his left hand, to pull it back toward his left side. This establishes the participant's necks in close proximity. Still holding the left arm, the right knee is pulled out to the right side (see Fig. 17-7B). Both the arm and knee are pulled as the client is rocked and turned from side to side. The breathing is again coordinated with the turning, with the therapist inhaling each time the arm is pulled.

Twist

Slowly, the right knee is moved toward the left side. Reaching under the left arm, the right hand positioned under the knee is placed with the left. Reaching over the shoulder, the upper right corner of the chest is held down by the right hand, while the left hand continues to pull the knee across the body (Fig. 17-8). Gradually and gently the spine is twisted/stretched, increasing the stretch slightly with each exhalation.

Knee Head

The right shoulder is released. The client's head is held with the right hand. The left hand is still under the right knee (Fig. 17-9). The therapist then plants his left foot forward and the right back, shifting his weight to rock slowly from foot to foot to "swing" the client forward and back.

Second Side

After completing the previous moves, the WATSU session flows into treating the other (left) side. The right knee is released and the heel of the left hand is placed under the left knee. Keeping the client's left arm under his left arm, the therapist slips his left shoulder under the head (Fig. 17-10). A mirror image of the previous moves is performed for the Arm Leg Rock,

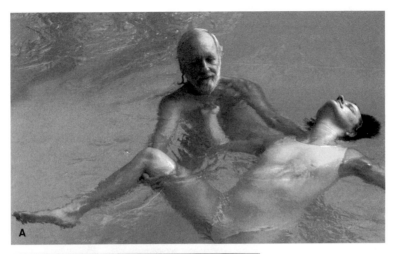

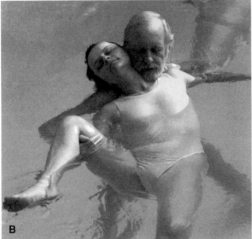

FIGURE 17-7. Arm-leg rock. (**A**) The client's neck is cradled. (**B**) The therapist pulls the client's upper left arm toward his left side, and pulls the client's right knee out to the right side.

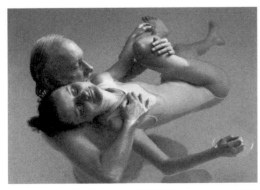

FIGURE 17-8. Twist.

Twist, and Knee Head from the left side. After "swinging" the client out and back, the left knee is released so the free hand can support the client under the sacrum.

Stillness

The client's head is held in the left hand and the sacrum in the right, with the right arm floating between the therapist and the client (Fig. 17-11). This is the Free Float position. Both arms and legs float freely. It is the best position in which to provide a moment of absolute stillness. The client is allowed to float perfectly still in

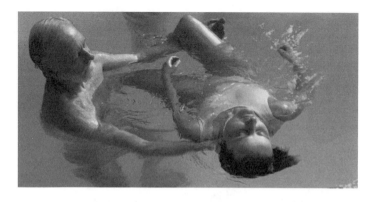

FIGURE 17-9. Knee head.

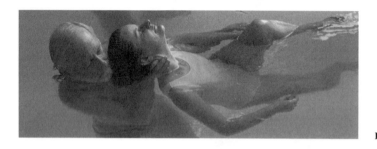

FIGURE 17-10. Second side.

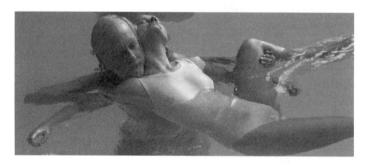

FIGURE 17-11. Stillness.

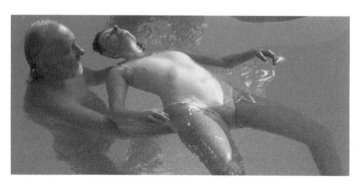

FIGURE 17-12. Free movement.

front of the therapist. If the client is heavy, the therapist can brace his right elbow against his right hip. If that does not alleviate the problem, or if the water temperature is less than ideal, the WATSU can progress into the next move, which embraces more of the Zen Shiatsu philosophy.

Free Movement

The stillness attained on the previous move should be focused in the body's "center," just below the navel. When the deepest point of that stillness is felt, energy may be released from that center in the form of waves or slow, dance-like movements (Fig. 17-12). Without intention, without directing movement with the arms, the body's "dance" from within will move the person in the therapist's hands ever more freely.

Hip Rock

As the free movement comes to completion, the therapist positions himself under the head and slips his left shoulder under the back of client's neck, staying low in the after to give as much support to the neck as possible. The hips are held with both hands, and they return to stillness for a brief moment. Without letting the lower back hyperextend, the client is moved from side to side like seaweed (Fig. 17-13). If the client is larger than the therapist and it is difficult to reach both hips, the right hand can be placed against the right hip while the left hand presses against the left side of the thorax.

Full Flow Only. After exploring movement in this position, the right hand remains under the right hip while the left hand reaches downward and slips the client's right arm behind the therapist's back to return to the first position.

Section II: Under the Far Leg, Shoulder and Hip

Simple Flow. The client's head is rested on the therapist's left shoulder, with the hips in the therapist's hands. The right hand slips the client's head off the shoulder and pulls it through the water. The left hand slips the client's left arm over the therapist's right arm, as he positions himself under the shoulder to perform Under Shoulder, Lengthening Spine, and Spine Pull (see subsections, later). The "float point" is used to move into the first position, and a mirror image of all of the moves is performed to return to the first side. The Water Breath Dance is repeated a third time, along with the Undulating Spine from Section III.

Simple Cradle. This can follow either the complex cradles or the Simple Flow. It requires less flexibility than the leg overs and can be done with clients of all sizes. After the basic moves, the far leg is rotated, and the client is turned and lifted so that the back of the right knee is positioned over the top of the therapist's left leg. The therapist then lifts the left knee in the crook of his right elbow, stretching the legs apart as he rocks side to side. The right knee is laid over the therapist's right leg as the rocking continues. Stabilizing the client's left shoulder with his right forearm and left hand, the therapist's right hand is free to treat the face, head, and neck. Treatment of these areas can continue as the head is cradled in the therapist's right elbow. Both hands are used to hold the occiput as the therapist rocks from side to side, lifting the head. The therapist then positions the head on his left arm and lifts the client's torso toward his chest, step-

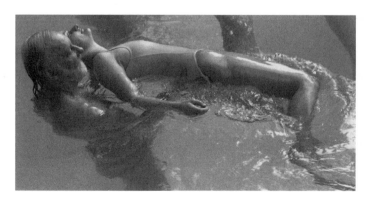

FIGURE 17-13. Hip rock.

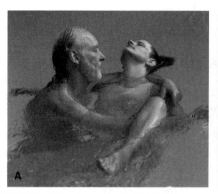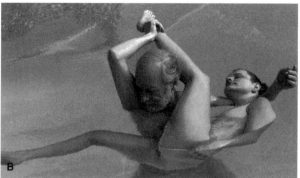

FIGURE 17-14. Far leg over. (**A**) The therapist scoops up the client's far leg with the crook of his elbow under the knee. (**B**) The therapist grasps the client's left leg just above the ankle with his right hand, lifting the leg higher than the therapist's head.

ping back to roll the client into the first position (lifting up under the sacrum with the right knee).

Far Leg Over

The basic moves are repeated. The near leg is abducted and rotated out to its fullest. The therapist removes his right arm out from under the near leg. Without breaking the rhythm of the rotation, the therapist leans forward to scoop up the far leg with the crook of his elbow under the knee (Fig. 17-14A). The far leg is rotated in the same counterclockwise direction as the near leg, flexing the knee as close as possible to the far shoulder. The body should move freely. When the therapist's arms are in their most open position during the last rotation, he reaches out with his right hand to hold the client's right leg just above the ankle. The leg is then lifted to a position higher than the therapist's head, thus creating a space, or a "window" between the

back of the leg and the therapist's arm (see Fig. 17-14B). The therapist slowly passes his head through this space. As the leg is lowered, the therapist wraps it around the back of his neck. (It is important that the therapist face away from the client's head to avoid pressure on his throat from the client's leg.) While his left hand keeps the head high enough to prevent the client's nose from going under, the therapist keeps his shoulder low enough to minimize the amount of weight on it.

Leg Push

The therapist holds the client's upper back behind the "heart center" using his left hand, with his left arm still supporting the head. With his right hand just above the knee, the therapist abducts the right leg (Fig. 17-15). As the leg is slowly pushed, the therapist turns clockwise so that the resistance of the water aids in stretching the leg.

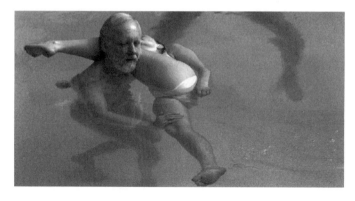

FIGURE 17-15. Leg push.

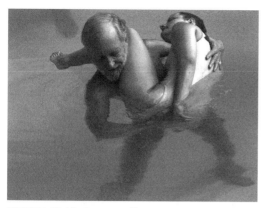

FIGURE 17-16. Sacrum pull.

Sacrum Pull

The client's knee is flexed and the right leg is depressed in front of the therapist so that it is positioned across his abdomen, and around his waist. The back of the right knee should be snug against the therapist's side. The client is in a side-lying position. The therapist uses one hand to pull the upper back and press the chest as close to the knees as possible, then hooks his fingers onto the superior aspect of the sacrum to pull downward to stretch the lumbar spine (Fig. 17-16). Counter pressure is applied with the right hand against the left hip. The left hand is used to lay the client back into the water without letting the head fall into too much extension. The "float point" is held under the upper back with the right hand as the therapist slips his left shoulder out from under the left leg by lowering himself in the water.

Under Shoulder

Staying low in the water, the therapist moves under the client's shoulder with his right shoulder and, reaching up around the other side of the neck, places his right hand on the "heart center." The right elbow remains elevated under the client's head, with the therapist's body positioned low in the water to prevent the neck from hyperextending (Fig. 17-17).

Lengthening Spine

The client's sacrum is supported by the therapist's left hand. As soon as the client exhales, the body is allowed to sink a little. As both participants inhale, the therapist slowly lifts the client up and away from him, using his left hand

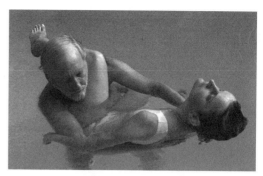

FIGURE 17-17. Under shoulder.

against the top of the sacrum (Fig. 17-18). This sinking and lifting is repeated with each breath. The therapist uses his right hand to apply very light pressure on the client's chest with each exhalation and sinking phase, while maintaining contact with the chest to provide traction to the spine each time pressure is applied to the sacrum.

Spine Pull

The therapist supports the client's occiput with his right hand as he straightens his right arm and moves down to the client's side, so that his left shoulder is positioned just under the left hip (Fig. 17-19). This is the Under Hip position. The therapist then hooks his left fingers onto the top of the sacrum, and pulls to stretch the whole spine.

Undulating Spine

The therapist remains low in the water, close to or just under the left hip, with his left hand, palm up, under the sacrum (Fig. 17-20A). Bouncing

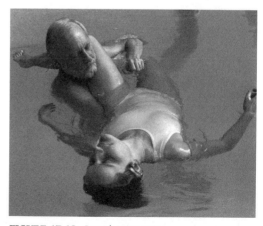

FIGURE 17-18. Lengthening spine.

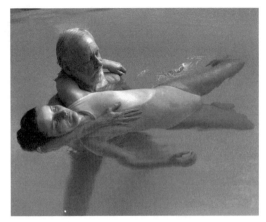

FIGURE 17-19. Spine pull.

on his feet, the therapist initiates wave movements up the client's spine, including the neck, which is loosely supported in the right hand (the right arm is still positioned in extension under the shoulder; see Fig. 17-20*B*). Again, the left hand supports the "float point," and occipital support is provided by the slightly flexed right elbow. The therapist then reaches over the

client's left arm to move into the first position on the second side.

Second Side

The basic moves are performed on the second side. The far leg is rotated and a mirror image of the previous moves (Far Leg Over through Undulating Spine) is completed. On return to the first side, the Water Breath Dance is repeated. If it appears that the client would not be comfortable in the next cradle, Heart Home and the Completion are performed.

Section III: The Near Leg Cradle

Near Leg Over

The basic moves are repeated. While rotating the near leg to its fullest, the therapist takes hold of it just above the ankle with his right hand (Fig. 17-21*A*). Staying low in the water, the therapist wraps the near leg around his neck, similar to the movement with the far leg in the last section

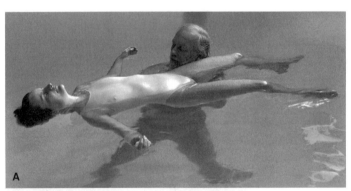

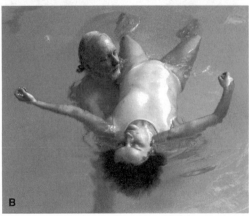

FIGURE 17-20. Undulating spine. (*A*) The therapist stands with his left hand, palm up, under the client's sacrum. (*B*) Bouncing on his feet, the therapist initiates wave movements up the client's spine.

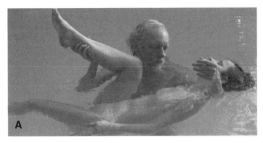 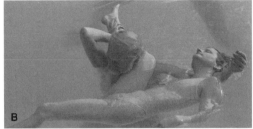

FIGURE 17-21. Near leg over. (***A***) While rotating the near leg to the fullest, the therapist holds it just above the ankle with his right hand. (***B***) The therapist wraps the near leg around his neck.

(see Fig. 17-21*B*). The occiput is supported by the left hand.

Down Quads

Starting at the proximal end of the far leg, the therapist grips the quadriceps muscles between the fingertips and heel of the right hand (Fig. 17-22). The leg is rolled, slowly working distally over the knee.

Leg Down

While slowly turning clockwise to stretch the far left leg, the therapist guides the leg away from him with his right hand. Depressing the left leg with his right hand, the therapist uses his left hand to support the neck and upper back, swinging the torso upward toward a vertical position (Fig. 17-23). (If the pool is so shallow that the left foot would hit the bottom, the knee can be flexed before depressing it.) The left knee is caught against the inside of the therapist's right leg just above his knee. The client rests his forehead against his right knee, which is still over the therapist's left shoulder; the therapist's right

hand supports the mid-back. Replacing his right hand with the left, the therapist reaches his right hand over the client's left shoulder to support his neck. The therapist then leans into the lowered knee with his right leg while pulling the upper back toward him to stretch the whole body. The cervical region can be massaged or worked with the right hand in this position, decreasing the likelihood of irritating the hamstring tendons through movement of the therapist's left shoulder. The right arm is also in proper position to receive the neck when the client is lowered in the next move.

Leg Pass

The therapist assumes a stance with the left leg behind the right, which is still supporting the client's left leg. The client's leg is allowed to rise toward the surface along the therapist's left side.

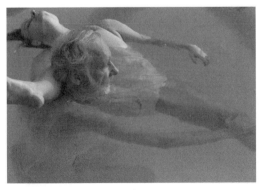

FIGURE 17-22. Down quads.

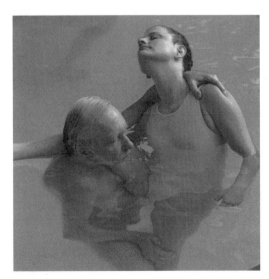

FIGURE 17-23. Leg down.

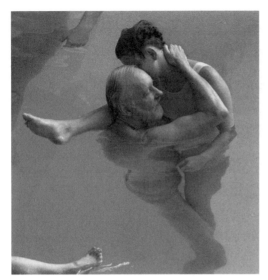

FIGURE 17-24. Massaging the neck just before the leg pass.

The neck is lowered into the crook of the therapist's right elbow (Fig. 17-24).

Arm

The client's right knee is still supported on the therapist's left shoulder. The therapist can adjust his shoulder position slightly to allow comfortable positioning of the hamstrings. With the client's right arm in front of him, the therapist uses both hands to squeeze the arm and pull it in opposite directions (Fig. 17-25). Gently tugging the left thigh with the left hand causes the right leg to slip off the therapist's shoulder, thus returning to the first position on the second side.

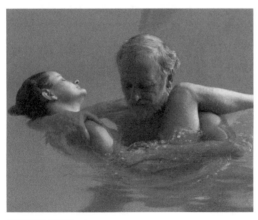

FIGURE 17-25. Arm.

Second Side

The basic moves are performed on the second side. The near leg is rotated and a mirror image of the previous moves (Near Leg Over through Arm) is completed. After returning to the first side, the Water Breath Dance is repeated. If it appears that the client would not be comfortable in the next cradle, the Simple Cradle and Heart Home can be performed.

Heart Home

The client is returned to the first position on the first side and gently rocked. Resting the side of his head on the client's "heart center" (facing away from the client with the head over the sternal region), the therapist continues rocking with the breath (Fig. 17-26A). After lifting his head, the therapist reaches under the near leg with his right arm and places his right hand on the sternum to continue the rhythm of the rocking (see Fig. 17-26B).

Completion

In the following closure, the client is leaning back against the wall. If there is no suitable wall, the pool steps or ledge or the shore can be used. If none of these is accessible, the client can stand in the middle of the pool, supported by the therapist's hands on the anterior and posterior thorax, over the "heart center," until the client is ready to stand alone. It is important to orient clients beforehand so that when they are repositioned at the wall (or steps, ledge, or shore), they know the WATSU is completed. A clear separation at this point is equally important, as is the proximity of the therapist when the client opens his eyes.

Wall Return

When the WATSU is near completion, the therapist slips his right forearm under both knees and brings them as close to the client's chest as possible. The therapist stands high in the water with the client's head resting on the left side of his chest, and rocks slowly. Gradually they approach the wall. When the client's back (still vertical) meets the wall, the client is set on the therapist's left knee, which is positioned along the wall (Fig. 17-27). The client's far leg is allowed

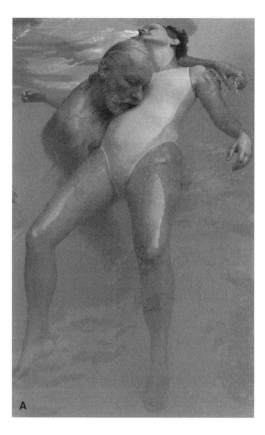

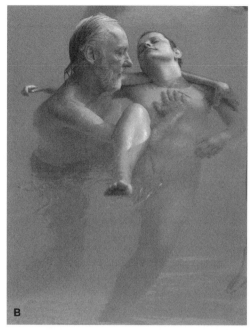

FIGURE 17-26. Heart home. (*A*) The therapist rests his head over the client's "heart center." (*B*) The therapist reaches under the near leg with his right arm and places his right hand on the sternum.

to slip off the right arm; the therapist gently pushes it out and away, and pulls the near leg toward him to create a wide base of support. Holding the neck and occiput with the left hand, the therapist positions the spine to a neutral, vertical orientation. With the left hand still at the base of the head, the therapist places his right hand on the "heart center" and moves in front of the client, providing additional support at the client's knees and feet with his own. This posture is held a moment, allowing both bodies to settle comfortably in the water.

Lift Off

The therapist gradually slips his left hand out from behind the neck, ensuring that the client's head is capable of being supported independently. With the right hand still on the "heart center," the therapist places his left hand lightly on the client's head, the heel over the "third eye" (the forehead) and the fingertips just touching the "crown chakra" on the top of the head (Fig. 17-28*A*). After a moment, the therapist slowly lifts both hands up. The therapist slips his hands back into the water to lift the client's hands slowly toward the surface. The therapist draws his own hands together out of the water and rocks back to withdraw contact from the client's knees and feet (see Fig. 17-28*B*).

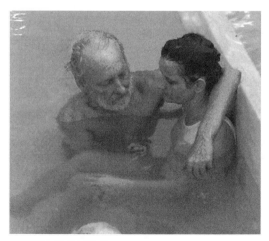

FIGURE 17-27. Wall return.

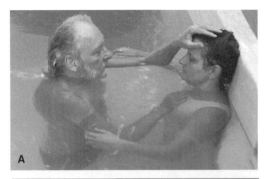

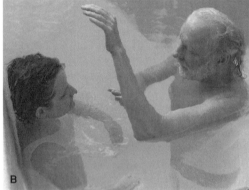

FIGURE 17-28. Lift off. (**A**) The therapist places his left hand lightly on the client's head. (**B**) The therapist lifts up both hands.

Honoring the Space

Staying low in the water, the therapist continues to step away from the client, honoring the "heart space" between them, and remaining in position until the client's eyes open (Fig. 17-29).

Expanding the Transition Flow

Before beginning the Expanded Flow, the Transition Flow should be mastered. The Expanded Flow presents additional bodywork that can be performed in each of the three sections of the Transition Flow. In this section, the moves as described in the Transition Flow are simply listed by title, if unchanged; in some cases, a variant sequence is described. The moves that are newly introduced in this section are numbered.

Expanding the First Section

The Expanded Flow consists of another variation of a continual sequence of transitional movements, beginning with the Head Cradle.

Capture or Variant Capture

Another way of moving the client into the head cradle from the first position is to float him, holding the far arm. During the final basic move, while rotating the near leg up toward the far shoulder, the therapist is positioned with his right arm under the client's knee. The therapist then takes hold of the upper left arm with his right hand, floats the client away from him, and slides his left arm out from under the neck. With his left hand, the therapist takes the right arm out from behind his back and places it between their bodies. Holding the head in his left hand, the therapist releases the left arm and slides his own arm along the back of the knee until the

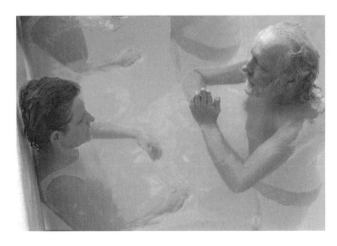

FIGURE 17-29. Honoring the space.

heel of his right hand is fitted between the hamstring tendons of the client's right knee. Maintaining this hand position on the knee, the therapist lowers his right shoulder under the client's head. The client's right arm should still be positioned under the therapist's right arm.

Arm Leg Rock

1. Arm Leg Rock II

After rocking the client from side to side, alternately pulling the right knee and the left arm, the therapist can create a more intense rock by maintaining the pull to the opposite side. Specifically, both the knee and the arm are pulled, while the therapist turns from side to side. This, too, can be performed to the rhythm of the breathing, as previously described.

2. Arm Opening

Holding the upper left arm with his left hand, the therapist squeezes and shakes the arm, slowly working distally to the left hand, to free the whole arm. The therapist holds the client's left hand and raises the arm toward an overhead position, stretching the whole body by pulling the right knee at the same time.

3. Chest Opening

The therapist reaches under the client's left arm and hooks his fingers into the upper corner of the chest, near the pectoral insertions. He then pulls back to stretch and expand the chest.

4. Shoulder Rotation

With a firm hold over the glenohumeral joint, the therapist rotates the left shoulder with his left hand.

5. Shoulder Blade

The therapist places his thumb between the mid-thorax and the scapula. Lifting the thumb rhythmically, he works distally along the medial border.

6. Bladder Meridian

With the client still in a relatively supine position, the therapist works down the line of points (bladder meridian) between the vertebrae, an inch to an inch and a half to the left of the midline. Each point is held with the left thumb as the body is rocked into the thumb. This process continues distally to the sacrum, to the point just to the left of the coccyx. The therapist hooks his left middle finger into this point and continues rocking.

7. Wall Knee

Still holding the knee, the therapist slowly backs up to the wall. The therapist straightens his left leg to brace his back against the wall. The right knee is flexed and lifted up into the client's lower back (to the right of the spine just above the sacrum). The therapist's left hand is positioned on the "hara" just below the navel to press down and hold. (Caution should be taken to avoid putting pressure against the kidney.) To "lengthen" the spine, the right knee is pulled toward the chest while the therapist's knee continues to press against the superior border of the sacrum (to the right of the spine). With the knee repositioned to the right of the coccyx, the therapist gently pushes the right leg downward, and continues with movements from the Transition Flow:

Twist
Knee Head Rock
Second Side

The WATSU continues with the Free Float:

Stillness
Free Movement

The transition is made to the Under Head position:

Hip Rock

8. Hara Rise

The right hand is placed under the sacrum with the left hand on the hara. The left hand pushes downward with each exhalation; the right pushes upward with inhalation. This is continued for several breaths, making sure the client's feet do not touch the bottom during exhalation. This maneuver should not be performed if the therapist cannot reach the client's sacrum.

9. Buttock Rock

Holding a buttock in each hand, with the head still on the client's left shoulder, the therapist slowly moves the client through the water. Moving and rocking from side to side, the therapist lifts alternate buttocks. More innovative, rapid movements can be explored to release tension in buttocks and back. After this, a moment of stillness is observed.

10. Slide Up Back

The therapist braces the heel of the right hand against the superior aspect of the sacrum and slowly slides the heel of the left hand superiorly along the lumbar spine, "lifting" vertebra by vertebra. The fingers of the left hand are directed toward the feet. This process is paused in the mid-thoracic region and repeated from the sacral level. With the third repetition, the therapist continues to the level of occiput, repositioning the hand so the fingers are directed superiorly. A traction force can be applied to the occiput and sacrum, "stretching" the spine.

11. Side Change

Pulling the head through the water with the left hand, the therapist simultaneously applies force to the lateral aspect of the near hip with the right hand. The hand position is reversed under the head and the opposite hip receives an upward force as the client is returned to the first side. If not difficult, this procedure can be repeated several times, alternating sides while pulling the body through the water by the head.

12. Forearm Lift

Supporting the head at the occiput with both hands, elbows directed toward the feet, the therapist applies a distraction force. Instead of pushing up against the hip, as described earlier, the therapist raises one forearm between the spine and scapula, and slowly rolls the client toward the opposite side. By lifting under the other side with the opposite forearm, the client is returned to the first side. This alternating movement is continued while gently gliding the head through the water, stretching the cervical region. The therapist moves his body to the right and slips the client's right arm behind his back to return to the first position.

Expanding the Second Section

Far Leg Over
Leg Push

1. Down Back

The therapist holds the client between the scapula and spine with the left hand while the right, reaching over the buttock, works Bladder Meridian points running distally from the upper to lower back, rocking the body into the fingers. The therapist holds the bladder point at the top of the leg firmly with the right thumb and rocks the client from head to toe. Still holding the upper back with the left hand, the therapist glides the right leg into abduction. The therapist then turns in the direction the water's resistance, helping to stretch the leg.

2. Foot

The therapist flexes the client's right knee and places the tibial shaft across the hara below the therapist's navel. The client's right foot is in the therapist's right hand. The therapist then makes a pincer with the thumb and finger to hold the ankle while rotating and stretching the foot with the forearm. The acupuncture point, kidney 1 (in the midline one third of the way down from the toes) is held in the therapist's right thumb. The foot is worked freestyle.

Sacrum Pull
Under Shoulder
Lengthening Spine

3. Twist Over

After elevating the sacrum upward, the therapist reaches over the near leg and under the far knee. The therapist pulls the far leg across the trunk while simultaneously stabilizing the left shoulder. The therapist then gradually and gently twists and stretches the client's spine.

4. Figure Eight

The therapist releases the far knee and quickly reaches under the near leg. The therapist then holds the far leg just above the ankle and glides it under the near leg and up to the surface. As the client's hip rotates, the therapist pulls (do not push) the leg all the way under to the other side. The therapist then repeatedly inscribes this figure-eight motion. The therapist is reminded to keep the left elbow raised enough to prevent the client's neck from being strained.

5. Lower Back

The therapist should release the far leg when it has reached its farthest position under the near leg. Before the client lays back, the therapist presses the forearm into the side of the lower back turned toward the therapist. The client is then rocked onto the therapist's forearm, which continues pressing between the sacrum and the rib cage. No pressure is to be placed directly on the spine.

The transition is made to the Under Hip position.

Spine Pull
Undulating Spine

6. Thigh Rock

Next, the therapist reaches over the near leg and, holding the buttock with the left hand, clasps the left thigh tightly to the therapist's waist. The occiput is held in the therapist's right hand. The therapist rhythmically turns away from the client so that the therapist's body "tugs and rocks" the thigh clasped to the therapist's side, releasing tension in the near hip.

7. Bow

The therapist reaches under the near thigh and over the far thigh to hold the middle of the far thigh in the left hand. The buttocks are braced against the therapist's side and the far leg is brought into extension, gently arching the whole body.

8. Lift

If the client is not too heavy or inflexible to lift out of the water, the therapist should slip the upper left arm under the client's knees. The therapist them flexes them to the chest and clasps the client's upper far arm in his left hand. The client's trunk is then elevated, the near arm still over the therapist's right shoulder, the side of the buttock propped on the therapist's hip. The therapist stands high enough out of the water to allow the client's head to fall forward (without the nose going under) and release any tension that the previous position might have built up in the neck. The therapist then holds the upper right arm loosely in the left hand. If easily accessible, the therapist can work the neck with the right hand. While the client is still upright, the therapist slips the right arm over the client's left arm and lowers the client back into the first position (still on the second side).

9. Neck Pull

Using his stronger arm, the therapist cradles the client's neck in the first position on the second side. Next, the therapist uses the left forearm against the client's upper thoracic spine while stretching and working the neck with the right arm.

From second side, repeat all of the above to return to the first side.

Expanding the Third Section

Near Leg Over
Down Quads

1. Up Liver

The therapist works quadriceps distally from the client's hip to below the knee, and then presses the heel of the right hand against the medial thigh immediately proximal to the knee. The therapist maintains a static stretch, and rocks the client's leg and gradually works proximal along the medial thigh (Liver Meridian) toward the hip.

2. Down Bladder

The therapist presses the right thumb into the posterior thigh immediately below the client's buttock. Repeatedly lifting the thumb, the therapist slowly works the midline of the posterior thigh, knee, and calf (Bladder Meridian). Avoid pressing up under the knee. The therapist then turns, gliding the far leg away from the therapist's body.

Leg Down or Variant—Both Knees Over

The therapist stands with the client's near leg over the therapist's shoulder, drapes the client's other leg over the therapist's other shoulder, and then bring the client (from the side) to a vertical position. The therapist then holds the client by pressing the client's upper back with one hand and works the client's neck with the other. This position can also be used as a transition.

Leg Pass
Arm

3. Freeing the Arm

The therapist releases the client's arm and squeezes, shakes, and moves it freely. The therapist's right hand can stay in one place, squeezing and mobilizing the client's upper arm (or left shoulder, if the therapist's other arm is not long enough to reach under the neck to the arm). The therapist works wrist, hand, and fingers. The therapist then "tugs" the client's left thigh with his left arm to slip the right leg off the therapist's shoulder. The participants return to the first position.

Second Side
Heart Home

4. Hara Rock

The therapist slides the right hand downward to just below the client's navel, clasps the hara between the thumb and fingers, and rocks. The therapist gently squeezes the hara each time the client exhales. (If it is not readily apparent, the therapist can place an ear close to the client's mouth to hear/feel the breath.) The therapist gently tugs or pulls the hara with each inhalation. The therapist then places the right hand on the heart center and continues the Water Breath

Dance, bringing both knees to chest and finishing as at the end of the Transition Flow.

Worldwide Aquatic Bodywork Association

The Worldwide Aquatic Bodywork Association is a nonprofit association that has been founded to explore the benefits of giving and receiving aquatic bodywork, and to make it available to everyone. The author has donated his teaching facility, The School of Shiatsu and Massage at Harbin Hot Springs, Middletown, California, to it. Schooling in WATSU and other bodywork techniques is available through the association.

REFERENCES

1. Morris DM. Aquatic rehabilitation for the treatment of neurological disorders. *Journal of Back and Musculoskeletal Rehabilitation.* 1994;4:297–308.
2. Dull H. *WATSU: Freeing the Body in Water.* Middletown, Calif: Harbin Springs Publishing; 1993.

P A R T

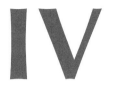

PRACTICE
MANAGEMENT

18 Facility Design

Marilou Moschetti

Aquatic rehabilitation is one integrant in a vast number of therapy programs. Whether patrons swim using traditional swimming strokes or vertically stand in the therapy pool, their musculoskeletal or neurologic injury may be treated in the aqueous medium. Successful rehabilitation is a result not only of a competent therapist, but a carefully designed aquatic facility.

It is estimated that there are hundreds of facilities providing aquatic therapy and rehabilitation programs in the United States, and the number is growing yearly (Osinski A, personal communication, December, 1994). This chapter defines elements and considerations throughout the preplanning, design, construction, and postconstruction phases of a center used for aquatic physical therapy, rehabilitation, and wellness.

Why Water?

Aquatic therapy is used for treatment of a variety of symptoms, including pain with movement, limited movement, decreased strength, or edema.[1-3] With an increase in the understood benefits of an aquatic therapy program, many individual practices, hospitals, and clinics have started or considered construction of their own aquatic facility.

Adding a pool to an existing practice's facility may provide the edge over other traditional therapy interventions and modalities. The existing client populations of the private practice, clinic, or hospital determine the size of the basic aquatic facility project.[4] Many clinics and hospitals considering the addition of therapy pools in existing space must also consider the acquisition costs and necessary adjunct services.

Development Phase

The initial step in the planning process is to analyze adequately the prospective service area.[5] Necessary steps to be taken in the early planning phase are (1) defining the user population, (2) determining the demand for service, and (3) evaluating resources.[6-8]

In planning to match the health requirements of a growing population, "wellness centers," many with pools, have become the focus of many communities, shifting health care responsibilities to the individual participant rather than the medical community. The current population is living longer and is more physically active than previous generations, and the aspect of maintaining wellness has become an increasing social concern.[9,10] Further, large corporations are building on-site fitness centers, including swimming pools, in an attempt to reduce health care costs among employees, while increasing the demand for aquatic programming across the nation.[11]

Increases in aquatic programming are not confined to corporate on-site fitness centers. Aquatic physical therapy as a procedure is found to increase referrals to for-profit and nonprofit hospitals, public entities, foundations, and private physical therapy practices.[12,13] Physicians can clearly document medically necessary aquatic therapy services.[14,15]

The wide spectrum of user populations (ambulatory, nonambulatory) requires careful consideration in treatment and facility design. To ensure patron comfort and treatment ease, accessibility to the aquatic wellness center must be considered a vital part of the preplanning phase.[16-18]

Preplanning Phase

The project planner must conceptualize complete programming requirements for the facility. During the initial analysis, the following should be identified: (1) the primary function of the intended users, (2) programs the facility will offer, and (3) how the facility will provide the services. A preplanning questionnaire is developed to narrow the focus of the project in an attempt to match the primary service requirements and treatment atmosphere of both provider and patron base.[19–22]

The facility design might reflect a broad base of programs in addition to aquatic therapy. Recreational wellness programs, water fitness programs, swim lessons, synchronized swimming, adapted aquatics, scuba diving, and lap swimming are options that encourage potential use by the community (Dunlap E, personal communication, Timpany Center, San Jose, California, 1994).[4,5,23–27] One thing to remember is that aquatic centers rarely are converted to another activity; therefore, it is important to get it right the first time. The pool may be open 16 hours a day and offer alternate programs every hour, and therefore need flexibility and durability in design.[28] Design features for the aquatic wellness center must account for water depth and temperature, support spaces, patron load, and access to the pool from either existing buildings or new infrastructures[10] (see Appendix 18-A).

Prebuilding Budget Development and Cost Analysis

Cost and budget estimates for construction, administration, and design are generated during the initial preplanning phase.[7] Site-specific feasibility studies are of critical importance. Site suitability is examined for zoning concerns, geotechnical and soil features, and load-bearing capabilities. General physical setting, existing land, economic impact, and economic resources provide limits to the size in square footage of the proposed project.[29] Financing is raised in a build–lease back plan, bond or capital fund raising, or donation campaign.

The appointed planning chair selects members of the planning team: aquatic consultant, provider, aquatic director, architect, contractor, pool builder, and local health and safety official (Box 18-1). A newly formed group, the International Association of Aquatic Consultants, publishes an annual directory of available experts in related specialized fields of aquatics. The areas they specialize in include Feasibility Study and Concept Development, Design and Construction Management, Program Development and Marketing, Lifeguard Training, and Risk Management. An aquatic consultant can troubleshoot problems in design and help prevent potential problems before construction.[30]

The planning team then gathers and analyzes information from site surveys and questionnaires. (By examining other aquatic therapy facilities of varying size, the planning team might collect relevant collateral information.[31]) In an effort to complete predesign information gathering, an open meeting can be held to allow the public affected by the proposed construction to voice concerns. Once this information is collected and analyzed, a more specific construction cost estimate can be generated.[4,21] Operating cost and revenue projections, along with insurance reimbursements, are taken into account in developing the initial annual budget.[7]

Based on findings of the planning team, the planning chair selects an architect who has considerable experience in pool design. The architect is responsible for schematic floor plans, facility access points, elevation plans, general operating efficiency, and a study model.[32,33] The architect uses the Uniform Building Code, used in California and most western states, or the Standard Building Code to define all concerns related to occupancy, building envelope, structural systems, structural materials, nonstructural materials, building services, special devices, conditions, and standards for the building and swimming pool tanks.[6] Barriers for swimming pools and hot tubs, site accessibility, ventilation, energy conservation, waterproofing, masonry, lighting, plumbing, flood-resistant construction, excavating and grading are all covered in the Uniform Building Code (see Appendix 18-B). By applying the recommendations of the planning team and architect, design, production, and construction elements are finalized. Bidding and other negotiations between the owner and contractors commence, and a time line for project development and completion is drawn for provider approval.

The architect and a technical survey team identify problems in subsoil, water table height, soil, and rock at the prospective building site. A construction checklist is developed to keep

BOX 18-1. Design Team

Aquatic Consultant

An aquatic specialist is familiar with equipment, products, materials, and all aquatic systems. The aquatic consultant assists in budget development, establishes costs, and critiques construction documents for design, hazards, code compliance, and common practices in the aquatic industry. He or she makes recommendations and sets priorities and goals for the planning team.

Architect

The architect is responsible for design of the space, estimates of project costs, and specifications and drawings from which the general contractor works. The architect observes construction and verifies the work is completed and meets with all specifications of the plan.

A design engineer works under the architect and is responsible for design of the building structure; mechanical equipment; and machinery and building systems, including electrical, plumbing, mechanical, heat, ventilation and air conditioning, and other operational systems. The design engineer checks finished work for compliance with industry and manufacturing performance standards.

Contractor/Pool Builder

Both the contractor and pool builder must be licensed and bonded by the state in which the facility is built. They purchase supplies, materials and equipment for the construction project, construct the facility, install all needed equipment, and follow installation specifications. Both are responsible for all subcontractors who work on the project, work schedules, and permits and inspections, in addition to the follow-up on inspection of equipment warrantees.

Health and Safety Official

The local county department has jurisdiction over the completed facility and helps in the design process, so the facility's plans and specifications meet all necessary regulations. A checklist of requirements is written to meet all local, state, and federal health and safety requirements.

Adapted from Allison Osinski, PhD, Aquatic Consulting Services, Inc.

the project on target. The Construction Specification Institute checklist for estimating and record keeping is used to estimate geographic cost modifiers. These are used by architects and engineers for construction specifications, and must be completed by the contractors. They consist of 16 divisions and provide specific performance standards for all general building materials and finished appliances used in development requirements for construction of the project (Box 18-2). In addition to providing a general outline for construction performance standards, the Construction Specification Institute performance checklist provides the planning team with manageable cost breakdown information for the type and size of the pool facility.

Cost of an "ideal" aquatic wellness center may vary from $75 to $155 per square foot, based on location (consult an architect for building cost assistance). For instance, the illustrated center (see Appendix 18-C) may cost $4,185,000 based on $155 per square feet on the high end (27,000 square feet × $155 a foot), and $2,025,000 on the lower end (27,000 square feet × $75 a foot).

After preplanning budgets, fees and permits,

BOX 18-2. Construction Specification Institute Checklist of Performance Standards Written for Each Division of:

General work
Site work
Concrete
Masonry
Metals
Carpentry
Moisture protection
Doors, windows, glass
Finish work
Specialties
Equipment
Furnishing
Special contruction—pool equipment
Conveying systems
Mechanical systems
Electrical systems

Adapted from Construction Specification Institute.

construction expenses, miscellaneous expenses, and preconstruction information, including geographic cost modifiers, are taken care of, construction documents are drawn up detailing the building. During construction, "build as" drawings, change requests, and change orders are formulated. The documents must be kept for the life of the building, showing all electrical, plumbing, and ventilation diagrams and layouts, in the event of equipment failures or building expansions. On the final approval of the design team and local, county, and state authorities, the construction phase of the aquatic wellness center may commence (see Appendix 18-B).

Postconstruction Phase

Near the end of construction and before facility opening, the planning chair hires an aquatic facility manager, director of aquatic physical therapy, maintenance chief, and office personnel. This early hiring ensures a smooth transition to the preoperation phase.

The main focus during the preoperation phase is development of training, personnel, and procedure manuals in each department. Furthermore, along with the design team, all managers, supervisors, or directors must participate in the final inspection and approve equipment relating to everyday operations in their departments. This includes chemical, filter, pump, ventilation, heating, plumbing, electrical, lighting, computer, and all other pieces of equipment in the facility. Equipment deficiencies are identified and corrected at this time.

When final inspection for the entire project is completed by local health and safety officials, the general contractor, and provider, approval is given and a certificate of completion and operating permit are issued. The final operating permit must be posted in the building.

There are three postconstruction phases used to sign-off the facility from contractor to owner. The first, or *warrantee phase* consists of an inspection after 11 months of daily operation. Notification is given to the contractor of any mechanical deficiencies during this time period. In the second phase, a *construction bond* (performance bond is based on finances of the project) is obtained by the contractor before the beginning of construction. The bond cost usually does not exceed 1% of construction (this is not a steady rate). The bond is held for 1 year to cover

repairs of faulty equipment. It is very important that deficiencies noted in the warrantee inspection be corrected before the expiration of the bond, or a claim must be filed. The third phase includes *postoccupancy evaluation* as a process of evaluating how the facility is operating after the first year. Records from all departments are compiled and the design team draws conclusions on operations.

An evaluation also is conducted as to how each piece of equipment has functioned during the first year, and what was done regarding repairs to mechanical, filtering, heating, or ventilation systems. A complete list should be kept by the maintenance chief on how each system was repaired. This is an optional additional service for architects, but it helps other developers analyze project outcomes as well as assists the owner in determining what changes should be made after a year's experience in operating the facility.

The "Ideal" Aquatic Wellness Center

All information in the description of the "ideal" aquatic wellness facility is in reference to the design in Appendix 18-C.

Considerations for the Project Floor Plan

The design for the "ideal" aquatic facility includes a functional floor plan that addresses the needs of both staff and patrons.[33] Balancing conflicting needs of competitive, physical education, recreation, and therapy programs determines the form the pool design will follow. Justifying design specifications, equipment, and personnel is vital to avoiding operation pitfalls. A two- or three-pool complex may be considered to serve the largest user population. A small therapeutic warm water pool (92°F to 94°F), hot-water spa (102°F to 104°F), and a larger, multiuse pool (82°F to 85°F) are illustrated in the planning design (see Appendix 18-C)

The floor plan for the "ideal" aquatic wellness center includes the following basic rooms and spaces: reception and lobby area, pool management and director offices, classroom, male and female dressing areas, family dressing rooms, staff, first aid and lifeguard office, mechanical and chemical rooms, support equipment storage, and janitorial and supplies cubicle. The multiuse center may also include a library, day care, and community center, attracting more users than just those interested in aquatics (not illustrated in Appendix 18-C).[34]

The *reception and lobby* area must be close to the parking lot, and allow the patrons easy check-in. Access must not be barred by obstacles for wheelchair users.[19] Potted plants, extra chairs, magazine racks, narrow doorways, or heavy doors all cause difficulty in negotiating the treatment area. Essential equipment in the reception area includes computer stations, necessary office machines, a video surveillance camera of the pool area, and an intrabuilding communications system.

For easy access and supervision, the *manager's office* is located between the dry and wet areas. The room must be well ventilated with all furnishings in the office constructed of rust-resistant materials to counteract the effects of humidity. The office has an observation window directly into the pool area, a direct line to emergency medical services, and an intrabuilding communication station. The manager can instantly analyze all computerized sanitation, filtration, and ventilation systems through a summary report station located on the office wall or displayed on a personal computer.[20]

The *classroom* ideally accommodates 25 to 30 people. Inservice staff meetings and patron education sessions are aided by pull-down projection screen, additional audiovisual equipment, a bulletin board, basic kitchen appliances, counter space, and storage cupboards. Mats, chairs, and low tables are also stored in the classroom and made available for dry physical therapy treatment sessions.

Dressing rooms are a major planning fault in most swimming pool designs.[35] Building code regulations specify that each person be given 5 square feet to be used for dressing. However, a well planned facility allows up to 20 square feet for dressing per person. Lavatories, toilets, and showers are required fixtures by code. Extras, such as indirect lighting, full-length mirrors, soundproofing, clocks, phones, graphics, plants, background music, and a diaper changing station, all add to facility design and patron comfort.[35–37] Hair dryer plug, counters, benches, and lockers are considered minimum amenities.

Privacy is maintained by planning and constructing changing areas with adjacent single-shower and dressing compartments, with either nylon curtains or doors, removing the "group" shower approach. Both private and group areas may be planned for the aquatic center.

Rust resulting from the use of ferrous metals must be avoided for floor brackets, door frames, ceiling and ventilation fixtures and units, and all other dressing room components.

Strategically placed towel hooks, coat hangers, extra deep or tall lockers, nonabrasive floor mats, disinfectant foot baths (check with local health and safety requirements, because many states have outlawed foot baths), paper towel and toilet paper dispensers, shampoo and soap dispensers, waste receptacles, low-flow shower heads, wall-mounted hand and hair dryers, disposable plastic bag holders, automated flush toilets with revolving sanitary seat protectors, automated infrared hand-washing faucets, diaper changing stations, and emergency pull cords or buttons, all enhance functionality for patrons and make maintenance easier for staff. A water extraction unit, used to squeeze out excess moisture in bathing suits, is desirable in both male and female dressing rooms. Odor control is satisfactory when cleanliness and ventilation are maintained in the facility's dressing areas.[38,39]

Family dressing rooms are included in the plan. The rooms are for use by couples, people requiring the assistance of a pool attendant, or those with specific privacy concerns. The family dressing rooms also double as a treatment room for those who must have immediate evaluation from the aquatic physical therapist. Amenities in the family dressing room include a toilet, sink, lavatory, counter space, padded folding plinth, diaper changing station, emergency pull cords, bench, and chair. All dressing rooms must meet Americans With Disabilities Act requirements. Showers in the room are wheelchair accessible. Direct access to the pool area is provided through the family dressing rooms.

Flooring options for the dressing areas are textured tile, raised-grid interlocking tiles (treated with fungicide), injection-molded polyvinyl chloride flexible interlocking tiles, vinyl tread matting, textured coatings, high-density nylon carpet, and roll-out carpet runners for wet areas. Extra ventilation in dressing rooms allows for periods of drying-out between heavy use, and after daily routine maintenance.

The *first aid room and lifeguard office* is adjacent to the pool area. The area is a combination work station and equipment and supply area.

Desk and tabletop space for staff to document treatment or swim sessions is provided. A padded plinth folds up on the wall. A complete first aid kit with supplies should be within easy reach of staff. In addition, a blood-borne pathogen protection kit, extrication collars, hand-powered suction unit, head immobilizer, rescue spine board, and resuscitation kit are all stored in this space. Required lifeguard equipment includes a ring buoy, rescue rope and tubes, and shepherd's crook, placed in appropriate locations around the pool.[40] The rescue tubes, located directly on the deck or lifeguard stands, are easily within reach of staff and lifeguards.[41]

The pool's *mechanical and chemical room(s)* contains the circulating water pump, filters, chemical controllers, vacuum system, disinfectant system, water heater, dehumidification system, and chemicals. The heater and dehumidification unit may be in the pool mechanical room or a separate room. The well planned mechanical room eases the maintenance burden.[42–44] The room should have direct access to the outside of the building, where there is a service drive. This allows for easy access for repairs and preventive maintenance.

The chemical storage room must meet federal, state Occupational Safety and Health Administration (OSHA), state health and safety, and local building code regulations for chemical storage. Goggles, full-face shields, splash-guard aprons, Neoprene boots, respirators, disposable latex gloves, and one-way cardiopulmonary resuscitation pocket masks must be purchased and worn by staff when needed for safe use in the chemical room.[45] Material safety data sheets are to be posted in the chemical room.[44] They are obtained from chemical manufacturers, importers, and distributors for products used in the facility for maintenance. The training of all staff on the proper use of all chemicals used or stored in the facility should be recorded and kept in a safety log in the facility manager's office.

Security of filter and chemical rooms must be a priority. Mixing of chlorine and acid results in immediate toxic gas formation. When water is poured over powdered chlorine, a spontaneous explosion could occur. Alternatives to chlorine are available. Another option is ozone (O_3), a form of oxygen (O_2), which is produced when an electric spark is passed through oxygen, creating a powerful oxidizing agent used to sterilize pool water. Bromine and chlorine generation systems are options pool operators can investigate.[46]

Warm pool or spa water necessitates sustaining the proper chemical balance.[47,48] Low residual chlorine levels, "breakpoints," foaming, and mineral staining must be monitored and recorded in daily logs by a certified pool operator during pool operations.[49,50]

Another important consideration in planning is the placement of dehumidification and ventilation systems for the building. If a dehumidification system is selected for use, the equipment should not be located on the roof of the building unless there is no practical alternative; 60% of one manufacturer's units are exterior to the building (ie, roof or ground mounted).[51] Exposure to the elements can deteriorate equipment quickly, and maintenance will be difficult. Humidity can cause wood to rot, decay the building, and escalate energy bills. Any ventilation system should be well designed to prevent dampness, rust, mold, and mildew.

New designs in equipment to prevent humidity are available nationwide. Because heating, ventilation, and air conditioning may account for 25% of the new facility's cost, preplanning and research in the specific needs of each site are important.[52,53] Dehumidification systems control humidity in an indoor building. Ultimate comfort for patrons in an indoor pool results when the relative humidity is between 50% and 60% and the air temperature is 82°F. However, in a therapy setting, an air temperature of 82°F and a water temperature of 88°F to 90°F create a chill for patrons leaving the warm-water pool. An air temperature of 85°F is recommended.[54] The mechanical engineer must work with the design team to overcome problems in ventilation and dehumidification. Up-front equipment costs may be less than those of future repairs for indoor pool structures.

The mechanical and chemical room may also include the pumping and circulation systems. By tracking the condition of the pool and its mechanical systems throughout the maintenance process, small problems can be tackled before they become big ones, and further problems can be prevented. A condensed, detailed rendition of the original construction plans should be mounted in the pool's equipment room, providing step-by-step instructions for equipment operation. Manufacturers should provide cutaway illustrations of equipment. Automatic chlorinators, filtration systems, heaters, and pumps must be cleaned frequently, including the exhaust fans and blowers. Frequent maintenance and visual inspections, temperature tests, gas pressure measurements, venting system checks, and burner inspections allow longer operational life.[55,56]

Once the facility has been constructed and signed-off by the general contractor, responsibility for maintenance and repair procedures becomes entirely the sponsor's and aquatic staff's. All scheduled maintenance inspections for water chemistry, water temperature and heat, air temperature regulation, chlorination, water depth adjustments, filter cleaning, deck cleaning, vacuuming, rust protection, and other work orders must be documented on a frequency of maintenance sheet. The follow-up procedures demonstrate that the proprietors have done everything possible to ensure safety in the aquatic environment, avoiding potential exposure to injury and subsequent lawsuit.

The *pool equipment storage room* must be constructed so that none of the hand-held and flotation equipment used for in-pool activity is stored on the floor. To increase equipment shelf life, hooks, racks, mesh storage bins, rope hoists, shelving, and rolling polyvinyl chloride pipe utility storage units are useful.[57] Equipment such as fins, buoyancy belts, Neoprene wraps, snorkels and masks, paddles, weights, Styrofoam equipment, Lycra or Neoprene gloves, water shoes, swim bars, and other support devices must be allowed to dry thoroughly before the beginning of each work day. This prevents cracking of products covered with liquid vinyl or Lycra material. Pool devices and flotation equipment can be periodically washed with a mild soap to counter the harsh effects of sanitizing chemicals. It has been suggested that a mild hair conditioner be applied to Neoprene and Lycra products to soften the material between use. Lane line racks, accessory hoses, cleaning brushes, garbage cans, lifeguard chairs, or other movable equipment can be placed in the storage room when not in use.

The janitorial supplies must be kept in a separate closet in the storage room. All hazardous materials must be labeled and meet all OSHA chemical storage regulations.[40] The closet should be large enough to store brooms, mops, buffing machines, blowers, brushes, cleaning products, hoses, and high-pressure hose nozzles.

Multiple hose bibs are installed around the pool deck, the men's, women's, and family dressing rooms, storage area, and chemical and mechanical rooms for easy maintenance.

Deck Specifications

The *pool deck* is constructed of nonskid materials. All decking, coping, or overflows should have a wet coefficient of friction greater than 0.70 with reference to bare feet, skin, and footwear. Sandpaper-type finishes are dangerously abrasive in the event of a fall, and must be avoided in a therapy setting.[36]

Several wheelchair parking spaces are found adjacent to the ramp and lift area. The deck space must be as wide as possible, preferably 15 to 20 feet, directly adjoining the pool.[20] Local health and safety codes vary from region to region; however, universally accepted aquatic emergency evacuation practices and procedures require the pool deck to be free of obstacles in the event of patron evacuation.[41,43]

Multiuse Pool and Gutter Specifications

The *multiuse pool* is 75 feet long, and 45 feet wide, with an average temperature range of 82°F to 85°F. A double-wide ramp allows wheelchair entrance with a drop ratio of 1 to 24 inches (1 : 24; 1-foot grade for every 24 feet in length). The therapist can use the ramp to kneel, lay, or cradle the patron for treatments.

Bump stairs rise 4 inches and have a 22-inch platform. The stairs are constructed next to the ramp. Patrons can sit, lie, stretch, and enter the pool on the stairs. The stairs can also be used for emergency evacuation from the pool by loading the spine board up or down as necessary. Grab-bar hand rails must be placed along both sides of the stairs for patron safety.

Attached beside the stairs is a long *seated bench*, with small grab-bars located on the seat. The seat depth is 22 inches, with varying heights of 16, 22, and 30 inches. Hydrojets located at varying heights for cervical, lumbar, shoulder, and knee massage are constructed within the bench back and seats. The hydrojet pressures are adjustable.

Patrons use a grab-bar hand rail along limited areas of the pool wall. The rails are placed 4 inches away from the wall, and are 1.5 inches in circumference. If the grab-bars are too close to the wall, hands and arms may become lodged in between them.

There are two types of *gutter systems* suggested for the wellness center pools. The gutter system for the multiuse pool is unique. The pool edge consists of a wall 24 inches wide and 18 inches high. Water constantly flows over the wall and into the gutters that are located in the deck outside the wall. This system allows wheelchairs to park alongside the wall for patrons to transfer directly from the chair to the wall. The overflowing water skims the surface of floating debris, and ensures a completely flat, calm surface. Round swivel seats, 24 inches in diameter, placed at intervals around the pool on top of the wall, make it more convenient for wheelchair users to enter the water. This gutter system is popular in Europe, New Zealand, and Australia, but is not widely used in the United States.

A *lift* is located near the ramp. The lift requires staff supervision for patrons' personal safety. There are several types of lifts: hydraulic, electric, mechanical, and pneumatic. The type of lift selected must meet the patrons' comfort needs and maximize staff safety. Many are fitted with both a stretcher and chair, and several models have interchangeable parts.[58] After the patron is transferred into the pool, the wheelchair must be removed immediately from the lift area so as not to obstruct movement around the pool deck.

A *graded pool bottom*, gradually sloping down to the desired variable depth, is recommended. The "ideal" wellness center pool has depths from 3 feet 6 inches to 7 feet. Water depths ranging from 2 feet to 4.5 feet are ideal for most types of therapy and recreation programs. However, deep water of 6.5 to 7 feet is also advantageous.[2,59,60]

Warming Pool and Gutter Specifications

A *small warming pool* measuring 20 by 20 feet is used for specialized water treatments, such as Bad Ragaz ring method or WATSU.[58] The *gutter system* for the warming pool is constructed with an overflow lip and allows excess water to drain back for heating and recirculating. Care in construction of the gutter system must be taken to reduce noise. Noise caused by water splashing through the overflow rim is a problem for patrons with sensory disabilities. Minimizing the auditory feedback by using good acoustic materials on the ceilings and walls helps cut pool area noise.[61,62]

Bump stairs allow patrons to walk into the pool, whereas a lift is used to move the patrons onto the deck from the water when necessary.

The water temperature is 92°F to 94°F in the warmer pool. Water is 3.5 to 4.5 feet deep. A bench with hydrojets is placed along the bump stair entrance. The hydrojets are placed in a variety of heights along the bench seat, and are designed to provide varying degrees of pressure to the cervical, thoracic, and lumbar spine or upper and lower extremities.

In lieu of a large, warmer pool, a tank-type pool may be substituted in the facility. There are several models with such features as bidirectional, multispeed in-floor treadmills; retractable floor (eliminating the need for a lift); multidirectional, variable-speed jets; variable water temperatures; computerized documentation for client sessions; fasteners for tethered swimming; and more.

Additional Features of the "Ideal" Aquatic Wellness Center Pool

Eye hooks (lane line rope anchors) placed at different vertical heights along the shallow wall in both pools are used so rubber tubing or a swim leash can be tied at desired heights for strength training. The hooks can be placed along both shallow and deep water walls.

A *swim flume* may be placed at either the shallow or deep end of the multiuse pool, providing an adjustable, broad, smooth water current of quantifiable resistance. The countercurrent is created for swimming and water walking or running.[63]

An *automatic retractable security pool cover* seals the pools, reducing heat and humidity during nonuse hours. *Underwater viewing windows* on the side wall of both pools are used to see the exact exercise techniques the patrons perform or to analyze the patrons' swim strokes. Underwater performance may also be viewed by a periscope and video camera. A proprietary system called Coach Scope is available at a lower cost than underwater windows, but is not a substitute for underwater windows because of its limited viewing capabilities.

Submerged plinths allow for fixation of patrons who are severely paralyzed or in pain. The plinth can be hooked over the hand rail lying at an angle below the surface of the water. Plinths range from half-body to full-body sizes, and are portable so they can be lifted out of the pool.[64]

A large *towel warmer* can be placed on the

pool deck near the dressing room entrance for patrons to retrieve their towels after the treatment sessions. A *detachable massage hose* placed on the hydrojet lip is used by the therapist to concentrate specific soft tissue massage to either upper or lower extremities, allowing the patron to lie, sit, or stand during treatment.

A *"dry dock,"* or treatment bay, allows the instructor or therapist to stand at the same level as the patron for instruction from outside the pool. The walkway is constructed on the side of either the multiuse pool or the warming pool (not illustrated in Appendix 18-C).

Ropes with rings are attached to the ceiling. They are removable, and are lowered into the water during treatments for spinal distraction, mobilization of the upper extremities, and other strengthening exercises.

A removable *gait training rack* drops from the ceiling into the shallow area of the pool. Pulley hoists secure the gait rack close to the ceiling when not in use.

Mirrors on the wall opposite the therapy pool allow patrons to check their form without leaving the water.

Deckside *video and computer capabilities*, underwater video cameras, and heart rate telemetry monitoring systems may be additional components.[58]

Safety Considerations for the Pool

Safety markings communicate to the pool user important information regarding hazards such as breakpoints between shallow and deep water and underwater steps and ledges. The point of separation of shallow and deep water is indicated by a black line 4 inches wide, placed on the pool bottom 12 inches from the shallow bendline. This allows the patrons to see where the shallow depth drops off. A double lifeline is hooked above the black line and attached to the gutter.[20,65]

Along the underwater ledges, a strip of contrasting color from the pool finish marks the end of the pool for underwater swimmers. A large "plus" (+) sign 6 inches wide is placed on the walls approximately every 6 feet.

The bump stairs are identified with bright red or dark blue strips to contrast against the pool finish. The strip of color should be 3 inches wide, and placed on each stair edge.

"No diving" zones are coded in bright red coloring along the deck surface in a wide strip. The letters must be 10 inches in height by 3 inches in width. The words "NO DIVING" must be printed along the deck surface at 15-foot intervals. Depth markings are painted on the deck in either red, yellow, blue, or green. The letters must be 10 inches tall and 3 inches wide, and allocate the specific depth in 10- to 15-foot increments around the pool.[43]

All *safety lines* must be constructed with continuous cylindric buoys on a coated stainless steel cable. An eye-hook rope anchor must be recessed into the pool wall to avoid obstruction along the pool wall.[66]

Caution signs must be placed in appropriate locations around the pool to communicate hazards to patrons. Warning signs convey specific messages to patrons. There are four of them: (1) *behavioral hazards*, such as running, unauthorized after-hour use, diving, or jumping; (2) *physical dangers*, including cloudy water, wet and slippery deck surfaces, broken fences, deep water, or other dangers; (3) *chemical dangers*, such as liquid chlorine and acid storage, and locations of cleaning chemicals; and (4) *environmental hazards*, such as electrical or power lines, communications equipment, or other elements. Federal, state, regional, and local bathing codes outline specific areas for pool operator compliance.[67]

Lighting on the pool deck must be at a minimum intensity of 100 foot-candles. Electric fixtures used must meet the National Electric Code. Many new pool complexes are using up to 200 foot-candles for lighting the pool area. Water surface reflections must be avoided, with lighting fixtures directed away from the surface. Sodium lighting may present a gloomy atmosphere. Head-injured clients find fluorescent lighting emissions irritating.[28] Metal halide bulbs give the most attractive color of light for the natatorium. Use of natural light creates an enjoyable atmosphere for patrons. Skylights or clerestory windows may be used as long as glare across the water is reduced or avoided. Lighting fixtures hanging directly over the pool water need special equipment to change the light bulbs. During the planning process, this problem should be addressed by the architect.

Underwater lighting must be placed along the side walls, and not at the end walls of the swimming lanes. The *Illuminating Engineering Society Handbook* recommends a minimum of 100 lamp lumens per square foot of pool surface for indoor pools. The underwater lights must be covered in such a way that patrons will not touch the glass and burn themselves.

At the deep end of the pool, the drain cover must not be removable by swimmers, and must be securely attached. Pool stepladders must be recessed into the pool wall, and grab-bars installed. A black, blue, or red stripe 3 inches wide should be painted on each step, and visible to those descending into the pool. The tread on a stair step must be 1 foot wide, rise 6 inches, and be constructed of a nonslip material.

If a traditional pool gutter is selected and not the specific gutter illustrated in Appendix 18-C, there should be four sets of standard stepladders for patron egress from the pool, in addition to the bump stairs.

The *acoustics* in indoor pools must be designed to reduce mechanical room noise, splash noise, multiple voices, and other distracting noises emitted in the area. The reverberative atmosphere of many indoor pools inhibits the clarity of amplified voices or music. It has been suggested that distributed systems with 8-inch coaxial speakers be placed throughout the building; this provides good frequency ranges. Speakers are sprayed with a Silicone protectant to inhibit humidity.*[68]

In the event of an emergency evacuation, an intrabuilding *public address system* is extremely important. Instructions can be given to groups simultaneously in all locations of the facility.

Selection of practical door hardware, door closures, circuit breaker location, alarm, lock and key systems, equipment and supply loading and unloading areas, and fire and emergency control systems must be considered by the planning team. In addition, security system design for prevention of break-ins, graffiti, and theft is essential. Towel theft can be reduced by installation of a towel sensor system.

Training manuals for facility personnel need to address not only pool maintenance and operations, but also procedures for dealing with unruly patrons, dressing room safety, and theft.

---

* It has been suggested by consultants and therapists alike that the pump room be made as soundproof as possible. Many patrons recovering from head injuries find the noise directly associated with the pumping equipment irritating, and it can make their treatment sessions difficult.

Cost Recovery Estimates and Potential Revenue for an Aquatic Center

An estimated income statement helps determine cash flows and net profit.[10] Humidity control is a high priority for indoor pools, and is very costly. In addition, selection of gas, solar energy, or cogeneration of electricity to heat the pool's water must be considered. Efficient operations can pull the plug on high energy consumption, resulting in lower operational costs for the facility and making a crucial difference in the facility's budget. In profit determination, a facility's programming has several components that must be considered.

Budget planning is based on daily, weekly, or monthly program fees. By dividing all components into significant cash flow surplus or cash-negative programs, the project planner, aquatic consultant, or budget development committee can evaluate financing expectations. Personnel are the single highest-expense item. Utilities are second, and general and liability insurance third. The project's aquatic consultant can prepare a detailed finance sheet to outline costs versus expenses.

Basic budgeting for startup and move-in costs for the facility are divided into six categories:

1. Operations cost estimates, including insurance, utilities, water, electricity gas, and telecommunications
2. Maintenance, including custodial supplies, paper products supplies, repair supplies, repairs and maintenance services, and landscaping
3. Full-time professional personnel such as pool manager, maintenance chief, director of physical therapy and rehabilitation, and professional support staff
4. Part-time personnel such as lifeguards, water safety instructors, building attendants and custodians, cashiers, and babysitters
5. Commodities, including office supplies, printing, postage, pool supplies, pool chemicals, program supplies, recreation supplies, staff uniforms, and awards
6. A professional and special services division involving advertising, publications, special activities, lifeguard safety audits, medical memberships, travel, meetings, training, education development, and other fees.[7]

Miscellaneous overhead includes payroll taxes (unemployment and Social Security), property taxes, capital acquisition, and debt retirement. During the first operation year, exact figures are calculated to plan for future budgets. An inflation factor of 5% is suggested in budget planning.[7] All aquatic program offerings are inclusive in budget planning.

The initial programming and services offered at the aquatic facility include therapy, recreation, and instructional and fitness programs. Funding and income sources are admission fees, lessons, rental of facility, concession sales, fund raising, donations, public funds from lottery, and taxes or local recreation tax revenues. Corporate support in the categories of sponsorships, special events, discount coupons, promotions, and contracts helps add to revenue generation for the facility.[32]

Treatments for aquatic physical therapy, according to the California Workers' Compensation Medical Fee Schedule, may be outlined as follows: (1) aquatic physical therapy for an initial 30-minute treatment; (2) aquatic physical therapy and prescribed aquatic activity for a 45-minute treatment; (3) aquatic physical therapy and prescribed aquatic activity for 60 minutes. (4) aquatic physical therapy and swim modification for 60 minutes; and (5) individual independent water exercise. Each activity is billed at a different rate. Excused broken appointments, broken appointments, or special written reports are other miscellaneous budget figures included in cost planning in the cost recovery budget.[32]

Recreation activity costs vary. The Bay Area Pool Operators Association, located in the greater San Francisco Bay Area, consists of over 100 municipal, county, and private facilities.[69] A survey done in 1990 reports the cost of a daily swim at between $0.75 and $2.50. Punch tickets, group discounts, senior discounts, family passes, and age-determined individual passes were used in the survey analysis. Lap swim, water exercise, swim lessons, private swim lessons, and all other activities have additional varying fees.

Provisions for a "sinking fund" must be planned for the aquatic wellness center. The fund is a special allocation designed for replacement of building components over the life of the building. Capital expenditures for broken equipment, major maintenance projects, and upgrades are all considered in the special allocation provisions (Dunlap E, personal communication, Timpany Center, San Jose, California, 1994).

Aquatic Therapy Facilities in Current Operation

Interviews conducted with currently operating aquatic therapy facilities revealed budget planning and design to be most important during the development of a pool center. To give proper perspective regarding diversification in facility design, two locations were selected to illustrate design variations.

New Haven Hotel, New Haven, Connecticut (Figs. 18-1 through 18-4)

This facility provides complete medical services. Within the facility are two stainless steel pools. The large lap pool is 75 × 32 feet, heated to 86°F to 88°F. The depth of the lap pool is 4 feet. The warm-water therapy pool is 20 × 20 feet and has a 4- to 7-foot depth. Both pools are located on the second floor of the building and were constructed as suspended pools.

The men's and women's dressing rooms have 3 showers, 40 lockers, and 2 toilets, in addition to a water extraction machine for bathing suits. There is an emergency cord in each bathroom and shower. The mirrors and sinks provide modest amenities, with hair dryers attached to the wall outlets to reduce electrical hazards.

The pool gutters and deck are constructed in mauve and gray mosaic tile. Pool area walls have tile up to the ceiling. Ceilings are of different heights, creating an optical illusion, with halogen lights tucked around the ceiling perimeter. Huge plants adorn the decks in the pool area.

A hydraulic lift is available for patron use. The facility is well equipped with 6 × 10-foot storage closets. Rolling basket bins are placed intermittently along the pool deck, allowing equipment to dry after daily use. Deck width is 15 feet on one side and 10 feet wide around the remaining pool perimeter. A wheelchair ramp is available, leading into both lap and warm pools, in addition to stairs. Two railings are used as grab-bars on each side of the stairs.

The lap pool contains stainless steel equipment, consisting of treadmill, Nordic track, and stair master. Rescue equipment on the pool deck includes collars, back board, and complete first aid kit.

All staff are certified in basic water rescue, first aid, and cardiopulmonary resuscitation. There

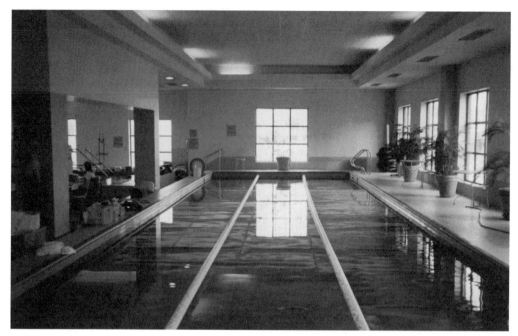

FIGURE 18-1. New Haven Hotel—Rehabilitation Unit therapy pool, New Haven, Connecticut. (Courtesy of Alvin D. Greenberg, MD.)

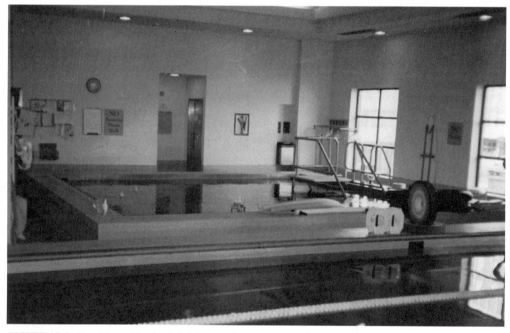

FIGURE 18-2. New Haven Hotel—Rehabilitation Unit therapy pool, New Haven, Connecticut. (Courtesy of Alvin D. Greenberg, MD.)

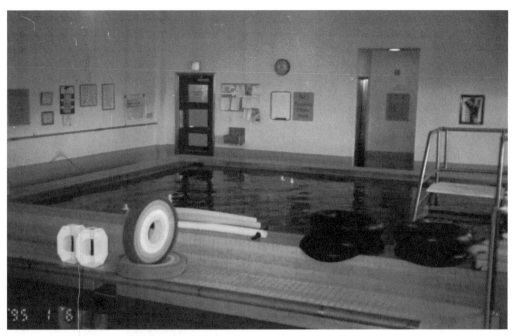

FIGURE 18-3. New Haven Hotel—Rehabilitation Unit therapy pool, New Haven, Connecticut. (Courtesy of Alvin D. Greenberg, MD.)

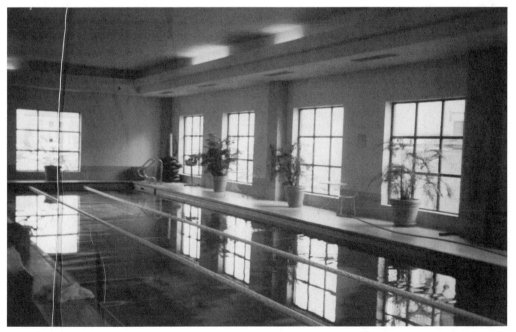

FIGURE 18-4. New Haven Hotel—Rehabilitation Unit therapy pool, New Haven, Connecticut. (Courtesy of Alvin D. Greenberg, MD.)

are six to eight aquatic staff, including an aquatic physical therapist, available to treat patrons. The staff usually sees 50 to 60 individuals daily. The facility offers underwater massage by a certified massage therapist. Additional programs include senior aerobics, target heart rate program for cardiac patrons, and arthritis foundation classes.

The Michael Hanley, D.C. Therapy Pool and Spa, Redding, California (Figs. 18-5 and 18-6)

The newly constructed building contains a lobby, office, and six treatment rooms, in addition to a small pool. In the interior of the building the pool uses forced-air heating ventilation during the winter months, and open fresh-air ducts located directly to the outside for summer cooling. The small pool has direct access from the exterior parking lot.

The pool dimensions are 15 feet wide by 25

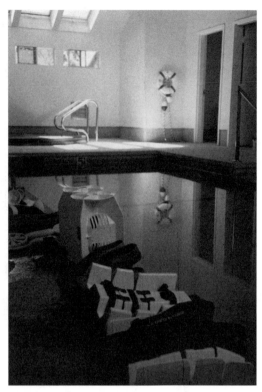

FIGURE 18-6. Michael Hanley, D.C., Therapy Pool and Spa, Redding, California. (Courtesy of Michael Hanley, D.C.)

feet long. The stairs are modified bump stairs, 24 inches wide with two railings on each side. The platform step drops 6 inches and is 18 inches deep. A rescue spine board does not fit between the hand railings. Pool depth ranges from 4 to 6 feet deep, featuring a level bottom with drop-off to the deep-water section. Railings on two pool walls provide grab-bars for patrons to grasp when in the water receiving treatment.

Deck space is 5 feet wide on three sides and 12 feet wide where the small hot-water spa joins the pool. Two, small, 7-square-foot dressing rooms each contain a shower, chair, and small storage unit. The toilets and sinks are outside the pool area adjacent to the hallway. An emergency exit is available directly to the outside parking lot.

The pump and heating equipment are located outside the building, reducing noise in the treatment area. No equipment storage units are available, and devices are stored on the pool deck. Pool water may be removed to a storage tank outside the building to allow depth reductions of 3 feet 6 inches without disrupting pool skimmers.

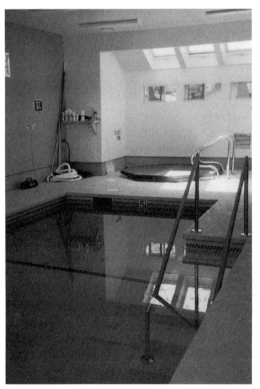

FIGURE 18-5. Michael Hanley, D.C., Therapy Pool and Spa, Redding, California. (Courtesy of Michael Hanley, D.C.)

Summary

The aquatic wellness center planning team must investigate the design and planning of the facility by considering the size, layout, programming, and use of the pool. Accurate demographic information gathered by visiting other facilities and interpretation of survey questionnaires gives the team data regarding construction costs, revenue recovery from programs, and needed budget analysis for daily operations. Without the preplanning information, the facility may be built with insufficient space, and costly planning errors may occur.

Acknowledgments
The author thanks David G. Thomas, MS, Professor Emeritus, State University of New York, Binghamton, New York, and Richard Scott, AIA, Counsilman/Hunsaker & Associates for editing a portion of the manuscript.

REFERENCES

1. Champion MR, ed. *Adult Hydrotherapy: A Practical Approach*. Hydrotherapy in Neuro Rehab. London: Heinemann Medical Books, 1990.
2. McWaters GJ. *Deep Water Exercise for Health and Fitness*. Laguna Beach, Calif: Publitec Editions; 1988.
3. Bloomquist L. *University of Rhode Island Adapted Aquatics Program Manual*. 2nd ed. Washington, DC: Department of Education; 1987.
4. Dieffenbach L. Aquatic therapy services. *Clinical Management*. 1991;11:14–19.
5. Hunsaker DJ. Pools from the ground up. *Athletic Business*. October 1990:37–43.
6. Osinski A. *Designing and Developing a Successful Aquatic Therapy Center*. Presented at the Aquatic Therapy Symposium, Charlotte, North Carolina, October 13, 1994.
7. Wiggins J. Building a budget. *Athletic Business*. August 1993:61–66.
8. Athletic Institute and American Alliance for Health, Physical Education, Recreation and Dance. *Planning Facilities for Athletics, Physical Education, and Recreation*. Reston, Va: American Alliance for Health, Physical Education, Recreation, and Dance; 1985.
9. Reister VC, Cole AJ. Start active, stay active in the water. *Journal of Physical Education, Recreation, and Dance*. January 1993:52–54.
10. Kacius JJ. Tide turns in pool design. *Athletic Business*. December 1990:71–75.
11. Visnic M. Aquatic therapy comes of age. *Aquatic Physical Therapy Report*. 1994;(4):6–8.
12. Aboulian K. Physical therapy plus. *Aquatic Physical Therapy Report*. 1994;1(4):11.
13. Hauss DS. How to buy aquatic therapy programs. *Rehabilitation Today*. January 1994:22–24.
14. Cirullo J. Aquatic therapy's rising tide. *Rehabilitation Management*. August/September 1992:74.
15. Becker BE, Cole AJ. Swimming onward: the future of aquatic rehabilitation. *Journal of Back and Musculoskeletal Rehabilitation*. 1994;4:309–314.
16. Long L. Obesity, weight control and swimming. *Aquatic Physical Therapy Report*. 1993;1(1):10–11.
17. Osinski A. Modifying public swimming pools to comply with provisions of the Americans With Disabilities Act. *PALAESTRA*. 1993;9(4):13–18.
18. American College of Sports Medicine. *Health and Fitness Facility Standards and Guidelines*. Champaign, Ill: Human Kinetics; 1992.
19. *Americans With Disabilities Acts Accessibility Guidelines*. Washington, DC: U.S. Senate Subcommittee on Disability Policy.
20. Gabrielsen AM, ed. *Swimming Pools: A Guide to Their Planning, Design, and Operation*. 4th ed. Indianapolis, Ind: Council for National Cooperation in Aquatics; 1987.
21. Gabrielson M, Mittelstaedt A. Advance planning: step-by-step supervision facilitates pool construction. *Aquatics*. July/August 1990:16–22.
22. Goldman D: State-of-the-art pools: design follows function. *Aquatics International*. March/April 1994: 10–16.
23. Berg R. The leisure pool challenge. *Athletic Business*. October 1993:37–42.
24. Fuerst CF. Rebirth of the pool. *Athletic Business*. October 1992:30–38.
25. Hunsaker DJ. European approach: aquatic leisure centers can be all things to all people. *Aquatics*. March/April 1991:10–14.
26. Spannuth JR. Promoting water walking step by step. *Aquatics*. November/December 1990:27.
27. Osinski A. Staying in step: water walking sets a new pace. *Aquatics*. November/December 1990:26–31.
28. American Red Cross. *Adapted Aquatics*. Washington, DC: American Red Cross; 1977.
29. Jackson E. Money matters: outside resources boost aquatic facilities budget. *Aquatics*. January/February 1991:14–22.
30. Osinski A. *Aquatic Facility Design Checklist*. Presented at the 3rd annual meeting of the Aquatic Exercise Association, San Diego, California, 1990.
31. Jackson E. Experts in the field: aquatic consultants offer assistance in all areas of design and operation. *Aquatics International*. November/December 1994: 10–15.
32. Clayton RD. Dollars and sense: proper budgeting is the key to efficient management. *Aquatics*. September/October 1989:12–16.
33. Byrne D. Problems, problems. *Athletic Business*. August 1992:38–40.
34. Jackson E. Pool of the future: today's needs dictate tomorrow's facilities. *Aquatics International*. January/February 1993:10–15.
35. Jackson E. Total automation: computers enhance managers' effectiveness. *Aquatics International*. January/February 1994:18–22.
36. Osinski A. Behind closed doors: locker rooms should uphold facility's image. *Aquatics*. May/June 1990: 20–23.
37. Baggett R. Dressing in style: San Francisco YMCA revenates locker rooms. *Aquatics International*. January/February 1993:27–32.
38. Jackson E. Country club living: member locker rooms satisfy upscale image. *Aquatics International*. March/April 1994:23–26.
39. Goethel P. The operative word is clean. *Fitness Management*. January 1992:32–35.
40. Moschetti M. Aquatics: risk management strategies

for the therapy pool. *Journal of Back and Musculoskeletal Rehabilitation.* 1994;4:265–272.

41. Osinski A. Risk management issues for aquatic physical therapy. *Orthopedic Physical Therapy Clinics of North America.* 1994;3:111–136.

42. Cirullo JA. Considerations for pool programming and implementation. *Orthopedic Physical Therapy Clinics of North America.* 1994;3:95–110.

43. Collopy C. *Aquatic Center Safety Manual.* San Jose, Calif: San Jose State University, Environmental Health and Safety; 1992.

44. Osinski A. Hidden problems: a step-by-step guide to pool/spa equipment room troubleshooting. *Aquatics International.* March/April 1993:23–29.

45. Jackson E. Hidden assets: well-planned mechanical rooms ease the maintenance burden. *Aquatics International.* July/August 1992:10–16.

46. Occupational Safety and Health Administration (OSHA). *Hazardous Waste Operations and Emergency Response.* Washington, DC: U.S. Government Printing Office; 1992.

47. Van Rossen D. Crystal clear: sanitizing alternatives make pool water sparkle. *Aquatics International.* January/February 1993:20–26.

48. Walsh M. Filter out your pool problems. *Parks and Recreation.* July 1993:58–64.

49. Devlin PM, Hwang JC, et al. Automated hydrotherapy pool water treatment system. *J Burn Care Rehabil.* 1989;10:74–78.

50. Zura RD, Groschel DH, Becker DG, et al. Is there a need for state health department sanitary codes for public hydrotherapy and swimming pools? *J Burn Care Rehabil.* 1990;11:146–150.

51. Osinski A. Safe and clean: amenities need special care to ensure guest satisfaction. *Aquatics International.* September/October 1992:20–28.

52. Wilson G, Kittler R, Teskoski J, Coursin K. Controlling indoor environments for comfort, structure protection. *Aquatics International.* November/December 1991:19–27.

53. Popke M. Behind enemy lines. *Athletic Business.* December 1993:71–74.

54. Chivetta C. Air power. *Athletic Business.* August 1993: 43–48.

55. Goldman JD. Planned repairs prevent lengthy pool closings. *Aquatics International.* November/December 1992:10–12.

56. DeRose R. A good start: proper opening procedures safeguard pool investment. *Aquatics.* March/April 1990:21–25.

57. Frantz JP. Keep it clean: proper maintenance protects pool filtration systems. *Aquatics.* February 1989: 25–28.

58. Davis BC, Harrison RA. *Hydrotherapy in Practice.* New York, NY: Churchill-Livingstone; 1988.

59. Wilder RP, Brennan DK. Fundamentals and techniques of aquatic running for athletic rehabilitation. *Journal of Back and Musculoskeletal Rehabilitation.* 1994;4:287–296.

60. McWaters GJ. For faster recovery: just add water. *Sports Medicine Update.* 1992;7(2):4–5.

61. Young E. Proper acoustics make a sound indoor pool. *Aquatics.* March/April 1989:10.

62. Cunningham J. Historical review of aquatics and physical therapy. *Orthopedic Physical Therapy Clinics of North America.* 1994;3:83–94.

63. Cunningham J. Applying the Bad Ragaz method to the orthopaedic client. *Orthopedic Physical Therapy Clinics of North America.* 1994;3:251–260.

64. Goldman JD. Big ideas: lap pools and artificial currents extend possibilities for exercise. *Aquatics International.* January/February 1992:8–12.

65. Goldman JD. Therapy pool settings promote positive outlook. *Aquatics International.* September/October 1991:8–13.

66. County of Santa Cruz Environmental Health Service. *Swimming Pool Plan Check Sheet.* Santa Cruz, Calif: County of Santa Cruz Environmental Health Service; 1994.

67. National Spa and Pool Institute. *Standard dimensions for public swimming pools. Athletic Business.* February 1994:272.

68. YMCA of the USA. *Aquatics for Special Populations.* Champaign, Ill: Human Kinetics; 1987.

69. Gerson V. Enhancing profits: pools can boost club revenues and creativity increases profits. *Aquatics International.* September/October 1993:26–29.

Appendix 18-A:
The Preplanning Budget

Before building a pool facility, a preplanning budget should be developed to establish costs of the project.[†]

A. Budget Development
  1. Office or rental space
     a. Computer
     b. FAX
  2. Maintenance
     a. Cleaning
     b. Supplies
  3. Insurance
     a. Liability
     b. Property damage
  4. Utilities
     a. Telephone
     b. Water
     c. Electricity
     d. Heat
  5. Support staff
     a. Wages
     b. Benefits
  6. Program development and daily operation analysis
     a. Project fiscal impact
     b. Program opportunities
     c. Probable operating costs
     d. Potential revenue sources
B. Preconstruction Expenses for Pool Site
  1. Site feasibility appraisal
  2. Civil/mechanical engineering

[†] Adapted from Wiggins,[7] Clayton,[32] Sport Management Group, and ELS Architects, Inc.

3. Zoning compliance
4. Land costs—own, lease
5. Power and communications installation
6. Environmental impact fees
7. Land development fees
8. Assessments

C. Preconstruction Costs for Development
   1. Aquatic consultant fees
   2. Architect fees—renderings, scale models
   3. Engineering fees
   4. Permit fees

D. Construction Costs*
   1. Demolition/improvements to existing work area
   2. Erosion control—earthwork, fill, slope protection
   3. Concrete paving, curbs
   4. Water, gas distribution
   5. Storm sewerage
   6. Sanitary sewerage
   7. Cast-in-place concrete work
   8. Access roads
   9. Signs
   10. Inspection fees
   11. Landscape
   12. Asphalt parking areas
   13. Communication, electrical lines
   14. Building Construction costs per foot

E. Miscellaneous
   1. Construction bond
   2. Interest on construction loan
   3. Support staff before, during, and after construction
   4. Inflation projections of 5%
   5. Attorney/accountant fees

Appendix 18-B: Project Construction Checklist

This check sheet is a partial list based on the California State Building Code Title 22 Regulations.[†]

Additional information taken from Means Repair and Remodeling Cost Date—Commercial/Residential—Construction Specification Institute Master Format, National Construction Estimator, Uniform Building Code (see Resources). It requires any person constructing, reconstructing, or altering a swimming pool, auxiliary struc-

---

* Regional costs vary by the square foot anywhere from $75 or less to $155 or more.
† Check local county construction requirements prior to building.

ture, or equipment, to submit legible plans and specifications to the enforcing agent for review and written approval before commencing work or issuance of necessary building permits [Section 65595]. The following must be submitted:

- Drawings to scale of the pool
- Drawings to scale of the equipment room
- Drawing to scale of all plumbing, electrical, and deck areas
- Drawings to scale of all drainage, fencing, gates, hose bibs, and drinking fountain locations
- Drawings to scale of restrooms, showers, and locker areas
- Drawings to scale of all pumps, filters, skimmers, chlorinators, heaters, flow meters, separation tanks, lights
- Drawings to scale of hand rails

All must be signed and dated by pool contractor and designer.

1. Acoustics
2. Accessory pool features
3. Compliance with Americans With Disabilities Act barrier removal and accessibility
   Entrances
   Corridors and aisles
   Stairways
   Clear floor Space for wheelchairs
   Protruding objects
   Telephones
   Countertops
   Electrical systems/lights
   Drinking fountains
   Restrooms
   Showers and lockers
4. Bathing codes
5. Building envelope insulation and heating requirements
6. Chemical balance and control systems, heating, disinfectant systems
   Type of unit
   Make and model
   Skimmer/gutters
   Flow meter—number of flow meters, make and model
   Range of pressure gauge—influent, effluent
7. Deck area
8. Facility overall design
9. First aid standards
10. Hazardous materials regulations
11. Illumination
12. In-pool equipment
13. Locker rooms

14. Plumbing systems and equipment
Pump—make, model, horsepower, number of pumps, turnover rate, hair and lint catcher, GPM system head loss
Filter—type, make, model, area in square feet, number of filters
Hydrostatic relief valve and assembly
15. Pool dimensions, construction, signage, markings:
Length
Width
Diameter
Surface area
Minimum depth
Maximum depth
Average depth
Volume in gallons
Odd configurations? (see plans)
Color
Return inlets—number, size, adjustable
Outlet bottom drain—safety cover, diameter, size of piping
Suction line size
Builder must furnish the following information or install listed items as indicated:
Depth markers—maximum/minimum depth, each end, break in slope, perimeter at 25-foot increments, vertical wall of pool at water line, vertical wall of pool and on deck surface, markers are _____ inches in height

Break markings:
Pool has break in slope at _____ feet
Flush-mounted devices for fastening safety rope and buoys across pool are installed _____ yes/_____ no
Break-in depth slip-resistant 4-inch tiles _____ yes/_____ no
Pool steps, stairs, ladders, fails:
Pool is at shallow end
Riser height of stairs _____
Number of safety rails _____
Height of rail above deck _____ inches
Number of ladders _____
Clearance between ladder and pool _____ inches
16. Pool/deck alarm systems
17. Pool finish
18. Pool office
19. Relative humidity and condensation control
20. Rescue/safety equipment
21. Site topography and microclimate analysis
22. Ventilation unit

Appendix 18-C: "Ideal" Aquatic Wellness Center

Drawings by David G. Thomas, M.S. Professor Emeritus, State University of New York, Binghamton, New York.

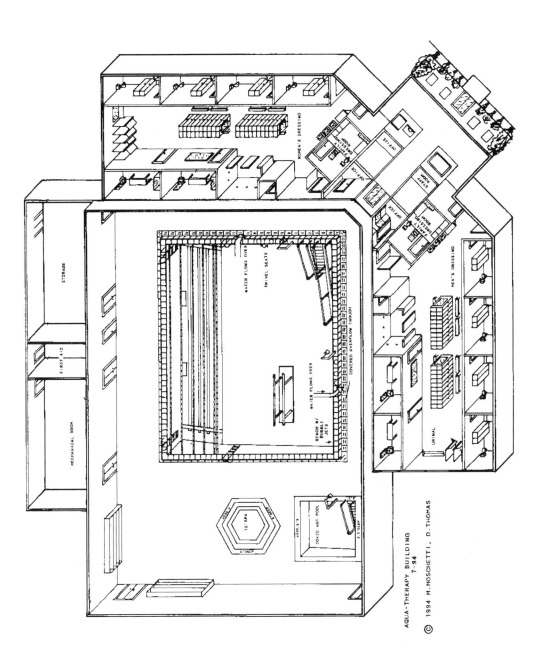

AQUA-THERAPY BUILDING
7-94

© 1994 M.MOSCHETTI, D.THOMAS

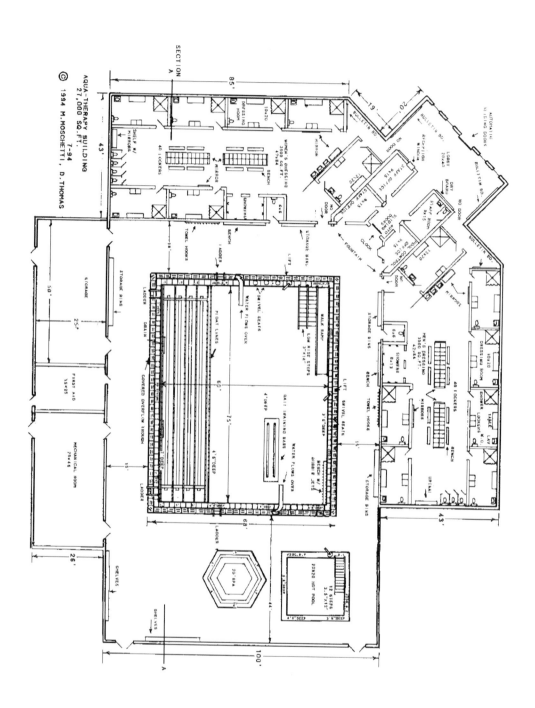

CHAPTER

19 Risk Management

Annie Clement

When health care professionals use a swimming pool, spa, or other specific areas containing water for rehabilitation, they assume all of the risks and responsibilities of both aquatic specialists and rehabilitation health care professionals. Health care professionals include but are not limited to physical, occupational, and recreational therapists, physicians, nurses, athletic trainers, exercise physiologists, and various aquatic specialists. Aquatic environments are risk environments. Where risk exists, injuries may occur—and when severe injury or death occurs, litigation often follows.

This chapter provides the aquatic rehabilitation professional with an understanding of the legal theories directly related to serving and managing aquatic programs; assists in establishing appropriate standards of care; and recommends a means for managing risks.

Of the 18,000 public accidental deaths reported in the United States in 1992, 3300 or 18% were drownings. Swimming injuries in public accidents in 1992 numbered 130,362. Contrast these figures with the injury rate of 5000 (27%) from falls.[1]

It is believed that approximately 66,200,000 people participated in aquatics in 1992. Among home accidents, drowning accounted for 700 deaths.[1]

Although swimming is listed as number one or two in participatory sports in the United States, well over 50% of the population cannot swim. Lanctot[2] found that 70% of the United States Marine Corps recruits at Paris Island were nonswimmers or had no knowledge of formal stroke mechanics. "Drowning is the third leading cause of accidental death to children under five years of age."[3] Head-first entry into the shallow water of swimming pools accounts for many aquatic injuries and about 10% of all spinal cord injuries.[4,5] Review of injury records suggests that the victim is usually male. With the exception of spinal cord injuries, these accidents have occurred in a setting in which there was no supervision.

In the middle 1980s, a number of swimmers were rendered quadriplegic as a result of hitting their head on the bottom of 3- or 3.5-foot swimming pools after a stretch dive from a speed swimming racing block. These accidents occurred under the supervision of coaches and were a first in physical activity litigation: serious injuries in an organized, supervised, and competitive atmosphere. Results of these accidents have inspired aquatic professionals to gain the level of knowledge of biomechanics needed to make informed decisions about movements into and in the water.

Analysis of drowning incidents reveals that few occur in supervised swimming pools. Although there are reports of litigation in aquatic rehabilitation environments, electronic case searches failed to reveal such cases. Also, evidence suggests that the physician recommending the rehabilitation program, rather than the therapist, is sued.

In traditional aquatic accidents, lifeguards, instructors, owners, and managers may be or have been named in lawsuits. Aquatic rehabilitation health care workers are usually carrying out the instructions of a physician. When accidents occur in aquatic rehabilitation situations, the physicians who ordered the therapy may be the only ones considered liable. When the aquatic rehabilitation specialist is providing direct service, he or she is liable.

Why would the aquatic rehabilitation professional be sued? If a client, under your direction, sustains a serious injury or aggravates an existing injury and the client believes that you contributed to his injury, you will be held accountable for your actions.

Risk Management: A Solution

Risk management is the identification, evaluation, and control of loss with regard to property, clients, employees, and the public. An understanding of law and applicable legal theories and an appreciation of the standard of care to be provided by the aquatic rehabilitation health care provider are skills essential to creating a successful risk management system. The following sections discuss law and legal theories most often found in the practice of aquatics and rehabilitation. The law is identified and explained; when applicable, an example is provided.

Law and Legal Theories: Practice

Knowledge of laws and legal theories found in litigation in aquatics, physical activity, and rehabilitation enables the professional to recognize the need for risk management and to communicate with members of the insurance and legal communities. The following provides a definition of each law and legal theory and, in some instances, one or more models of its use in aquatic rehabilitation. The law and legal theories applied to the professional's standard of care describe actions in the work environment. Defenses involve the actions of the plaintiff, the person suing. Damages are the awards, usually money, that the court gives to one of the parties; they are called judgments.

Negligence

Negligence occurs when a professional does (or fails to do) an act that either a "reasonable person" or another professional would not (or would) be expected to perform. It is behavior that falls beneath the standard established by law for the protection of others against harm, or established by a professional organization as a standard or duty of care. The elements of negligence are:

1. A legal duty of care
2. Breach of the legal duty
3. Breach of the legal duty is the cause of the injury
4. Substantial damage

For liability to exist, all four elements must exist. Negligence is the type of litigation found most often in published cases in physical activity.

Legal Duty of Care

The legal duty of care is the level of care expected of a reasonable person or the standard of care established by members of a profession. When minimum standards have been placed in writing and formally accepted by members of the profession, they are considered to be the standard of care for that profession. When state statutes mandate a standard, that standard is the recognized standard of care. When organizations recommend guidelines, professionals are not required to follow the guidelines; however, it is wise for professionals to be aware of the guidelines and to be able to explain why they have rejected their use.

In many areas of physical activity, standards or guidelines do not exist. In these situations the court looks to accepted practice in the field.

Breach of the Legal Duty

Breach of the legal duty means that the courts, judge, and jury, with knowledge of the legal duty of care, examine the facts of the incident and injury, and determine whether the defendant has failed to adhere to his or her duty of care.

Breach Is Proximate Cause of Injury

When it has been determined that the defendant failed to adhere to the duty of care, the court determines the relationship between the failure and the injury. For liability to be found, the failure to meet the standard of care must be the cause of the injury.

Substantial Damage

Significant physical or psychological damage must exist.

Degrees of Negligence

The seriousness of negligence is identified in degrees, with negligence, gross negligence, and willful and wanton neglect as the categories.

Negligence is "an absence of that degree of care and vigilance which persons of extraordinary prudence and foresight are accustomed to use or . . . a failure to exercise great care" (p 211). An example of negligence is the failure of a professional to inspect the pool ladder to ensure it is secure.

Gross negligence is "failure to exercise even that care that a careless person would use" (p 212).[6] An example of gross negligence would be failure to secure the ladder when the therapist or lifeguard knew that the ladder was not secure and that it could present danger to participants.

Willful, wanton, and reckless misconduct is "an intentional act of an unreasonable character in total disregard of human safety" (p 587).[7] An example would be the failure to prevent a danger of which the professional was aware, such as allowing people to enter a pool when the water is so cloudy the bottom cannot be seen. Examples of willful, wanton, and reckless misconduct are

"1) failure, after knowledge of impending danger, to exercise ordinary care to prevent the danger;

"2) failure to discover a danger which could have easily been discovered by the exercise of ordinary care; and

"3) failure to inspect the installation of new equipment or determine that it has been properly installed or that persons qualified to install the equipment have certified that it is properly installed" (p 31).[8]

Defenses to Negligence

Defenses often used in response to a negligence claim are contributory negligence and assumption of risk. Contributory negligence means that the injured person is in some way responsible for his or her injuries; they either created or contributed to the event that caused the injury. An adult who fails to warm up properly before activity is an example. A "challenged person" who fails properly to take care of a prosthesis could be an example of contributory negligence. A client hiding important medical facts from a therapist is contributorily negligent. One who enters the pool in a manner contrary to instruction is contributorily negligent. A refusal to acquire basic aquatic survival skills might be considered contributory negligence.

Assumption of risk means that the participant consented to the risk involved in the rehabilitation program. The consent may have been express (verbal), in writing, or inferred. When the consent is in writing it can be drafted in contract terms and used under contract law. A contract is the only method for transferring a risk. In light of the fact that minors cannot be held to a contract, the rights of minors cannot be signed away. Consent may be inferred when an adult, for example, chooses to participate in a particular activity. Assumption of risk can be used only when the parties:

1. "Know the risk exists,
2. Understand the nature of the risk, and
3. Freely choose to incur the risk" (p 34)[8]

Comparative Negligence

Comparative negligence is negligence based on percentages of fault. It is a system in which the injured person's contributory negligence and assumption of risk are used to reduce the injured person's recovery—money damages—from the defendant. This reduction is in proportion to the injured person's relative fault. For example, a client who fails to follow instructions, or tries pool tricks or stunts they have not executed for years or ones their grandsons engage in, may have contributed to his injuries at the time of the accident.

An example of comparative negligence is the court arriving at a negligence ratio based on the defendant's negligence in failing to warn the participant of the danger of the reoccurrence of a shoulder injury in training for the back crawl swim stroke, and the contributory negligence of the participant in swimming a continuous 100 yards of back crawl when he or she was cautioned to execute the skill for 20 yards or less.

A client who knowingly enters the water without a fully fastened life vest is contributorily negligent, whereas a therapist who fails to notice that the vest is not fastened is also negligent. This situation could find a defendant 60% negligent and a plaintiff 40% negligent.

Where Negligence Is Found

Negligence is found most often in aquatics with:

1. Faulty equipment and facilities
2. Failure to supervise

3. Malpractice or faulty instruction
4. Failure to provide or faulty emergency care

Faulty Equipment and Facilities

Equipment and facilities account for many aquatic injuries. Early lawsuits often dealt with cloudy water and swimming pool chemical balance problems. Today, facilities and equipment suits tend to be "failure to warn" incidents—for example, failure to warn clients that they could ingest water, or failure to warn of problems in entering and leaving the pool. When treadmills, steps, and other exercise equipment are placed in the water, clients should be warned of the dangers they could encounter if they were to lose their balance and hit the equipment. Exercise equipment powered by electricity presents many problems and preventive measures require that only approved equipment be purchased. This equipment must be inspected continuously and repaired immediately.

Failure to Supervise

Failure to supervise is often listed as the leading form of negligence in aquatic accidents. The presence of lifeguards is the most important element in the aquatic environment. The lifeguards' attention to participants and their speed in determining a victim in need of assistance is within the area of supervision.

Malpractice

Malpractice or faulty instruction and practice include the improper use of modalities and exercise sequences. They include all aspects of applied physiology and biomechanics. Of particular importance in aquatics are the provisions made to ensure that the client can sustain himself or herself under water and return to an above-water position without assistance, or using the plan of assistance created to enable the person to move to the surface. Rehabilitation modalities and routine aquatic skills are the areas in which malpractice might occur.

Failure to Provide for Faulty Emergency Care

Aquatic facilities must have an emergency rescue plan. In addition to instructions and preparation, and immediate and temporary care in the water and on the deck, professionals must be prepared for a water rescue. The emergency plan must be in writing and rehearsed periodically by employees, and evidence of the rehearsals documented.

Intentional Torts

An intentional tort is a deliberate act or failure to act. The professional is liable for an intentional tort when he or she intended to do an act even though he or she may not have intended to harm someone. When the court finds an intentional tort, the defendant is automatically liable. Horseplay is an intentional tort often found in sport activities; throwing a person into a swimming pool for fun is an intentional tort.

Until recently, administrators and insurance companies found it difficult to consider the commission of an intentional tort in a learning environment or as part of a rehabilitation process. Acts of sexual harassment, misconduct, and molestation are intentional torts and are appearing in many settings. Case law demonstrates these acts to be prevalent among psychological therapists and counselors.

Damages

Courts award two types of damages in tort cases, compensatory and punitive. Examples of compensatory damages are medical expenses, lost wages, and the cost of maintaining a physically challenged person. Punitive damages are dollar awards assessed in an effort to deter defendants from continuing to engage in the unsafe behavior that caused the injury. The objective is to assess an amount that will cause the defendant to hesitate to engage in the behavior that caused the injury. The defendant's assets or wealth, not the cost of the plaintiff's injuries, determine the amount of the award. Punitive damages are awarded in negligent actions deemed willful and wanton negligent conduct, and in intentional torts.

Law and Legal Theories: Management

Aquatic administrators need to be aware not only of the legal theories relating to lifeguards and therapists but those important to managers.

Legal theories important to managers include those pertinent to employment relationships, vicarious liability, safe working environments, product liability, and contracts. Statutes significant to aquatic management at local, state, and federal levels are noted, including the Americans With Disabilities Act (ADA) and the Occupational Safety and Health Act (OSHA).

Employment Relationships

Employment relationships in aquatic rehabilitation settings tend to be regular employer–employee, independent contractor, and leased employee. The basic differences in these employment relationships have to do with contract, supervision, liability, and responsibility for state and federal taxes and withholdings from wages. The Internal Revenue Service and the courts play major roles in disputes in this area. Relevant legal theories include vicarious liability, safe working environments, and contracts. Product liability is addressed here because of the need for management to be highly sensitive to this issue in the activity setting.

Regular Employee

In a regular employment relationship, the employee answers to the employer or to someone in the employer's chain of command. Job responsibilities, work performance, and evaluation are controlled by the employer. In this relationship, the employer is responsible or vicariously liable for the torts of the employee. A regular employee is assured an equitable hiring process, a safe working environment, and an evaluation based on the job description. The employer dictates job tasks and controls the method of carrying out the tasks from hiring to termination. A regular employment relationship exists when the parties agree to the relationship, know that the employee is acting on behalf of the employer, and that the employer has agreed to pay the employee.

Vicarious Liability

Under the legal theory *respondeat superior*, an employer is responsible or *vicariously liable* for torts committed by employees in the work environment. An administrator, for example, is vicariously liable for the torts of lifeguards and therapists. Aquatic administrators are expected to verify the employee's background and credentials. Also, the employer is personally responsible for hiring an incompetent lifeguard or therapist. Managers are not responsible for employee torts that are beyond the employee's job responsibilities. They become liable when an employee is asked to commit an intentional tort or to carry out a task beyond his or her job responsibilities. Corporate insurance carriers deny coverage when an employee's intentional torts or negligence are beyond the job requirements.

Volunteers are held to the same vicarious liability as salaried employees. The expertise of the volunteer, not the wage of the employee, determines the liability or standard of care expected.

Independent Contractor

When an employer has only a contract right to the results of the job, the employment relationship is called an independent contractor relationship. The relationship is characterized as one in which the employer requests a service or product, identifies a level of quality, and agrees to pay a lump sum for the service. An employer agreeing to an independent contractor status does not control the people who carry out the contract, and is not responsible for wages, insurance, compensation, or employee benefits. Also, the employer is not liable for the torts of the employee; the employee retains that responsibility. The employer is, however, liable for general working conditions, including the safety of the work environment.

Leased Employee

Leased employees are regular employees of the leasing firm and work as members of the leasing firm's independent contractor relationship with the agency. Leasing firms hire, evaluate, and terminate their employees. Also, they pay wages, insurance, and benefits and withhold appropriate state and federal taxes. Leasing firms are independent contractors with the agencies for whom the work is done. Therefore, employees of leasing firms are independent contractors while on the job, and regular employees of the leasing company.

Health agencies were among the first to make use of leasing firms; many exercise scientists working in hospitals and corporate fitness are employees of leasing firms.

Court Analysis of Employment Relationships

On occasion, management will establish an independent contractor relationship in an effort to save the cost of record keeping and to avoid liability. When a manager chooses an independent contractor employment relationship, he or she needs to understand that a court of law or the Internal Revenue Service may deny the status if an examination of the facts fails to warrant an independent contractor status. A business whose independent contractor status is denied automatically becomes liable for the torts of the independent contractor and their employees, and is subject to unpaid federal and state employee taxes and withholdings.

If challenged by a court or the Internal Revenue Service, the employer has to prove most of the following points:

A. The independent contractor understood the written, signed agreement.
B. The independent contractor employed, evaluated, and fired the workers; the employer was not involved in these events.
C. The independent contractor was paid in a lump sum.
D. Requests for specific employee certifications and other credentials were part of the initial agreement or an addendum to the agreement.

In spite of an independent contractor agreement, an employer "may be personally liable for the following:

1. Selecting a contractor with a history of carelessness.
2. Allowing a hazardous situation to exist.
3. Failing to perform a duty that cannot be delegated by law.
4. Allowing the party to do inherently dangerous work" (pp 100–101).[9]

For further information on independent contractor and employee concerns, the reader can consult general discussions of master–servant relationships and vicarious liability.[8,10,11]

Safe Working Environment

Employers are to provide a safe physical and psychological working environment. When a safe working environment cannot be guaranteed, employees must be warned, before accepting a position, about dangers that cannot be eliminated. Employers need to be sure that the employee knows, understands, and is willing to accept the risk. When risks become evident after an employee has accepted a position, the employer is to inform the employee immediately and provide as safe an environment as possible. When the purchase of special clothing or safety equipment is required by law, the employer must provide the equipment. If special equipment or clothing is recommended, the employer should make the purchase by employees easy by finding a supplier.

Product Liability

Product liability is the responsibility of the manufacturer, wholesaler, retailer, and supplier for defective products placed on the market. A product may be defective when it fails to function according to written specifications or advertising brochures, or the manufacturer fails to warn of dangers in the use of the product. Special conditions for product repair also need to be placed in writing. The professional using the product must adhere to all written conditions from the manufacturer, and must pass on to clients all instructions provided by the company. Failure to inform or follow the instructions makes an aquatic rehabilitation professional a party in a product liability lawsuit.

Vendors in the exercise equipment business usually provide the materials mentioned, assemble the equipment, and give inservice training to staff who will be using the equipment. When bids are placed for large amounts of equipment, these services need to be mentioned in the proposal. Swimming pool vendors are under product liability and need to be held to the aforementioned standards.

Contracts

A contract is an agreement between two or more people in which one party makes a promise, a second party accepts the promise, and consideration passes between the parties. The promise may be to do or not do an action; the second party accepts the promise and usually provides the consideration. Consideration can be a promise to do something or the conveying of a sum of money. When a party fails to live up to the agreement, the party is said to have breached or broken the contract. Legal action may be taken to ensure that all parties are treated fairly. Contracts are to be drafted by legal counsel.

Agreements are often used by the health care aquatic professional. The following sections describe two instances in which contracts are used, in the leasing of a facility and as a waiver of legal liability.

Leasing of a Facility

In the leasing of a facility, one party agrees to lease the facility and a second party accepts the lease. Usually the accepting party provides the consideration or money: facility A leases or sells their space to agency B, who wishes to use the space for therapy, recreational play, and so forth. Money is exchanged.

When the contract is a lease, city and state laws may dictate parts of the agreement. The specificity of a lease is determined by the needs of the parties. Often, it is wise to consider a wide range of factors in the leasing arrangement. The agency leasing the facility needs to consider the problems associated with a drowning when their facility is being operated by an outside agency. What harm could come to their reputation and the public's feeling of safety in the facility? As a result of these concerns many aquatic facilities require that outsiders leasing their facility use resident lifeguards.

The written agreement contains the promises and the details of care and responsibility for the facility. The following are a few suggestions for use in creating the list.

1. Physical condition of the facility at the time of receipt and return
2. Keys exchange and security
3. Time in use
4. Safety (ie, types and certification of lifeguards)
5. Emergency plan for handling a serious accident

Leases are to be drafted by competent legal counsel.

Waiver of Liability

A range of statements and agreements are used in aquatics to educate and inform participants about the risks involved in using water as a vehicle for rehabilitation and exercise. These documents are excellent educational tools and should be used whenever possible. The value of informed consent documents in a court of law is to demonstrate that the parties were clearly informed about the risks, understood the risks (provided the form withstands the scrutiny of the court), agreed to encounter the risks, and signed a statement acknowledging their understanding of the risks. Statements need to be so specific that the participant has an estimate of the probability of sustaining a loss, and what the loss might be. Informed consent documents enhance an assumption of risk argument under comparative negligence.

Courts have upheld defendants in negligence when the plaintiff had signed a waiver of liability that fully conformed with the legal requirements of a contract. The release must be clear, unambiguous, explicit, and concise. In addition to the contract requirements, it should be noted that only adults can enter into a contract; parents cannot sign away the rights of their children, but parents can sign away their own rights to a cause of action for their children.

Releases used in the setting of general negligence (intentional tort and gross misconduct) may be considered by the courts to be so offensive to society that parties are not permitted to sign away their rights and to endure such treatment.

Again, all documents used as educational tools and waivers of liability are to be drafted by legal counsel and must consider relevant local and state statutes.

Local and State Statutes

Local and state laws relating to public and, in some cases, private swimming pools and spas, exist in all parts of the country. Some of these standards relate to construction and include electrical, plumbing, and sanitation codes. Enforcement of local building codes is fairly well supervised during construction periods. Sanitation codes appear to be enforced with diligence in some states and communities. Responsibility for enforcement of these codes rests with the various agencies whose enforcement personnel are expected routinely to verify adherence to the code.

Standards for supervision of pools open to the public or membership groups are found in most states and some municipalities. They include, among other items, swimmer-to-lifeguard ratios and types of certifications required by professionals.

Federal Statutes

Federal statutes are numerous; each statute, unlike those previously discussed, covers the entire United States. Examples of two federal statutes, ADA and OSHA, are outlined. Both federal statutes were enacted relatively recently and are of interest to aquatic professionals.

Americans With Disabilities Act

The Americans With Disabilities Act of 1990 has had a profound impact on all people associated with aquatics. President Bush, on July 26, 1990, signed the ADA into law with the statement, "Let the shameful walls of exclusion finally come tumbling down." Forty-three million Americans with disabilities were specifically assured equal opportunity and access to the mainstream of life.

The Americans With Disabilities Act provides the same civil rights protection to people with disabilities as those provided to people on the bases of race, color, sex, and national origin. The Civil Rights Act of 1964 and Section 504 of the Rehabilitation Act have played a significant role in the creation of the ADA.

The ADA is separated into three titles: employment, state and local government services, and places of public accommodation. Title I, employment, is the responsibility of the Equal Employment Opportunities Commission. Title II, state and local government services, and Title III, public accommodations, are the responsibility of the Department of Justice. ADA applies to all public facilities and to all private facilities that own, lease from or lease to, or operate a place of public accommodation. If the public is invited to a facility, that facility falls under Title III of ADA. Private clubs and religious entities are excluded.

Requirements of accessibility are of two types: those required for design and construction of new facilities and for major alteration of existing buildings, and those required of all existing structures. New buildings and major renovations are under the technical specifications of the American National Standards Institute and the ADA. Architects and planners must incorporate these requirements in all facilities coming on line after July 26, 1992. The Internal Revenue Code, as amended in 1990, allows a deduction of up to $15,000 per year for expenses associated with the removal of qualified architectural and transportation barriers.

The purpose of Public Law 101-366, 104 Stat. 327, July 26, 1990, effective 1992, is:

(1) to provide a clear and comprehensive national mandate for the elimination of discrimination against individuals with disabilities;

(2) to provide clear, strong, consistent, enforceable standards addressing discrimination against individuals with disabilities;

(3) to ensure that the Federal Government play a central role in enforcing the standards established in this Act on behalf of individuals with disabilities; and

(4) to invoke the sweep of congressional authority, including the power to enforce the fourteenth amendment and to regulate commerce, in order to address the major areas of discrimination faced day-to-day by people with disabilities" (Section 2 [b]).[12]

The term "disability" for the purposes of the Act means, with respect to an individual, "a physical or mental impairment that substantially limits one or more of the major life activities of such individuals" (Section 3 [2]).[12]

Title III of the Act, Public Accommodations and Services Operated by Private Entities, specifically covers swimming pools and spas. A manager studying the Act will note the phrase "readily achievable," a term that can easily be misinterpreted by an agency with limited resources; it means easily accomplishable and able to be carried out without much difficulty or expense. In determining whether an action is readily achievable, consideration is given to:

1. "The nature and cost of the action . . . .
2. Financial resources of the facility and number of persons involved . . . and
3. Overall financial resources of the entity" (Section 301 (9)).[12]

Specific prohibitions of discrimination under construction are as follows:

1. "Application of eligibility criteria that screen out or tend to screen out an individual with a disability . . . .
2. a failure to make reasonable modifications in policies, practices, or procedures, when such modifications are necessary to afford services, privileges, advantages, or accommodations to individuals with disabilities . . . .
3. a failure to take such steps as may be necessary to ensure that no individual with a disability is excluded, denied services, segre-

gated or otherwise treated differently than other individuals because of the absence of auxiliary aids and services.
4. a failure to remove architectural barriers, and communication barriers that are structural in nature, in existing facilities, and transportation barriers in existing vehicles" (Section 302 (b) [2a]).[12]

The Act is enforced by the Attorney General of the United States and may grant the following forms of relief:

Injunction
Demand that a modification be made
Assess a civil penalty in an amount of:
    $50,000 or less for first violation
    Not exceeding $100,000 for subsequent violations

A checklist for examining an existing facility for minimum compliance with ADA is provided in the risk management plan.

Occupational Safety and Health Act

On August 1, 1991, the Comprehensive Occupational Safety and Health Reform Act[13] was introduced in both the Senate and House. The Act was originated in the 1970s. All standards went into effect in 1992. By 1994, agencies under OSHA needed a safety committee, a comprehensive plan including all hazards, and arrangements for an annual meeting. The standards are to address exposure monitoring, medical surveillance, and ergonomics. Penalties for failure to adhere to the standard my be as high as $10,000 to $50,000 per day.

Two portions of the Act, the hazardous chemicals legislation and the exposure to blood-borne pathogens legislation, are of primary interest to aquatic rehabilitation professionals. The hazardous chemicals portion of the Act covers all work with swimming pool chemicals. The blood-borne pathogens portion of the Act has created misunderstandings as to its coverage in the aquatic industry. Some believe that lifeguards and people administering cardiopulmonary resuscitation are not under OSHA because the major portion of their job does not involve these hazards. Others differ! The choice of which standard an agency adopts must be made with the guidance of the respective state OSHA agency and retained counsel, because one aquatic rescue could cause an agency to be under the law.

Employers have a responsibility to provide a safe working environment for their employees. Even if OSHA does not find the agency under their statute, a court of law will want to know why the agency did not protect the employees from a blood-borne pathogen exposure. The following guidelines will assist a professional in meeting OSHA standards.

Policy: A Department of Labor Specification

1. Create a policy and procedure of exposure control for each area and put the plans in writing.
2. List the names of employees whose duties involve reasonably anticipated exposure to chemicals, blood, or other infectious materials. Identify the anticipated exposure for each employee. Also, list all jobs in which such exposure could be anticipated (eg, lifeguards and people administering cardiopulmonary resuscitation).
3. Create a plan to reduce or eliminate the exposure. This may include an opportunity for employees to obtain a free hepatitis B vaccination within 10 days of taking the job.
4. If exposure cannot be avoided, devise a plan of barrier precaution when exposure is anticipated. Protective equipment should fit and be free to employees. Employees are expected to use equipment. Those refusing to use equipment are asked to sign a statement of their refusal.
5. In the event of an equipment failure or inability to protect, employees must be warned of the dangers and must be provided with safety measures in the event of an exposure. Hand and eye wash kits and facilities are to be readily available. When regular washrooms are used for clean-up after an exposure, they are then contaminated and cannot be used by the public.
6. All surfaces exposed to blood or chemicals are to be wiped clean immediately with an appropriate disinfectant.
7. A system is designed and used for the removal or laundering of waste and contaminated protective equipment.
8. Complete records must be kept of an exposure incident, including the circumstances surrounding the incident, controls in use, protective equipment used, and policy in action. An incident must be reported to supervisors immediately.
9. Post-exposure evaluation and follow-up:

a. Determine circumstances of exposure.
b. Employees must undergo a complete evaluation, from a physician, with results provided in writing. All findings are confidential.
c. Complete records on each incident are kept for the duration of victim's employment plus 30 years.
d. If the business has more than 10 employees, the employer must post the exposure incident (Department of Labor rule).

Labeling

1. A list of all hazardous chemicals and their locations exists.
2. Containers used to store and transport chemicals are marked according to law.
3. Material data sheets exist and are retained. State and federal laws dictate what the sheets are to contain and how long they should be retained.

Information and Training

All employees with exposure possibilities shall, annually, be provided a training program at no cost, during normal working hours. Training is to include:

1. OSHA standards
2. Explanation of hazards
3. Explanation of exposure control
4. Information on protective equipment
5. Actions to take in the event of an exposure
6. Explanation of signs
7. Opportunity for questions and answers

Records of the training, including dates, names and job titles of participants attending, and content of meetings should be kept.

Records

1. Medical records for each exposure
2. Department of Labor posting when 10 or more employees exist
3. Training records
4. Nonuse of personal equipment
5. Refusal to take vaccine, if appropriate
6. If business ceases, contact OSHA to turn over records

If an employee reports the employer to OSHA, the employer cannot punish or discriminate against the employee.

Risk Management

Risk management is the identification, evaluation, and control of loss to property, clients, employees, and the public. Components of a risk management system include:

1. Audit, the identification of all risks
2. Evaluation of risk
   a. Probability: high or low
   b. Severity: serious or minor
   c. Magnitude: many or few people involved
3. Establishment of controls that:
   a. Eliminate risk activities
   b. Provide alternative programs for risk activities
   c. Retain risk activities and cover with additional safety precautions, warnings, and insurance

Risks are usually identified through a comprehensive audit. An aquatic rehabilitation program audit includes an analysis of local, state, and federal codes; professional guidelines; facilities; equipment; personnel; supervision; leasing; therapy and instruction; participants; and the emergency action plan. This is not an all-inclusive list; the audit identifies all aspects of a specific ongoing program that have the potential for risk. Each item in the audit is evaluated and a decision is made to retain, alter, or eliminate. This system is unique to an agency and should be designed by the agency management in conjunction with the insurance company and the attorney who will represent the agency in litigation.

One cannot prevent a lawsuit; anyone can be sued. The professional can, however, build an effective defense. People engaged in risk activities need to prepare for a lawsuit, just as they prepare to work with serious injuries. A strategy for working with a lawsuit is prepared, rehearsed, and used when needed.

Safety Committee

A safety committee is recommended and becomes essential as health care aquatic professionals become more involved with OSHA and other federal statutes. The committee should include representatives from management, public relations, therapy, professional staff, and maintenance. Safety committee members play a major role in the creation of the audit, assist in analyzing the results of the audit, and help establish the methods of control. Committee members meet periodically to consider the efficiency of the entire risk management plan, make recommendations, and monitor the results of change.

Some experts recommend that an external consultant be used in the creation of the original audit and about every 5 years to assess the system.

Standard of Care

The standard of care for all aspects of the program is the minimum performance that should be expected. Anyone operating below that standard should be dismissed; facilities or equipment failing to meet the standard should be taken out of use. Many professions have placed standards in print; health care providers are among them. Physical activity specialists have been hesitant to place standards in print; they rely on the acquisition of college course content through heavily supervised professional program experiences. Aquatic professional have, however, come to a fairly common set of standards.

When printed standards are available, the courts use them in establishing a standard of care. When printed standards are not available or are too difficult for the lay person to understand, experts are used by the court to guide them in the establishment of a standard of care.

Aquatic rehabilitation specialists, in many cases, have to rely on expert opinion. Therefore, it is recommended that they arrive at a clear understanding of the minimum duty or standard they must meet at all times, and identify a considerably higher standard toward which they continuously strive.

Aquatic rehabilitation health care professionals should first look to the following for guidance in establishing a standard of care:

1. State and federal statutes
2. Certification programs provided by agencies such as the American Red Cross, YMCA, Ellis Associates, and others
3. Guidelines from professional organizations
4. Professional opinion, or the standard established by experts
5. Literature in the field

Preparing the Audit

The following are suggestions for preparing an audit for an aquatic rehabilitation program. Also, many of the statements serve as recommendations for an agency examining the program. This is not a comprehensive check sheet, but merely examples of topics that might be considered.

Local, State and Federal Codes

1. Identify local, state, and federal codes that affect aquatics and rehabilitative services provided by the agency. Facility codes include swimming pools and spas; electrical and plumbing systems; maintenance standards; and others.
2. Programs are influenced by codes relating to qualifications of categories of employees and supervision of the pool. All employees licensed by a state are under a specific code for their respective licensure. Most states have a minimum standard for swimming pool supervision; that standard tends to be at least one lifeguard on duty at all times. Note state requirements and competencies for certification and testing of employees.
4. Retain a copy of codes that directly affect the operation of the facility and the program. Bring them up to date yearly.

Americans With Disabilities Act Recommended Standards for Buildings Built Before 1992

1. One accessible entrance from the parking lot or street to the building is provided. If possible, the entrance should be the one used by the general public. Entrance door is to be 36 inches wide with maneuvering clearance for a wheelchair. Exterior door weight is not to exceed 8.5 pounds; interior, not over 5 pounds. Floor surfaces are to be stable, firm, and slip resistant. When floor surface levels change more than one-fourth inch, a ramp must be provided.
2. Parking spaces are identified for rear and side exits from vans. One of every 25 parking spaces is to be handicapped accessible.
3. At least one bathroom is wheelchair accessible. An accessible bathroom must have an entry door to the toilet 36 inches wide that swings out. The toilet is to be 17 to 19 inches high and have grab-bars, automatic flush, and an automatic paper dispenser.

4. At least one shower, tub, and sink must be handicapped accessible. The sink must be mounted 34 inches above the floor for wheelchair knee clearance.
5. All buildings with three or more floors must have an elevator.
6. All activities must be available to anyone with special needs.
7. Signs must be large, at eye level, raised, have Braille characters, and be pictorial. There should be contrast for ease of viewing. The international symbol of accessibility is used to designate all accessible areas.
8. One pay phone must be accessible.

Professional Guidelines

1. Recognize the difference between a code and a guideline. A code must be followed; one has a choice in following a guideline. Failure to follow a code can result in civil punishment; failure to follow a guideline does not result in civil punishment. However, when an agency chooses to ignore a popular guideline, a court may ask why that decision was made. Guidelines must be studied, and when decisions are made to reject or ignore them, the reasons should be placed in writing.
2. Determine all professional organization guidelines that might impact the agency. Examples are American Red Cross, YWCA, YMCA, American College of Sports Medicine, and organizations with professional members. Obtain and examine guidelines.
3. Be sure employees are aware of and follow codes. Provide a process of verifying knowledge and practice.
4. Physicians' specifications and orders are to be followed as directed. Recommendations of sports skills, including swimming and aquatic art skills used in therapy, need to be made with a clear understanding of biomechanics.

Facilities

1. Facilities are routinely inspected. Emphasis is placed on the identification of hidden hazards. Appropriate people conduct the inspections.
2. The facility inspection system is checked for accuracy and consistency.
3. Protocols for repair, follow-up, and closing of a facility in need of immediate repair are created and used.

4. Lighting and illumination meets National Electrical Code and state and local codes.
5. Water depth markings are obvious and meet or exceed code.
6. Basic pool chemistry is maintained; chemicals are stored properly.
7. Pool temperatures are often in the 70°F to 80°F range. A temperature of 82°F to 88°F is preferred for pools used for therapy. General pool maintenance courses, texts, and general health information tend to be for pools maintained at a temperature of 70°F. Chemical pool suppliers, public health officials, and aquatic planners can guide a facility in raising the temperature while maintaining appropriate bacteria counts.
8. Head-first entries into the water are controlled, and locations for entries are clearly marked.
9. Local health standards are maintained.

Equipment

1. Rescue equipment meets acceptable standards and is clean, accessible, well maintained, and ready to use.
2. Equipment used for rehabilitation, instruction, supervision and rescue is inventoried and routinely inspected. Many of these inspections are performed daily.
3. Lifeguard chairs and stations permit full pool visibility.
4. Equipment is maintained, repaired, and used according to manufacturers' specifications. Instructions and warnings provided by the manufacturer are obvious to participants.
5. Emergency power for pool, locker rooms, halls, and stair wells is available in the event of a power failure.
6. Diving board and exercise equipment are routinely inspected for wear.

Personnel

1. Employment guidelines are followed, with emphasis placed on the avoidance of discrimination in hiring.
2. Comprehensive job descriptions exist for each position.
3. Certification and qualifications essential to success on the job are established and made known to applicants. For example, a specific lifeguard system such as Ellis, American Red Cross, YMCA or others, is identified. All lifeguards have the lifeguard certification or

credential. Basic water safety or teaching credentials are not adequate unless lifeguard training has been incorporated into the preparation. These certificates must be current when a person is employed and are maintained up to date throughout the period of employment.

4. Employees are asked to sign a statement acknowledging their understanding of the need to maintain an up-to-date specific certification and that failure to do so will result in automatic termination.
5. Applicants understand expectations created when they present certain credentials. They know what the literature and training guides have defined as their responsibilities.
6. Orientations are provided for personnel.
7. Periodic testing of rescue and other qualification skills is conducted.
8. Professionals are encouraged to maintain fitness levels needed to be assured of the energy essential for water rescues and the demands of continuous work in the water. Equipment and opportunities are available to maintain these skills.
9. Policy manuals containing detailed information on emergencies and injury protocol are studied. Employees are asked to sign a statement that they have read, understand, and will comply with the policies and procedures contained in the manual.
10. Inservice emergency preparedness training, including simulation of accidents, is provided new employees; updates are provided periodically.
11. Staff are informed on insurance coverage and legal responsibilities.
12. The work environment is safe for employees (see OSHA standards).
13. Employees are encouraged to report unsafe conditions.

Supervision

1. A recognized system for supervision is used. The system in use is documented in detail.
2. The lifeguarding system ensures that at least one person is scanning the water at all times. That person is to be fully and currently certified as a lifeguard.
3. Employees know their responsibilities.
4. Horseplay is prohibited.
5. Standards are maintained at all times.

Leasing

1. External facilities used by an agency and the loaning of an agency facility to an outside group always involve written contracts.
2. The contract identifies exactly how the facility is to be opened and closed. Lifeguard arrangements, including credentials, are noted. Some facilities require that external contractors maintain agency standards.
3. The leasing facility should provide information about the nearest emergency facility and hospital, and information pertinent to accidents. Responsibility for an emergency action plan is with the leasing group.

Therapy and Instruction

1. Professional guidelines, recommendations, and appropriate techniques are followed.
2. When the professional is permitted to select content, content is selected with the needs of each individual in mind. The aquatic professional is able to justify all aspects of instruction. Goals and objectives of each task are examined to be sure that the methods of satisfaction are appropriate for all learners. For example, the necessity that a person is able to support his or her body in water over the head could be accomplished in various ways by people who are challenged. This area is wide-open for creative ideas. Knowledge of biomechanics becomes important in the selection of experiences for all learners.
3. Planning is documented. Therapy protocols, courses of study appropriate to expertise of employees and expectations of clients, and progressive learning sequences are on file.
4. Participants are aware of all safety tips given in each session.
5. Records of specific benchmark achievements exist and are available on request. Computer printouts are used when possible. Client progress and readiness for advanced work are documented and retained on file.
6. Documentation shows that clients were properly warmed up for activity.
7. Documents demonstrate that appropriate safety techniques were used in the activity.
8. Methodologies used by teachers meet the test of peer scrutiny.

9. Preassessment is used to qualify participants for certain activities.
10. If possible, use individualized assessment and teaching.

Participants

1. Professionals have reviewed client health records and physician prescriptions and are prepared to work with routine concerns.
2. Clients understand the risks involved in aquatics. Written statements may be required to ascertain this knowledge.
3. When appropriate, consent, warnings, and waivers are used. They serve to inform the public about the risks involved.
4. Agency rules are posted and participants are made aware of the rules through written information provided the client before the first session.
5. Opportunity exists for clients to report unsafe conditions.

Emergency Action Plan

All accidents requiring emergency squad or emergency room attention require a full investigation. Accidents reported after the fact that have involved emergency room attention or have been considered significant by medical authorities must receive the same attention. The following are among the items to be addressed in preparing an emergency action plan. Care needs to be taken to ensure that all unique characteristics of the agency have been included in the plan. No two plans are the same.

1. A detailed written plan must exist. In addition to the injuries anticipated in a physical skill setting, it must include fire, tornado, earthquake, and other hazards.
2. The plan is rehearsed often. Orientation is provided to all new staff before they become responsible or work their first day.
3. Immediate and temporary care is identified, with assignments of those qualified to give the care. Those responsible practice often.
4. Telephones, regular and cellular, are provided. A telephone emergency message is attached to or above each telephone. It contains the address, location of injured party in building, and the best method of entering the

building. Also, the caller should be ready to identify the victim by age, sex, vital signs, and nature of the injury.
5. Cooperation with emergency medical personnel is obtained in the creation of the emergency plan. Personnel follow predesigned plans.
6. Emergency medical staff are briefed on the incident, the extent of immediate and temporary care provided, and length of time lapsed since injury.
7. A plan for working with the media exists and is implemented.
8. The emergency action plan is known by all, and has been rehearsed periodically.
9. When the victim refuses follow-up care and appears to be making rational decisions, ask the victim to sign a statement that first aid was given and the victim was released to his or her own care or the care of a parent or legal guardian. A form to this effect is available with the accident report. Always advise the victim to see his or her physician.

Accident Report

1. Freeze the incident by making a mental "snapshot" of the entire situation, including witnesses. Record the incident. Also record, if possible, any observations before the incident. Only the immediate care of the victim is more important than recording the incident.
2. Provide immediate and temporary care, then fill out incident report.
3. Know when the agency will close down the pool or the building and when they expect to maintain the program in spite of an incident. If the pool is to be closed, designate one person to work with the media and one or more people to close down the pool; the rest of the staff becomes involved in the accident report and preliminary investigation. When the facility remains open, some members of the staff are assigned to the accident report and the investigation.
4. Obtain verbatim statements from witnesses. Record the names of all witnesses and people in the vicinity of the incident.
5. Obtain statement from victim, record the statement verbatim, and ask victim to sign or initial statement. Have a witness present to verify the statement later and assist in determining the victim's mental state at the time of the statement.

6. Be kind, but protect all parties. Do not admit anything at any time.
7. Accident reports should be readily available and prepared under direction of retained counsel.
8. Accident reports should be provided to administrators within 1 hour of accident. Telephone calls to key administrators should be made right after emergency call if staff is sufficient, or immediately after departure of emergency vehicle.

Investigation

After the victim has been transferred to a medical facility or released to his or her own care, and the accident report has been completed, an investigation of the incident is conducted. Knowledge of how the insurance company and retained attorney expect the investigation to be conducted is vital. The following are suggestions to be used in creating the plan.

1. Record time and date of incident. Mention weather and any other condition that might be significant.
2. Diagram the scene.
3. Obtain pool maintenance logs for the day.
4. Identify personnel directly and indirectly involved in the incident. Note the dates and contents of each of their certificates, inservice training, and safety rehearsals.
5. Debrief all personnel, employed and volunteers, before they leave the building on the day of the incident. All interviews are individual and in the presence of a witness. If possible, the witness should not have been in the vicinity of the incident or hold administrative authority. Taped interviews are used only when people interviewed has granted permission.
6. Have all witnesses sign statements.
7. Notify insurance company, attorney, and all people in the liability chain. Some accidents and health problems are required by law to be reported to authorities.

Evaluation

When the audit is complete, each item is evaluated for potential risk. The factors of probability, severity, and magnitude affect the way the potential risk is evaluated. Is the probability of the risk high or low? What is the national incident ratio on the risk? Has the risk become reality in the agency? If so, how often? If an incident occurs around the risk, will the injury be serious or minor? If death is anticipated, the item needs to be addressed differently from an injury that allows the victim to return to activity the following day. Should an incident occur, how many people will be affected?

Control

Once the risk has been evaluated, decisions are made to control the risk. The risk can be eliminated, a change can be made in the activity, or the risk can be retained and covered by insurance. Often, safety precautions and warnings can be helpful in controlling risks.

Summary

Rehabilitative health care aquatic professionals must be competent in their specialty, understand the needs of the aquatic environment, and be able to document that competence. Knowledge of laws and legal theories that affect their responsibilities are used to create an effective risk management program, a program they use continuously and systematically. When a serious accident occurs, the professional is ready to meet the incident with the highest level of professional competence.

REFERENCES

1. National Safety Council. *Accident Facts*. Itasca, Ill: National Safety Council; 1993.
2. Lanctot B. Americans fail in swimming ability. *Aquatic International*. March/April 1992; 4(2): 4.
3. Elder J. *Human Factor Analysis, Child Drowning Study*. Bethesda, Md: United States Consumer Product Safety Commission; 1987: 1.
4. Samples P. Spinal cord injuries: the high cost of careless diving. *The Physician and Sports Medicine*. July 1989; 17(7): 143.
5. Present P. *Diving Study: Report on Injuries Treated in Hospital Emergency Rooms as Result of Diving Into Swimming Pools*. Washington, DC: United States Consumer Product Safety Commission; 1989.
6. Keeton WP, Dobbs DD, Keeton RE, Owen D. *Prosser and Keeton on Torts*. 5th ed. St. Paul, Minn: West Publishing Company; 1984.
7. Restatement of the Law (Second) of Torts. St. Paul, MN: American Law Institute, 1977.
8. Clement A. *Law in Sport and Physical Activity*. Dubuque, Iowa: Brown/Benchmark; 1988.

9. Clement A. #7, Sports Law: product liability and employment relations. In: Parkhouse B, ed. *The Management of Sport*. St. Louis, Mo: Mosby-Year Book; 1991: 97–106.

10. Restatement of the Law of Agency (Second), Section 220.

11. Urquhart JR III. *Independent Contract Agreements*. Irvine, Calif: The Fidelity Publishing Corporation of America; 1989.

12. *Americans With Disabilities Act of 1990*, Public Law 101-366, 104 Stat. 327, July 26, 1990.

13. *Occupational Safety and Health Act* 29, CFR, 1910.

CHAPTER

20

Exercise Equipment in the Aquatic Environment

Cheryl S. Fuller

Water is becoming an increasingly popular rehabilitative and conditioning environment. Health care professionals are becoming interested, educated, and skilled in the field of aquatic exercise and rehabilitation. With greater understanding of the physical properties and hydrodynamics of water, health care professionals are making the most of this unique medium.

Water's physical properties alone provide an environment for exercise in which there is little need for elaborate or expensive equipment. The property of buoyancy provides support and may serve to facilitate movement, reduce pain, and promote independence, making it possible to perform exercises that might be difficult or even impossible on land. Also, muscle strengthening and cardiovascular conditioning are possible because of the resistance offered by water. The physical properties of water, along with the positioning of the body and limbs, the length of the lever arm, the range of motion, and the speed of movement, can be used to enhance aquatic exercise. To enhance further the benefits of exercise in water, one may use equipment designed to take advantage of water's physical properties.

The growing popularity of aquatic exercise and rehabilitation has led to the emergence of a new industry for the manufacture of exercise equipment designed exclusively for the water. The history of aquatic equipment actually began with the development of devices designed to train or condition swimmers, as well as make the swimming experience more pleasurable. These early devices included swim mitts, paddles, and pull buoys for isolated strengthening of the arm stroke, along with kickboards and fins to assist in conditioning the lower extremities. It was not until the early 1980s that equipment was designed and marketed specifically for exercise and rehabilitation in the aquatic environment. As the popularity of aquatic exercise and rehabilitation grew among health care professionals, manufacturers of exercise equipment have emerged not only from the fitness industry, but from the medical industry. These manufacturers have made a natural transition, developing and marketing products ranging from personal water fitness gear to aquatic rehabilitation tools designed to increase the benefits of water exercise.

Equipment Principles and Benefits

Aquatic exercise and rehabilitation equipment is usually designed for one of several purposes: to offer needed support, increase the intensity of an exercise, add variety to a program, or make the exercise more challenging and enjoyable. The use of equipment for support and balance is not only beneficial but often essential. Movements learned in gravity may seem awkward on entering water. Therefore, activities must be presented in such a manner that adjustments to the new environment are facilitated. With the use of flotation aids, a participant's fear of water may be alleviated, creating a more comfortable and secure environment. Another benefit of this support is that the health care professional is not required to support the full weight of the person, which permits easier positioning and handling. As the participant improves and becomes more confident in the water, flotation aids used for support may be removed and other equipment may be used to increase the intensity of an exercise. Devices may be used that challenge balance, increase resistance, or target endurance. Aquatic equipment can also make exercise more enjoyable by adding variety to a routine. A wide array of equipment can keep participants interested in their exercise program as well as motivating them to work harder.

There are two basic classifications of aquatic exercise equipment. First are devices that use the effect of buoyancy to alter positioning or movement. Flotation devices (Fig. 20-1) are those items that increase the effect of buoyancy to provide support, decrease compressive forces or lessen impact, assist movement to the water's surface, and increase resistance in movement away from the water's surface. In contrast, weight equipment (Fig. 20-2) decreases the buoyant effect. This is often useful in obtaining proper body position, providing for a person's stability, furnishing a means of traction, graduating compressive forces, assisting movement away from the water's surface, and increasing

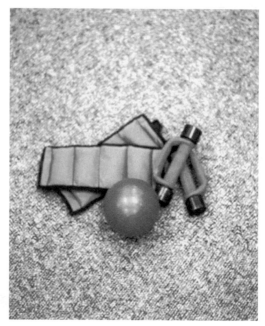

FIGURE 20-2. Weight equipment.

resistance in movement toward the water's surface.

Buoyant and weight equipment are most often used for support and to progress weight-bearing activities. However, they can also be used for isolating resistance. Using buoyant or weight equipment for resistance is particularly useful to protect a joint from a specific motion or to isolate the strengthening of a particular muscle group. Examples of this principle include protecting a sprained medial collateral ligament during standing straight leg hip abduction and adduction. With the use of an ankle weight, the leg can be abducted toward the water's surface with increased resistance. The weight then assists with adduction to protect the compromised ligament from possible stress due to the resistance of the water. Another example illustrates how to isolate strengthening of the hip adductors during rehabilitation of a client with patellofemoral syndrome. Here a buoyant ankle cuff is used. This cuff assists standing hip abduction to eliminate strengthening of the lateral musculature, yet increases the resistance for hip adduction to stimulate proper muscle balance and improved patellar tracking.

Most water exercise involves only concentric muscle contractions because of the resistance of the water encountered by any motion. This is especially true when resistance equipment

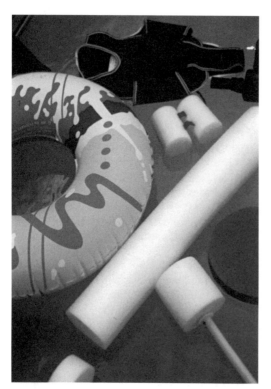

FIGURE 20-1. Flotation devices.

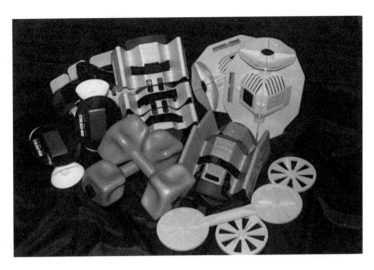

FIGURE 20-3. Aquatic products that increase resistance.

based solely on the principle of drag is used. However, with buoyant equipment, eccentric muscle contraction can occur as the limb moves toward the surface of the water and the antagonists try to control the buoyant force. Eccentric contractions may also occur with the use of weight equipment as the antagonists control motion toward the pool floor. This is important because many functional activities involve eccentric muscle contractions.

The second basic classification of aquatic exercise equipment includes products that simply increase resistance by increasing the surface area that is pulled or pushed through the water (Fig. 20-3). These devices are based on the principles of drag and movement through the water. The larger the surface area, the greater the drag forces are that increase the resistance. There are three factors that determine the amount of resistance these products encounter. The first factor is the size of the piece of equipment or the space it takes up in the water. Drag is increased as an object takes up more space in the water because it interrupts the flow of a greater number of water molecules. This type of resistive drag is called form drag.

The second factor that determines the amount of resistance a piece of equipment encounters is the shape the object presents to the water. A tapered shape produces the least amount of drag in the water because it allows the direction of water molecules to change gradually as they pass around it. An object that presents a large, flat surface to the direction of movement through the water greatly increases resistance not only as a result of form drag, but because

of frictional and wave drag. When an object's shape is such that water molecules cannot change direction gradually and continue to move around the object, it is considered unstreamlined. When water molecules come in contact with a flat surface, they rebound away in random directions, producing a wide pattern of turbulence that greatly increases the pressure in front of the object. If the rear of the object is not tapered, but also flat, it keeps the flow of water separated for a longer time after the object's passage. This creates a larger area of eddy currents, considerably reducing the pressure behind the object. This pressure differential produces significant resistive drag.

The other major factor that influences resistance or drag is the speed of movement of the piece of equipment through the water. As the speed of movement through water increases, drag force increases, and therefore the resistance increases. Some aquatic equipment is designed so that it may be moved in a streamlined pattern for decreased resistance or an unstreamlined pattern for greater resistance and strengthening. However, because the size and shape of most items is predetermined, altering the amount of resistance is primarily a function of the object's speed of movement.

Products Available

Pools

Aquatic equipment used for exercise and rehabilitation can range from a custom-designed swimming pool to a wide array of accompany-

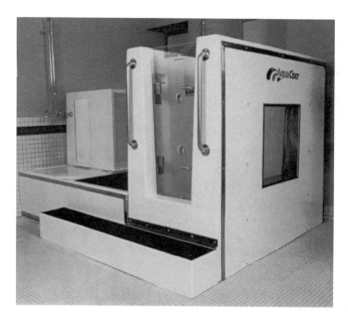

FIGURE 20-4. Custom therapy pool.

ing equipment to enhance the physical properties of water. Where there is no access to a full-size, in-ground swimming pool, a customized therapy pool is an alternative (Fig. 20-4). These pools come in various sizes as well as price ranges. An advantage to using these pools is the ability to adjust the depth and temperature of the water for the needs of each client. Some of the pools include swim jets that provide a variable current for resistance. Other options available include a flotation device and tethering system for nonweight-bearing activities, a built-in treadmill with variable speeds, a patient lift for easy access, and a glass wall for underwater visibility.

Treadmills

In addition to the treadmills that are part of a self-contained unit, there are also portable underwater treadmills that have been designed for use in existing pools. An attractive feature of an underwater treadmill is the control over variables such as speed and water depth, which are reproducible. This is not only an advantage for documenting a client's progress, but is essential for research.

Access Equipment

The passage of the Americans With Disabilities Act in 1990 led to innovations in pool access equipment. This law requires that all public places, including swimming pools, be easily accessible to the disabled. There are three basic types of pool access equipment available. The appropriate device for a facility depends on the pool structure as well as the pool participants. There are portable stairs with hand rails to provide access for those people who are able to ambulate up and down steps. Portable ramps with safety rails are another option that may provide access for those who are mobile enough to walk into the pool, as well as clients in wheelchairs. The third type of access equipment is the pool lift. Pool lifts, which are available in manual or automatic models, can facilitate both independent and assisted transfers into the pool. They provide optimum pool accessibility as well as a measure of safety for participants and staff.

Regardless of the type of pool access equipment chosen, it should be functional and safe. The equipment should be rustproof and slip resistant. There should be safety hand rails for support, and the weight restriction should always be observed.

Another device that may be used for Americans With Disabilities Act compliance is a movable pool floor system that can provide deck-level access to the pool. This system is designed to enhance a pool facility's flexibility. It provides the ability to adjust the pool depth at any time, and even create a variable-depth pool. Movable floor systems can be installed in new or existing pools. Motors hydraulically raise and lower the pool floor or some portion of it, changing the pool depth at an average of 1 foot per minute. For security, the movable pool floor can also serve as a cover for the pool at deck level when the pool is not in use.

Flotation Equipment

There are many flotation devices that are designed to keep a person buoyant while working out in deep water or lessen impact while working out in shallow water. The Wet Vest and Wet Belt (Fig. 20-5) are just two examples of devices designed to suspend the user in a vertical position, submerged to neck level. Buoyant vests and belts come in various sizes and designs as well as price ranges.

Buoyant barbells, called swim bars or trainers (Fig. 20-6), may be used for balance and support while gait training in shallow water, as well as flotation tools in the deep water. They consist of a light-weight bar with rubber or Styrofoam discs attached on each end. They use the principle of buoyancy to provide support and may also provide resistance when moved against the force of buoyancy.

A set of Hydro-Fit equipment (Fig. 20-7) also capitalizes on the principle of buoyancy. The set includes a buoyant belt, buoyant ankle cuffs, and buoyant barbells that are used for flotation and resistance for the upper and lower extremities. In addition, the ankle cuffs, when attached to one another, may be used as a flotation belt.

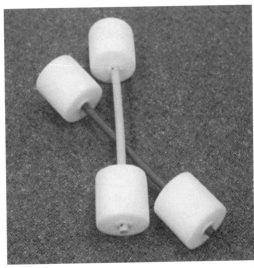

FIGURE 20-6. Swim bars or trainers offer balance and support.

This equipment is made from a closed-cell foam and covered with a colored nylon fabric.

Kickboards (Fig. 20-8), usually made of Styrofoam, were originally designed as a swimming aid. Their use is once again based on the concept of buoyancy. The kickboard is now being replaced with other Styrofoam devices of various shapes and sizes that are designed expressly for aquatic exercise.

Other useful flotation devices include balls, neck supports, and inner tubes (Fig. 20-9). Balls are often used for balance and coordination activities in the pool. Inflatable neck supports are invaluable for comfortable support of a person in the supine position in the water. Inner tubes of various sizes provide an inexpensive flotation device for deep-water activities, as well as serving as positioning aids for supine activities.

Weights

Weights are often used in the pool for traction or upper and lower extremity strengthening. Most weights on the market are not suitable to use in the water because they rust and cause staining of the pool surface. Therefore, weights used in the pool must be of a type designed for water exercise. Many manufacturers of aquatic equipment are now designing ankle and hand weights in various sizes for pool use.

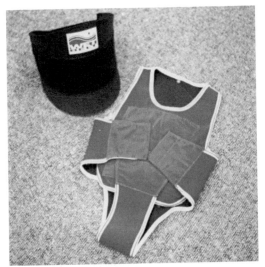

FIGURE 20-5. Wet Vest and Wet Belt both suspend the user in a vertical position.

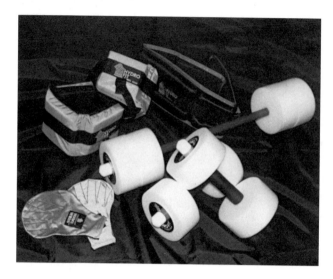

FIGURE 20-7. A set of Hydro-Fit equipment.

Resistance Equipment Based on Drag

Fins

The types of equipment based on the concept of drag to produce resistance are as varied as buoyant equipment. Fins and the benefits they provide in increasing range of motion and strengthening of the ankle, knee, and hip are not new to aquatic professionals. Manufacturers, however, are creating modern designs that differ slightly in fit and mechanics.

Gloves and Hand Paddles

For upper extremity strengthening, webbed gloves (Fig. 20-10) have become a popular item. They are based on the principle of increasing the surface area of the hand to produce greater resistance. They are snug-fitting gloves made of colorful Lycra or rubberized material. Hand paddles, which were originally designed for swimmers, are also being marketed in conjunction with webbed gloves as an upper extremity resistance device. They are flat plastic paddles that attach to the wrist and middle finger with rubber tubing.

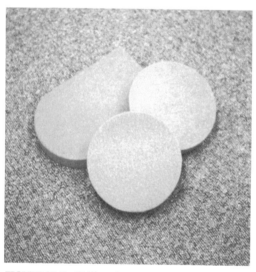

FIGURE 20-8. Kickboards.

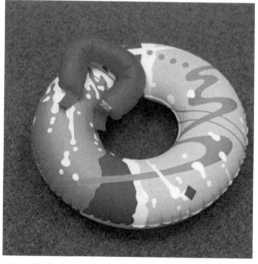

FIGURE 20-9. Assorted flotation devices.

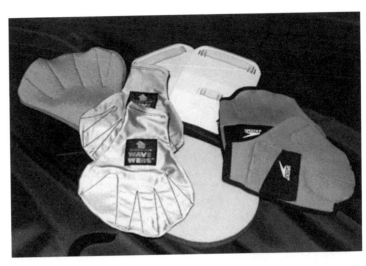

FIGURE 20-10. Webbed gloves are used for upper extremity strengthening.

Aquatoner

The Aquatoner (Fig. 20-11) is a resistance device with three paddles or blades that can be adjusted to create a fan with variable surface area. The Aquatoner can be hand held for upper extremity exercises, or attached to the ankle or leg for lower extremity exercises.

Hydro-Tone

A unique piece of aquatic resistance equipment on the market is the Hydro-Tone system (Fig. 20-12). The system consists of lower extremity boots and upper extremity hand-held bells that have a three-dimensional design. They are constructed from colorful hard plastic and, although buoyant, capitalize on the principle of resistance. The Hydro-Tone equipment significantly increases drag, making any exercise more challenging.

Tether System

A resistance tether is a miscellaneous piece of equipment used for jogging or swimming in a small pool. A tether system is simply rubber tubing that is attached to the participant by a belt around the waist and then attached to the pool wall. The system keeps a person in place while running or swimming, and eliminates the constant need to change directions in a small pool. It may also be used to increase the intensity by increasing the force the subject must overcome.

Underwater Exercise Stations

Portable exercise stations are larger pieces of equipment targeted for total-body workouts. These devices are based on existing land aerobic exercise machines, but are designed for pool use. Four machines currently on the market include a cross-country ski machine, lateral skate machine, treadmill, and parallel bars. They incorporate the same movements as the land-based machines, but use the principle of drag for resistance.

Aquatic exercise steps (Fig. 20-13) may also be used as an exercise station. These steps are designed and built specifically for use in the water. They are light weight, yet stay firmly in place on the bottom of the pool. The aquatic

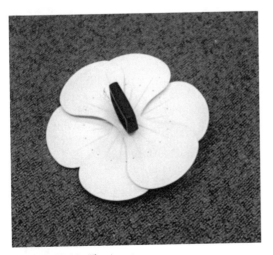

FIGURE 20-11. The Aquatoner.

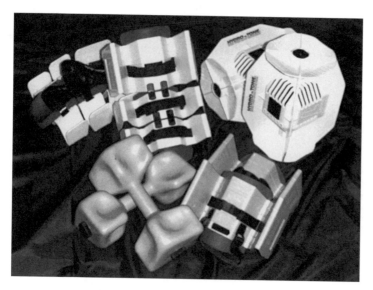

FIGURE 20-12. The Hydro-Tone system.

exercise steps can provide a means of performing dynamic closed-chain activities for lower extremity strengthening as well as cardiovascular conditioning.

Toys, Games, and Recreational Equipment

Various aquatic toys, games, and recreational items may be used for balance and coordination activities, relaxation techniques, socialization skills, endurance activities, and for enjoyment. Games are often an important aspect of an enjoyable aquatic experience. They provide a pleasant atmosphere that encourages participation. Aquatic toys and recreational items are designed for skill development as well as for fun.

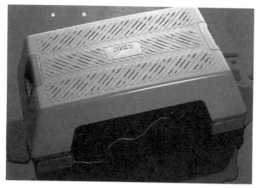

FIGURE 20-13. Aquatic exercise steps.

Safety Equipment

An aquatic facility is responsible for providing the necessary safety and rescue equipment to meet the minimum standards established by local and state ordinances. The type and amount of safety equipment required are determined by the size and type of facility.

A first aid kit is a basic safety item for the pool area. First aid kits are designed to provide everything needed to give fast and efficient emergency first aid care. A kit that is kept at a pool should be an all-weather kit with a rubber gasket seal to protect the contents from moisture. A first aid kit should be checked and restocked routinely.

An alarm or warning system to summon help needed in the pool or surrounding area is a highly recommended piece of equipment. Ideally, the alarm should be accessible from anywhere in the pool because a person in distress can quickly become a drowning victim if it is necessary to leave the pool for help.

The following rescue equipment is used to assist a person in a distress or drowning situation. A reaching pole or shepherd's crook should be available at the pool side. A reaching pole is a long, straight pole that is extended to a victim in distress. A shepherd's crook is a long, straight pole with a large, blunt hook. It may be used as a reaching pole or to encircle a person's body during a rescue.

A heaving line is an excellent rescue device for active victims. It is a rope with a length of one to one and a half times the length of the pool that is usually attached to a ring buoy. This is thrown to the victim to provide flotation as the rescuer pulls the person to safety.

A rescue tube is a rectangular foam float that has a 4- to 6-foot rope and shoulder strap attached. The tube is flexible and may be wrapped around the body and secured. It is designed with sufficient buoyancy to support two people. A backboard should be a standard piece of rescue equipment at all aquatic facilities. They are often made from aluminum, a heavy plastic material, or ¾-inch plywood. They need to have hand holds along each side as well as a head immobilizer and torso straps. In addition, cervical extrication collars in various sizes should be available.

The primary concern of any aquatic professional is the safety of the person using the pool facility. Adequate and accessible safety and rescue equipment is essential at all pools. In addition, all staff should be competent in its use.

Aquatic Apparel

There are a variety of aquatic apparel options (Fig. 20-14) on the market that are not only stylish, but provide a comfortable fit and are very durable. Swimwear includes recreational and competitive swim suits as well as garments designed for the aquatic professional. These items include tights, leotards, wetsuits, bodysuits, and jumpsuits. There are also disposable suits and wrap-around suits designed for people who have difficulty dressing. Swimwear is now being made of Lycra, which offers optimum protection from pool chemicals, so they last much longer than the cotton blends.

Aquatic shoes (Fig. 20-15) are highly recommended for aquatic exercise. There are many styles and colors on the market. Shoes that are designed to be worn in the water have several purposes, the most important of which is to protect the feet from the bottom of the pool. These shoes are also designed to provide better traction and prevent slipping, both in the water and on the wet deck. Wearing shoes in the water tends to increase drag, which in turn increases the intensity of a workout. The design of aquatic shoes has been improved to provide more support and cushioning.

Goggles are an item invaluable for any underwater activities. They protect the eyes from irritating pool chemicals and improve underwater

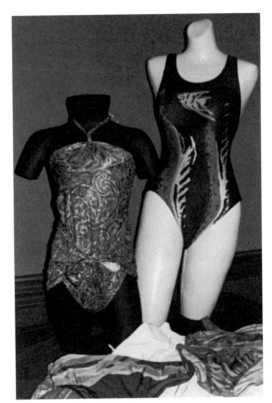

FIGURE 20-14. Aquatic apparel.

vision. Goggles come in different styles, shapes, sizes, and colors. Other features available include variable adjustments for a more customized fit, antifog lenses, and prescription lenses.

Other items that may make underwater activities more comfortable and enjoyable include earplugs and nose clips. These may be found at most sporting goods stores.

Special populations may require various hygiene products to enable them to enter the pool safely. Many conditions that were once considered contraindications to entering a pool are now only considered precautions. Beginning in the 1980s, many new products have been developed and marketed that enable people with open wounds to safely enter a pool. An occlusive dressing such as Duoderm, or a semiocclusive dressing like Op-Site, Bio-occlusive, or Tegaderm may be used to cover wounds for pool activity.

Plastic wraps are also available to protect bandages or casts from water during bathing or swimming. Waterproof casts (Fig. 20-16) are the latest development that permits water activity. A waterproof cast consists of Gore Cast Liner (a

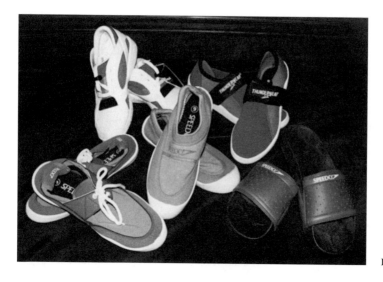

FIGURE 20-15. Aquatic shoes.

waterproof cast padding from W. L. Gore and Associates, Flagstaff, AZ—the makers of Gore-Tex fabrics), which is then covered by fiberglass casting tape (Fig. 20-17). The product can be safely immersed in water.

Diapers and plastic undergarments are two hygiene products that make it possible for people who are incontinent to enter the pool. Swim diapers may be purchased for children, which eliminates the need for plastic pants. However, if swim diapers are not used, plastic pants should be worn over a standard as well as a disposable diaper.

Measuring Devices

Measuring devices can aid aquatic health care professionals in determining the effects of exercise in water. A pace clock at the pool side can be a useful tool; it is a large clock with a second hand and a minute hand. A pace clock is helpful for timed exercises, rest periods, interval work-

outs, and pulse checks. There are also measuring devices that have been specifically designed for underwater use. Water-resistant heart monitors are available for a more accurate and continuous pulse check. In addition, dynamometers to measure strength and provide biofeedback are currently entering the marketplace. These measuring devices enable the health care professional to monitor a client's progress in the water, which is valuable for documentation and research.

Choosing Equipment

Aquatic exercise and rehabilitation equipment present an almost overwhelming array of options. There are vests and belts that help to keep the body floating in a vertical position for deep-water jogging, as well as weights designed to

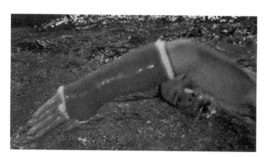

FIGURE 20-16. A waterproof cast permits water activity.

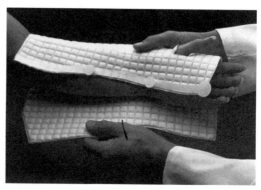

FIGURE 20-17. Waterproof cast liner.

counter the buoyant force of the water. There are also hand paddles, webbed gloves, and other devices that effectively increase the surface area of the hands, arms, feet, and legs to increase the resistance factor during exercise, thus improving the overload effect on the working muscles. With the wealth of aquatic exercise products on the market today, the aquatic professional should have no difficulty finding the right piece of equipment to fit any need. When selecting equipment, the following factors should be taken into consideration. The first consideration should be the client or participant population and the types of activities to be conducted. Buoyancy and weight equipment designed for support and body positioning might be more appropriate for a therapy setting, whereas resistance equipment designed for strengthening and endurance might be more appropriate for a sports or fitness setting.

Another important consideration when choosing aquatic exercise and rehabilitation equipment is the construction and durability of the product. The equipment should be well constructed with materials that are durable and can withstand the pool environment. Common materials used in the construction of pool products include foam, rubber, plastic, various fabrics, and metal. Foam items should be made from a closed-cell foam so they do not absorb water, even if cut or punctured. Some rubber, plastics, and fabrics do not hold up well in the pool environment because they absorb water, so it is important to choose these items carefully. Many companies now use fade-resistant and chemical-resistant fabrics and materials to enhance the durability of equipment subjected to pool chemicals. Also, any piece of equipment that is metal must be constructed of a high-grade stainless steel to prevent the item from rusting. The fit and comfort of the equipment as well as the equipment's flexibility are also important factors to take into consideration before purchasing an item. Equipment must fit correctly to be used properly. It should be comfortable so as not to irritate the skin. Ideally, equipment also should be flexible and versatile so that it not only is adjustable to accommodate various body sizes, but adaptable to different purposes, as well as changing levels of proficiency.

The price of equipment is always a factor that must be considered before purchasing an item. However, cost should never be an issue when it comes to safety. Equipment that ensures the safety of staff and patrons should be provided at any cost. By considering all of the factors discussed—program needs, fit and comfort, durability, flexibility and versatility, safety, and of course price—the aquatic health care professional can select the most beneficial and cost-effective aquatic exercise and rehabilitation equipment.

Equipment used for aquatic exercise and rehabilitation may be obtained directly from most manufacturers. In addition, the manufacturers often include a satisfaction-guaranteed return policy as well as instructional brochures or exercise cards and videos demonstrating their products. Many items that are out on the market may also be purchased from retailers such as pool supply companies, sporting goods stores, discount chains, drug stores, and specialty shops.

When making equipment recommendations for people interested in exercising in the water, it is important to consider the person's needs and abilities. To determine the type of equipment, the aquatic health care professional should first consider the age of the person and the goals that are desired. The person's physical condition should then be considered, including any known medical conditions or disabilities. The aquatic professional assesses the person's comfort level in water as well as their natural buoyancy, taking into consideration any limitations in balance, range of motion, strength, or endurance. The equipment recommended is affordable and accessible as well as suited to the person's needs. Finally, the proper fit is ensured, if required, as well as the person's knowledge of proper use and care of the equipment.

Proper Care of Equipment

As with all new equipment, proper care enhances the durability and extends the useful life of the product. This includes establishing and maintaining a properly designed storage area for all equipment, to prevent mold and mildew. Nothing should be stored on the pool deck, nor should equipment be stacked. Ideally, equipment should be stored in such a manner that it may dry easily. There are storage systems currently on the market, or one can easily be designed using polyvinyl chloride pipe or wall grid storage systems, so equipment may hang freely. This not only allows the equipment to dry quickly, but provides an attractive and convenient storage area for easy access to each piece of equipment.

Routine cleaning and safety inspections of all aquatic exercise and rehabilitation equipment should be performed daily. Equipment should be washed with warm soapy water, and then disinfected. A dilute solution of sodium hypochlorite and water may be used for this purpose. As the equipment is being cleaned, it should also be inspected for any damage that may compromise its safety. Any faulty equipment should promptly be repaired or discarded and replaced to ensure the safety of those who may use it.

Liability

Liability issues regarding equipment are not only the responsibility of the manufacturer, but also the health care professional who may provide or recommend equipment for another person's use. Manufacturers usually indicate how to use their product correctly, as well as warn of possible injury with use of the product. They also usually specify proper care and repair of the equipment. The health care professional must ensure that the equipment is used only for the purpose intended by the manufacturer, as well as explain any manufacturer's warnings to the person using the equipment. The health care professional should also educate the client on the proper care of the equipment. Failure to provide this information could be considered negligence on the part of the professional.

Summary: Future Equipment Needs

As aquatic exercise and rehabilitation has increased in popularity, so has the amount of equipment available for aquatic programs. Although water is a unique medium that provides natural resistance for exercise, equipment designed specifically for aquatic exercise and rehabilitation can enhance the overall benefits. Exercising in water is excellent for the injured, older, pediatric, prenatal, and overweight populations, as well as the top-conditioned athlete. The advantages include reduced pressure on joints in a medium that increases flexibility, muscular strength and endurance, proprioception, and cardiorespiratory fitness. With the use of proper equipment, aquatic exercise and rehabilitation can not only be more enjoyable, but more beneficial to the participant. As research and new techniques in aquatic exercise and rehabilitation advance, new equipment should be designed and developed based on sound hydrodynamic principles.

Index

Page numbers followed by *f* indicate figures; those followed by *t* indicate tables; those followed by *b* indicate boxes.

403

for the therapy pool. *Journal of Back and Musculo-skeletal Rehabilitation.* 1994;4:265–272.

41. Osinski A. Risk management issues for aquatic physical therapy. *Orthopedic Physical Therapy Clinics of North America.* 1994;3:111–136.

42. Cirullo JA. Considerations for pool programming and implementation. *Orthopedic Physical Therapy Clinics of North America.* 1994;3:95–110.

43. Collopy C. *Aquatic Center Safety Manual.* San Jose, Calif: San Jose State University, Environmental Health and Safety; 1992.

44. Osinski A. Hidden problems: a step-by-step guide to pool/spa equipment room troubleshooting. *Aquatics International.* March/April 1993:23–29.

45. Jackson E. Hidden assets: well-planned mechanical rooms ease the maintenance burden. *Aquatics International.* July/August 1992:10–16.

46. Occupational Safety and Health Administration (OSHA). *Hazardous Waste Operations and Emergency Response.* Washington, DC: U.S. Government Printing Office; 1992.

47. Van Rossen D. Crystal clear: sanitizing alternatives make pool water sparkle. *Aquatics International.* January/February 1993:20–26.

48. Walsh M. Filter out your pool problems. *Parks and Recreation.* July 1993:58–64.

49. Devlin PM, Hwang JC, et al. Automated hydrotherapy pool water treatment system. *J Burn Care Rehabil.* 1989;10:74–78.

50. Zura RD, Groschel DH, Becker DG, et al. Is there a need for state health department sanitary codes for public hydrotherapy and swimming pools? *J Burn Care Rehabil.* 1990;11:146–150.

51. Osinski A. Safe and clean: amenities need special care to ensure guest satisfaction. *Aquatics International.* September/October 1992:20–28.

52. Wilson G, Kittler R, Teskoski J, Coursin K. Controlling indoor environments for comfort, structure protection. *Aquatics International.* November/December 1991:19–27.

53. Popke M. Behind enemy lines. *Athletic Business.* December 1993:71–74.

54. Chivetta C. Air power. *Athletic Business.* August 1993:43–48.

55. Goldman JD. Planned repairs prevent lengthy pool closings. *Aquatics International.* November/December 1992:10–12.

56. DeRose R. A good start: proper opening procedures safeguard pool investment. *Aquatics.* March/April 1990:21–25.

57. Frantz JP. Keep it clean: proper maintenance protects pool filtration systems. *Aquatics.* February 1989:25–28.

58. Davis BC, Harrison RA. *Hydrotherapy in Practice.* New York, NY: Churchill-Livingstone; 1988.

59. Wilder RP, Brennan DK. Fundamentals and techniques of aquatic running for athletic rehabilitation. *Journal of Back and Musculoskeletal Rehabilitation.* 1994;4:287–296.

60. McWaters GJ. For faster recovery: just add water. *Sports Medicine Update.* 1992;7(2):4–5.

61. Young E. Proper acoustics make a sound indoor pool. *Aquatics.* March/April 1989:10.

62. Cunningham J. Historical review of aquatics and physical therapy. *Orthopedic Physical Therapy Clinics of North America.* 1994;3:83–94.

63. Cunningham J. Applying the Bad Ragaz method to the orthopaedic client. *Orthopedic Physical Therapy Clinics of North America.* 1994;3:251–260.

64. Goldman JD. Big ideas: lap pools and artificial currents extend possibilities for exercise. *Aquatics International.* January/February 1992:8–12.

65. Goldman JD. Therapy pool settings promote positive outlook. *Aquatics International.* September/October 1991:8–13.

66. County of Santa Cruz Environmental Health Service. *Swimming Pool Plan Check Sheet.* Santa Cruz, Calif: County of Santa Cruz Environmental Health Service; 1994.

67. National Spa and Pool Institute. *Standard dimensions for public swimming pools. Athletic Business.* February 1994:272.

68. YMCA of the USA. *Aquatics for Special Populations.* Champaign, Ill: Human Kinetics; 1987.

69. Gerson V. Enhancing profits: pools can boost club revenues and creativity increases profits. *Aquatics International.* September/October 1993:26–29.

Appendix 18-A:
The Preplanning Budget

Before building a pool facility, a preplanning budget should be developed to establish costs of the project.[†]

A. Budget Development
   1. Office or rental space
      a. Computer
      b. FAX
   2. Maintenance
      a. Cleaning
      b. Supplies
   3. Insurance
      a. Liability
      b. Property damage
   4. Utilities
      a. Telephone
      b. Water
      c. Electricity
      d. Heat
   5. Support staff
      a. Wages
      b. Benefits
   6. Program development and daily operation analysis
      a. Project fiscal impact
      b. Program opportunities
      c. Probable operating costs
      d. Potential revenue sources
B. Preconstruction Expenses for Pool Site
   1. Site feasibility appraisal
   2. Civil/mechanical engineering

[†] Adapted from Wiggins,[7] Clayton,[32] Sport Management Group, and ELS Architects, Inc.

Summary

The aquatic wellness center planning team must investigate the design and planning of the facility by considering the size, layout, programming, and use of the pool. Accurate demographic information gathered by visiting other facilities and interpretation of survey questionnaires gives the team data regarding construction costs, revenue recovery from programs, and needed budget analysis for daily operations. Without the preplanning information, the facility may be built with insufficient space, and costly planning errors may occur.

Acknowledgments
The author thanks David G. Thomas, MS, Professor Emeritus, State University of New York, Binghamton, New York, and Richard Scott, AIA, Counsilman/Hunsaker & Associates for editing a portion of the manuscript.

REFERENCES

1. Champion MR, ed. *Adult Hydrotherapy: A Practical Approach*. Hydrotherapy in Neuro Rehab. London: Heinemann Medical Books, 1990.
2. McWaters GJ. *Deep Water Exercise for Health and Fitness*. Laguna Beach, Calif: Publitec Editions; 1988.
3. Bloomquist L. *University of Rhode Island Adapted Aquatics Program Manual*. 2nd ed. Washington, DC: Department of Education; 1987.
4. Dieffenbach L. Aquatic therapy services. *Clinical Management*. 1991;11:14–19.
5. Hunsaker DJ. Pools from the ground up. *Athletic Business*. October 1990:37–43.
6. Osinski A. *Designing and Developing a Successful Aquatic Therapy Center*. Presented at the Aquatic Therapy Symposium, Charlotte, North Carolina, October 13, 1994.
7. Wiggins J. Building a budget. *Athletic Business*. August 1993:61–66.
8. Athletic Institute and American Alliance for Health, Physical Education, Recreation and Dance. *Planning Facilities for Athletics, Physical Education, and Recreation*. Reston, Va: American Alliance for Health, Physical Education, Recreation, and Dance; 1985.
9. Reister VC, Cole AJ. Start active, stay active in the water. *Journal of Physical Education, Recreation, and Dance*. January 1993:52–54.
10. Kacius JJ. Tide turns in pool design. *Athletic Business*. December 1990:71–75.
11. Visnic M. Aquatic therapy comes of age. *Aquatic Physical Therapy Report*. 1994;(4):6–8.
12. Aboulian K. Physical therapy plus. *Aquatic Physical Therapy Report*. 1994;1(4):11.
13. Hauss DS. How to buy aquatic therapy programs. *Rehabilitation Today*. January 1994:22–24.
14. Cirullo J. Aquatic therapy's rising tide. *Rehabilitation Management*. August/September 1992:74.
15. Becker BE, Cole AJ. Swimming onward: the future of aquatic rehabilitation. *Journal of Back and Musculoskeletal Rehabilitation*. 1994;4:309–314.
16. Long L. Obesity, weight control and swimming. *Aquatic Physical Therapy Report*. 1993;1(1):10–11.
17. Osinski A. Modifying public swimming pools to comply with provisions of the Americans With Disabilities Act. *PALAESTRA*. 1993;9(4):13–18.
18. American College of Sports Medicine. *Health and Fitness Facility Standards and Guidelines*. Champaign, Ill: Human Kinetics; 1992.
19. *Americans With Disabilities Acts Accessibility Guidelines*. Washington, DC: U.S. Senate Subcommittee on Disability Policy.
20. Gabrielsen AM, ed. *Swimming Pools: A Guide to Their Planning, Design, and Operation*. 4th ed. Indianapolis, Ind: Council for National Cooperation in Aquatics; 1987.
21. Gabrielson M, Mittelstaedt A. Advance planning: step-by-step supervision facilitates pool construction. *Aquatics*. July/August 1990:16–22.
22. Goldman D: State-of-the-art pools: design follows function. *Aquatics International*. March/April 1994:10–16.
23. Berg R. The leisure pool challenge. *Athletic Business*. October 1993:37–42.
24. Fuerst CF. Rebirth of the pool. *Athletic Business*. October 1992:30–38.
25. Hunsaker DJ. European approach: aquatic leisure centers can be all things to all people. *Aquatics*. March/April 1991:10–14.
26. Spannuth JR. Promoting water walking step by step. *Aquatics*. November/December 1990:27.
27. Osinski A. Staying in step: water walking sets a new pace. *Aquatics*. November/December 1990:26–31.
28. American Red Cross. *Adapted Aquatics*. Washington, DC: American Red Cross; 1977.
29. Jackson E. Money matters: outside resources boost aquatic facilities budget. *Aquatics*. January/February 1991:14–22.
30. Osinski A. *Aquatic Facility Design Checklist*. Presented at the 3rd annual meeting of the Aquatic Exercise Association, San Diego, California, 1990.
31. Jackson E. Experts in the field: aquatic consultants offer assistance in all areas of design and operation. *Aquatics International*. November/December 1994:10–15.
32. Clayton RD. Dollars and sense: proper budgeting is the key to efficient management. *Aquatics*. September/October 1989:12–16.
33. Byrne D. Problems, problems. *Athletic Business*. August 1992:38–40.
34. Jackson E. Pool of the future: today's needs dictate tomorrow's facilities. *Aquatics International*. January/February 1993:10–15.
35. Jackson E. Total automation: computers enhance managers' effectiveness. *Aquatics International*. January/February 1994:18–22.
36. Osinski A. Behind closed doors: locker rooms should uphold facility's image. *Aquatics*. May/June 1990:20–23.
37. Baggett R. Dressing in style: San Francisco YMCA revenates locker rooms. *Aquatics International*. January/February 1993:27–32.
38. Jackson E. Country club living: member locker rooms satisfy upscale image. *Aquatics International*. March/April 1994:23–26.
39. Goethel P. The operative word is clean. *Fitness Management*. January 1992:32–35.
40. Moschetti M. Aquatics: risk management strategies